# NMS Q&A
# USMLE Step 2 CK

**4th** EDITION

# NMS Q&A
# USMLE Step 2 CK

**4th** EDITION

## EDITORS

**Kenneth Ibsen, PhD**
Emeritus Professor of Biochemistry
College of Medicine
University of California Irvine
Former Director Academic Development
National Medical School Review (NMSR)
Newport Beach California
Continuing Medical Education Director
Kaplan Medical, USA

**Nandan Bhatt, MBBS, MD, FRCS**
Physician & Surgeon
Department of Developmental Services
State of California
Former Faculty National Medical School Review (NMSR)
Newport Beach, California
Faculty, Kaplan Medical, USA

Wolters Kluwer | Lippincott Williams & Wilkins
Health
Philadelphia • Baltimore • New York • London
Buenos Aires • Hong Kong • Sydney • Tokyo

*Acquisitions Editor:* Susan Rhyner
*Product Manager:* Stacey Sebring
*Marketing Manager:* Joy Fisher-Williams
*Manufacturing Coordinator:* Margie Orzech
*Designer:* Holly Reid McLaughlin
*Compositor:* Aptara, Inc.

Fourth Edition

**Library of Congress Cataloging-in-Publication Data**

NMS Review for USMLE Step 2 CK / Editors Kenneth Ibsen &
Nandan Bhatt – 4th ed.
    p. ; cm. – (National medical series for independent study)
    USMLE step 2 clinical knowledge
    Rev. ed. of: NMS review for the clinical skills assessment exam /
Erich A. Arias. c2001.
    Includes bibliographical references and index.
    Summary: "During the past decade, the first, second and 3rd editions of the NMS Review for USMLE Step 2 have served as important adjuncts for students preparing to take the USMLE Step 2 Examination. This the 4th edition of NMS Review for USMLE Step 2 CK reflects the fact that it only relates to the CK (clinical knowledge) component of the current two-part Step 2 Examination. In providing this knowledge, it continues the traditions of relevance and excellence established by the previous editions"–Provided by publisher.
    ISBN 978-0-7817-8739-0 (pbk. : alk. paper)
    1. Physicians, Foreign–Certification–United States.  2. Clinical competence–Study guides.  I. Ibsen, Kenneth.  II. Bhatt, Nandan. III. Arias, Erich A. NMS review for the clinical skills assessment exam. IV. Title: USMLE step 2 clinical knowledge.  V. Series: National medical series for independent study.
    [DNLM: 1. Clinical Competence.  2. Foreign Medical Graduates. 3. Medical History Taking–methods.  4. Physical Examination–methods. WB18]
    R697.F6A75 2011
    610.76–dc22                                  2011003429

DISCLAIMER

Care has been taken to confirm the accuracy of the information present and to describe generally accepted practices. However, the authors, editors, and publisher are not responsible for errors or omissions or for any consequences from application of the information in this book and make no warranty, expressed or implied, with respect to the currency, completeness, or accuracy of the contents of the publication. Application of this information in a particular situation remains the professional responsibility of the practitioner; the clinical treatments described and recommended may not be considered absolute and universal recommendations.

The authors, editors, and publisher have exerted every effort to ensure that drug selection and dosage set forth in this text are in accordance with the current recommendations and practice at the time of publication. However, in view of ongoing research, changes in government regulations, and the constant flow of information relating to drug therapy and drug reactions, the reader is urged to check the package insert for each drug for any change in indications and dosage and for added warnings and precautions. This is particularly important when the recommended agent is a new or infrequently employed drug.

Some drugs and medical devices presented in this publication have Food and Drug Administration (FDA) clearance for limited use in restricted research settings. It is the responsibility of the health care provider to ascertain the FDA status of each drug or device planned for use in their clinical practice.

To purchase additional copies of this book, call our customer service department at **(800) 638-3030** or fax orders to **(301) 223-2320**. International customers should call **(301) 223-2300**.

Visit Lippincott Williams & Wilkins on the Internet: http://www.lww.com. Lippincott Williams & Wilkins customer service representatives are available from 8:30 am to 6:00 pm, EST.

## Dedication

*We are very proud to dedicate this edition to the thousands of students and physicians who have benefitted from our previous endeavors and to those who will follow. We wish each and every one of you every success.*

*We also wish to dedicate this edition to the following:*

*Dr. Ibsen, to his wife Marilyn, who has been his strong support; and Dr. Bhatt, to his mother Radha Bhatt and his late father, Wing Commander S.K.R. Bhatt, Fighter Pilot, IAF.*

## Note from the Editors

We have been encouraged by the overwhelming response to our previous collaboration and are humbled by it. We both hope that this iteration, now in its fourth edition featuring many more questions, and additional tests on the web will be equally if not more useful to thousands of students worldwide.

This book and the material on the web is a source of review not only for those preparing for USMLE Step 2 CK, but to those requiring background information for USMLE Step 3, those preparing for board examinations in some other disciplines, and for specialist physicians who need to take the SPEX examination as well. As will be apparent, we have incorporated basic science information that we feel will provide a strong foundation for the practice of medicine, which is in keeping with the guidelines set forth by USMLE as well. The first edition of this review was made possible due to the vision of Dr. Victor Gruber, Director National Medical School Review.

*Students are strongly advised to review the information in the preface and the study guide before taking the tests in this book and on the web.*

## Acknowledgements

We are very grateful to Lippincott Williams & Wilkins, and especially to Sirkka Howes, for her forbearance and understanding. We all put in long hours and despite illnesses, computer glitches, and the attendant frustrations, we are proud of this product that has now come to light.

Lastly, this edition could not have been completed without the patience and support of our wives, Marilyn Ibsen and Yuling Bhatt.

*Kenneth Ibsen*                                                                                      *Nandan Bhatt*

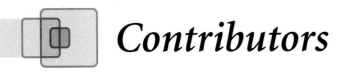

# *Contributors*

**Nandan Bhatt, MBBS, MD, FRCS**
Physician and Surgeon
Department of Developmental Services
State of California
Faculty, Kaplan Medical, USA

**William G. Cvetnic, MD, FAAP**
Board Certified in Pediatrics and
Neonatal-Perinatal Medicine
Faculty, Kaplan Medical, USA
Jacksonville, Florida

**Kenneth Ibsen, PhD**
Emeritus Professor of Biochemistry
College of Medicine
University of California Irvine
Irvine, California
Former Director Academic Development
NMSR/Kaplan Medical
Continuing Medical Education Director
Kaplan Medical, USA

**Christine E. Koerner, MD, FAAP, FACEP**
Associate Professor of Emergency Medicine
University of Texas Health Science Center at
Houston Medical School
Chief, Division of Pediatric Emergency Medicine
Lyndon B. Johnson General Hospital
Houston, Texas

**Elmar P. Sakala, MA, MPH, MD, FACOG**
Professor of Gynecology and Obstetrics
Clinical Clerkship Director
School of Medicine
Loma Linda University
Loma Linda, California
Director, Obstetrics and Gynecology
Kaplan Medical, USA

**Roderick Shaner, MD**
Clinical Professor of Psychiatry
Keck School of Medicine
University of Southern California
Medical Director
Los Angeles County Department of
Mental Health
Los Angeles, California

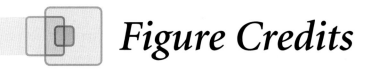

# Figure Credits

**Test 2 Question 34**

Adapted from Goldschlager N, Goldman M. *Principles of Electrocardiography*, 13th ed. Norwalk, CT: Appleton & Lange, 1989. Used with permission from McGraw-Hill.

**Test 4 Questions 28, 29, 31**

From Fleisher GR, Ludwig S, Baskin MN. *Atlas of Pediatric Emergency Medicine*. Philadelphia: Lippincott Williams & Wilkins, 2004.

From Oski F.A. (Ed.). *Principles and Practice of Pediatrics*. Philadelphia: J.B. Lippincott, 1990.

From Becker KL, Bilezikian JP, Brenner WJ, et al. *Principles and Practice of Endocrinology and Metabolism*, 3rd ed. Philadelphia: Lippincott Williams & Wilkins, 2001:196, with permission.

**Test 5 Question 6**

From Rubin E, Farber JL. *Pathology*, 3rd ed. Philadelphia: Lippincott Williams & Wilkins, 1999.

**Test 6 Questions 8, 19, 47–50**

Adapted from Goldschlager N, Goldman M. *Principles of Electrocardiography*, 13th ed. Norwalk, CT: Appleton & Lange, 1989. Used with permission from McGraw-Hill.

From Fleisher GR, Ludwig S, Baskin MN. *Atlas of Pediatric Emergency Medicine*. Philadelphia: Lippincott Williams & Wilkins, 2004.

From Rubin E, Farber JL. *Pathology*, 3rd ed. Philadelphia: Lippincott Williams & Wilkins, 1999.

**Test 10 Questions 14, 19**

Adapted from Goldschlager N, Goldman M. *Principles of Electrocardiography*, 13th ed. Norwalk, CT: Appleton & Lange, 1989. Used with permission from McGraw-Hill.

From Rubin E, Farber JL. *Pathology*, 3rd ed. Philadelphia: Lippincott Williams & Wilkins, 1999.

**Test 13 (online) Questions 4, 16, 24,**

Photo courtesy of Centers for Disease Control and Prevention.

Photo courtesy of George A. Datto, III.

From Fleisher GR, Ludwig S, Baskin MN. *Atlas of Pediatric Emergency Medicine*. Philadelphia: Lippincott Williams & Wilkins, 2004.

**Answers 31, 39**

From Eisenberg RL. *An Atlas of Differential Diagnosis*, 4th ed. Philadelphia: Lippincott Williams & Wilkins, 2003.

From Klossner NJ, Hatfield N. *Introductory Maternity and Pediatric Nursing*. Ambler, PA: Lippincott Williams & Wilkins, 2005.

**Test 14 (online) Questions 5, 19**

From Fleisher GR, Ludwig S, Baskin MN. *Atlas of Pediatric Emergency Medicine*. Philadelphia: Lippincott Williams & Wilkins, 2004.

From Goodheart HP. *Goodheart's Photoguide of Common Skin Disorders*, 2nd ed. Philadelphia: Lippincott Williams & Wilkins, 2003.

### Test 15 (online) Questions 12, 18, 35

From Dean D, Herbener TE. *Cross-Sectional Human Anatomy*. Baltimore: Lippincott Williams & Wilkins, 2000.

From Tasman W, Jaeger E. *The Wills Eye Hospital Atlas of Clinical Ophthalmology*, 2nd ed. Philadelphia: Lippincott Williams & Wilkins, 2001.

From Smeltzer SC, Bare BG. *Textbook of Medical-Surgical Nursing*, 9th ed. Philadelphia: Lippincott Williams & Wilkins, 2000.

### Test 16 (online) Answer 5

Porth CM. *Pathophysiology Concepts of Altered Health States*, 7th ed. Philadelphia: Lippincott Williams & Wilkins, 2005.

### Test 17 (online) Questions 4, 39–42

From Goodheart HP. *Goodheart's Photoguide of Common Skin Disorders*, 2nd ed. Philadelphia: Lippincott Williams & Wilkins, 2003.

Figures were from Test 17 in the 3rd edition; no credits were provided.

### Test 18 (online) Answer 6

From Rubin E, Farber JL. *Pathology*, 3rd ed. Philadelphia: Lippincott Williams & Wilkins, 1999.

### Questions 7, 12

From Gold DH, Weingeist TA. *Color Atlas of the Eye in Systemic Disease*. Baltimore: Lippincott Williams & Wilkins, 2001.

Figure was from 3e Test 17; no credit was provided.

### Test 19 (online) Questions 1, 7, 18, 23, 26

From Rubin E, Farber JL. *Pathology*, 3rd ed. Philadelphia: Lippincott Williams & Wilkins, 1999.

MacDonald MG, Seshia MMK, et al. *Avery's Neonatology Pathophysiology & Management of the Newborn*, 6th ed. Philadelphia: Lippincott Williams & Wilkins, 2005.

Photo courtesy of Kathleen Cronan.

From Rubin E, Farber JL. *Pathology*, 3rd ed. Philadelphia: Lippincott Williams & Wilkins, 1999.

Photo courtesy of Esther K. Chung.

### Test 20 online Questions 16, 43, 46

From Rubin E, Farber JL. *Pathology*, 3rd ed. Philadelphia: Lippincott Williams & Wilkins, 1999.

From Eisenberg RL. *An Atlas of Differential Diagnosis*, 4th ed. Philadelphia: Lippincott Williams & Wilkins, 2003.

From Boder E, Sedgwick RP. Ataxia-telangiectasia. In Goldensohn ES, Appel S (Eds.). *Scientific Approaches to Clinical Neurology*. Philadelphia: Lea & Febiger, 1977.

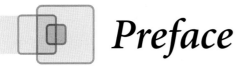

# *Preface*

## About This Edition

During the past decade, the first, second, and third editions of the *NMS Review for USMLE Step 2* have served as important adjuncts for students preparing to take the USMLE Step 2 Examination. This, the fourth edition of *NMS Q&A: USMLE Step 2 CK,* reflects the fact that it only relates to the clinical knowledge (CK) component of the current two-part Step 2 Examination. In providing this knowledge, it continues the traditions of relevance and excellence established by the previous editions.

- All items (an item is defined as a clinical vignette, with distractors, answers, and explanations) have been replaced with new ones or updated to conform to current clinical practice.
- All distractors, correct and incorrect, are explained.
- The style of the items closely reflects that presently found on the USMLE.
- All tests have 50 items, approximately 80% of which are of the one-best-choice variety and remainder are multiple choice.
- Content is highly relevant to that asked on the examination.
- The questions cover the various clinical disciplines in a random fashion, as they do in the USMLE.
- A simplified subject-item index is included, making it possible to study each discipline independently. The approximate total percentage of items per discipline is as follows: medicine, 32%: pediatrics, psychiatry, and surgery, 15%; obstetrics and gynecology, 14%; and preventive medicine and public health, 8%.
- Explanations, often detailed, are provided for the incorrect choices, as well as for the correct answer, thus helping the student understand why he or she chose an incorrect distractor and also increasing the breadth of coverage related to a given question.
- This edition also has a key word index to help students find specific topics of interest.

**A study guide is provided to help students optimize their preparation for the examination and to more effectively use this edition.**

## USING THIS BOOK

### The Book's Structure

The authors of this book have taken great efforts to create a product that simulates the questions used in the USMLE Step 2 CK Examination in terms of analytical prowess required and format. However, as a whole, the difficulty level may be a bit higher than that of the real examination. A total of 1,000 questions are arranged into twenty 50-question examinations in which the subject material is arranged in a random fashion, requiring the test taker to practice the mental gymnastics of rapidly switching from topic to topic. Six hundred of these questions are published in the book, and the remaining 400 are found on the web. As in the real examination, the initial 75%–80% of the questions are of the one-best-choice variety, while the remainder are matching sets. In addition to providing the correct answer, the correct and incorrect distractors and unused matching distractors are explained, often in detail. A subject index at the back of the book describes the subject of each question in terms of the six major clinical disciplines—medicine, obstetrics and gynecology, pediatrics, preventive medicine and public health, psychiatry, and surgery. Most of the many topics included in the USMLE description of the examination are included as belonging to one or another of these six disciplines. For example, dermatology and ophthalmology are considered subdisciplines of medicine and surgery, respectively.

### Suggested Ways to Use This Book

**In Preparation for the USMLE.** You can use the items in this book as a tool for increasing your knowledge base, for developing the analytical skills that will be required, and as a measure of your readiness to take the examination. It is suggested that, during the very early phases of your study, you randomly select 10 to 15 questions for 5 to 10 days, setting aside a period equal to 1 minute per question for the question selected. At the end of each of these mini-tests, study both the correct and incorrect responses to try to understand why the correct answer is correct and the others are incorrect. These items can also be used for discussion in your small study group during following days.

After this period, you should be ready to test yourself more seriously. Now, set aside an hour and take one of the 50-question examinations. This will give you an average of 72 seconds to answer each question, a time on a par with the real examination. Pace yourself, and make sure you answer all the questions, even if you have to guess to finish on time; in other words, make believe you are under the same constraints as you will be when the big day arrives. When you finish, study the answers as before, but also calculate your overall percentage score and the percentage obtained in each of the six disciplines. Don't worry if you are not getting 100%; remember that correctly answering 60%–70% of the questions on the real examination should be a passing score, while answering 75%–80% correctly will result in a score that is at or above the mean. However, if your score in one of the disciplines is remarkably below your average, devote extra time for study in that area. For each question, be sure you understand why the correct answer is correct and the incorrect one is not. Once you feel that you have gleaned all the information you can from that examination, repeat the experience using a second 50-question examination. After that, repeat the same process, but set aside 2 hours and answer 100 questions found in two examinations. This time, it should be easier to finish all the questions in the allotted time, and your percentage score should improve as you gain additional knowledge and better hone your test-taking skills.

Ideally, your next step is to simulate taking the full 9-hour examination. Try to arrange your affairs so that you can set aside an uninterrupted 9-hour day in which you take eight 1-hour examinations (400 questions) with 1 hour of free time disbursed in the way you think will be most efficient. In addition to providing further study, this will help you get used to the stress and fatigue factors and serve as a model to guide your future distribution of free time. During this 9-hour period, follow the rules prescribed by the NBME. After finishing, relax and limit your thinking to how you might have better used your free time; for example, were you too tired toward the end, and might you have done better if you had saved more free time to refresh yourself? On the following day, dissect your performance in more detail; once again, make sure you understand why correct answers are correct and wrong ones wrong; determine if your score could be in the passing range or above average; determine if there are topic areas in which you are weaker than average. Then, spend time taking appropriate remedial action. Finally, repeat the process, once again taking advantage of what you learned and using the final 400 questions.

Except for the first 100–150 questions taken randomly for the earliest mini-tests, the program outlined does not require using the same question more than once. However, in the unlikely event that you still do not feel ready to take the examination, you might wish to test yourself further. If so, select a minimum of 50 questions from one of the earlier examinations and repeat the trial test process under timed conditions, followed by analysis. You should see further improvement. Don't assume that it is because you have memorized the questions and answers, since there is little chance that a repeated question will be more than vaguely familiar after the passage of a couple of weeks filled with other study materials.

Try hard to set aside the suggested two 9-hour days. However, if for personal reasons, this is impossible, set aside an equivalent series of uninterrupted sequences, always making certain that you obey the time restrictions established by the NBME.

**As a Tool for Study During or for Review of Clerkships and Other Related Examinations.** The format of asking clinically relevant questions followed by detailed explanations of the correct and incorrect answers makes this book a potentially valuable tool for study during clerkships for third and fourth year students. It will take only minimal effort to select questions in a specific discipline for self-evaluation and/or study.

## Examination Study Guide

### STEPS TO LICENSURE AND THE STRUCTURE OF THE USMLE STEP 2 CK EXAMINATION

**Background.** During the past few decades, the National Board of Medical Examiners (NBME) has transformed the United States Medical Licensing Examination (USMLE) from the multiple-choice Steps 1 and 2 of the 1980s and early 1990s to the present four-step process—Step 1, Step 2 CK (Clinical Knowledge), Step 2 CS (Clinical Skills), and Step 3. In doing so, they also changed the process from one that primarily required recall of facts into a process that better tests the application of knowledge and skills to the solution of realistic clinical problems. Of these four steps to licensure, the Step 2 CS examination requires examinee interaction with live simulated patients, while the step 3 examination has a computerized clinical examination component. In contrast, the Step 1 and Step 2 CK retain a multiple-choice format, but the examiners have developed more sophisticated modes of presentation, requiring analytical problem-solving abilities that better replicate those required of practicing physicians. During this time period, the examinations also have evolved from pencil-and-paper examinations to the contemporary computerized ones. Although passage of all three multiple-choice examination steps requires application of similar types of cognitive skills, each step requires a more sophisticated level of understanding of clinical principles at the following levels:

- The USMLE Step 1 tests how well the examinee understands the application of the basic sciences to clinical situations at a level expected of a U.S. student who has just finished the second year of medical school.
- The USMLE Step 2 CK is designed to test the basic elements of biomedical and clinical knowledge at a level that will permit the student to care for patients under close supervision.
- The USMLE Step 3 is designed to assess the same elements, but now at a level permitting safe care of patients under unsupervised conditions and with greater emphasis on management of the ambulatory patient.

Although the steps are designed to be taken in sequence, if you are a student or graduate of a school accredited by the Liaison Committee on Medical Education (LCME) or the American Osteopathic Association (AOA), you may take the Step 1, Step 2 CK, and Step 2 CS examinations in any order. However, if you are an international medical graduate (IMG), you may take the Step 2 CK examination prior to the Step 1 examination, but you must have passed the Step 1 examination before being permitted to register for the Step 2 CS examination. Generally, it is wisest to take these three examinations in the suggested sequence; an exception to this generality may be foreign graduates who had been practicing physicians and who, because of their already developed clinical acumen, may find it easier to slide into the USMLE examinations at the Step 2 CK level. All persons must have passed Step 1 and both parts of Step 2 before being permitted to take Step 3. In general, the Step 3 examination is taken toward the end of the first year of residency. However, several states permit students to take this examination before being admitted into a residency program.

## Structure and Content of the Step 2 CK Examination

### STEP 2 CK TEST QUESTION FORMATS

Only the essential highlights will be provided here, since the reader can obtain a detailed and continuously updated description of the examination on the USMLE website (USMLE.org).

### CONTENT

The Step 2 CK examination has two types of questions: The single one-best-answer question and matching sets. The former type predominates, as it does in this book, in which this form represents about 80% of all the questions.

**Single One-best-answer Question.** As described in the USMLE website, this format consists of a statement or question followed by three to twenty-six options that are in alphabetical or logical order. In this book, most questions only offer five options: the "one best" answer, plus four distractors; however, a significant minority has additional distractors, each of which (as well as the one best answer) is explained in some detail. Most of these questions stand as independent entities, but several are in the so-called *sequential item sets*, in which a single patient-centered vignette is associated with two to three consecutive questions. In this review, these sequential item sets are limited to two questions and are primarily found in the web component (i.e., in tests 13–20). In the real examination, you must click "Proceed to Next Item" to view the next item in the set; once you click on this button, you will not be able to add or change an answer to the displayed (previous) item.

**Matching Sets.** This format consists of a series of questions related to a common topic. As described on the USMLE website, all matching sets contain set-specific instructions, a list of lettered response options, and at least two questions with between four and twenty-six response options. As in the actual examination, you are directed to select the one best answer for each question in the set. In this book, each of the potential choices, whether used as a correct choice or not, is further explained. As mentioned previously, 20% of the questions in each test are in this format. This is likely to be a higher proportion than you will find in the actual examination.

## Structure of the Examination, Timing During the Examination, and Scoring of the Examination

In the third edition, the editors attempted to provide a summary of the structure, timing, and scoring of the examination. However, they are now succinctly covered, with guaranteed accuracy and detail, on the USMLE website. Therefore, only a few points deemed particularly pertinent will be repeated here:

- *Scoring.* The score you receive is based upon the total number of correct answers. Incorrect answers are not counted against you, so it behooves you to answer all questions, even if you must randomly guess to finish within the allotted time.
- *Score reporting.* Each person takes a different examination, but all examinations are designed to be at an equivalent difficulty level. The three-digit score you will receive is calculated by a formula that includes your percentage score and your percentile compared with those of recent examinees. You will also be provided with the mean score and the standard deviation of recent examinations, as well as the minimum passing score. The latter may change from year to year and has been raised for the past few years; presently (November 2010) it is set at 189. A two-digit score is also reported. This score is in reality an anachronism used so that a score of 75 can be reported as the minimal pass, as required by some institutions. Students sometimes mistakenly assume that this is a percentage score, but it has no innate meaning, since it is derived from the three-digit score. Although the two- and three-digit scores report equivalent information, the three-digit scale provides a better assessment of performance, since scores are condensed in the two-digit system.

Graphical performance profiles are also shown. These summarize your relative strengths and weaknesses and are not reported to any other party.

## Preparation for and Taking the Examination

### DEVELOPING BASIC KNOWLEDGE

Each of you has a unique set of academic strengths and weaknesses that will affect what and how you should prepare for the examination. In addition, you each are influenced by a set of nonacademic factors including personal relationships and financial resources that influence the time and modes available for study. These factors, plus your innate genetic constitution, also influence the psychologic and physiologic resources you can make available for preparation, as well as for taking the examination itself. This makes it impossible to lay out one set of study rules that will fit everybody. Nonetheless, several generalities fit most students preparing for the USMLE. Each student must decide how to best weigh these generalities and make decisions concerning scheduling study time and selecting topics to study, materials to use, and study and learning modes, and how to best care for themselves as they proceed. However, some ideas that will be germane for most students are provided here:

- *Limit isolated passive study.* Reading and highlighting textbooks and/or lecture notes is a way to become familiar with basic terminology, but continually rereading the same material, trying to make the subject matter sink in, will almost guarantee failure. Even when studying in isolation, you should make the process more active by asking yourself questions; for example, by writing important terms down on flash cards and then testing yourself with them.
- *Use a study group to help formulate central concepts.* As your understanding of the basic terminology increases, you will subconsciously be formulating central concepts. These concepts will permit you to extrapolate information derived in a given situation to a different one, a function required to successfully interpret many of the questions on the examination. Concept formulation is even better facilitated by the exchange of ideas that occurs in study groups of four or five persons, in which you are exposed to differing opinions. To avoid the fatal error of formulating false concepts, you must be an active participant in your group and not be afraid to freely share your thoughts, even if it means you might demonstrate your ignorance. To not share your thoughts is only a half-step up from studying in isolation and will still run the risk of fortifying fallacious central concepts. However, the converse is equally true: You must not try to dominate the group because, in addition to making yourself unpopular, you will not hear what others are saying. How these study groups are best created depends in large part upon your background.

If you attend medical school in the United States or are a U.S. student from an offshore medical school, you probably have such a study group composed of classmates. In addition, you may be able to participate in short review courses provided by your school. Besides highlighting important concepts, such review courses serve as organized study groups.

However, if you are an international medical graduate, you probably do not have a preexisting study group available; thus, you should seek out like persons with whom you can share information and feelings. Often, this is most easily and efficiently done by participating in a commercially available review course in which the material reviewed is presented either via lecture or video. Although these can be expensive, the experience is usually worth the cost. In either case, the opportunity to interact with fellow students can be as important as exposure to the material presented.

Book- or computer-based studies present an effective way to test yourself as your studies progress. Additionally, if a study group of four or five students works in unison using the same study material, they have in effect established a mini-review program; for example, a group can agree beforehand to individually answer $y$ questions in test $x$ and then subsequently meet as a group to discuss the questions and answers. In this way, those who have trouble with a concept can see how those who do not have a problem came up with the correct response. It also provides a chance to discuss ramifications among yourselves and even—rarely, one hopes—decide that the information provided is in error.

## CONFIRMING YOUR ACADEMIC ABILITY TO TAKE THE EXAMINATION

The study activities described in the preceding paragraphs will increase your familiarity with an ever-increasing number of terms that you will be able to associate with an ever-increasing number of relevant conditions, and this will help you consolidate some central concepts. However, it will still be necessary to answer simulated USMLE test questions. This will further consolidate your knowledge, increase your test-taking skills, and confirm your readiness to take the examination. To truly test your readiness, you have to take practice examinations that not only probe your knowledge base but also test your ability to apply this knowledge to taking the real examination. Basically, there are two ways to obtain realistic testing experiences:

- *Take the real examination on a trial basis.* Since you can repeat the examination without a failure counting against you as far as testing associations are concerned, this may seem to be reasonable option. ***However, it is not recommended because the attempt will be entered into your record,*** and if you pass, you will be forever burdened with a score that may not reflect your true potential. An additional burden is that, when it comes to licensing after passing Step 3, every state has a different guideline on how many attempts are admissible for all three tests for one to be licensed. If one exceeds the stated limit set by that state, then one cannot be licensed in that state. Some states require you to make only one attempt at each step, others allow you a few more, and very few allow you unlimited attempts. Given these factors, it is not a good idea to take the examination as a trial, or to figure out what it is all about. In addition to the financial and emotional cost, you will needlessly diminish your ability to be licensed to practice medicine in some states.
- *Take commercially available USMLE-style examinations available in books or as computer programs.* Such commercially available examinations are of variable quality. Often, they consist of a mix of questions that can be answered by rote, along with questions on par with those used in the USMLE. Further value will be obtained if such programs explain both the correct and incorrect responses; this expands the breadth of the question, often clarifies why you chose the incorrect response, and helps you understand relationships between related conditions; for example, how to distinguish among different diseases to be considered as part of a differential diagnosis. Not surprisingly, we recommend this publication.

## IMPROVING YOUR TEST-TAKING SKILLS

Doing well on multiple-choice type examinations requires developing a set of test-taking skills. Most U.S. students have been exposed to multiple-choice examinations since childhood, whereas many IMG students have had minimal experience with them. Although this does provide the U.S. student with an advantage, surprisingly, the playing field has become more level with the advent of the new type of USMLE examinations, because these require many of the analytical skills used in an oral or essay examination. A practical example of the change is in the advice that can be given concerning the most efficient way to answer questions. The classic response to answering the older single-best-choice question was to simply read the first and last sentences of the stem to determine what the question is about and what is asked and then to look for the most logical distractor. Typically, that minimal effort would put you in a good position to select the best choice among the distractors. However, contemporary Step 2 CK questions usually require that you also understand the significance of the information imparted in the body of the vignette before attempting to answer the question. Consequently, it is recommended that, while using USMLE-type practice examinations to test your knowledge, you hone your question-answering skills by using the following approach: (1) Look at the last sentence in the vignette and determine what discipline is involved (pediatrics, surgery, medicine, etc.) and what the question asks—is it diagnosis, the next best step in management, pathology, etc.? (2) Carefully read the vignette, and in your mind, formulate the underlying central concept by asking yourself what of the description is truly relevant to the question asked. (3) Carefully read the distractors, looking for the one that most clearly relates to the central concept you formulated and also answers the question asked. You should be able to identify the one best choice.

Often, a second choice will seem as if it too might be correct; perhaps there is a distractor that would be correct under special circumstances, or one that relates to a factoid in the vignette not relevant to the central concept. Having read the vignette carefully, you should be able to identify the one that is the best choice, but if you are still in doubt, don't waste time deliberating; make a choice and move on to the next question. Realize that, although this might seem like making a guess, because you did think about it, it is an educated guess, and your choice is most likely the correct one. Resist the temptation to brood over a subtlety you may find. This will cause you to waste time, perhaps forcing you to make wild guesses on other questions in the last few seconds before time is up. Moreover, if you do finish before the allotted time is up, you should learn to refrain from going back and changing your first response on the basis of lingering doubts; odds are that your first response was the correct one.

After finishing your practice tests, go back to look at questions over which you debated between two possible choices and see if your instinctive response was correct. More often than not, it would be surprising if it wasn't. Furthermore, by analyzing the explanation provided, you may be able to understand why you were tempted by the wrong choice. A corollary to this approach is to carefully control the time factor; learn to spend no more than 72 seconds, preferably less, on each question.

The previous paragraphs focus on the one-best-choice type of question. These will constitute the majority of questions on the examination. The remaining ones will be of the matching-set variety. In these, you are faced with up to 26 optional choices, each to be matched with a brief question. A suggested approach for efficiently answering such matching item sets is the following: (1) First read the question; (2) glance at the options to get an idea of the type and range of possibilities; (3) read the first question vignette; (4) think of an option of the type listed that seems logical; (5) look through the list and choose the one that most closely agrees to the one in your mind. Odds are you will find one close match, and this will be the correct choice. However, if you can't come up with a matching choice, attack the problem in the reverse manner and eliminate choices that are obviously wrong; even if this won't necessarily provide one clear choice, it will reduce the number of possibilities, making a correct guess more likely. After completing this cycle by answering the question raised in the first vignette, do the same with the second one, then the third, and so on. Remember that a given option may be used once, more than once, or never, so don't try to eliminate a choice on the basis of its prior use.

Both types of questions may involve a list of clinical laboratory values, and as a rule, the only ones relevant to the question are among those that are abnormal. Although you will be able to refer to a table of accepted values to identify abnormal ones, this will take time. Thus, it will behoove you to memorize some of the normal ranges of laboratory values of several of the more common disease states. Although the reference range of normal values used at various hospitals or clinics may differ to a slight degree from those provided by the USMLE, these differences are too small to influence an answer. In the real USMLE, the clinical values are readily available via a computerized list. Since this is not possible in a written format, the correct values are provided in this NMS edition along with the question.

## IMPROVING YOUR PSYCHOLOGIC AND PHYSIOLOGIC ABILITY TO TAKE THE EXAMINATION

Your psychologic and physiologic status can be as important as your intellectual readiness. There is no escaping the fact that spending almost 9 hours in an intimate relationship with a computer is stressful. Consequently, you need to prepare yourself as well as possible. Some ideas include the following:

- Once you have studied enough to achieve a basic working vocabulary, start answering USMLE-style questions by taking USMLE-style mini-examinations using suitable USMLE-type question-and-answer materials. These mini-examinations serve several purposes. As discussed above, they enhance your examination-taking skills (increase your sense of timing, etc.). They increase your knowledge base directly by exposing you to new information and indirectly by providing feedback to help guide your studies. The consistent improvement you are bound to show will boost your confidence. This can be of critical importance for students who suffer from excessive test anxiety.

- At first, these mini-examinations should be composed of a relatively small number of questions because you should still be expanding your knowledge base, and much of your time should be spent analyzing why you missed what you did. If you determine that most of your errors were due to ignorance, go back to your earlier phases of study. If you tend to primarily miss questions in a given area, focus on that area. However, more than likely, you will find that you more often miss questions because you misinterpreted the question and/or one or more distractors and consequently jumped to an incorrect assumption. Realizing this and making a conscious effort to reread and interpret this type of question, coupled with practice, should reduce your tendency to make such erroneous snap judgments, even under the pressure of limited time. Increase the number of questions in your practice sessions as your scheduled time to take the examination draws nearer. At least 2 weeks before the examination, you should try simulating a full 9-hour examination. Then, about a week later, simulate taking the full examination again, even if you must use the same practice examination. Don't worry—unless you have a photographic memory, the improvement you show will be because you learned something, and this improvement will once again heighten your confidence. As mentioned above, the real examination consists of eight 1-hour examinations. This edition that has 12 examinations in the book and 8 on the web, provides enough test material including full simulated examinations.

- From the beginning, time yourself. You will have exactly 60 minutes to answer up to 50 questions on the real test. To make the process a bit more challenging, assume only 50 minutes are available. Thus, you should allot 50 minutes for a 50-question test, 25 minutes for 25-question test, etc. You are better off timing the whole group of questions rather than individual ones; not only is this easier to do since you need only set your timing device once, but it will help you develop an intrinsic sense of proper pacing.

- Review the tutorial on the official USMLE CD-ROM, then re-review it until you have memorized the operational key strokes required to navigate from screen to screen and the types and locations of information on the screens. The operational aspects of the program should be second nature for you by the time you take the examination. This again will lead to a feeling of confidence at the start of the test and will also permit you to use most of the 15-minute tutorial session provided to answer questions rather than playing with the computer.

- Establish beneficial sleep habits. Begin by going to bed early and getting up early at least a month before your scheduled examination date. This will adjust your circadian rhythm to match that required when the real day comes. It will also improve the odds that you will get a good night's sleep and be able to wake up refreshed and prepared to remain alert during that long examination day that not only will include the 9-hour examination, but also time to eat breakfast, get dressed, travel, etc.

- Plan on getting to the Prometric Center about 30 minutes earlier than your scheduled time. Although this will extend the length of your day, it will provide a margin of safety in case of unexpected travel delays and will give you time to relax and acclimatize yourself.

- Watch your diet; practice eating a good breakfast that will maintain you into noon. If possible, get into the habit of having a bowel movement after breakfast and before the time you will need to leave to take the examination; you don't want to waste examination time sitting on the toilet. If early hunger becomes a problem, experiment with a power bar or some such supplement that satisfies you, that can be readily consumed, and does not stick to your teeth to distract you afterward. Also, get into the habit of packing light but nutritious lunches that satisfy, are not messy, are easy to carry around, and will sit well in your stomach.

- As much as possible, adjust personal arrangements to reduce stress. Discuss your need for a peaceful interlude with your spouse, significant other, or those in any other close relationships. Get your finances under control; make sure there will be no financial crises arising during the week prior to the examination.

- At least a day before the examination (and ideally earlier if travel is not a major obstacle), go to the Prometric Center where your examination is scheduled. Make sure you know how to get there and how long it will take. Go inside and familiarize yourself with personnel, procedures, and the computer setup.

- If the drive to the Prometric Center from your residence is excessive, make arrangements to spend the night before the examination in a comfortable and quiet place closer to the Center.

- On the night before the examination, lay out what you will need the following day, your clothes, lunch, anything you might want as a snack, and any other personal items, such as your watch, glasses, and a pen or pencil. You will also want to lay out the items required for admission to the examination, including your photo identification, scheduling permit, and confirmation ticket and number. Also make arrangements to wake up in time; ask for a wake-up call or better still, set an alarm clock. Not only will that get you started on time, but also it is likely to help you sleep better because you will not subconsciously be worried about waking up. Don't forget transportation. If you are going by public transportation, be sure of the schedule and have the proper change for carfare. If you are going in your own car, make sure it has enough fuel and is otherwise in proper operational order. Also determine ahead of time what parking facilities are available and allow for extra transportation time if there is inclement weather.

- On the day before the examination, you will be nervous. Rather than trying to do last-minute cramming that is liable to be ineffective at best and will only make you more nervous, try to relax. Go someplace special with a loved one, who very likely has been feeling neglected, or at least take a walk, commune with nature—in short, do something peaceful and pleasant, even if part of your day must be spent in travel. Whatever you do, don't use alcohol or drugs as a tool to help you relax; you want to be clear-headed the following morning.

## Taking The Examination

After having a relaxing day and a good night's sleep, you arrive 30 minutes before your scheduled time at the designated examination site, nervous but bright-eyed and bushy-tailed. After checking in, you then make good use of any free time remaining by taking a brief walk in anticipation of sitting for a long time. Also make a prophylactic trip to the bathroom. The momentous moment arrives; you enter your cubicle and face the computer. Now it is up to you to manage the next 9 hours at maximal efficiency and demonstrate what you really know.

- *Managing your scheduled free time.* You are provided with a total of 9 examination hours, which include eight 1-hour blocks of uninterruptible test time, 45 minutes of free time, and 15 minutes of optional tutorial time. Since you have practiced the tutorial at home ad infinitum, there is no reason for you to do so again. Thus, you can use this 15 minutes as extra free time in any manner you like. Remember that the computer will continue to count time even if you depart from your cubicle during an hour scheduled as examination time. This not only shortens the time available for test taking, but the departure will be logged in as a potential irregularity; so use the free time to prevent a need for an interruption, as well as a way to refresh yourself so that you can function well during these intense sessions. We suggest that you use about 30 minutes of the available hour of free time in short 5- to 10-minute breaks between testing blocks to unwind after finishing an intense hour. During these brief intervals, stretch your legs and exercise your arms by doing pushups against the wall. If you are hungry, eat a small bite; if possible, go outside and breathe fresh air, and go to the bathroom. Use the remaining 30 minutes of free time after the fourth or fifth examination block as a longer break during which you eat your prepacked light lunch and then relax. Above all, remember to keep track of your free time; once you use it up, there will be no more breaks, no matter how fatigued you are. Moreover, any nonexamination time you might take in excess of the allotted hour is subtracted from the final hour of examination time. Conversely, by completing an examination block in less than an hour, you in effect buy additional free time that may come in handy later in the day.

- *Managing your examination time.* Remember that you will have exactly 1 hour in which to finish a question block. When time is up, the computer will switch off. There will be no last seconds to fill in unanswered questions, as in the typical paper-and-pencil examination. Consequently, it is best to answer questions one at a time, in the order presented, proceeding at a measured pace and always keeping an eye on the clock so that no question will be left unanswered when the program terminates. Should it appear that you will not finish on time, increase the pace, and, as a last resort, guess. An incorrect response is no worse than no response. If there are about 20 minutes remaining, and you still have not finished answering the one-best-choice type of questions, quickly glance at them, make your best guess; mark these as questions you may wish to return to, and then start answering the matching questions. Generally, one can answer these faster than the one-best-choice variety. Moreover, the odds of guessing a correct answer are 20% for the typical five-distractor one-best-choice questions and 10% or less for matching questions; thus, guessing is apt to have better returns for the former. If, after finishing the matching questions, extra time still remains, go back to the first one-best-choice that began the guessing sequence and proceed as if it were the first time you saw it; under these circumstances, changing an answer after making a guess is permissible, since this is not the same as changing an answer on questions that you had time to think about. Make a habit of using the question-marking function, but do it very conservatively; use it only on those items for which your guesses were not made on the basis of due deliberation. If you made an "informed" guess, odds are that your first response was the proper one anyway. If you feel a rising sense of panic during an examination time, stop for a moment, take a series of deep breaths, think about the successes you had during your practice sessions, and remember that nobody is asking you to be perfect. Odds are that you will pass even if you miss one of every three questions, and you might be doing better than average if you are answering 25% of the questions incorrectly.

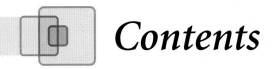

# Contents

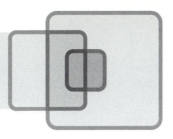

# test 1

# Questions

**Single Best Choice Directions:** *This section consists of numbered statements or questions followed by a list of potential answers; you are to select the ONE best answer.*

**1** A 24-year-old man who had been alcoholic since his early teens underwent rehabilitation therapy during which he suffered severe withdrawal symptoms, including a seizure. Subsequently, he had seizures on a regular basis, during which he would turn pale, feel nauseous, become rigid, stop breathing, lose consciousness, and fall to the ground. After a minute, his body would jerk in a violent fashion for an additional 3 or 4 minutes; he would then lapse into a period of flaccid coma, which lasted 30 to 60 minutes more. After recovering consciousness, he had a headache, was disoriented and confused, felt nauseated, and had sore muscles but could remember nothing concerning his seizure. Following a detailed diagnostic workup including electroencephalography, he was put on medication. Which of the following drugs was most likely used in his initial treatment?

(A) Felbamate
(B) Topiramate
(C) Phenytoin
(D) Ethosuximide
(E) Tiagabine

**2** A 14-year-old boy comes to the office because his breasts have recently become tender and slightly swollen. He is worried that he is undergoing feminization and will grow up to become a "freak." Upon examination a tender, 2-cm mass is found to be palpable in the subareolar region of both breasts. Which of the following describes the best course of action?

(A) Excise the masses by performing a subcutaneous mastectomy.
(B) Incise and drain the masses.
(C) Treat the masses with topical steroids.
(D) Aspirate the masses for culture and cytology.
(E) Leave the masses alone.

**3** A 20-year-old woman had her ears pierced when she was 16 years old. Since that time, she has had only two pairs of earrings, both given to her by her parents; both were 18 karat gold. Last week her 21-year-old boyfriend gave her a new pair of earrings for St. Valentine's Day, which she started to wear immediately. Three days later, she developed localized areas of erythema and vesicle formation where she had pierced her ears. The mechanism responsible for this reaction most closely resembles which of the following?

(A) Type I hypersensitivity
(B) An Arthus reaction
(C) A positive purified protein derivative (PPD) skin reaction
(D) Antibody-dependent cell-mediated cytotoxicity
(E) An immune complex disease

**4** A 32-year-old woman, gravida 4, para 4, consults a physician because for the past 6 months she has had abnormal vaginal bleeding that occurs intermittently between her predictable menstrual cycles. The bleeding is not associated with cramping, but there are often larger clots of blood. She has to wear panty protection and even a tampon when the bleeding is heavy. She underwent a tubal sterilization after her last delivery 5 years ago. She denies use of any medications other than multivitamins. She also is unaware of a history of bleeding disorders in any family member. A urine β-hCG test result is negative. On physical examination, she is well developed and well nourished. Results of a general examination are unremarkable. Pelvic examination reveals normal external genitalia and vagina. No cervical abnormalities are seen. The uterus is slightly enlarged but mobile and nontender. Pelvic imaging studies reveal uterine leiomyomata. Which of the following locations of leiomyomas would be most associated with the kind of bleeding seen in this patient?

(A) Submucosal
(B) Subserosal
(C) Intramural
(D) Intraligamentous
(E) Parasitic

**5** A forensic pathologist obtained cerebrospinal fluid (CSF) from three cadavers who died shortly before the samples were taken. One of the individuals died from a heart attack, the second from a self-inflicted gunshot wound, and the third from an intentional overdose of barbiturates. Metabolites derived from which of the following compounds are most likely to be found at a lower concentration in the cadaver who died from the gunshot wound than in the cadavers who died from a heart attack or a barbiturate overdose?

(A) Serotonin
(B) Protein
(C) Norepinephrine
(D) Glucose
(E) Epinephrine

**6** Twenty-four hours after an elective cholecystectomy, a 5 foot 2 inch (1.57 m) 155 lb (70.3 kg), 45-year-old woman develops a temperature of 101.6°F (38.7°C) and suffers pain and difficulty upon inspiration. Radiologic examination shows elevation of the right diaphragm. Which of the following is the most likely cause of these symptoms?

(A) A wound infection
(B) A urinary tract infection secondary to catheterization
(C) Pulmonary embolus
(D) Intravenous (IV) catheter–related sepsis
(E) A spontaneous pneumothorax
(F) Atelectasis

**7** A 65-year-old man complains of increasing sadness and inability to find pleasure in anything. He cannot even watch a TV program with his wife without getting so bored he starts fidgeting; he usually gets up and leaves before the end of the program. He has recently been forced to retire from his job, and he has been diagnosed with hypertension, diabetes mellitus, and glaucoma. Which of the following symptoms is most likely to suggest he may be at risk of committing suicide?

(A) Feelings of hopelessness
(B) Tearfulness
(C) Sleep disturbance
(D) Lassitude
(E) Anorexia

**8** A 23-year-old married woman comes to the office after recent exposure to a person with active hepatitis A. She has a long history of recurrent sinopulmonary infections and bronchial asthma. In addition, after her last pregnancy, she received a blood transfusion for severe postpartum hemorrhage. After receiving an intramuscular dose of immune serum globulin as prophylaxis against hepatitis A, she develops an anaphylactic reaction. Which of the following is the most likely cause of this patient's reaction?

(A) Immunoglobulin A (IgA) deficiency with anti-IgA antibodies
(B) A hemolytic transfusion reaction
(C) Contaminated immune serum globulin
(D) A type IV hypersensitivity reaction against a protein in the immune serum globulin
(E) A febrile reaction

**9** A 47-year-old man recently consulted a physician about developing weakness, particularly in his right hand. Upon providing a history, the man explained that he does house repair and has been working on a neighborhood rehabilitation project for the past several months. In doing this, he sandblasts and sands and scrapes by hand to remove the old paint. These homes were first constructed in the 1920s and since have been covered with several layers of paint. He also revealed that he habitually ate his lunch at the work site, which he described as being dusted with old paint particles. In addition to the weakness in his arm, he admitted to sporadic stomachaches, constipation, and said his wife had complained that he is always irritable. He also states that, until recently, he had been in good health. Upon examination, he was found to be 6 feet (19.7 m) tall and to weigh 170 lb (77.1 kg). His heart, lungs, and abdomen were normal, as were most analytical values, but he did show signs of right wristdrop consistent with radial nerve palsy and his complete blood count (CBC) showed a microcytic anemia; his serum iron levels were found to be normal. Which of the following diagnostic tests would provide the most useful information regarding the appropriate treatment?

(A) Nerve conduction velocity (NCV) study of the right arm
(B) Radiography of the right arm and wrist
(C) Magnetic resonance imaging (MRI) scans of the right arm and wrist
(D) Urine screen for heavy metals (lead, mercury, arsenic)
(E) Screening for diabetes mellitus

**10** A 14-year-old girl, a recent immigrant from Southeast Asia, is diagnosed with uncomplicated pulmonary tuberculosis. She is placed on a three-drug combination regimen, with two of the drugs administered daily and one of the agents administered twice weekly. Because of this drug therapy, the patient is also given pyridoxine on a daily basis, and she must undergo periodic tests of ocular function. During her drug treatment, a red–orange coloration of sweat and lacrimal secretions is noticed. Results of her liver function tests are normal. This patient is taking which of the following three drugs?

(A) Bismuth, metronidazole, tetracycline
(B) Ethambutol, isoniazid, rifampin
(C) Clarithromycin, isoniazid, streptomycin
(D) Ethambutol, isoniazid, rifabutin
(E) Isoniazid, pyrazinamide, rifampin

**11** A 34-year-old woman has a long history of difficulty forming close interpersonal relationships because she fears rejection. She has an unwarranted low self-esteem and often becomes anxious in the presence of others. According to psychodynamic theory, which of the following best describes her problem?

(A) It is a response to environmental pressure.
(B) It most likely developed after she left the shelter of her family.
(C) It is caused by childhood problems.
(D) It is unlikely to be responsive to treatment.
(E) It is innate.

**12** A 25-year-old woman of African descent who recently immigrated from Jamaica to the United States presents with intense pain in both hips. A radiograph of her pelvis shows bilateral hip deformities with increased density of the bone, while electrophoresis of a red cell hemolysate reveals predominantly hemoglobin S (HbS), slightly more than the normal amounts of fetal hemoglobin (HbF), and the presence of HbA$_2$, but no HbA. Which of the following is the most likely diagnosis?

(A) Osteomyelitis caused by *Staphylococcus aureus* infection
(B) Aseptic necrosis of the femoral heads
(C) Pathologic bone fracture
(D) Osteoarthritis
(E) Legg-Calvé-Perthes disease

**13** A 33-year-old anthropologist from New York had been doing research in a desert region of Arizona for about 6 months. After returning home, he visits his physician complaining of an influenza-like illness with cough, mild chest pain, and occasional fever. He says that the illness started during the last few weeks of his stay in Arizona. Red, tender nodules are present on his shins. Chest x-rays fail to reveal evidence of pulmonary infiltrates or pleural effusion. Which of the following is the most appropriate next step in the management of this patient?

(A) Delay treatment until culture results are obtained.
(B) Begin treatment with fluconazole.
(C) Begin treatment with amphotericin B.
(D) Aspirate bone marrow and culture.
(E) Institute immediate isolation.

4 • *USMLE Step 2 CK*

**14** A 40-year-old man complains of attacks of fear, agitation, a sense of being unable to breathe, and feelings of impending doom. Mental status examination reveals a hyperalert, restless, dysphoric individual. There is no evidence of cognitive impairment, hallucinations, illusions, delusions, or disorganized thinking. Which of the following is the most likely diagnosis?

(A) Delirium
(B) Depersonalization disorder
(C) Dysthymic disorder
(D) Panic disorder
(E) Schizoaffective disorder

**15** A 59-year-old man has a body mass index (BMI) of 42. As might be expected, his fasting blood glucose level is high, 210 mg/dL, as was his HbA1c level, 9.8%. In addition, he suffers from hypertension and dyslipidemia. His physician advised him to lose weight both for his general well-being and to help control his diabetes. Consequently, for the past 4 years, he has desperately tried to lose weight. He worked his way through an alphabet of popular and fad diets, from the Atkins diet to the Weight Watchers diet. If he lost a few pounds while on a particular diet, he gained back the pounds lost, plus a few more within a few months of terminating the diet. Finally, he and his physician decided he should try bariatric surgery, the Roux-en-Y gastric bypass procedure. A week after leaving the hospital, his fasting blood glucose level was 100 mg/dL. Three months later, it was 96 mg/dL and his HbA1c was 6.0%. Which of the following choices is most likely to explain this remarkable improvement is his diabetes?

(A) The reduction in level of his circulating glucagon-like peptide-1 (GLP-1)
(B) The reduction in level of his circulating peptide YY (PYY)
(C) The reduction in his mass of adipose tissue
(D) The reduction in the level of his circulating ghrelin
(E) The reduction in the level of his circulating leptin

**16** A 37-year-old man, an illegal immigrant from Guatemala, presents to the emergency room with vomiting and abdominal distension. He reports that he has not had a bowel movement in over a week. Rectal examination reveals the absence of stool in the rectal vault with a dilated colon. He also has a low-grade fever derived from what was diagnosed as Chagas disease. Further examination would most likely also demonstrate which of the following conditions?

(A) Diverticula
(B) Hirschsprung disease
(C) Adenomatous polyps
(D) Inflamed colon
(E) Anal fistulas

**17** A 48-year-old man complains of a 5-month history of memory impairment; he is afraid of losing his job as a waiter because he has some difficulty in speaking clearly, has difficulty in doing the few complex maneuvers required, such as folding napkins properly, and he is losing tips because he can no longer recognize regular customers. Mental status examination reveals an alert and attentive patient with an average vocabulary. He remembers one of three objects after 5 minutes and has marked difficulty with reasoning and abstraction. Which of the following is the most likely diagnosis?

(A) Delirium
(B) Amnestic disorder
(C) Dementia
(D) Major depressive disorder
(E) Mental retardation

**18** A 23-year-old African American man presents to the emergency room with swollen lips, eyelids, and palms and blotchy swellings in his buttocks and genitalia that itch and are painless. He also complains of colicky abdominal pain. He has a history of similar recurrent attacks since his early teens. His family history is strongly positive for a similar problem on his paternal side. Physical examination reveals a young man in apparent respiratory distress due to swollen lips and tongue. He has large, blotchy, nontender lesions with indistinct margins in the gluteal areas, and obvious diffuse swelling of his eyelids and hands. Examination of his chest reveals a few scattered rhonchi and rales. His abdomen is soft, but diffusely tender. There is no rigidity, and bowel sounds are present. Which of the following assays would be the best screen for this disease?

(A) C3 complement assay
(B) Quantitative immunoglobulins assay
(C) C4 complement assay
(D) Serum antinuclear antibody assay
(E) Sweat chloride assay

**19** A 32-year-old woman, gravida 1, para 0, with a history of infertility, underwent ovulation induction resulting in a twin pregnancy, now at 31 weeks' gestation. An early obstetric sonogram at 7 weeks' gestation showed dichorionic placentation. She has a positive group B β-hemolytic streptococcus vaginal culture. Because of epigastric pain, vaginal bleeding, and uterine contractions, she is evaluated at the maternity unit. An obstetric sonogram shows twin A to be a female fetus in breech presentation and twin B to be a male fetus in transverse lie with the back down. The sonogram also shows a marginal anterior placenta previa. Her initial vital signs are as follows: temperature, 37.2°C (99.0°F); pulse, 95/min; respiration, 18/min; blood pressure, 165/115 mm Hg. Her urine dipstick test shows 2+ glucose and 3+ albumin. Which of the following is a contraindication to tocolysis in this case?

(A) Multiple gestation
(B) Marginal placenta previa
(C) Severe preeclampsia
(D) Early gestational age
(E) Positive group B β-hemolytic streptococcus vaginal culture

**20** A 67-year-old man who had been successfully medicated for hypertension for the past 15 years develops a diastolic pressure of 110 mm Hg. At that time, he was taking hydrochlorothiazide, acebutolol, clonidine, and doxazosin mesylate for his blood pressure and metformin for type 2 diabetes. A serum panel was unremarkable, except that his creatinine level was 4 mg/dL (normal, 0.6–1.2 mg/dL), and his blood urea nitrogen (BUN) was 28 mg/dL (normal, 8–20 mg/dL). In an attempt to lower his blood pressure, his physician added enalapril; the patient rapidly developed renal failure. Which of the following choices represents the most likely diagnosis?

(A) Renal arterial stenosis due to fibromuscular dysplasia
(B) Acute renal artery occlusion
(C) Renal vein thrombosis due to a malignant occlusion
(D) Malignant hypertension
(E) Renal arterial stenosis due to occlusive arteriosclerotic disease

**21** A 29-year-old nulligravida complains of severe pain with menses for the past 3 years. Her last menstrual period was 10 days ago. She has been married 7 years and has used an intrauterine copper contraceptive system/device until the last couple of years, when she and her husband decided to start a family. Intercourse is painful with deep penetration. In spite of 15 months of unprotected twice-weekly intercourse she has been unable to conceive. Her menarche began at age 15, and her menstrual periods have been regular. She is employed as a nurse in a local doctor's office. She has had normal annual Pap smears. Findings of her general examination are unremarkable. On pelvic examination, external genitalia are without lesions. Her vagina is moist and supple. Her cervical os reveals clear, watery mucus. Her uterus is retroverted, tender to palpation, and there is nodularity of the uterosacral ligaments on rectovaginal examination. Which of the following will be the most helpful in confirming the diagnosis for this patient?

(A) History
(B) Laparoscopy
(C) Physical examination
(D) Hysterosalpingography
(E) Culdocentesis

**22** An 86-year-old woman is taken to the emergency room by her granddaughter because she has become disoriented, confused, and in general is not acting normal. In taking a history, with the aid of the granddaughter, the physician was able to ascertain that the patient complained of ringing in her ears, pain in her stomach, and dizziness. In addition, it was ascertained that in the days leading up to this incidence she had been taking two 325-mg aspirin tablets every 4 hours because of arthritic pain. Vital signs were: temperature 101.6°F (38.7°C), respiration 14/min, heart rate 150/min, blood pressure 85/45 mm Hg, and a plasma glucose level of 175 mg/dL. An electrolyte panel shows an anion gap of 18 mEq/L. Salicylate poisoning was suspected, and blood gases were analyzed. Which of the following arterial blood patterns most clearly points to salicylate poisoning?

|  | pH | Paco$_2$ | Bicarbonate |
|---|---|---|---|
| Normal range | 7.35–7.45 | 33–44 mm Hg | 22–28 mEq/L |
| (A) | 7.28 | 53 | 25 |
| (B) | 7.38 | 22 | 12 |
| (C) | 7.29 | 58 | 30 |
| (D) | 7.48 | 70 | 46 |
| (E) | 7.53 | 30 | 20 |

**23** A 30-year-old woman seeks treatment for persistent anxiety that has increased since she joined a law firm 4 years ago. She describes worry and rumination that she is inadequate in social situations, concern that she will not be granted partnership next year, and fears that her life will turn out badly. She also complains of difficulty sleeping, trouble concentrating, tenseness, and irritability. She denies any other significant medical problems, any substance abuse, or any history of psychosis. However, she admits to worrying a lot since childhood; for example, if her parents left her with a babysitter, she would fear that they would not come home and would be awake until they did. Mental status examination reveals an anxious woman. She is appropriately dressed, and her thought processes are logical. There is no evidence of hallucinations or delusions. She shows no psychomotor retardation. Her conversation includes no suicidal rumination or feelings of hopelessness. Which of the following is the most appropriate initial pharmacologic treatment for this patient?

(A) Modafinil
(B) Zolpidem
(C) Risperidone
(D) Alprazolam
(E) Venlafaxine

**24** A 28-year-old primigravid woman comes to the outpatient prenatal clinic at 34 weeks' gestation with a twin pregnancy. Her fundal height is 40 cm and the orientation of the fetuses in the uterus is cephalic–breech presentation. She was standing in the kitchen when she experienced a sudden gush of fluid that soaked her underwear and created a pool of fluid on the floor. Since then, she has had intermittent watery vaginal discharge for the past few days. She has had to wear a perineal pad for comfort. She denies dysuria or urinary burning but admits to urinary frequency. She is having occasional uterine contractions, up to three per hour. Which of the following is the most appropriate next step in the management of this patient?

(A) Nitrazine paper on the perineum
(B) Speculum examination for vaginal pooling
(C) Sonogram for amniotic fluid volume
(D) Urinalysis for urinary tract infection
(E) Digital examination for cervical dilation

**25** A 56-year-old indigent man had been sent home after undergoing an operation. However, 9 days later, he returns to the hospital's emergency room because of severe abdominal pain that has been getting progressively worse for the past week and has now become totally unbearable. On examination, the emergency physician observes an overweight male who looks much older than his stated years. His blood pressure is 88/68 mm Hg. He has a marked tenderness in the epigastric region along with "bruising" in that area. Laboratory analyses show an elevation of serum amylase. Which of the following is the most likely cause of his symptoms?

(A) A reaction to anesthetic drugs
(B) Hypovolemia
(C) Total parenteral nutrition (TPN)
(D) A common bile duct exploration for gallstones
(E) Postoperative infection

**26** A 19-year-old man who fell while playing basketball fractured the shaft of the right radius and ulna and subsequently underwent closed reduction and application of a cylindrical cast. He now presents with complaints of pain in the right index finger; there is no tingling sensation. Clinical examination reveals no diminution in capillary refill time and no hypesthesia. Cyanosis is absent. Passive movement of the finger elicits pain. The cast appears intact. Which of the following would be the most appropriate next step in the management of this patient?

(A) Reassure the patient
(B) Prescribe analgesics
(C) Prescribe corticosteroids
(D) Cleave the cast
(E) Leave the cast intact and elevate the arm for 24 hours

**27** A 65-year-old patient develops aspiration pneumonitis after general anesthesia. Twenty-four hours later, there is a rapid onset of dyspnea, tachypnea, cyanosis, and intercostal refractions. A chest radiograph shows diffuse, bilateral infiltrates with both an interstitial and an alveolar pattern. There is sparing of the costophrenic angles. Air bronchograms are noted. The arterial blood gases (ABGs) on 30% $O_2$ show a pH of 7.20 (normal, 7.35–7.45), a $PaCO_2$ of 74 mm Hg (normal, 33–44 mm Hg), and a bicarbonate of 28 mEq/L (normal, 22–28 mEq/L). This patient's clinical and laboratory findings are most likely the result of which of the following mechanisms?

(A) Depression of the respiratory center
(B) Intrapulmonary shunting
(C) Increased compliance of the lungs
(D) Increased elasticity of the lungs
(E) Respiratory alkalosis

**28** A 28-year-old man who was in an automobile accident is brought to the emergency department by paramedics. The patient is conscious. Clinical examination reveals no sensations below the level of the umbilicus and absent superficial and deep tendon jerks. Which of the following would be an expected finding in this patient?

(A) Hypertension and tachycardia
(B) Hypotension and bradycardia
(C) Hypertension and bradycardia
(D) Hypotension and tachycardia
(E) Normal blood pressure and normal pulse rate

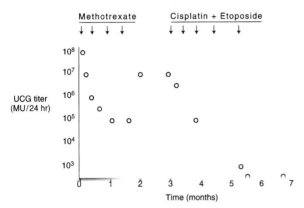

**29** The graph above represents two courses of chemotherapy of metastatic choriocarcinoma in a patient monitored by urinary chorionic gonadotropin (UCG) titer (mU/24 h). Both courses represent regimens of drug treatment in a pulsatile mode (indicated by downward arrows). In each course, the drug doses were maximized to the toxicity limit of a 2-log decrease in blood platelets. Which of the following statements about these data is correct?

(A) The effects of chemotherapy on UCG titer bear no relation to cell kill.
(B) The maximal effect of methotrexate is a 2-log decrease in UCG titer.
(C) The drug-induced changes in UCG titer are directly proportional to decreases in platelet count.
(D) The use of UCG titer as a guide to therapy in choriocarcinoma is less valuable than use of chest x-ray films.
(E) The maximal effect of cisplatin plus etoposide is greater than a 4-log decrease in UCG titer.

**30** A woman at 7 months' gestation presents for a prenatal examination. She has a history of mild hyperthyroidism, and despite her advanced pregnancy, she is found to have lost 4 lb since her last visit a month ago. She also has developed a fine tremor of her fingers. Her resting heart rate is 120 beats/min, and her thyroid gland is noticeably larger than it was at the time of her last office visit. Management of this patient's condition would be best achieved by treatment with which of the following?

(A) Lugol's solution
(B) Radioactive iodine ($^{131}$I)
(C) Iodide followed by surgical removal of the gland
(D) Propylthiouracil
(E) Propranolol

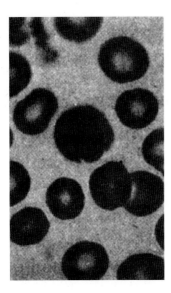

**31** The cell depicted in the peripheral smear illustrated above is representative of the majority of cells in an afebrile 75-year-old male with generalized, non-painful lymphadenopathy, hepatosplenomegaly, and petechiae and ecchymoses scattered over his body. His complete blood count (CBC) shows a hemoglobin of 9.0 g/dL (normal for males is 13.5–17.5 g/dL), his red blood cell (RBC) indices are normal, his platelet count is 70,000 cells/μL (normal is 150,000–400,000 cells/μL), and his leukocyte count is 90,000 cells/μL (normal is 4500–11,000 cells/μL). Eighty-five percent of the leucocytes are lymphocytes that are morphologically indistinguishable from small normal lymphocytes. Which of the following scenarios should be expected?

(A) The patient will develop a monocytopenia.
(B) The patient's disease will progress into an acute myelogenous leukemia.
(C) The leukocytes represented in the peripheral smear illustrated above have Auer rods.
(D) Bone marrow infiltration by the cells represented in the peripheral smear illustrated above is manifested by paratrabecular lymphoid aggregates.
(E) Diffuse bone marrow and lymph node infiltration is suggested by the cells represented in the peripheral smear illustrated above.

**32** A 61-year-old man comes to a family physician for the first time after recently moving into town. In providing a history, he reveals that he has osteogenesis imperfecta (OGI), a condition that has been in his family for several generations. As a consequence, he has had at least a dozen major fractures, all in various long bones. He also discloses he is diabetic and takes metformin, 850 mg, twice daily and that the last time he had a hemoglobin A1c determination, about a year earlier, the value was 5.9%. Additionally, he has been diagnosed as hypertensive and is taking 25 mg hydrochlorothiazide once daily, and 20 mg enalapril, as well as 200 mg acebutolol twice daily. At this time, his only complaint is various aches and pains, which are particularly bad in his left wrist and ankle, both of which had suffered at least one break. Upon awakening in the morning, he feels stiff and has minor pain, but as the day progresses the pain grows worse and, particularly if he had been on his feet for an extended period, the pain in his left ankle becomes excruciating. Examination yielded the following data: temperature 37°C (98.6°F), blood pressure 128/85 mm Hg, respiration 12/min. There was clearly discernible limitation of motion in both the left ankle and wrist, but neither joint was warm to the touch. Examination of his heart and lungs disclosed no abnormalities. At this time, which of the following tests is most likely to lead to a treatment protocol that will provide long-term beneficial results?

(A) A bone density determination
(B) Blood test for the rheumatic factor
(C) Radiographic studies
(D) A complete blood count
(E) An erythrocyte sedimentation determination
(F) Blood test for antinuclear antibodies
(G) Arthrographic examination of the affected joints

**33** A 75-year-old homeless man develops painful swelling of the right parotid gland 10 days after cholecystectomy. His physician cannot help noticing that he has a bad case of halitosis and that his teeth seem to be poorly cared for. The painful swelling of the right parotid gland is most likely secondary to which of the following?

(A) *Staphylococcus aureus*
(B) Duct obstruction by a stone
(C) A viral infection
(D) Hemorrhage
(E) An immunologic reaction

**34** A 29-year-old man is brought to a marriage counselor by his wife, who complains that her husband refuses to attend PTA meetings, neighborhood gatherings, and social functions with her. The husband confesses during the interview that he has feelings of extreme anxiety when in social situations. He realizes that, as a result, he avoids social gatherings, feels lonely, is not promoted in his job, and is liable to lose his wife. He feels helpless. Which of the following is the most appropriate initial treatment?

(A) Assertiveness training
(B) Implosion therapy
(C) Psychodynamic psychotherapy
(D) Lorazepam
(E) Systematic desensitization

**35** A 52-year-old woman presents to the emergency department because of the recent onset of hallucinations and delirium. Approximately 1 month ago, she was diagnosed with type 2 diabetes, and her physician prescribed 250 mg of chlorpropamide daily. At that time, the patient told her physician that she was worried about starting a lifetime drug regimen because she had no health insurance and a limited income. Results of physical examination are unremarkable. Her skin turgor is normal. Laboratory studies indicate the following values: serum sodium concentration, 120 mEq/L (normal, 135–147 mEq/L); serum potassium concentration, 3.2 mEq/L (normal, 3.5–5.0 mEq/L); serum chloride concentration, 90 mEq/L (normal, 95–105 mEq/L); serum bicarbonate concentration, 21 mEq/L (normal, 22–28 mEq/L); serum glucose concentration, 140 mg/dL (normal, 70–110 mg/dL); and serum blood urea nitrogen (BUN) concentration, 5 mg/dL (normal, 7–18 mg/dL). Random urine sodium level is 80 mEq/L (normally >20 mEq/L indicates increased loss; <20 mEq/L indicates increased reabsorption). A computed tomography (CT) scan of her head showed small lateral ventricles consistent with cerebral edema. No bleeding was observed. Which of the following would be most appropriate in the management of this patient?

(A) Treat her with a selective serotonin reuptake inhibitor (SSRI).
(B) Restrict sodium from her diet.
(C) Substitute metformin for the chlorpropamide.
(D) Increase her water intake.
(E) Add sodium to her diet.
(F) Administer demeclocycline, an antidiuretic hormone (ADH) inhibitor.

**36** A 2-week-old, term infant presents to the pediatrician for a well-child check. According to the mother, the patient is a healthy baby; she has been feeding and growing well. Physical examination is pertinent for a slightly jaundiced infant, which after the review of the birth history and laboratory data is attributed to breastfeeding. The total bilirubin is 18 mg/dL (normal is <7 mg/dL), and the direct bilirubin is 0.8 mg/dL (normal is 0–0.4 mg/dL). Which of the following is a true statement about jaundice associated with breast-milk jaundice?

(A) It is seen in the first few days of life.
(B) There is a significant elevation of conjugated bilirubin.
(C) Serum bilirubin falls slowly if breastfeeding is discontinued.
(D) The mother should stop breastfeeding completely.
(E) Mild breastfeeding jaundice requires no intervention.

**37** A 26-year-old nulligravid woman comes to the office complaining of increased facial and general body hair. She states that she had no problem until 6 months ago, when she began noticing prominent, coarse, dark hair on her upper lip and chin. She says her bra is fitting her much more loosely than it used to. Her menses have always been regular every 30 days, but now she reports her periods are irregular. She is sexually active with her husband of 5 years. She states her libido has increased over the past few months. She denies any family history of excessive body hair. On examination, she presents as a well-nourished, muscular woman with a deep voice. She has copious pubic hair with a male-appearing escutcheon. Examination of her external genitalia reveals clitoromegaly. On bimanual examination a 4 × 5 cm mass is palpated in the left adnexa. Which of the following is the most likely diagnosis?

(A) Granulosa-theca cell tumor
(B) Brenner tumor
(C) Sertoli-Leydig cell tumor
(D) Fibroma
(E) Dysgerminoma

**38** A 43-year-old woman becomes listless and apathetic after a series of setbacks in her life. She no longer tries to make her life better, and spends 12 to 14 hours per day in bed. Mental status examination reveals moderate psychomotor retardation, soft speech, and difficulty concentrating. Which of the following is the most accurate behavioral explanation for her symptoms?

(A) Faulty cognitive framework
(B) Object loss
(C) Inadequate exposure to light
(D) Learned helplessness
(E) Double-bind communication

**39** A 58-year-old woman presents with vaginal bleeding, which started 1 week ago. Her last menstrual period was 7 years ago, and she has not had any bleeding since that time. She has never been married and has never had any children, nor has she ever used any form of contraception. She is 160 cm (63 in) tall and weighs 86 kg (190 lb). She states she has always been overweight and has a difficult time exercising regularly. Ten years ago, she was diagnosed with type 2 diabetes mellitus for which she has been managed with oral hypoglycemic agents. She does not check her blood glucose values regularly. She is taking hydrochlorothiazide for chronic hypertension, which was diagnosed 5 years ago. Which of the following is the diagnostic method of choice in this patient?

(A) Pap smear
(B) Endometrial biopsy
(C) Pelvic examination under anesthesia
(D) Laparoscopy
(E) Colposcopy

**40** A 35-year-old woman, gravida 3, para 2, underwent a spontaneous vaginal delivery at 39 weeks' gestation of a 3,295 g (7 lb 4 oz) male neonate who has done well. She had a prolonged third stage of labor, resulting in an attempted manual removal of the placenta. The placenta was not completely removed, and bleeding progressed to hemorrhage. Ultimately, she underwent an emergency total abdominal hysterectomy due to placenta accreta. She received 5 units of packed red blood cells (PRBCs). Her blood pressure was in the hypotensive range for 30 minutes during the procedure. Which of the following pituitary hormones is most likely to be affected by her clinical course?

(A) Adrenocorticotropic hormone (ACTH)
(B) Prolactin
(C) Thyroid-stimulating hormone (TSH)
(D) Follicle-stimulating hormone (FSH)
(E) Antidiuretic hormone (ADH)

*Directions for Matching Questions (41 through 50): Each set of matching questions is preceded by a list of 4 to 26 lettered options followed by a brief explanation of the required task and then by a series of numbered statements. For each lettered statement, you are to select ONE lettered option that best fulfills the task as it relates to that statement. Remember that each of the listed options might be correctly selected once, more than once, or not at all.*

## Questions 41–45

(A) 47XX + 21
(B) 47XYY
(C) 45X
(D) 47XXY
(E) 47XY + 13

*Match the ONE indicated chromosomal aberration listed above with the phenotype described below.*

**41** Children born alive failed to develop the normal formation of the frontal cortex, a condition called *holoprosencephaly*. They also have a cleft lip and palate, midfacial abnormalities, peculiar punched-out scalp defects, and polydactyly.

**42** A male child developed normally. Although somewhat taller than expected, he otherwise is a phenotypically normal man. However, his parents fear he may become a criminal since males with this chromosomal pattern are found in a higher than expected frequency in mental or penal institutions.

**43** A female baby is born with a flattened face and occiput, upward slanting eyes, an extra skin fold at the medial aspect of the eyes, a large tongue, and small ears. In addition the newborn is hypotonic.

**44** This boy appeared normal at birth and through childhood until puberty, when it became evident that he had small testes and postpubertal gynecomastia that did not resolve.

**45** A teenage girl is brought to the pediatrician by her mother because she has not started her menstruation. The child and her family recently immigrated to this country, and the mother says that although the patient's immunizations are current, she was not routinely seen by a physician. Pertinent on physical examination is that the girl appears short for her age, has a webbed neck, and underdeveloped breasts with widespread nipples due to a shield-shaped chest.

## Questions 46–50

(A) Fractured talus
(B) Tear of the Achilles tendon
(C) Fracture of the calcaneus
(D) Tear involving muscle fibers of the plantar flexors
(E) Torn lateral ligament in the ankle
(F) Fractured metatarsal shafts

*Choose the ONE lettered type of injury from the list above that best relates to the symptoms described in the numbered vignettes below.*

**46** A 27-year-old woman running to catch a bus is wearing shoes with 3-inch heels when her heel strikes a pebble and she twists her ankle. As a consequence, she can no longer walk without pain.

**47** A 46-year-old man has been running for several hours each day in preparation for a local marathon. As a result, he has developed some slight pain in the back of the right leg just above the heel. Since it doesn't bother him too much, he agrees to play a game of tennis with his girlfriend. She lobs the ball over the net, forcing him to run in close, and then she returns it over his head, making him back up and twist on his right foot. At that moment, he hears a pop and feels a sharp pain in his ankle. Subsequently, the ankle becomes swollen, and he can only limp along in pain.

**48** A 42-year-old ex–minor league pitcher who now makes his living selling insurance was pitching in a pick-up game during a fourth of July picnic. He succeeded in striking out all the opposing batters until there were two out in the 7th inning. By now, he was becoming acutely aware that he no longer was in A-1 physical shape. As he pressed on and was throwing a hard fastball, he suddenly heard a popping sound in his hind leg (the one he rears on to get force and then extends behind him as he lunges his body and the ball forward). He later says that it felt as if somebody hit him on the calf muscle with a stick followed by rather severe pain that radiated up to his knee and down to his ankle. Within hours, the same area was bruised and swollen.

**49** A 19-year-old man was washing windows on the second floor of a house when his ladder slipped and he fell to the ground feet first. When he picked himself up he found that he could not bear weight on the right foot, and he is unable to evert that foot.

**50** A 73-year-old man decided that walking would be good for his cardiovascular system and started a program of daily walks, increasing the distance regularly. By the second week, he developed a pain behind the second toe on his right foot. Figuring he could walk through it, he continued walking, but on stepping out of his house during the fourth week, he felt a crackling sensation and the pain intensified. His primary care physician found a tender area on the second metatarsal about an inch below the toe. An x-ray film was negative.

# Answer Key

| | | | | |
|---|---|---|---|---|
| 1 C | 11 C | 21 B | 31 E | 41 E |
| 2 E | 12 B | 22 B | 32 A | 42 B |
| 3 C | 13 A | 23 E | 33 A | 43 A |
| 4 A | 14 D | 24 B | 34 A | 44 D |
| 5 A | 15 D | 25 D | 35 C | 45 C |
| 6 F | 16 B | 26 D | 36 E | 46 E |
| 7 A | 17 C | 27 B | 37 C | 47 B |
| 8 A | 18 C | 28 B | 38 D | 48 D |
| 9 D | 19 C | 29 E | 39 B | 49 C |
| 10 B | 20 E | 30 D | 40 B | 50 F |

# Answers and Explanations

### 1 The answer is C *Medicine*

Some 0.5% of the population in the United States is afflicted with some form of epilepsy, in which seizures generally start between 5 and 20 years of age. Most cases have no known cause, but several types of known triggers also exist; among these, as in the case described, is withdrawal from drugs or alcohol after a period of addiction. Two broad subtypes of epilepsy exist, partial and generalized seizures. The partial seizures are categorized as either simple or complex, whereas generalized seizures include absence (petit mal), atypical absence, myoclonic, and tonic-clonic (grand-mal). In the latter case, seizures may be isolated, recurrent (with an interval of days, weeks, months, or even years between attacks), serial (with a short period of hours or less between attacks), or repeated (with new sets of convulsions without recovering consciousness in between). This latter condition is known as *status epilepticus* and is a medical emergency. For patients with recurrent forms of epilepsy, the goal is to prevent further attacks by administration of an antiepileptic drug. The best drug for initiation of treatment depends upon the type of seizure, and continued use of the same drug depends upon effectiveness and tolerance of side effects by the patient. The symptoms provided in the vignette consist of tonic-clonic seizures clearly suggesting grand mal epilepsy, and phenytoin (choice **C**) is commonly used as the drug of first choice. The advantages of this drug include that it is effective in most cases of grand mal usually within 10 days of the initial dose, its side effects can generally be tolerated, and a single daily dose provides the required blood level of 10 to 20 $\mu g/\mu L$. The latter is important because the less often a drug needs to be taken, the greater the compliance.

Felbamate (choice **A**) can also be used to treat tonic-clonic seizures but is not approved for use as a first-line drug because of the risk of aplastic anemia and hepatic dysfunction. Topiramate (choice **B**) is only approved for adjunctive treatment in cases of partial seizure and secondary generalized seizure; in addition, somnolence and potential blindness are discouraging side effects; in addition, it must be administered twice daily, which increases the chance of nonadherence. Use of ethosuximide (choice **D**) is generally reserved for treatment of petit mal, whereas tiagabine (choice **E**) is an anticonvulsant primarily used as monotherapy for partial seizures.

### 2 The answer is E *Surgery*

The patient has gynecomastia, the development of breast tissue in males, which is normal in the neonate, pubertal boy, and elderly male. Increased estrogen stimulation (hyperestrinism) of breast tissue is the common factor in all cases of gynecomastia.

Adolescent gynecomastia is usually bilateral, and the tissue averages 2 to 3 cm in diameter. The breast enlargement is transient and most often subsides within 1 year; as a consequence the gynecomastic breast usually should be left alone (choice **E**). The boy should be reassured that he is normal and does not have to worry about developing breasts.

However, if the mass is greater than 5 cm or does not regress by 16 to 17 years of age, a subcutaneous mastectomy should be performed (choice **A**). Incision (choice **B**), aspiration (choice **D**), and topical steroids (choice **C**) are not indicated under any circumstances. Gynecomastia in a postpubertal, adult male younger than 70 to 80 years is not normal and hyperestrinism should be suspected. Hyperestrinism in an adult male is most commonly due to decreased catabolism of estrogen due to liver cirrhosis, most often induced by alcoholism. However, hyperestrinism also can be due to increased synthesis secondary to an adrenal or testicular tumor; increased human chorionic gonadotropin (HCG) from a testicular tumor; the hyperplastic Leydig's cells in Klinefelter syndrome; decreased androgen activity, which leaves estrogen unopposed (e.g., caused by hypothalamic or pituitary disorders); and by several drugs.

**3** **The answer is C** *Medicine*

It seems highly probable that the earrings given to her by her boy friend were not 18 karat gold, but rather a cheaper alloy containing nickel, and she developed contact dermatitis. Contact dermatitis is a common inflammatory disorder of skin that is associated with exposure to various antigens and irritating substances. Four types have been described—allergic contact dermatitis, irritant contact dermatitis, contact photodermatitis, and contact urticaria. Allergic contact dermatitis, of which this case is an example, is a cell-mediated type IV hypersensitivity reaction. Three conditions must be present for this reaction to occur; namely, a genetic predisposition, absorption of sufficient antigen through the skin surface, and a competent immune system. Antigenic substances of low molecular weight penetrate the skin, are phagocytized by Langerhans' cells, and are then transported to regional lymph nodes, where they are presented to T lymphocytes. The T lymphocytes release cytokines that are responsible for the inflammatory response in the tissue. Antigenic substances include rhus (found in poison ivy and poison oak), nickel (jewelry such as earrings, hair dyes), potassium dichromate (household cleaners, leather, cement), formaldehyde (cosmetics, fabrics), ethylenediamine (dyes, medications), mercapto-benzothiazole (rubber products), and paraphenylenediamine (hair dyes, chemicals used in photography).

Because allergic contact dermatitis is a type IV hypersensitivity reaction, the positive purified protein derivative (PPD) skin reaction (choice **C**), which involves the interaction of T cells and macrophages, most closely resembles the mechanism of inflammatory response observed in this patient. Irritant contact dermatitis is not a cell-mediated immune response. It is due to the local toxic effect of the chemical on the skin. Contact photodermatitis is similar to allergic contact dermatitis except that reaction depends on ultraviolet light. Contact urticaria is a wheal-and-flare reaction that may be secondary to a type I hypersensitivity (immunoglobulin E [IgE]-mediated) reaction or a nonimmunologic reaction. The clinical presentation of contact dermatitis, regardless of the mechanism, ranges from localized areas of erythema with vesicle formation to erythematous plaques of thickened skin in chronic disease. The treatment involves removal of the offending agent along with the use of wet compresses with Burow's solution in acute disease, followed by local application of steroid cream to suppress inflammation. Subacute or chronic cases should be treated with local steroid creams without the compresses. Extensive disease may require the use of systemic corticosteroid therapy.

In terms of the other mechanisms listed in the question, type I hypersensitivity (choice **A**) involves the interaction of IgE antibodies developed against specific antigens and mast cells. Reexposure to the antigen causes mast cell degranulation, with the release of histamine and other chemical mediators that produce increased vessel permeability, tissue swelling, and an inflammatory reaction. An Arthus reaction (choice **B**) is a localized immune complex disease (type III hypersensitivity) that activates the complement system to produce anaphylatoxins and chemotactic agents that cause the inflammatory reaction. An example of an Arthus reaction is farmer's lung, in which exposure to thermophilic actinomycetes in the air results in a localized immune complex deposition in the alveoli, with subsequent inflammation and hypersensitivity pneumonitis. Systemic immune complex diseases such as systemic lupus erythematosus (SLE) or serum sickness are also associated with immune complex deposition in various tissues, including the joints, skin, and vessels in the skin and glomerulus. Antibody-dependent cell-mediated cytotoxicity (ADCC) (choice **D**) is a variant of type II hypersensitivity. It involves the presence of antibody against a target tissue, which attracts killer cells, natural killer cells, or macrophages. These cells interact with the antibodies and destroy the target tissue. Warm autoimmune hemolytic anemia (AIHA), with destruction of immunoglobulin G (IgG) antibody-coated red blood cells (RBCs) by macrophages in the spleen, is a classic example of an ADCC reaction. An immune complex disease (choice **E**), such as serum sickness, is a type III hypersensitivity disease.

**4** **The answer is A** *Obstetrics and Gynecology*

The urine β-hCG (i.e., the free β subunit of human chorionic gonadotropin) test rules out the most common cause of abnormal bleeding, pregnancy. Anovulation, another common cause of abnormal vaginal bleeding is associated with unpredictable menstrual cycles rather than predictable ones, as in this case. The history of bleeding between normal predictable menses is classic for a genital tract anatomic lesion. The normal vaginal and cervical examinations rule out lower genital tract lesions. Upper tract lesions include endometrial polyps and submucosal leiomyomas. The latter lesion (choice **A**) causes bleeding by distorting the overlying endometrium, altering its normal response to hormonal changes through the menstrual cycle. This change can lead to abnormal bleeding. Visualization of anatomic lesions of the uterine cavity can be by hysterosalpingogram (using radiopaque dye) or saline vaginal sonogram (using a catheter to instill 10 cc of saline into the uterine cavity). The method of choice is hysteroscopy, which is not only diagnostic but also therapeutic because resection of the lesion can be carried out immediately on diagnosis.

Subserosal myomas (choice **B**) alter the external contour of the uterus, giving the lumpy, bumpy shape but do not cause bleeding. Intramural myomas (choice **C**) located within the myometrial wall are the most common kind of myomas and are generally asymptomatic. Intraligamentous myomas (choice **D**) bulging into the round ligament, and parasitic myomas (choice **E**) attaching to abdominal viscera have no direct impact on uterine bleeding.

### 5 The answer is A *Psychiatry*

In postmortem studies, levels of 5-hydroxyindole acetic acid (5-HIAA), a metabolite of serotonin, were found to be lower in the cerebrospinal fluid of victims of suicide by violent means, but not in victims who die by more passive means, such as by drug ingestion or nonviolent events such as a heart attack.

No other biochemical findings (e.g., altered levels of protein [choice **B**], norepinephrine [choice **C**], glucose [choice **D**], or epinephrine [choice **E**] have been consistently found in such studies). Some investigators believe that these findings provide evidence that a low level of central nervous system serotonin activity is causally related to depression. However, the relationship to violent suicide is unexplained.

### 6 The answer is F *Surgery*

Atelectasis (choice **F**) is the most common cause of fever in the first 24 hours of the postoperative state. Atelectasis refers to collapse of the lung distal to an area of obstruction in the airway. In the postoperative state, the dry secretions imposed by anesthesia and pain-restricted clearance of pulmonary secretions predispose the patient to segmental atelectasis and a nidus of inflammation, resulting in fever. Loss of lung mass leads to elevation of the diaphragm on that side. Prevention is the best strategy to avoid post operative atelectasis. Early recovery from anesthesia, sparing use of narcotics, encouraging coughing and deep breathing exercises, incentive spirometry, early ambulation, and use of nebulizers and chest physiotherapy are all part of the regime.

Wound infections (choice **A**) are more common in the 5- to 10-day postoperative period. Urinary tract infections from indwelling catheters (choice **B**) are common but do not usually cause fever unless pyelonephritis is a complication. Pulmonary embolus (choice **C**) is incorrect; symptoms usually occur within a few days following surgery, rather than soon after. Moreover pulmonary embolus may present with non-characteristic symptoms such as dyspnea and palpitations, or with characteristic symptoms such as cough, hemoptysis, tachypnea, and tachycardia. There may be evidence of deep venous thrombosis in the lower extremities. *Candida albicans* is a common cause of intravenous (IV) catheter-related sepsis (choice **D**) and would have a different set of symptoms. A pneumothorax (choice **E**) is usually not associated with fever and is not a common postoperative complication.

### 7 The answer is A *Psychiatry*

The presence of hopelessness (choice **A**) as a component of depression greatly increases the chance of suicide. Another high-risk finding would be a suicide plan.

Tearfulness (choice **B**), sleep disturbance (choice **C**), lassitude (choice **D**), and anorexia (choice **E**) are associated with the syndrome of depression, but are not as strongly associated with suicidal behavior.

### 8 The answer is A *Medicine*

Immunoglobulin A (IgA) deficiency is the most common immunodeficiency. It occurs in 1 in 500 individuals. There is an intrinsic defect in the differentiation of B cells committed to synthesizing IgA. Although most persons are largely asymptomatic because of a compensatory increase in secreted IgG and IgM, both circulating and secretory IgA are deficient, leaving these patients susceptible to mucosal problems, such as recurrent sinopulmonary infections, allergies, and diarrhea secondary to *Giardia* and other organisms. There is also an increased incidence of autoimmune disease. In some patients, an additional selective deficiency of the IgG subclasses $IgG_2$ and $IgG_4$ predisposes them to bacterial infections. Exposure to blood products containing IgA (through blood transfusion) often sensitizes these patients to IgA, and they develop antibodies against IgA (choice **A**). Reexposure to IgA causes an anaphylactic reaction. IgA deficient patients should not receive blood products containing IgA. If transfusions are necessary, blood from IgA-deficient patients must be used.

A hemolytic transfusion reaction (choice **B**), contamination of the immune serum globulin (choice **C**), a type IV hypersensitivity reaction (choice **D**), and a febrile reaction (choice **E**) are not associated with the administration of immune serum globulin and would not explain the patient's history of sinopulmonary disease and asthma.

**9** **The answer is D** *Medicine*

His work removing old paint and eating on site very likely exposed him to fine particles of paint that, judging by the age of the buildings, would have been lead-based, so lead toxicity is a likely cause of his weakened state. Moreover, lead is a known inhibitor of heme synthesis, causing a microcytic anemia but not affecting circulating iron levels. Typical early symptoms of lead toxicity include colicky abdominal pain, constipation, headache, irritability, and motor neuropathy, the potential cause of his wrist drop. Thus, lead toxicity is suspect, and a urine screen for heavy metals (lead, mercury, arsenic) (choice **D**) will confirm lead poisoning, permitting treatment with disodium calcium edetate (EDTA), dimercaptosuccinic acid (DMSA), or British anti-Lewisite. Animal studies suggest that high levels of ascorbic acid may enhance the effects of these chelating agents.

A nerve conduction velocity (NCV) study (choice **A**) would only confirm the clinical diagnosis of motor neuropathy, not give the cause. X-rays (choice **B**) and magnetic resonance imaging (MRI) scans (choice **C**) would give uninformative structural information. Diabetes mellitus (choice **E**) is the most common cause of neuropathy and involves the sensory, rather than the motor fibers. Moreover, his age and relatively lean physique makes type 2 diabetes unlikely, and his claim of having been in good health would tend to rule out type 1 diabetes.

**10** **The answer is B** *Medicine*

Ethambutol potentially causes a dose-dependent optic neuritis that may be reversible, whereas the metabolites of rifampin impart a characteristic red–orange color to body fluids. Thus, the need for periodic ocular tests and the presence of a red–orange coloration of sweat and lacrimal secretions indicate that both ethambutol and rifampin were administered, and only choice **B** uses both these compounds. When isoniazid is used in the treatment of tuberculosis, the coadministration of vitamin $B_6$ prevents the development of neurotoxicity without interfering with the antibacterial action of the drug.

Choices **A** and **D** do not include rifampin, therefore these are incorrect. Moreover, bismuth, metronidazole, and tetracycline (choice **A**) are not used in the treatment of tuberculosis, and the only approved use for rifabutin (choice **D**) is in the treatment of infections due to *Mycobacterium avium-intracellulare*. Pyrazinamide used in choice **E** produces hepatotoxicity, which is not evident in this patient; moreover, this combination of drugs does not explain the need for ocular examinations. Clarithromycin (choice **C**) is not used in tuberculosis, but the drug is useful for prophylaxis and treatment of infections caused by *M. avium-intracellulare* in AIDS and HIV patients as well as pharyngitis, tonsillitis, sinusitis, bronchitis, and atypical pneumonias associated with *Chlamydia pneumoniae*. Streptomycin is recommended to be added as a fourth drug until drug sensitivity is established in a regime containing rifampin, isoniazid, and pyrazinamide, in order to increase the chance of preventing the growth of drug-resistant *M. tuberculosis*. It is also used as a second-line drug in cases where other drugs are not tolerated.

**11** **The answer is C** *Psychiatry*

Symptoms that include long-term difficulties with interpersonal interaction and distorted self-image are suggestive of personality disorder. Psychodynamic theory postulates that the adult personality is, in large part, the product of early childhood experiences (choice **C**). Personality pathology results from various kinds of emotional traumas and conflicts that occur during development. Specific kinds of childhood trauma result in specific kinds of personality disorders.

Psychodynamic theory does not suggest that long histories of difficult interpersonal relationships and low self-esteem are innate (choice **E**), will be unresponsive to treatment (choice **D**), or are a response to environmental pressure (choice **A**). Psychodynamic theory suggests that interpersonal problems often develop during the period when a child is raised within the family, not after leaving the shelter of the family (choice **B**).

**12** **The answer is B** *Medicine*

This patient clearly has sickle cell disease. Electrophoresis of red cell lysates from patients with sickle cell disease reveals HbS as the predominant Hb; in HbS, valine is substituted for glutamic acid at the sixth position of the β chain. Small quantities of HbF, in which a γ chain occurs in place of the β chain, and $HbA_2$, in which δ chains replace the β chains, but no HbA (the predominant normal adult Hb) will be found. Sickle cell disease is a recessive condition that becomes a chronic multisystem disease with eventual death from vital organ failure. With good supportive care, death generally occurs in the fourth or fifth decade. Cells in which HbS is the primary Hb tend to sickle when in a low-oxygen environment. Such sickled cells gather in aggregates, causing vaso-occlusion that reveals itself as acute pain, low-grade fever, and organ necrosis. A common site of sickle cell occlusion is in the marrow of the long bones, resulting in aseptic necrosis in 10% to 25% of patients. The hip joint is most commonly affected, causing bilateral aseptic necrosis of the femoral heads (choice **B**). Heterozygous persons are said to have sickle cell trait, a relatively benign condition in which patients are usually clinically normal, only expressing acute painful episodes under extreme conditions.

In sickle cell disease, as with the other hemoglobinopathies, *Salmonella* osteomyelitis is ten times more common than osteomyelitis caused by other organisms, and ischemic necrosis is 50 times more common than osteomyelitis as a cause of bone pain, consequently choice **A** is not the most likely choice. A pathologic bone fracture commonly results from osteoporosis or metastatic disease to bone and does not commonly occur in sickle cell disease (choice **C**). Osteoarthritis commonly occurs in weight-bearing joints, usually in older individuals, due to chronic wear and tear and is by no means a hallmark of sickle cell disease (choice **D**). Legg-Calvé-Perthes disease is an avascular necrosis of the femoral head that shows a predilection for boys between 4 and 10 years old, not teenage females suffering from sickle cell disease (choice **E**). Legg-Calvé-Perthes disease is characterized by the insidious development of a limp, with pain in the groin, anterior thigh, or knee initially bringing the patient to a physician. The process is self-limited, and its cause is unknown. Approximately 55% of patients have a full recovery with revascularization of bone; 45% of patients have a permanent hip deformity.

### [13] The answer is A  *Medicine*

This patient most likely has a fungal infection of the lung due to *Coccidioides immitis,* an airborne fungus endemic to dry regions of the southwest United States. Infection of the lungs is often asymptomatic, but after a 10- to 30-day incubation period, about 40% of infected individuals develop an influenza-like illness. In either case, in an otherwise healthy patient, no drug treatment is indicated unless there are lung lesions or disseminated disease. Thus, treatment should be delayed until culture results are obtained (choice **A**) confirming the disease and until an assessment of the patient's clinical status can be made. The painful leg nodules are erythema nodosum, which is a delayed (cell-mediated) hypersensitivity response to fungal (or bacterial) antigens and is a favorable prognostic sign. No organisms are present in the lesions; therefore, erythema nodosum is not a sign of disseminated disease.

If treatment is indicated, intravenous (IV) amphotericin B (choice **C**) is the drug of choice for severe cases. An oral azole such as fluconazole (choice **B**) is used in milder cases and as continuation therapy after an initial positive response to amphotericin B. A bone marrow aspirate with culture (choice **D**) is primarily reserved for ruling out systemic fungi as a cause of fever of unknown origin. Isolation is not required (choice **E**) because the condition is not contagious.

### [14] The answer is D  *Psychiatry*

This patient's symptoms are most suggestive of the anxiety attacks that characterize panic disorder (choice **D**). Other symptoms of panic attacks include hypervigilance, motor tension, and autonomic symptoms such as dyspnea, tachycardia, and diaphoresis. Anxiety can also occur during the course of the other conditions listed; however, additional symptoms are also present.

In delirium (choice **A**), impairment of consciousness is present. In depersonalization disorder (choice **B**), there are illusions involving body distortion. In dysthymic disorder (choice **C**), persistent depression is present. In schizoaffective disorder (choice **E**), both psychotic symptoms and prominent mood symptoms are present.

### [15] The answer is D  *Medicine*

Bariatric surgery has shown a remarkable ability to not only reduce the risk of diabetes but to also apparently cure it. For example, in one controlled study, 84% of patients who underwent Roux-en-Y gastric bypass surgery were cured from diabetes and a third of these went into remission before leaving the hospital. This response is far too fast to be accounted for by reduction in his mass of adipose tissue (choice **C** is incorrect). One of the prevailing hypotheses for this remarkable response to bariatric surgery is that the level of circulating ghrelin is reduced (choice **D**). Ghrelin is a so-called hunger hormone produced by the stomach that not only signals a person to eat more but also inhibits the secretion of insulin. By removing a portion of the stomach Roux-en-Y gastric bypass surgery decreases ghrelin production and disinhibits insulin production. (Although not relevant to this question, ghrelin also is produced in the hypothalamic arcuate nucleus, where it stimulates secretion of growth hormone by the anterior pituitary gland and has other functions.)

Changes in the level of circulating GLP-1 have also been implicated in this effect of bariatric surgery. However, in this case, it would be the increase in the level of GLP-1 not the reduction (choice **A** is not correct) that controls the diabetes. The concept is that, after surgery, food is brought to the distal end of the small intestine more quickly than normal; this is where GLP-1 is synthesized by L-cells, the idea being the more rapid exposure of the L- cells to food stimulates GLP-1 synthesis and since GLP-1 stimulates insulin production this has an antidiabetic effect. PYY is another hormone involved in appetite control and obesity. Like GLP-1, it is synthesized in the L-cells. It functions to suppress appetite; thus, if it has a role in attenuating symptoms of diabetes, circulating levels would once again be increased not decreased (choice **B** is incorrect). Leptin is a circulating polypeptide that reduces appetite. It is produced by adipoid cells and basically works in opposition to ghrelin. Contrary to logical expectations, obese individuals have increased levels of circulating leptin; it is hypothesized that obese individuals are resistant to the hormone in a manner analogous to the resistance of diabetics to insulin. In any case, there is no evidence that bariatric surgery has a direct affect on circulating leptin levels, let alone that such an affect helps moderate diabetic symptoms; thus, reduction in the level of his circulating leptin is incorrect, as is choice **E**.

### 16 The answer is B *Surgery*

Constipation, absence of stool in the vault, and a dilated colon (megacolon) suggest Hirschsprung disease (choice **B**), which is caused by an absence of ganglion cells in the myenteric plexus of the rectum. In this condition, stool is unable to pass the aganglionic segment, thus producing an obstruction that distally leaves the rectal vault free of stool and causes megacolon due to proximal dilatation of the bowel with concomitant constipation. Classic Hirschsprung disease is a congenital condition in which babies are born without these ganglionic cells, and such newborns with this disorder are frequently unable to pass their meconium. However, Hirschsprung disease can also occur in adults, particularly in association with Down syndrome, Chagas disease, spinal cord injury, Parkinson disease, and abuse of some narcotics. Chagas disease is due to *Trypanosoma cruzi* and is endemic in South and Central America and is the probable cause of Hirschsprung disease in this patient.

The other choices are not accompanied by symptoms similar to those described in the case vignette. Diverticula (choice **A**) produce no symptoms unless inflamed, causing diverticulitis, which is characterized by left flank pain. Adenomatous polyps (choice **C**) also produce no symptoms unless they transform into a carcinoma and the cancer causes problems. An inflamed colon (choice **D**) is more typical of ulcerative colitis. Anal fistulas (choice **E**) may arise from many causes, and although they can be serious, usually they are not.

### 17 The answer is C *Psychiatry*

The symptoms are most suggestive of dementia (choice **C**), which is characterized by memory disturbance coupled with other cognitive disturbances, such as difficulty with abstraction, aphasia (difficulty with articulation), apraxia (loss of ability to execute complex motor behaviors), and agnosia (failure to recognize people or objects). Dementia is often associated with central nervous system damage and is likely to have a protracted course. Although Alzheimer disease is very unlikely at this age, the dementia could be due to other causes, such as early Parkinson disease, vitamin $B_{12}$ deficiency, vascular dementia, and hypothyroidism, all of which need to be ruled out.

Delirium (choice **A**) is distinguished from dementia by the additional presence of impaired awareness and attention. It usually has a shorter course than dementia, and symptom severity may fluctuate. Amnestic disorder (choice **B**) is characterized by memory impairment with preservation of awareness and other aspects of cognition. Major depressive disorder (choice **D**) may include complaints of difficulties with memory; however, cognitive testing does not usually reveal marked deficits. Mental retardation (choice **E**) may be characterized by difficulties with reasoning and abstraction. However, vocabulary is usually limited, and a specific complaint of a short history of memory impairment is unlikely.

### 18 The answer is C *Medicine*

This young man has hereditary angioedema, a condition marked by periodic swelling of mucosal tissues, most often involving oral organs but sometimes elsewhere often including the genitals. It is frequently accompanied by urticaria and abdominal pain, as in the case described. Urticaria is marked by the eruption of wheals or hives on the skin. Angioedema is a urticaria-like condition that involves edema in deeper tissues. The most common causes of angioedema is an allergy or adverse drug reaction. Hereditary angioedema is rare, occurring in less than 0.4% of all cases of angioedema. It is an autosomal dominant disease characterized by the symptoms and family history described in the vignette; these symptoms generally first start early in the second decade and as a rule life expectancy is normal, although early death can occur due to asphyxiation caused by uncontrolled laryngeal edema. The abdominal pain is due to edema of the mucosa of the gastrointestinal tract. An angioedema episode usually lasts about 2 to 3 days. The urticarial lesions associated with angioedema typically have indistinct borders. This disease is caused by an inherited C1 complement esterase inhibitor deficiency. The complement system consists of nine proteins, C1 through C9. Activation of C1 starts a cascade that results in the use of some of other members of the complement family. Normally, C1 esterase inhibitor acts as a monitor, preventing runaway activation of this system. Absence of this inhibitor results in excessive stimulation of the system, resulting in the release of breakdown products that cause the release of histamine and other vasodilators. These vasodilators increase vessel permeability, resulting in swelling of soft tissue. During the ensuing activation, C4 and C2 are consumed. As a consequence, the best screen is a C4 complement assay (choice **C**). Since C4 complement levels are low in these patients even when they are in a quiescent period, a normal C4 assay value essentially excludes the disease. The diagnosis is confirmed with a C1 esterase inhibitor assay. In acute attacks, maintenance of the upper airways is the most important factor. Recently, concentrates of the C1 esterase inhibitor have become available and are used to treat attacks. In its absence, fresh frozen plasma (which supplies the inhibitor) is used. Prophylactic treatment may also be obtained using ε-aminocaproic acid (a nonspecific serum protease and esterase inhibitor) and/or certain synthetic androgens (e.g., danazol or stanozolol) that have immunosuppressive properties and also stimulate the synthesis of C1 esterase inhibitor.

Quantitative immunoglobulin assay (choice **B**), C3 complement assay (choice **A**), serum antinuclear antibody assay (choice **D**), and the sweat chloride assay (choice **E**) for cystic fibrosis are not indicated with this clinical history.

### 19 The answer is C *Obstetrics and Gynecology*

This twin pregnancy is complicated by preterm contractions and placenta previa, as well as preeclampsia. All three of these entities are increased with multiple pregnancies. Over 12% of all infants born in the United States are preterm, and they account for up to 70% of neonatal morbidity and mortality. Thus, prevention of preterm birth is a high priority unless there are reasons that make tocolysis (i.e., delaying or inhibiting delivery) unsafe for either mother or fetus. Preterm multiple gestation (choice **A**) and preterm placenta previa (choice **B**) are indications for tocolysis. However, if severe preeclampsia (choice **C**) is present, the mother's life and health are jeopardized by prolonging the pregnancy; therefore, tocolysis is inappropriate. Early gestational age (choice **D**) and a positive group B β-hemolytic streptococcus culture (choice **E**) are not contraindications for tocolysis.

### 20 The answer is E *Medicine*

In the general population, fewer than 5% of the cases of hypertension result from renal arterial occlusion. However, renovascular occlusion accounts for 70% of the cases of hypertension in patients over the age of 60 who have a diastolic blood pressure above 105 mm Hg and a serum creatine value above 2 mg/dL; moreover 80% to 90% of these cases are due to occlusive arteriosclerotic disease (choice **E**). If both kidneys are occluded, provision of an angiotensin-converting enzyme (ACE) inhibitor, such as enalapril, tends to provoke acute renal failure because the ACE inhibitor decreases angiotensin II production, which is required for effective renal circulation. This is noted on renal function tests by a rising creatinine level.

About 10% to 15% of the cases of renal arterial stenosis are due to fibromuscular dysplasia (choice **A**); renal stenosis is almost unique among the renal diseases in that it is not accompanied by proteinuria, since the glomerulus is intact and renal arterial pressure is decreased. However, these cases primarily occur in females who are between the ages of 30 and 50 years. Renal vein thrombosis due to a malignant occlusion (choice **C**) presents with severe back pain and hyperproteinuria. Symptoms of malignant hypertension (choice **D**) include rapid and extreme increase in systolic blood pressure (over 200 mm Hg), blurred vision, headache, shortness of breath, chest pain, proteinuria, and sometimes seizures. Such an acute attack occasionally occurs for no apparent reason, usually in a person who was being treated for hypertension. It is the extreme increase in systolic pressure that induces the other symptoms, which will get worse the longer the pressure remains elevated. Consequently, this is a medical emergency; the pressure must be reduced immediately, usually by IV administration of antihypertensive agents.

Even though an arthrosclerotic artery is more readily occluded than a healthy one, by definition acute renal artery occlusion (choice **B**) differs from occlusion due to stenosis in that the latter is a chronic event. However, other difference between an acute occlusion and an occlusion due to stenosis are that the acute occlusion generally is unilateral, whereas stenosis is bilateral 70% of the time, and acute occlusion presents with backache and blood in the urine, whereas stenosis presents with hypertension. An occlusion generally occurs after major surgery or trauma affecting the abdomen or side or in individuals with atrial fibrillation or mitral or valve disease.

### 21  The answer is B  *Obstetrics and Gynecology*

The scenario in this question is characteristic of endometriosis, a benign condition in which endometrial glands and stroma are located outside of the endometrial cavity. The pathophysiology is probably related to retrograde menstruation through the fallopian tubes into the peritoneal cavity. The history of secondary dysmenorrhea, dyspareunia, and infertility is classic. This condition affects up to 15% of all women in the United States. Although a history (choice **A**) and pelvic examination (choice **C**) may be suggestive of endometriosis, only a laparoscopy (choice **B**) is definitive. Visualization of the characteristic "powder burns" is typical, along with adhesions, particularly in the cul-de-sac, which cause the fixed, retroverted uterus along with uterosacral ligament nodularity.

A hysterosalpingogram (choice **D**) is not helpful because the findings are extrauterine, and one would not expect an abnormality of the endometrial cavity. A culdocentesis (choice **E**) has been used for identifying nonclotted cul-de-sac blood in cases of ruptured ectopic pregnancy but lacks specificity and sensitivity for diagnosing endometriosis.

### 22  The answer is B  *Medicine*

Salicylate poisoning can result from short-term ingestion of a large dose or by long-term ingestion of more salicylates than can be excreted. In 2000, more than 20,000 cases of salicylate intoxication were reported to poison control centers in the United States; these resulted in 55 deaths. Salicylate poisoning most commonly occurs in infants and in the elderly. In infants, the sources may seem innocuous such as salicylate-coated teething rings or even breast milk from mothers who use excessive amounts of topical analgesics containing a salicylate. In the elderly, long-term aspirin use coupled to decreased renal function and perhaps forgetfulness can raise plasma levels dangerously. Usually, one of the early signs is ototoxicity marked by tinnitus and dizziness. Other symptoms include central nervous effects ranging from mild confusion to coma, emesis, tachycardia, hyperventilation, hypotension, and early hyperglycemia followed by hypoglycemia; death is usually caused by pulmonary edema. Although a tentative diagnosis can be made on the basis of history, symptoms, and the finding of a metabolic acidosis with an increased anion gap, it is confirmed by measurement of serum salicylate levels; the arterial blood gas pattern can also be very revealing, since it is likely to show a mixed pattern, metabolic acidosis plus pulmonary alkalosis (not simply compensation). This is because, as the plasma levels increase, the central respiratory center is stimulated, causing hyperventilation and inducing respiratory alkalosis, while still further exposure to salicylate causes a cascade of metabolic abnormalities starting with the uncoupling of oxidative phosphorylation and progressing to inhibition of the Krebs cycle dehydrogenases. In turn, these events lead to accumulation of acetoacetate, acetate, and lactate and stimulation of gluconeogenesis, resulting in a metabolic acidosis with an increased anion gap, as well as initial hyperglycemia. The anion gap is defined as $[Na^+] - ([Cl^-] + [HCO_3^-])$, and any value above 14 is indicative of metabolic acidosis with a positive anion gap. Choice **B** shows a low normal pH and lower than normal $Pa_{CO_2}$ and bicarbonate level. The low bicarbonate level is compatible with both metabolic acidosis and respiratory alkalosis, whereas the lower than normal $Pa_{CO_2}$ value is compatible with metabolic acidosis and respiratory alkalosis. A double acidosis (respiratory plus metabolic) can be ruled out because the pH would be far below normal, and the anion gap data clearly show metabolic acidosis, a value greater than 14 mEq/L. The decrease in the $Pa_{CO_2}$ is a characteristic of respiratory alkalosis. Although respiratory alkalosis is to be expected as compensation for metabolic acidosis, the normal rule is compensation cannot bring the pH back to normal. This "above normal" compensation can best be explained by a mixed acid–base status, namely respiratory alkalosis with metabolic acidosis, a sequel expected in salicylate poisoning. Thus, **B** is the correct choice.

In choice **A**, the pH is less than 7.35, the $Pa_{CO_2}$ is elevated, and the bicarbonate value is in the normal range—results consistent with metabolic acidosis with respiratory compensation. Choice **C** also indicates acidemia, but in this case the $Pa_{CO_2}$ and bicarbonate values are greater than normal, indicating respiratory acidosis. In choices **D** and **E**, the pH values are above 7.45, indicating alkalemia. In choice **D**, the $Pa_{CO_2}$ and bicarbonate values are elevated, suggesting a metabolic basis, while in choice **E**, they are decreased, indicating a process driven by the respiratory system.

**23** **The answer is E** *Psychiatry*

The woman most likely suffers from generalized anxiety disorder. The diagnostic feature is poorly controlled anxiety lasting longer than 6 months. Onset is often in childhood and may continue long-term at a low level into adulthood, but the condition may flare up when exacerbated by stressful conditions. Venlafaxine (choice **E**) is an effective treatment, especially when accompanied by depressive symptoms such as rumination. Other antidepressants, buspirone, and longer-acting benzodiazepines, such as diazepam, may also be useful.

Modafinil (choice **A**) is used for disorders associated with excessive sleepiness and may cause anxiety. Zolpidem (choice **B**) is a short-term treatment for insomnia and may cause rebound anxiety. Risperidone (choice **C**) should be reserved for psychosis and manic episodes. Alprazolam (choice **D**) is a shorter-acting benzodiazepine with a higher potential for inducing dependence when used for extended periods.

**24** **The answer is B** *Obstetrics and Gynecology*

The clinical scenario strongly suggests premature rupture of membranes (PROM). Accurate assessment of PROM is essential because the outcome of pregnancy can be adversely affected by a positive diagnosis. This question addresses confirmation of PROM by examination, rather than with historic data. A speculum examination (choice **B**) is helpful in determining the extent of vaginal pooling.

Nitrazine paper on the perineum (choice **A**) assesses pH of the fluid. A blue color indicates alkaline pH. Although alkaline amniotic fluid will be Nitrazine positive, so can urine, which is often alkaline in pregnancy. Sonographic evidence of oligohydramnios (choice **C**) is often present with PROM; however, it has a low specificity and sensitivity for ruptured membranes. Urinalysis (choice **D**) is not relevant. Digital examination (choice **E**) should never be done until membrane rupture is ruled out, because of the potential increase in infectious morbidity from ascending vaginal flora into the uterus, leading to chorioamnionitis.

**25** **The answer is D** *Surgery*

It seems most likely that this man suffers from postoperative pancreatitis, which most commonly is seen after common bile duct exploration for a gallstone (choice **D**) during a cholecystectomy. Both the pancreatic duct and the common bile duct empty into the ampulla of Vater. Emptying is determined by the sphincter tone in the ampulla. Low obstruction in the common bile duct by a stone causes reflux from the bile duct into the pancreatic duct, which can lead to pancreatitis. Endoscopic retrograde cholangiopancreatography is also a cause of pancreatitis.

Anesthetic agents (choice **A**), hypovolemia (choice **B**), total parenteral nutrition (TPN) (choice **C**), and postoperative infection (choice **E**) do not predispose to acute pancreatitis.

**26** **The answer is D** *Surgery*

This patient has a compartment syndrome, which occurs as a result of external or internal compression of the neurovascular structures due to soft tissue swelling. Fractures of the leg and forearm region tend to have a high propensity for compartment syndrome; however, it can be found in fractures involving other areas, including those of the calcaneus. After the fracture, tissues begin to swell, but the fascial sheath covering the muscles is unyielding. This leads to pressure on the neurovascular structures, resulting in ischemia to the muscles. Failure to recognize the condition could lead to Volkmann's ischemic contracture causing hyperkalemia, myoglobinuria with renal failure, and even loss of limb due to vascular compromise. Typically, the patient complains of pain in the fingers or toes on movement. Paresthesias may be present. The pulse is normal until late in the process; therefore, viability of the pulse does not exclude impending complications. In cases of compartment syndrome, compartment pressure usually exceeds 35 mm Hg; however, compartment syndrome occasionally may be present with lower pressures. The most important diagnostic sign is the presence of pain on passive movement of the fingers or toes. Treatment involves cleaving (i.e., splitting the cast along its length) (choice **D**) to relieve edema, followed by elevation. Once the swelling has subsided, a full cast can be reapplied.

Reassurance (choice **A**) would be injudicious without concomitant treatment. Administering analgesics (choice **B**) would not address the problem; although it would relieve the pain, it would not in any way stall the relentless march of edema. Although corticosteroids (choice **C**) may initially relieve some of the swelling, they have no role in the management of this condition because the primary problem has to be addressed. Leaving the cast intact and elevating the arm (choice **E**) will help but is insufficient.

**27** **The answer is B** *Medicine*

Adult respiratory distress syndrome (ARDS) is marked by the rapid onset of dyspnea within 12 to 24 hours of an initiating event. Initiating events with an increased propensity for ARDS are sepsis (most common), aspiration of gastric contents (this patient), drug overdose, shock, burns, diffuse pneumonias, and oxygen toxicity, to name only a few. The mechanism of injury is primarily a neutrophil-related event in the lungs, with the release of protease, free radicals, and leukotrienes that produce pulmonary vasoconstriction and increased vessel permeability. The increased vessel permeability results in leaky capillaries, which liberate monocytes that release cytokines; these also contribute to the inflammatory process. Type II pneumocytes are damaged, thus decreasing the production of surfactant; this results in widespread atelectasis (alveolar collapse). Because atelectasis is a prominent feature of ARDS, the primary defect is intrapulmonary shunting (choice **B**) of blood, accompanied by profound hypoxemia.

Compliance (ability of the lung to expand) is decreased, not increased (choice **C**) by increased inflammation and edema in the interstitium of the lungs. Damage to elastic tissue support would induce a decrease, not an increase (choice **D**) in elasticity (the recoil properties of the lung). In this patient, the $PaCO_2$ is 74 mm Hg, a value typical in uncompensated respiratory acidosis; the bicarbonate value of 28 mEq/L, and the pH of 7.20 are also compatible with uncompensated respiratory acidosis, not respiratory alkalosis (choice **E**). The respiratory center is not directly involved (choice **A**).

**28** **The answer is B** *Surgery*

This patient will have hypotension and bradycardia (choice **B**) as a result of neurogenic shock. Sympathetic outflow is absent after spinal cord injuries. As a result of sympathetic paralysis, norepinephrine cannot act on blood vessels to induce vasoconstriction; thus, hypotension follows. Failed sympathetic function leads to unopposed parasympathetic action, which causes bradycardia.

A variable degree of hypertension with tachycardia (choice **A**) is seen in patients with acute severe pain; relief of pain lowers blood pressure and heart rate. The combination of hypertension and bradycardia (choice **C**) signifies raised intracranial pressure, as occurs in epidural hemorrhage. Cerebral perfusion pressure, which should be 50 mm Hg at a minimum, depends on the difference between mean arterial pressure and cerebrospinal fluid (CSF) pressure. As intracranial pressure rises, CSF pressure rises; the difference between mean arterial pressure and CSF pressure falls. To maintain the minimum level of cerebral blood flow, the systolic blood pressure has to rise. Bradycardia is a consequence of the resulting hypertension. Hypotension and tachycardia (choice **D**) are seen in hypovolemic shock, in which there is loss of extracellular volume into the third space or elsewhere. In the case of spinal injuries, there is no loss of blood from within the vascular compartment. The blood remains within the system but cannot be distributed due to lack of sympathetic function; hence, there is bradycardia rather than the more typical tachycardia. Furthermore, the treatment of neurogenic shock involves use of vasoconstrictors to drive the blood back into circulation, whereas hemorrhagic shock requires volume expansion. Choice **E** makes no sense in a person suffering such severe injuries.

**29** **The answer is E** *Medicine*

In questions that ask you to examine the data, do just that. This question includes several statements that may well be true. For example, the effects of chemotherapy may not bear any relationship to cell kill (choice **A**); however, no data concerning cell kill are provided, so the examinee is not in a position to make a judgment concerning the accuracy of the statement. Similarly, it is possible that evaluation of chest x-ray films may be more valuable than monitoring UCG titer as a guide to therapy (choice **D**). Once again, no data are provided to permit such a conclusion. Examining the data, it is clear that the effects of the drug regimens on UCG titer are variable. They cannot possibly be directly proportional to decreases in platelet count (choice **C**) because all drug doses were adjusted to a toxicity limit of a 2-log decrease in platelet count. The methotrexate regimen lowered UCG titer from $10^8$ to $10^5$, a 3-log decrease (not a 2-log decrease [choice **B**]). Cisplatin plus etoposide lowered UCG titer from $10^7$ to less than $10^3$, a more than 4-log decrease (choice **E**), the correct answer.

The seemingly small titer changes cause 2- or 4-log changes because the chemotherapeutic agent destroys normal cells as well as malignant ones. Consequently, the platelet count drops considerably. The combination of cisplatin and etoposide has a greater effect than one drug alone.

### 30 The answer is D *Medicine*

Treatment of hyperthyroidism during pregnancy depends in part on the severity of the disorder. Hyperthyroid females can often tolerate the mild exacerbation of the state that accompanies pregnancy without therapy, and there appears to be no increase in the incidence of fetal loss. If treatment is judged to be required, propylthiouracil (choice **D**) is usually preferred over methimazole, in part because the latter drug enters the fetal circulation more readily and has been reported to cause aplasia cutis. Propylthiouracil also inhibits 5′-deiodinase, decreasing formation of triiodothyronine ($T_3$). The primary objective of drug therapy is to maintain free thyroxine ($FT_4$) and thyroid-stimulating hormone (TSH) at high-to-normal levels using the lowest possible dose of propylthiouracil.

Lugol's solution (iodine and potassium iodide) (choice **A**) exerts only a temporary antithyroid effect. Propranolol (choice **E**) should not ordinarily be given as an adjuvant because it may cause fetal growth retardation and neonatal respiratory depression. Antithyroid agents carry less risk to the patient and the pregnancy than does surgery; in any event, surgery is contraindicated during the third (and first) trimester of pregnancy (choice **C**). Radioactive iodine ($^{131}I$) (choice **B**) should never be given during pregnancy.

### 31 The answer is E *Medicine*

This patient has chronic lymphocytic leukemia (CLL), a disease primarily affecting the elderly; 90% of patients are over 50, and the median age at presentation is 65 years. The primary clinical characteristic signifying CLL is lymphocytosis with white cell counts usually over $100,000/\mu L$, of which 75% to 98% are lymphocytes. Diagnosis can be confirmed by immunophenotyping in which the B lymphocyte lineage marker CD19 is expressed along with the T lymphocyte marker CD5. The Rai staging system grades CLL as follows: stage 0, lymphocytosis only, stage I, lymphocytosis plus lymphadenopathy; stage II, organomegaly; stage III, anemia; and stage IV, thrombocytopenia. In most cases, these lymphocytes are morphologically indistinguishable from normal small lymphocytes; the exception is a CLL variant disease known as *prolymphocytic leukemia*, in which the lymphocytes are larger and immature and the disease course is more aggressive. More typically, CLL follows an indolent pattern, and patients often present with a nonsymptomatic lymphocytosis discovered by chance (i.e., stage 0); other cases commonly first present with fatigue or lymphadenopathy (stage I). Obviously, this man with hepatosplenomegaly, anemia, and thrombocytopenia with petechiae and ecchymoses has already progressed to stage IV. As the disease progresses, the lymph nodes and bone marrow progressively become invaded by small lymphocytes, the latter eventually causing the anemia and thrombocytopenia. Thus, in the case described, diffuse bone marrow and lymph node infiltration by the cells represented in the peripheral smear illustrated (choice **E**) is to be expected. No therapy is required until the disease is well advanced into stage II and, of course, in stages III and IV. The median survival for patients first diagnosed in stages 0 or I is 10 to 15 years. Until recently, the mean survival of patients in stages III or IV has been less than 2 years. However, with newer regimens of fludarabine-based therapy, more than 90% of patients live beyond 2 years. Still, treatment of some 5% to 10% of patients becomes complicated by development of an autoimmune thrombocytopenia or hemolytic anemia or non-Hodgkin's lymphoma.

Nearly all patients with hairy cell leukemia develop a monocytopenia (choice **A**), which is encountered in almost no other disease, including CLL. Chronic myelogenous leukemia most commonly terminates as an acute myelogenous leukemia (choice **B**). Auer rods are splinter- to rod-shaped cytoplasmic inclusions seen in myeloblasts in acute myelogenous leukemia (choice **C**) and are not found in the smear illustrated. Paratrabecular lymphoid aggregates in the bone marrow are a characteristic manifestation of the non-Hodgkin's lymphomas (choice **D**); in CLL, lymphocyte invasion is diffuse.

### 32 The answer is A *Medicine*

Osteogenesis imperfecta is a hereditary osteoporosis due to defective type 1 collagen synthesis. Type I OGI is usually not debilitating, and there are often extensive family histories showing an autosomal dominant mode of inheritance. Fractures most often occur prior to puberty, but like everybody else, as patients age, their bone density decreases. Since their bone structure is less than optimal to start with, this puts them at a greater risk than average of developing age-induced osteoporosis, resulting in additional fractures. Among the general population, osteoporosis in the elderly is estimated to cause at least 1.5 million fractures annually in the United States. In age-induced osteoporosis, the rate of bone formation is usually near normal, but the rate of reabsorption is increased significantly. This results in a greater loss of trabecular bone than compact bone, accounting for the primary clinical features, namely crush fractures of the vertebrae and fractures of the neck of the femur and of the distal end of the radius. These fractures are a leading cause of morbidity among the elderly and indirectly also increase mortality; thus, diagnosis and treatment before fractures occur can be of great value. If he is found to have osteopenia or early osteoporosis, and this diagnosis triggers the start of treatment, the determination of bone density (choice **A**) will have a significant positive effect on his lifestyle and perhaps on his longevity. The most probable treatment regimen will be administration of a bisphosphonate that inhibits osteoclastic activity.

Blood test for the rheumatic factor (choice **B**) is not called for because there are no symptoms suggestive of rheumatic arthritis, such as symmetric joint involvement, prolonged stiffness, low-grade fever, hot joints, or fatigue. Radiographic studies (choice **C**) could be used to confirm that this patient's joint pain is osteoarthritis, but such studies really are not needed because clinical judgment alone should suffice to reach this conclusion. In any case, even if osteoarthritis were confirmed by radiography, it would not lead to a changed treatment modality. A complete blood count (choice **D**) and an erythrocyte sedimentation determination (choice **E**) could be of potential value if this were an inflammatory condition but are essentially irrelevant in this case. A blood test for antinuclear antibodies (choice **F**) has great value in ruling out a number of inflammatory conditions because of its great sensitivity; it is positive in some 30% to 60% of rheumatic arthritis cases, and in almost all cases of systemic lupus erythematosus, Sjögren syndrome, and diffuse and limited scleroderma (CREST) syndromes, as well as in polymyositis/dermatomyositis. However, this patient shows no signs suggesting that he may suffer from any these conditions. Arthrographic examination of the affected joints (choice **G**) is a procedure in which a liquid contrast medium is injected into a joint and its penetration is followed by radiography to see if there are any tears in the cartilage or other tissues. It is rarely used to diagnose a case of nontraumatic osteoarthritis.

### 33 The answer is A *Surgery*

The patient most likely has acute surgical parotitis (sialadenitis). Surgical parotitis usually occurs 1 week postoperatively in elderly patients who have poor dental hygiene and have been intubated. *Staphylococcus aureus* (choice **A**) is the organism isolated most commonly. Surgical drainage and antibiotics are required.

Acute and chronic sialadenitis can also result from sialolithiasis, which refers to calculi in the major salivary gland ducts, most commonly in Wharton's duct draining the submandibular gland (choice **B**); however, the vignette provides no suggestion that this might be the case. Mumps is a common cause of viral parotitis and may be bilateral. However, the advent of vaccination against it has made it very rare indeed (choice **C**). Hemorrhage (choice **D**) into the parotid gland is rare. Parotid gland enlargement is also associated with Sjögren syndrome, a collagen vascular disease characterized by immunologic destruction of minor salivary glands with subsequent development of dry eyes and dry mouth (choice **E**); rheumatoid arthritis is frequently present as well.

### 34 The answer is A *Psychiatry*

This patient's symptoms are most suggestive of social phobia, characterized by anxiety in social situations. Assertiveness training (choice **A**) is the treatment of choice for this disorder and involves education, role playing, and desensitization to feared social stimuli. Medications that are useful for social phobia include newer antidepressants such as paroxetine, and monoamine oxidase (MAO) inhibitors such as phenelzine. Buspirone is also used occasionally.

Implosion therapy (choice **B**) involves massive exposure to feared stimuli and is not effective for social phobia. Psychodynamic psychotherapy (choice **C**) may bring individuals insight into the reasons for their social phobia, but it has not been demonstrated to reliably decrease the associated symptoms. Lorazepam (choice **D**) and other benzodiazepines are usually ineffective in lessening social avoidance. Systematic desensitization (choice **E**) used alone is less effective than assertiveness training.

### 35 The answer is C *Medicine*

This woman clearly suffers from hyponatremia, which is defined as a sodium concentration below 130 mEq/L. A urine sodium concentration of 80 mEq/L indicates that the decrease in plasma sodium is due to excess loss into the urine. This typically is caused by hyperfunction of antidiuretic hormone (ADH), also known as vasopressin. Normally, ADH acts to limit water excretion. As a consequence, the normal physiologic response is to increase ADH activity only when the body senses increasing osmolarity, as in a hypovolemic state. This woman's skin turgor is normal, and there is a small decrease in concentration of electrolytes other than sodium and chloride, indicating that she is basically euvolemic. Thus, this increase in ADH activity is inappropriate, a condition known as the *syndrome of inappropriate ADH secretion* (SIADH). The question then becomes what is causing SIADH in this woman and what can best be done to alleviate this condition. In this case, the obvious solution is to prescribe some drug other than chlorpropamide to treat her diabetes (choice **C**). Although chlorpropamide is an inexpensive and effective long-acting hypoglycemic agent, it rarely is prescribed these days in part because it has a hyponatremic effect due to its propensity to react with kidney ADH receptors and thus enhance ADH activity. This may result in abnormal loss of sodium from the extracellular compartment, which creates an ionic gradient leading to the influx of water into cells throughout the body including the central nervous system, where it causes serious mental distress and accounts for the small vesicles seen on the CT scan.

Choice **A,** administration of a serotonin-reuptake inhibitor, is inappropriate because the cause of her mental problems is the influx of hypoosmotic fluid into the CNS, not a hormonal imbalance. Moreover, several dozen cases of SIADH caused by an SSRI have been reported, albeit mainly in the elderly. Restricting sodium from her diet (choice **B**) or increasing her water intake (choice **D**) makes no sense, since she is already hyponatremic. Adding sodium to her diet (choice **E**) superficially makes sense and might transiently increase circulating sodium levels, but because it does not get at the root cause, any effect provided would not be long lasting. Administering demeclocycline, an ADH antagonist; (choice **F**) is primarily used in patients in whom SIADH is caused by ectopic secretion of ADH by a tumor, such as a small-cell carcinoma, in which the underling mechanism of SIADH is overproduction of ADH.

### 36 The answer is E *Pediatrics*

Mild breastfeeding jaundice does not require either intervention (choice **E**) from the physician or that the mother stops breastfeeding completely (choice **D** is incorrect). Breast-milk jaundice may appear in 2% of term, breastfed infants after the seventh day of life. There is a significant elevation of unconjugated (not conjugated) bilirubin (choice **B**). Bilirubin may be as high as 10 to 30 mg/dL during the third week. If the mother continues breastfeeding, the hyperbilirubinemia gradually decreases and may persist for 3 to 10 weeks at lower levels. The serum bilirubin level rapidly (not slowly [choice **C**]) declines if nursing is discontinued for 24 to 48 hours. If nursing is resumed after 24 to 48 hours the serum bilirubin will not rise to its previously high levels. Breastfeeding jaundice (not breast-milk jaundice) is seen in the first few days of life (choice **A**) and is also associated with increased unconjugated hyperbilirubinemia (>12 mg/dL). Breastfeeding jaundice occurs in 13% of breastfed infants in the first week of life because of decreased milk intake with concomitant dehydration.

### 37 The answer is C *Obstetrics and Gynecology*

The scenario described a young woman undergoing virilization, not just hirsutism. Hirsutism is the development of male-pattern hair in a female, whereas virilization is development of male secondary sex characteristics in a female, including deepening voice, increasing muscle mass, and clitoral enlargement. Virilization requires a high level of peripheral androgens, most often from a tumor. The rapid onset, as in this case, is also consistent with a tumor of either the adrenal gland or the ovary. All the choices are ovarian tumors. The ovarian tumor that produces androgens is the Sertoli-Leydig cell tumor (choice **C**).

Another hormone-producing no-functional ovarian tumor is the granulosa cell tumor (choice **A**), which produces estrogen and promotes feminizing signs and symptoms. Brenner tumor (choice **B**), fibroma (choice **D**), and dysgerminoma (choice **E**) are not endocrinologically active.

### 38 The answer is D *Psychiatry*

This woman's symptoms are most suggestive of depression. Learned helplessness (choice **D**) is a behavioral theory of depression in which depression is viewed as a reaction to a perception of one's inability to improve a situation.

Faulty cognitive framework (choice **A**) is a cognitive theory of depression; object loss (choice **B**) is a psychodynamic theory of depression, and inadequate exposure to light (choice **C**) is a biologic theory of depression; none of these is a behavioral explanation. Double-bind communication (choice **E**) refers to incongruity between spoken and unspoken communication in a given exchange. It was a view of family dynamics in schizophrenia that is no longer considered valid.

**39** **The answer is B** *Obstetrics and Gynecology*

With any patient having postmenopausal bleeding, endometrial carcinoma must be ruled out; therefore, endometrial biopsy (choice **B**) is the diagnostic method of choice. Endometrial carcinoma is the most common gynecologic cancer and is most often diagnosed in stage 1 (confined to the uterus) because of vaginal bleeding, the most common symptom.

Cytologic screening by Pap smear (choice **A**) is used for cervical cancer screening, but it misses 60% of endometrial carcinoma cases. Pelvic examination under anesthesia (choice **C**) may be helpful in staging cervical cancer but is not diagnostic for any cancer. Laparoscopy (choice **D**) is useful for diagnosing benign pelvic disease such as endometriosis or pelvic adhesions but not for any kind of cancer. Colposcopy (choice **E**) is used for localization of cervical biopsy sites but is not used for endometrial cancer diagnosis.

**40** **The answer is B** *Obstetrics and Gynecology*

This patient is a candidate for developing Sheehan syndrome because of hypoperfusion of her anterior pituitary gland. The pituitary hormone most commonly affected is prolactin (choice **B**), resulting in the most common symptom, which is failure of lactation. Although all pituitary trophic hormones are at risk, usually only a few are affected. The sequence in frequency of loss is prolactin most commonly, followed by gonadotropins (follicle-stimulating hormone [FSH] and luteinizing hormone [LH]), with loss of thyroid-stimulating hormone (TSH) and adrenocorticotropic hormone (ACTH) only seen rarely.

If FSH (choice **D**) is involved, the woman will not resume menstrual periods and will experience secondary amenorrhea due to lack of estrogen. Severe involvement of ACTH (choice **A**) may lead to adrenal insufficiency including hypoglycemia, hypotension, and weakness. If TSH (choice **C**) is affected, the patient will experience hypothyroidism. Symptoms of ACTH and TSH deficiency are usually seen in chronic rather than acute Sheehan syndrome and may take months or years to manifest themselves. Loss of antidiuretic hormone (ADH) (choice **E**), is seldom seen.

**41** **The answer is E** *Pediatrics*

A karyotype is described by first listing the total number of chromosomes, followed by the sex chromosomes plus any abnormalities in number or structure. Normal euploid individuals have 46 chromosomes, of which two are the sex chromosomes; in other words they are 46XX or 46XY. Thus, 47XY + 13 (choice **E**) describes a male (XY) with 47 chromosomes, the extra one being chromosome 13. Expressed differently, he has three number 13 chromosomes, or trisomy 13. Approximately 1 in 15,000 newborn infants have trisomy 13, and about half of these will die within the first month of life. Those who survive are severely developmentally and mentally retarded.

**42** **The answer is B** *Pediatrics*

This is a male with one extra Y chromosome (choice **B**). There is no specific name for this condition, but it occurs in about 1 per 1,000 male live births, and surveys of mental and penal institutions found that the incidence among inmates was 4 to 20 per 1,000, raising the question of whether an extra Y chromosome may be causally related to aberrant behaviors. However, the magnitude of social pathology, if any, has not yet been determined.

**43** **The answer is A** *Pediatrics*

This is a description of a baby girl with Down syndrome due to trisomy 21 (choice **A**). The overall incidence of this disorder is approximately 1 per 750 live births, but it depends on the mother's age. The occurrence of trisomy 21 increases with maternal age (≥35 years), but because of the higher overall birthrate in younger women, they represent half of all mothers with Down syndrome babies. Therefore, all women should be offered prenatal screening (free β-hCG, unconjugated estriol, and α fetoprotein) for Down syndrome in their second trimester. In about 95% of the cases, the cause of Down syndrome is trisomy 21 due to errors in meiosis. An additional 4% of cases are due to an unbalanced translocation; the remaining individuals with Down syndrome are mosaics having both a 47 + 21 cell line as well as the normal euploid line. In addition to the unusual appearance described, children with Down syndrome will have growth retardation, have some degree of mental retardation, and will show signs of premature aging. They also have a risk of serious heart disease, a risk of serious gastrointestinal problems, and a greater-than-normal risk of leukemia, serious infections, cataracts, and thyroid abnormalities. Individuals who live beyond the age of 35 show signs of Alzheimer disease. The life expectancy for children with Down syndrome is approximately 50 years.

### 44 The answer is D *Pediatrics*

The Y chromosome usually carries the genes that code for maleness. As a consequence, this boy has a basic male phenotype, despite the fact he is XXY (choice D). However, the extra X chromosome does cause some feminization. This condition is known as Klinefelter syndrome, and it occurs in about 1 per 1,000 male births. In addition to having small testicles and possibly having enlarged breasts, such individuals are usually tall and thin and have arms and legs that are disproportionally long. The testicular tubules are hyalinized, and there is a failure to produce sperm, making them infertile. Despite these signs of feminization, superficially they are phenotypically male with perhaps some small but feminine breasts counterbalanced by a normal-sized penis. There is no mental retardation, although the IQ may be somewhat lower than expected. A few men have more than one extra X chromosome, and the greater the number of X chromosomes, the greater the likelihood of frank mental retardation. Their cells have Barr bodies, but at least some cells retain a viable X chromosome.

### 45 The answer is C *Pediatrics*

This girl has Turner syndrome due to the loss of one X chromosome (choice C), a condition that occurs in about 1 in 1,500 to 2,500 live births. It is estimated that 99% of concepti with Turner syndrome are spontaneously aborted. In addition to the characteristics noted in the case description, girls with Turner syndrome have an increased carrying angle at the elbow and cardiovascular and renal abnormalities. Newborn infants with Turner syndrome are noted to have lymphedema of the hands and feet. They may also have a short neck with extra skin folds, widely spaced nipples, and decreased femoral pulses.

### 46 The answer is E *Surgery*

This patient has a twisting injury to the lateral aspect of the ankle, resulting in a sprained lateral ligament (choice E). The lateral ligaments of the ankle consist of the posterior talofibular, the anterior talofibular, and the calcaneofibular ligaments. Although all three ligaments may be involved, usually the anterior talofibular ligament is most severely injured. Sprains are classified as grade I if the ligament involved is simply stretched and not torn, grade II if slightly torn, and grade III if severely torn or ruptured. The ecchymosis (bruising) and swelling in all three grades is due to bleeding from surrounding soft tissue. Injury to these ligaments may occur with or without an associated avulsion fracture of the base of the fifth metatarsal and/or the tip of the lateral malleous rarely, a fracture of the talus. The patient would also be unable to walk on this leg if there were ecchymosis on the dorsolateral aspect of the ankle. She would probably hop, using the good foot.

### 47 The answer is B *Surgery*

This patient has a tear of the Achilles tendon (choice B), just proximal to its insertion in the calcaneus. The prevalence of Achilles tendon tears increases 3 to 5-fold after the age of 40 years, and overall about 2% of Achilles tendon injuries result in a tear that may be partial or complete. Achilles tendon tears often follow tendinitis (patient's slight pain) and can then be caused by even minor additional stress. Patients complain of pain behind the ankle and have difficulty walking on tiptoe. A gap is felt when a finger is run over the skin at the point of tear, and plantar flexion following compression of the bellies of the calf muscles below and behind the knee is weak (Thomson test). There is no pain on compression of the calf muscles. Radiography is irrelevant to the diagnosis, which is clinical. This condition should be differentiated from tears involving the bellies of the calf muscles.

### 48 The answer is D *Surgery*

This patient has a tear involving some of the muscle fibers of the plantar flexors (i.e., gastrocnemius [most common] and soleus) (choice D). Such tears most commonly occur in males in their fourth to sixth decade. Often, these men are former athletes who are still well muscled but now no longer workout regularly, so-called "weekend warriors." The muscle tears in response to a sudden push-off of the foot, as might occur in hill running, jumping, tennis, or any other activity involving similar movements. Whereas stretching and tears in ligaments are called *sprains,* analogous muscle injuries are called *strains.* Patients who injure the plantar flexors have pain in the calf, and ecchymosis may be present in the overlying skin. Compression of the bellies of the calf muscles causes pain. Plantar flexion is normal with calf compression because most of the muscle fibers are intact, and the insertion to the posterior aspect of the calcaneus is not endangered. Therefore, no gap will be felt in that area. Patients can walk on tiptoe, although with pain. An x-ray film is noncontributory to the diagnosis, which is clinical. This condition should be differentiated from tears of the Achilles tendon.

**49** **The answer is C** *Surgery*

As a result of his fall, this patient has sustained a fracture of the calcaneus (choice **C**), which most commonly occurs from a foot-first fall from a height greater than 6 feet or from an automobile accident in which the patient had the feet firmly braced on the floor. Although the complaint often centers on just one foot, the injury may be unilateral or bilateral, and both legs should be investigated. Also, the force is transmitted to the lumbar spine, and often there is an associated compression fracture of the lumbar vertebra. Thus, one must suspect a compression fracture and obtain an x-ray film to exclude it. Failure to do so could have dire consequences, especially if the patient is moved, because an ensuing paraplegia would be irreversible. Due to the presence of fascial compartments restraining the muscles of the foot, which are in four layers in the plantar region, a compartment syndrome and even necrosis of the skin could also ensue. This is due to the edema resulting from trauma impeding blood flow to the tissues.

**50** **The answer is F** *Surgery*

This patient has a "march" fracture, which usually involves the shafts of the metatarsals (choice **F**), especially the second and third. This condition was initially noted in soldiers who had marched for long distances, hence the name. These patients complain of pain in the foot, which may not become worse with walking. Tenderness over the point of fracture is noted. Although the fracture cannot be seen on x-ray films, a bone scan will reveal the fracture and a second x-ray film taken about 4 weeks later will show the healing fracture.

Choice **A,** fracture of the talus, is incorrect. The talus is a small bone that sits between the calcaneus and the tibia and fibula, forming the subtalar joint. Although the talus may be broken by twisting an ankle, this is relatively rare. It is more commonly broken in falls, automobile accidents, and snowboarding accidents.

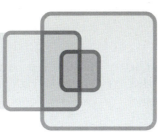

# test **2**

# Questions

*Single Best Choice Directions: This section consists of numbered statements or questions followed by a list of potential answers; you are to select the ONE best answer.*

**1** A 30-year-old woman visits her family physician for a routine physical examination. During her interaction with him, she stated that she had unprotected sex with a bisexual male about 6 months previously. At this time, she did not suffer from any tiredness, weakness, fever, or untoward health problems. However, she was concerned that she may have contracted acquired immune deficiency syndrome (AIDS) during that encounter. She felt that an AIDS test would be appropriate to assuage her fears. Which of the following parameters described in the standard 2 × 2 table below should be fulfilled by the test that was ordered by the physician?

|  | Disease Present | Disease Absent | Totals |
|---|---|---|---|
| Exposed to infection | *a* | *b* | *a* + *b* |
| Not exposed | *c* | *d* | *c* + *d* |
| Totals | *a* + *c* | *b* + *d* | |

(A) The value of *d* must be much less than that of *c*.
(B) The value of *d* must be much greater than that of *b*.
(C) The value of *a* must be much greater than that of *c*.
(D) The value of *d* must be much less than that of *b*.
(E) The value of *a* must be much greater than that of *b*.

**2** A 45-year-old war veteran made an appointment with a clinical psychologist seeking help to deal with recurring nightmares concerning horrific events that he witnessed and participated in during a war almost two decades ago. Lately, his reaction to these dreams had intensified; he wakes up screaming and damp from a cold sweat. When prodded by the psychologist, he admitted that he has come to feel emotionally distant from other people and uncomfortable in their presence. He states that he considers himself to be rejected by "society" and wants to seek out other veterans with similar experiences in an attempt to "relate." Which of the following is the most appropriate first step in the management of this patient?

(A) Begin psychodynamic psychotherapy to explore his guilt before considering unstructured meetings with other veterans.
(B) Cognitively reframe his experiences and focus on the present.
(C) Make arrangements for him to join a peer support group.
(D) Initiate therapy with a combination of clonazepam and paroxetine.
(E) Suggest that he meet with citizens and veterans from the nation he fought against to heal anger and guilt.

**3** A 30-year-old woman, gravida 3, para 1, abortus 1, is at 30 weeks' gestation by dates. She has been married for 7 years to the same husband. Her first pregnancy ended in a spontaneous first-trimester loss. Her second pregnancy was unremarkable until delivery at term, when she underwent an emergency low-transverse cesarean section because of double footling breech presentation. She has worked in a child day-care center for the past 5 years. She vacationed in Thailand for 2 weeks last year. On routine prenatal laboratory testing, you find that she is hepatitis B surface antigen positive, and anti-HBc IgM negative. She inquires about the significance of this finding concerning herself, as well as her baby. Which of the following statements best summarizes what you will say?

(A) Pregnancy accelerates the course of acute hepatitis B in the mother.

(B) Mode of delivery has no impact on maternal–neonatal hepatitis B transmission.

(C) Breastfeeding does not increase neonatal risk of hepatitis B.

(D) Neonates can be protected from hepatitis B by passive immunization at birth.

(E) Rapidity of hepatitis B progression is the same in mother and neonate.

**4** A 4-day-old, 1,500 g (3 lb 5 oz) premature infant recovering from a respiratory distress syndrome is noted to have bounding peripheral pulsations and a hyperactive precordium. A continuous machinery murmur is most audible at the left infraclavicular area. Left ventricle hypertrophy (LVH) is present on the electrocardiogram (ECG). The chest x-ray film shows slight enlargement of the heart and increased pulmonary venous markings. Which of the following is the most likely diagnosis?

(A) Patent ductus arteriosus

(B) Atrial septal defect (ASD)

(C) Ventricular septal defect (VSD)

(D) Pulmonic stenosis

(E) Tetralogy of Fallot

**5** A 49-year-old blue-eyed blonde woman was brought to the emergency room with a history of having come down heavily on the right leg while stepping off a curb. The paramedics reported that she had vomited once during the trip. The patient stated that she had had a dull ache in the right thigh for the past few weeks and had noticed a "boil" there. She had made an appointment to see her primary care physician for this and for recent onset of hot flushes (also called hot flashes). The emergency physician noted that she was in moderate distress. Her blood pressure was 90/60 mm Hg, pulse was 98/min regular and thready, her respirations were 22/min, and her temperature was 37.5°C (99.5°F). She had no cyanosis, but had pallor of the mucosa. Cardiovascular examination was unremarkable except for a sinus tachycardia and a capillary circulation longer than 2 seconds. Examination of the respiratory system revealed normal breath sounds bilaterally. Her right thigh was swollen, and she had lateral rotation and shortening of the leg. The right groin was tender to palpation, and movement of the leg induced severe pain. There was a raised papular lesion over anterior midthigh, surrounded by inflammation. The pelvis and the left leg were normal. Which of the following choices is the most likely reason for her problem?

(A) Chronic osteomyelitis

(B) Osteoporosis

(C) Stress fracture

(D) Osteogenesis imperfecta

(E) Metastatic bone disease

**6** A 75-year-old man was rushed to the emergency room of a local hospital after having collapsed at home. The patient's spouse related that he had complained of sudden severe pain over the left flank. She informed the physician that he had been complaining of backache for a few years, but did not want to see a physician, as he felt that it was "no big deal." Physical examination revealed a conscious male, in acute distress, with definite signs of hypotension, tachycardia, tachypnea, and hypothermia. He had mucosal pallor but no cyanosis. The abdomen was tender to palpation, and a pulsatile supraumbilical mass was present. Bowel sounds were diminished, and peripheral pulses were equal and moderately strong. The patient was given 100% oxygen by mask, at 10 L per minute. The cardiac monitor showed sinus tachycardia with mild ischemia. Which of the following mechanisms is most likely involved in the pathogenesis of this patient's clinical disorder?

(A) Cystic medial degeneration

(B) Defect in collagen

(C) Defect in fibrillin

(D) An immunologic reaction

(E) Atherosclerosis

**7** A child is at his pediatrician's office for a well-child check. The patient has been well according to the parents, and there are no complaints. On physical examination, no abnormalities are noted. Additionally, the pediatrician performs a developmental screen on the patient. He finds that the child is able to say his first and last name and play interactive games. The patient's mother reports that the patient is toilet trained and is able to pedal a tricycle. He is capable of copying a cross and a circle, but cannot copy a square or triangle. He is also not able to catch a bounced ball or dress without supervision. Which of the following is the most likely age of this child?

(A) 1 year old
(B) 2 years old
(C) 3 years old
(D) 4 years old
(E) 5 years old

**8** Some-town in the USA, has a population of 100,000. During 2010, there were 1,600 live births, 85 stillbirths, and 15 neonatal deaths. Among the births that year, there were 20 sets of twins and four sets of triplets, and four mothers died at the time of delivery. Which of the following represents the perinatal mortality rate in this town during 2009?

(A) 100/1,685
(B) 85/1,600
(C) 125/2,205
(D) 100/1,700
(E) 59/2,205

**9** A 37-year-old woman, gravida 4, para 4, underwent a routine cervical Pap smear during an annual examination. She has regular menstrual periods and underwent a tubal sterilization surgical procedure after her last delivery 5 years ago. She denies excessive pain with menses or intercourse. She has been watching her diet and exercises regularly at the local fitness center; as a result, during the past 6 months she lost 15 pounds. She underwent a divorce 3 years ago but has now remarried. Her present husband also was divorced after 10 years in a previous marriage. The cytologic evaluation showed a high-grade squamous intraepithelial lesion (HSIL). She was referred for colposcopy and directed biopsies. Which of the following findings would be an indication for a diagnostic cervical conization?

(A) Intraepithelial neoplasia on biopsy with satisfactory colposcopy
(B) Negative endocervical curettage with satisfactory colposcopy
(C) Cervical biopsy showing mild dysplasia
(D) Cervical biopsy showing carcinoma in situ
(E) Cervical biopsy showing stage IB invasive carcinoma

**10** A 24-year-old woman, gravida 4, para 1, abortus 2, is at 28 weeks' gestation by poor dates. She admits to intravenous (IV) drug use and having sex for drugs. She is unsure who is the father of this pregnancy. She has recently undergone treatment for syphilis identified by a positive venereal disease research laboratory (VDRL) test result and confirmed by a positive fluorescent treponemal antibody (FTA) test. On her last prenatal visit, she underwent human immunodeficiency virus (HIV) testing by enzyme-linked immunosorbent assay (ELISA), which was found to be positive and was confirmed with a positive Western blot assay. She inquires as to the significance of this finding for herself, as well as her baby. Which of the following statements best summarizes what you will say about her medical conditions?

(A) Pregnancy accelerates maternal progression from HIV positive to acquired immune deficiency syndrome (AIDS).
(B) Mode of delivery has a significant impact on maternal–neonatal transmission of HIV.
(C) Breastfeeding does not increase neonatal risk of becoming HIV positive.
(D) Neonates can be protected from HIV by passive immunization at birth.
(E) Rapidity of disease progression is the same in mother and neonate.

**11** A 40-year-old man with a 20-year history of schizophrenia, paranoid type, is brought in by police because local business owners complained that he spends all day outside a particular strip mall where his malodorousness and pacing were driving away customers. He lives in the alley behind the mall in a makeshift shelter. The man adamantly refuses hospitalization or any other help with his living situation. He demands to leave. Which of the following findings would provide the best legal support for hospitalizing the man against his wishes?

(A) He lives in a shelter made from wooden crates and cardboard, and receives money for food from begging.
(B) He believes that members of the central intelligence agency are following him.
(C) He believes that he hears the voice of Elvis Presley.
(D) He is disheveled and shows evidence of poor hygiene.
(E) He has a gun and has threatened to kill himself.

**12** An 85-year old woman who lives in a small rural Midwest town has always kept active despite her age, singing in her church choir, baby sitting her great-grandchildren, etc. However, for the past several months she has not felt well, not even able to muster sufficient energy to go to church on Sunday mornings, let alone go to choir practice. Also, she has problems sleeping, is extremely nervous with hand tremors, constantly anxious, sweats more than usual and can't stand having the heat on, has chronic diarrhea, and has the sensation that her heart races. When she mentions some of these observations to her local primary care provider, he basically shrugs them off, saying that no one of her age can expect to feel as they did when younger. He was worried however by the fact her systolic pressure rose from an average of 125 mm Hg to 185 mm Hg at the time of her visit; he prescribed hydrochlorothiazide and suggested she return in 3 months for a follow-up examination. However, in the meantime, she started to have trouble with her eyes: she had double vision and they appeared to her to be reddish and swollen; they also were itchy. Consequently her granddaughter took her to an optometrist who practised in a nearby town. After her initial examination, the optometrist became alarmed to such a degree that she arranged a visit to the Mayo Clinic in Rochester Minnesota. After giving her a thorough physical, the physicians there started her on a therapy with the aim of alleviating the underlying cause of her symptoms, including the problem with her eyes. Which of the following choices most probably describes an aspect of the treatment used to alleviate the underlying cause of her symptoms?

(A) Prescription of levothyroxine
(B) Injection of interferon-β 1a
(C) Watchful waiting
(D) Prescription of zolpidem
(E) Prescription of propylthiouracil

**13** A 55-year-old man presented to his family physician with fairly rapid progress of failing memory and impaired cognition. Recently, he developed difficulty in walking and jerky movements of his limbs that materialize spontaneously, usually in the morning but also occur during his sleep. The patient had been diagnosed earlier with coronary artery disease. In addition, a few years earlier, he developed visual problems in the right eye as a result of an ocular injury; this problem resolved after a corneal transplant. All his life, he lived and worked as a farmer in the San Joaquin Valley of California. The farthest he had traveled was to Nevada. Physical examination revealed a rather disheveled man who demonstrated features of moderate dementia. He had fasciculations of his upper extremities, and during the examination, his limbs jerked uncontrollably in a rapid manner. He also demonstrated cerebellar signs. Magnetic resonance imaging (MRI) shows bilateral areas of increased signal intensity in the caudate and putamen in T2-weighted images. An electroencephalograph (EEG) report showed periodic high-voltage sharp spikes. Which of the following is the most likely diagnosis?

(A) Creutzfeldt-Jakob disease
(B) Bovine spongiform dementia
(C) Parkinson disease
(D) Alzheimer disease
(E) Progressive multifocal leukoencephaly

**14** A 33-year-old man who had been morbidly obese underwent successful Roux-en-Y gastric bypass surgery 33 months earlier. However, recently, he has been having disturbing symptoms. These include insomnia, sensory disturbances such as numbness and tingling in his hands and feet, as well as an inflamed tongue, dizziness, and poor coordination and balance. In addition, he developed a strange way of walking, a stomping gait striking first heavily with his heel. He had not returned for 2 or more years after the gastric bypass operation to see a physician, but because of concern about these symptoms, he finally did. When quizzed about his dietary habits, he responded that he thought he ate a balanced diet of the type prescribed for post-gastric bypass surgical patients and that he generally, but not always, did take a daily multivitamin pill, but after the first half year or so he did not take any special supplements; he felt they were too expensive and unnecessary. The symptoms described and the patient's somewhat lackadaisical approach to his postsurgical diet leads the physician to believe that the patient's symptoms were almost certainly due to a nutritional deficiency. The deficiency that would most likely cause the symptoms described is which one of the following?

(A) Iron
(B) Vitamin $B_{12}$ (cobalamine)
(C) Folate
(D) Zinc
(E) Copper

**15** A 40-year-old man is obsessed with dressing in women's undergarments. Although he risks extremely negative reactions from his coworkers, he often wears such apparel beneath his office clothes. He is disturbed by his behavior but says that he cannot resist the sexual arousal associated with it. Which of the following is the best description of this man's behavior?

(A) Exhibitionism
(B) Frotteurism
(C) Gender identity disorder
(D) Transvestic fetishism
(E) Voyeurism

**16** A 13-year-old girl comes to the outpatient office complaining of bleeding irregularly for the past 3 months. She denies cramping, pain, nausea, vomiting, or diarrhea with her menstrual periods. She started breast budding 3 years ago, with development of pubic and axillary hair a year later. She underwent menarche 1 year ago and uses tampons regularly. She is a student at the local middle school and is doing well in her studies. Her height is 62 inches (1.57 m) and she weighs 130 lb (59 kg). On general examination, she appears well developed, well nourished, and in no distress. General and pelvic examinations are unremarkable. If an endometrial biopsy were performed on this girl, which of the following histologic findings would be most likely seen on microscopic examination?

(A) Serrated endometrial glands with inspissated secretions
(B) Tubular endometrial glands with many mitoses
(C) Back-to-back endometrial glands with prominent nuclei
(D) Decidual reaction forming around endometrial arterioles
(E) Hyperchromatism and loss of cellular polarity

**17** A 38-year-old man presents with bouts of severe, right retro-orbital pain lasting one-half hour or more, up to several times a day. The pain often occurs at night and is associated with nasal congestion on the right nostril and right conjunctival injection. Which of the following would be an effective short-term treatment in this patient?

(A) Sublingual nitroglycerin
(B) An alcoholic beverage
(C) Vigorous exercise
(D) Oxygen
(E) A warm pack over the eye

**18** A 25-year-old woman comes to the outpatient office complaining of a pruritic, painful vaginal discharge. She is sexually active with two male sexual partners but finds intercourse very uncomfortable because of her vaginal symptoms. For the past 8 months, she has been using the estrogen–progestin contraceptive patch. She exercises regularly by walking 2 to 3 miles a day. She is following a low-carbohydrate diet and takes a multivitamin preparation. Findings of her general examination are unremarkable. Speculum examination of the vagina shows a foul-smelling greenish, frothy discharge. Vaginal pH, using Nitrazine paper, is 6.5. A wet mount of vaginal secretions in a saline suspension reveals a highly motile organism. Which of the following pharmacologic agents would be the most appropriate treatment?

(A) Metronidazole
(B) Clotrimazole
(C) Miconazole
(D) Acyclovir
(E) Azithromycin

**19** While perusing a research article, a student came across a data set composed of the numbers 7, 5, 8, 2, and 8. Which of the following sets of numbers provides the correct range, mean, median, and mode in the appropriate order?

(A) 2, 7, 8, 6
(B) 8, 8, 7, 5
(C) 6, 7, 6, 8
(D) 5, 5, 7, 8
(E) 6, 6, 7, 8

**20** A teenage boy was seated in the waiting area of an emergency room when he suddenly became very agitated and had a bizarre look. He then cried out loudly, fell to the floor, and his body began to shake uncontrollably. His arms and legs kept flailing, and there was froth coming out of his mouth. The patient was unconscious and continued to shake. Which of the following choices represents the best initial intervention for this patient?

(A) Insert a tongue blade
(B) Administer an intravenous (IV) bolus of 50% dextrose
(C) Secure the airway
(D) Inject 2 mg of IV lorazepam followed by phenytoin infusion
(E) Induce pentobarbital coma

**21** An obstetric sonogram is performed on a 22-year-old woman, gravida 2, para 1, who is at 30 weeks' gestation by dates and confirmed by early first-trimester ultrasound crown–rump measurements 9 weeks' gestation. Her pregnancy is complicated by gestational diabetes diagnosed at 26 weeks' gestation, which is being managed by diet alone. Her home blood glucose monitoring shows the following mean values: fasting 85 mg/dL; 1 hour post-meal, <130 mg/dL. The sonogram reveals an anterior-fundal placenta and a normal amniotic fluid volume. There is a single fetus with the head in the right upper quadrant, with his back to the mother's left. Both fetal thighs are flexed and both legs are extended. In this case, which of the following is the correct fetal presentation?

(A) Transverse breech
(B) Complete breech
(C) Double-footling breech
(D) Incomplete breech
(E) Frank breech

**22** A 45-year-old woman with polyhydramnios delivers a full-term male infant with a birth weight of 6 lb 12 oz (3.06 kg). The infant's physical examination is pertinent for hypotonia, upward and slanted palpebral fissures and epicanthic folds, a simian crease, and a short fifth finger. A few hours after birth, the infant begins to vomit bile-stained fluid. On physical examination, the abdomen is not distended. Radiographs of the chest and abdomen were obtained, and the results revealed a "double-bubble" sign. Which of the following is the most likely diagnosis?

(A) Congenital pyloric stenosis
(B) Duodenal atresia
(C) An intussusception
(D) A diaphragmatic hernia
(E) A perforated viscus

**23** A 67-year-old man presents with headache, vomiting, blurred vision, difficulty with speaking and swallowing, and loss of balance. He also complains of numbness in his face. His past history is significant for diabetes mellitus and hypertension. The patient presently is on metformin for the former and a combination of an angiotensin converting enzyme (ACE) inhibitor and diuretic for the latter. The acute problem occurred approximately 2 hours prior to being seen in the emergency room. His blood pressure is 150/100 mm Hg, his pulse rate is 80/min with a few irregular beats, and his temperature and respiratory rate are normal. The patient is conscious, the left pupil is smaller than the right, and the eyeball appears to be sunken into the orbit. He also has partial closure of the left upper eyelid. He has no pain sensations over the left side of the face to pinprick. However, touch is preserved. His gag reflex is depressed, and the palate is noticeably lowered on the left side, with the uvula being pulled to the right when he was asked to say, "aaah." There was a noticeable nystagmus to the left, and he has poor coordination of his left upper and lower extremities. His gait is ataxic. When tested with a pin, he cannot feel pain in the right upper and lower extremities. However, the sensation of touch is preserved. A noncontrast computerized tomography (CT) of the brain was normal. Which of the following is the best means of immediate medical management in this patient?

(A) Heparinization and observation
(B) Right carotid endarterectomy
(C) Left carotid endarterectomy
(D) Thrombolytics
(E) Antiplatelet agents

**24** A 65-year-old woman went bicycling into the country near Lake Tahoe, California, with a few of her friends. She had not bicycled since her childhood growing up at the foothills of the Ural Mountains in Russia. The front wheel struck a pothole and she fell to the ground. While doing so, her chest struck the handlebar. She was immediately rushed to the local hospital. On arrival, she is conscious and appears to be in moderate distress. Her blood pressure is 140/95 mm Hg, pulse 96/min. Her respirations are shallow and rapid, at 22/min. Bruising over the left anterior hemithorax is observed upon examination of the chest. There is no jugular venous dilatation. The rest of her examination findings are unremarkable. Further examination would most likely yield which of the following?

(A) Increased breath sounds on the left
(B) Egophony on the left
(C) Increased timbre
(D) Increased width of intercostals on the left
(E) Mediastinal structures shifted to the left

**25** A 60-year-old man presents to the emergency room with a history of vomiting, increasing confusion, hearing voices, and blurred vision. The patient provided a history of congestive cardiac failure and reported he is being treated with an unnamed diuretic, enalapril, carvedilol, and digoxin. His blood pressure is 140/95 mm Hg; pulse, 88/min irregular; respirations, 22/min; and body temperature is normal. Physical examination confirmed altered mental status, an irregular cardiac rhythm to auscultation, and basilar rales on the left, but there is no cyanosis or pallor. The electrocardiogram shows left axis deviation and paroxysmal atrial tachycardia with block. A chest x-ray film confirms left ventricular hypertrophy with blunting of the left costophrenic angle and diffuse shadowing at the base. Effective management of cardiac dysfunction would include which one of the following?

(A) Raising the serum sodium level
(B) Raising the serum magnesium level
(C) Lowering the serum magnesium level
(D) Raising the serum calcium level
(E) Raising the serum potassium level

**26** A 38-year-old woman visits her family physician because of her concern about a lump in her left breast, which she noticed after a fall approximately 1 week previously. She does not smoke, drinks wine on social occasions, and takes birth control pills. She is a divorced mother of two and recently returned to the dating scene. There is no family history of breast cancer. Physical examination reveals a rather stocky woman with pendulous breasts. She has a moderate-sized, nontender, irregular lump in the lower outer quadrant of her left breast. The overlying skin appears thickened. No nipple discharge is present, and she has no axillary lymphadenopathy. The right breast and axilla are normal. Mammography reveals increased density in the affected region. Ultrasound-guided fine needle aspiration biopsy (FNAB) was performed. The pathology report was consistent with a diagnosis of fat necrosis. Which of the following is the most appropriate next step in the management of this patient?

(A) Excise the mass
(B) Repeat fine needle aspiration biopsy after 1 month
(C) Repeat mammography in a month
(D) Reassure the patient, and follow up in a few weeks
(E) Mastectomy

27 A 42-year-old man with hyperopia presents with a history of sudden severe pain in the right eye, associated with blurred vision, nausea, and vomiting. Examination of the eye reveals lid and corneal edema, conjunctival injection, and a shallow anterior chamber. Physical examination reveals the pupil to be mid-dilated and fixed. No discharge is present. The examining physician would expect to find which of the following?

(A) Intraocular pressure greater than 22 mm Hg
(B) Blood in the anterior chamber
(C) Corneal abrasion on slit-lamp examination
(D) Papilledema
(E) Bloodless arterioles and a cherry-red fovea

28 A 69-year-old man with a known history of coronary artery disease (CAD), atrial fibrillation, and hypertension presents with sudden onset of right facial weakness and numbness. He also complains of a roaring in the right ear. On examination, he has some difficulty with speech. He does not have a pronator drift, and his grip strength is normal. However, there is weakness of the face on the right side, including the orbicularis oculi. He is unable to appreciate taste on the anterior tongue on the right side. He has normal sensations on the face to touch and pinprick. Which of the following would best explain these findings?

(A) Upper motor neuron lesion
(B) Brainstem glioma
(C) Left middle cerebral artery embolus
(D) Hemorrhage within the left internal capsule
(E) Lower motor neuron lesion

29 A 55-year-old woman presents to the emergency room with a history of severe crushing retrosternal chest pain while she was moving some furniture around the house. Electrocardiography shows elevated ST segments in leads II, III, and aVF, consistent with an inferior myocardial infarction. This diagnosis is further supported by cardiac enzymes that test positive. The patient is hemodynamically stable. She is moved to the intensive care unit. A few hours later, she developed tachyarrhythmia. Treatment with intravenous (IV) boluses of lidocaine controls the arrhythmia only transiently—the arrhythmia disappears within 1 minute only to reappear within 4 minutes of each bolus dose. Plasma levels of lidocaine measured soon after each injection remained within the therapeutic range (1–5 mg/L). Which of the following statements is most accurate?

(A) Rapid metabolism of lidocaine is responsible for the short duration of its antiarrhythmic action after the bolus administration.
(B) Laboratory determinations of blood levels of lidocaine after IV administration are frequently in error.
(C) The elimination half-life of lidocaine is approximately 2 minutes.
(D) Lidocaine rapidly redistributes from blood to other tissues.
(E) Cardiac cells rapidly develop tachyphylaxis to lidocaine.

**30** A 30-year-old Caucasian man from Scotland met and married a 26-year-old French Caucasian woman. Both of them were healthy and lived a healthy lifestyle. They moved to California after their marriage and worked in the entertainment industry in Hollywood. Three years later, the woman gave birth to a child who had respiratory and gastrointestinal problems. The child was diagnosed with cystic fibrosis. Both parents are convinced that the disease was not inherited and are not concerned that subsequent children will have a substantial chance of acquiring the disease. They support this contention by pointing out that they are not related and there is no history of cystic fibrosis in either of their families. Which of the following statements is most likely true?

(A) The case described is a new mutation.
(B) The degree of penetrance is low; therefore, some of their relatives were genetically affected but did not express the disease.
(C) Both parents are carriers and each subsequent child will have a 25% chance of expressing the disease.
(D) It would be easy to determine if they are carriers using simple physiologic methods.
(E) DNA fingerprinting can be used to determine whether or not each parent carries the unique mutation that causes cystic fibrosis.

**31** The paramedics were called to a theme park to attend to a 75-year-old woman who suddenly took ill. She complained of headache and numbness and weakness on the left side of her body. She had a prior history of a mitral valve replacement and was on warfarin. She lapsed into coma on the way to the hospital. The emergency room physician observed a left hemiplegia, with hemi-neglect and conjugate ocular deviation to the right. Which of the following is the most appropriate emergent test to obtain?

(A) Magnetic resonance imaging (MRI) scan of the brain
(B) Computed tomography (CT) of the brain
(C) Electroencephalogram (EEG)
(D) Carotid duplex ultrasonography
(E) Spinal tap

**32** An anxious 33-year-old woman, gravida 3, para 1, abortus 1, is seen for her first prenatal visit at 10 weeks' gestation by dates. This was a planned pregnancy, and she discontinued the transdermal contraceptive patch 4 months ago. She is taking prenatal vitamins, including iron and folic acid. First-trimester bleeding that progressed to hemorrhage complicated her first pregnancy, necessitating a suction dilatation and curettage at 8 weeks' gestation. Her last pregnancy was uncomplicated prenatally. She went into spontaneous labor at 39 weeks' gestation, progressing normally in labor with a reassuring electronic fetal heart rate monitor pattern. However, after an uncomplicated spontaneous vaginal delivery with neonatal Apgar scores of 8 and 9 at 1 and 5 minutes, respectively, her female neonate died on the second day of life from overwhelming group B β-hemolytic streptococcal (GBS) infection. Which of the following statements best expresses what you will tell her about her current pregnancy?

(A) Most women with a positive vaginal GBS culture will have uninfected infants.
(B) A negative vaginal GBS culture means the fetus will not be at risk at delivery.
(C) Appropriate treatment for a positive GBS vaginal culture can eradicate the organism.
(D) The GBS organism is a pathologic bacterium in the female genital tract.
(E) Rapid nonculture assay tests are highly sensitive for the GBS organism.

**33** A 6-year-old presents to his pediatrician with left ear pain. His parents state that he had been in his usual state of good health until he went swimming in a lake a few days ago. The patient's vital signs are within normal limits for age. He is afebrile and appears nontoxic. Physical examination of the left ear reveals edema and erythema of the ear canal, as well as a greenish otorrhea. It is difficult to visualize the tympanic membrane. Pain is increased by manipulation of the pinna and pressure on the tragus. Which of the following is the most likely pathogen producing this patient's symptoms?

(A) *Haemophilus influenzae*
(B) *Pseudomonas aeruginosa*
(C) *Moraxella catarrhalis*
(D) *Streptococcus agalactiae*
(E) *Escherichia coli*

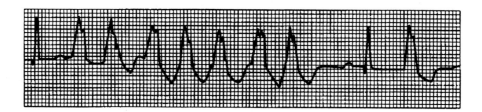

**34** The above electrocardiogram (ECG) is from a 65-year-old man with ischemic heart disease. Which of the following is the most likely diagnosis?

(A) Premature atrial contractions
(B) Atrial flutter
(C) Paroxysmal atrial tachycardia
(D) Ventricular tachycardia
(E) Sinus tachycardia

**35** A 65-year-old woman had a 5-year history of pain in the right hip that had gradually gotten worse. She had reached a point where she hobbled with the help of a cane. Nonsteroidal analgesics did not help her very much. She finally agreed to undergo surgery. An x-ray film of the right hip confirmed severe osteoarthritis. There was no osteoporosis. The orthopedic surgeon recommended hip arthroplasty, and she was admitted to the hospital. She was considered at high risk for deep venous thrombosis, and heparin prophylaxis was begun. Which of the following is the best test to monitor heparin therapy?

(A) Thrombin time (TT)
(B) Prothrombin time (PT)
(C) Prothrombin and proconvertin test
(D) Activated partial thromboplastin time (aPTT)
(E) Bleeding time

**36** A 34-year-old woman with major single-episode depressive disorder has responded well to sertraline after 1 month of treatment. There are no significant untoward effects, such as intolerable nausea or other gastrointestinal problems that selective serotonin reuptake inhibitors (SSRIs) sometimes cause. Which of the following is the most appropriate next step in management?

(A) Continue the sertraline for 6 months.
(B) Continue the sertraline indefinitely.
(C) Decrease the sertraline gradually until she is medication free, unless depression recurs.
(D) Stop the sertraline immediately.
(E) Switch to fluoxetine.

**37** A 58-year old male computer programmer presented to his physician for a routine check-up after his wife nagged him into it. This was his first visit to a physician in at least a decade. After work, he would come home, eat dinner, watch television, and go to bed. He spent his weekends watching sports on television. While doing so, he often ate peanuts, buttered popcorn, or potato chips and downed it with a couple of beers. When asked if this had always been his lifestyle, he replies that prior to turning 40 he played sports and enjoyed dancing with his wife. His subsequent physical examination and laboratory work did not uncover any abnormalities with his heart, lungs, thyroid hormone levels, or kidney function. On the other hand, three different blood pressure readings taken by both the physician and his assistant obtain similar results, namely, an average reading of 178/ 92 mm Hg. He is 5 feet, 9 inches (1.75 m) tall and weighs 204 pounds (92.5 kg). A fasting blood sugar and lipid profile show a glucose level of 124 mg/dL, total cholesterol (TC) level of 234 mg/dL, and low-density lipoprotein (LDL) level of 158 mg/dL. The most appropriate first line of management in this patient would be which of the following?

(A) Gastroplasty
(B) Prescription of an anorexic drug
(C) Prescription of gemfibrozil
(D) Persuade him to take his wife out dancing at least twice a week.
(E) Prescription of a dietary supplement containing ephedra
(F) Prescription of tolbutamide

**38** A young woman with phenylketonuria (PKU) who wants to become pregnant asks her physician if any special preparation is required before conception to ensure that her baby is healthy. Her physician tells her that women with PKU who are not on low-phenylalanine diets have a higher risk of spontaneous abortion than the general population and often give birth to infants with mental retardation, microcephaly, and other congenital anomalies; high levels of phenylalanine seem to be the cause of these problems. Therefore, prospective mothers who have PKU should be placed on a low-phenylalanine diet before conception. Which of the following values represents the highest blood phenylalanine concentration that provides a high probability of avoiding untoward complications?

(A) 1 mg/dL
(B) 6 mg/dL
(C) 11 mg/dL
(D) 16 mg/dL
(E) 21 mg/dL

**39** A 65-year-old man with a long history of coronary artery disease and recent history of myocardial infarction is seen in the emergency room with a history of sudden onset of pain in the right leg. The patient also complained of numbness in the leg. Physical examination revealed pallor of the right leg, the skin was cool to the touch, and the patient had difficulty in moving his toes. Raising his leg increased the pallor, and the dorsalis pedis pulse could not be felt. These symptoms most likely represent which of the following abnormalities?

(A) Superficial thrombophlebitis
(B) Herniation of a lumbar disk
(C) Arterial occlusion
(D) Deep venous insufficiency
(E) Hypovolemic shock

*Directions for Matching Questions (40 through 50): Each set of matching questions is preceded by a list of 4 to 26 lettered options followed by a brief explanation of the required task and then by a series of numbered statements. For each lettered statement, you are to select the ONE lettered option that best fulfills the task as it relates to that statement. Remember, each of the listed options might be correctly selected once, more than once, or not at all.*

## Questions 40 and 41

*Match each disorder with the ONE graph below that best describes the course of the disease described.*

**40** Cyclothymic disorder or depressive episodes. Cycling is often rapid.

**41** Bipolar II disorder

**42** Bipolar I disorder

## Questions 43–48

(A) Varicella-zoster virus
(B) Epstein-Barr virus
(C) *Rickettsia prowazekii*
(D) *Rickettsia rickettsii*
(E) Cytomegalovirus
(F) Herpes simplex

*Select the one infectious agent from the list above that is most likely responsible for the symptoms described in questions 43–48.*

**43** A 17-year-old high school junior has had her first sexual experience with the star quarterback football player, a senior. Four days later, she suffered from itching and tenderness in the genital area accompanied by a headache and mild fever. This itchiness rapidly progressed into pain and subsequently vesicles appeared on her external genitalia, labia majora, labia minora, and introitus. The vesicles then ruptured, leaving exquisitely tender ulcers. Her doctor told her there was no cure, but the symptoms should clear up within a month and he would write a prescription for a treatment that should help alleviate the symptoms.

**44** A 55-year-old man was hunting with his dog in Western North Carolina during late July. After the hunt, he spent some time digging ticks out from his dog's fur. A week later, he developed a severe headache, muscle pain, and loss of appetite. He then started to feel nausea with vomiting. He felt so badly, he made an appointment to see his primary care physician. By the time his doctor saw him 4 days later, he developed joint pain, abdominal pain, diarrhea, and a rash. The rash appeared as small, flat, non-itchy areas on his wrists, forearms, and ankles. The rash then spread to the palms of hands and inward toward his trunk.

45 During the interval between high school and college, an 18-year-old man spent a month at a coeducational camp where he was very active in sports and social events. Among the events he participated in were dances and various games, including spin the bottle. About 2 weeks after returning home, he began feeling unusually tired. After moping around for several days, his tiredness graduated into extreme fatigue and he developed a fever of 102.5°F (39.2°C), accompanied by a very sore throat. Worried, his mother took him to a doctor who confirmed upon examination that he had a temperature and his throat was red and raw with pus-like material at the back of his throat. He also noted that he had swollen lymph nodes in his neck. Upon palpitation of his abdomen, he also found his spleen to be slightly enlarged. After completing the examination, the doctor said that he was fairly sure what type of infection the young man has but he will run diagnostic blood work just to make sure. He added that there is no specific therapy but rest, but within about 2 weeks he should feel a lot better, although a feeling of tiredness may linger for a while longer. He also added that as long as he did not feel well, he should avoid any contact sport because his swollen spleen could rupture.

46 A 71-year-old Ethiopian immigrant woman was taken to an Emergency Facility in New York City. She was shivering, had a fever of 102.5° F (39.2°C) and pharyngitis. She complained about pain in her joints and muscles and a very severe headache. Examination showed her to have a papular rash on her legs and back. Physical and radiographic examination of her chest indicated an atypical pneumonia. Upon taking her history, she revealed that there had been a typhus epidemic in her village when she was 5–6 years old, and her parents and siblings were very sick but she only had a slight cold. The patient was treated with doxycycline, and her symptom cleared up within 10 days.

47 One morning, a 77-year-old woman woke up feeling vaguely unwell, with too little energy to get up and do anything. Later in the day, she developed a headache, and by bedtime, a low-grade fever. That night her, sleep was disturbed by an itch on the left side of her waist, and by morning, she felt an itchy, tingling, stinging, throbbing sensation interspersed with sharp stabs of an extreme, agonizing pain. Two days later, a hive-like rash appeared on her waist in the same area as the pain. The rash made a belt-like pattern in a stripe that started in the middle of her spine and extended to the left around her body to the midline of her stomach, completely confined to her left side.

48 A 20-year-old woman developed symptoms typical of mononucleosis. As confirmatory measures, her physician ordered a heterophil antibody test (a mono spot test) and a complete blood count (CBC). The result of the mono spot test was negative, and the CBC did not show reduced white cells or increased lymphocytes. Twelve days later, thinking that antibodies may not yet have had time to develop, her physician had the laboratory run another mono spot test; it too came back negative. Just to be sure she ordered an Epstein-Barr antibody test. It came back positive for both the viral capsid antigen and the nuclear antibody, indicting she had been infected with Epstein-Barr virus sometime in the past.

## Questions 49 and 50

(A) Conduct disorder

(B) Delirium

(C) Generalized anxiety disorder

(D) Obsessive-compulsive disorder

(E) Oppositional defiant disorder

(F) Panic disorder

(G) Separation anxiety disorder

(H) Social phobia

(I) Specific phobia

*Match each patient with the ONE correct associated anxiety disorder.*

49 The parents of a 4-year-old boy seek marital therapy because they have grown steadily apart since the birth of their only child. They state that they never do things together anymore. It has been years since they left their child and went out to dinner with friends or took a vacation. They have little romantic life. They tried to leave their son with a baby-sitter several times, but the child became so upset that they canceled the outing. The child sleeps in their bed every night. Occasionally, they have tried putting him in his own bed, but he cries or crawls into their bed later.

50 A 35-year-old single male librarian seeks therapy because he is lonely and unhappy. He describes a solitary life spent cataloguing books all day, then remaining alone at night and on weekends. He declines all invitations to dinners or get-togethers because he feels anxious around people. He says that he has tried to meet others but gets so uncomfortable that he goes home quickly.

# Answer Key

| | | | | |
|---|---|---|---|---|
| **1** C | **11** E | **21** E | **31** B | **41** B |
| **2** C | **12** E | **22** B | **32** A | **42** D |
| **3** D | **13** A | **23** D | **33** B | **43** F |
| **4** A | **14** B | **24** C | **34** D | **44** D |
| **5** E | **15** D | **25** E | **35** D | **45** B |
| **6** E | **16** B | **26** D | **36** A | **46** C |
| **7** C | **17** D | **27** A | **37** D | **47** A |
| **8** A | **18** A | **28** E | **38** B | **48** E |
| **9** C | **19** E | **29** D | **39** C | **49** ̶F G |
| **10** B | **20** C | **30** C | **40** C | **50** H |

# *Answers and Explanations*

**1** **The answer is C** *Preventive Medicine and Public Health*

In the case presented, the physician would first order a screening test, namely the enzyme-linked immunosorbent assay (ELISA) test (aka, enzyme immunoassay [EIA]), which is about 99.5% sensitive (i.e., it usually gives a positive value in the presence of serum samples containing the human immunodeficiency virus [HIV]). High sensitivity is the key feature required of a screening test. In the above 2 × 2 table sensitivity is mathematically defined as $a/a + c$, where $a$ = true positives (i.e., individuals with the disease who test positive) and $c$ = false negatives (i.e., individuals who have the disease who test negative). To have a high degree of sensitivity, $a$ must be much greater than $c$ (choice **C**). For example, when $c = 0$ (i.e., when there are no false-negatives [FNs]), $a/a + c = 1$ (i.e., 100% of the patients with the disease will test positive, or the test is 100% sensitive). However, this says nothing about the number of false-positives (FPs) *(b)*. If $b = 0$, there are no FPs. Although the ELISA is highly sensitive, it is not very specific. It provides a large fraction of FPs, or in terms of the 2 × 2 table, $b$ is a significant, finite number.

In testing for HIV, a positive ELISA result would typically be followed by a Western blot test. The ELISA is used as a sensitive screening test, and the Western blot test as a specific confirmatory test. A highly specific test is one that provides few FP results (i.e., one in which $b$ approaches 0). Specificity is conventionally defined in terms of the ratio $d/d + b$ (choices **B** and **D**). Thus, when $b = 0$, $d/d = 1$ (i.e., 100% of all individuals without the disease will test negative) (choice **B**). There is a limit regarding the lack of specificity that a screening test can tolerate. If $d = 0$, all individuals without the disease will test positive, and the test will have no specificity (i.e., it will be of no value). If $d = b/2$, one-half of the normal individuals will test positive; therefore, the test could possibly have value as a screening test (choice **D**).

The practical value of a screening test depends on several factors, including relative cost and the population being tested. Based on these factors, the ELISA is a practical screening test. The ELISA is easier to perform, less time-consuming, and significantly less expensive than the Western blot test. Because the ELISA has a very low specificity, it is only used when there is reason to believe that the person was exposed to the virus. In such populations, the total fraction of normals is lower; therefore, the specificity is higher. This principle carries over to all screening procedures.

Other parameters conventionally described by a 2 × 2 table include the positive predictive value, the negative predictive value, the odds ratio, and the prevalence. The *positive predictive value* is defined as the probability that a positive test result would actually be associated with a patient who has the disease. In mathematical terms, this is expressed as: $a/a + b$. Thus, as in choice **E**, where $a$ is much greater than $b$, if $b = 0$, the positive predictive value would be 100% (i.e., all cases would be true positives). *Negative predictive value* is defined as the probability that a patient who did not have the disease would test negative, or: $d/c + d$ (choice **A**). In this case, if $c = 0$, the negative predictive value would be 100%. The *odds ratio* is a measure of the probability that a positive test result would prove that the patient actually has the disease, or $a/a + c ÷ b/b + d$. Stated in words, the likelihood ratio is the true-positives (TPs) divided by all of the diseased cases, which, in turn, is divided by the FNs divided by the negatives. The likelihood of a positive test result being 100% dependable will then occur when $c = 0$ (no FNs) and when $d = 0$ (no FPs). The *prevalence* is simply a measure of the proportion of individuals with the disease in the total population. In terms of a 2 × 2 table, the negative + false-positives divided by the whole sample equals the fraction of positive cases in that particular population at that particular time. Mathematically, this is stated as $a + c/a + b + c + d$.

**2** **The answer is C** *Psychiatry*

This patient's symptoms are most suggestive of posttraumatic stress disorder (PTSD), characterized by persistent reexperiencing of traumatic events, coupled with anxiety and emotional numbing. The patient's desire to seek out other veterans with similar experiences is well advised. Peer support groups (choice **C**) permitting collective recall and discussion of traumatic experiences are often effective treatment. Although PTSD is historically associated with war veterans, it can be induced by any traumatic event, and symptoms can persist for a lifetime.

Psychodynamic therapy (choice **A**), cognitive behavioral therapy (choice **B**), as well as hypnotherapy are all acceptable means of nonpharmacologic therapy. However, in this case, the patient's expressed preferences for group therapy should take precedence. There is little to suggest that a combination of medications (e.g., clonazepam and paroxetine) (choice **D**) is useful for treating PTSD in the absence of specific symptoms of anxiety or depression, and individuals with PTSD are at higher risk for clonazepam and other benzodiazepine abuse. While meeting with citizens and veterans from the nation he fought against (choice **E**) may be helpful in the future, there is little to suggest that this would be a good initial plan or that it even would be possible to arrange.

### 3 The answer is D *Obstetrics and Gynecology*

Hepatitis B is a serious perinatal viral infection that can be vertically transmitted from mother to neonate, most often at birth. The neonate can be protected from hepatitis B by passive immunization at birth (choice **D**) using hepatitis B immune globulin (HBIG) followed by immunization thereafter. Confirmation of immunization in the infant is carried out approximately a year after birth by testing for HBsAg, anti-HBc, and anti-HBs. The hepatitis B virus is a double-stranded DNA virus that is transmitted via blood, saliva, vaginal secretions, semen, and breast milk, as well as across the placenta. Hepatitis B surface antigen (HbsAg) is the earliest marker of hepatitis B viral infection or carrier state. To clarify further, anti-HBc IgM should also be checked. It is the best marker of acute hepatitis B infection and is seen early. If this had tested positive in the mother, she has acute infection and is not a carrier of the disease. In the vignette presented, she is a carrier of the disease.

Pregnancy does not appear to accelerate acute hepatitis B in the mother (choice **A**). The main route of neonatal infection is by vaginal delivery (choice **B**). The virus also can be transmitted through breast milk (choice **C**). Neonatal infection has a higher likelihood of progression to active hepatitis than it does in the mother (choice **E**). Most pregnant women exposed to hepatitis B will become carriers with no active liver disease. However, in the neonate, the course of the infection often can be fulminant and lethal.

### 4 The answer is A *Pediatrics*

A patient with patent ductus arteriosus has a continuous machinery murmur (choice **A**). Bounding pulses with hyperactive precordium may be found on physical examination. Although the electrocardiogram (ECG) is usually not helpful, it may show left ventricular hypertrophy (LVH).

Patients with atrial septal defect (ASD) (choice **B**) have a widely split and fixed second heart sound. Patients with ventricular septal defect (VSD) (choice **C**) have a harsh holosystolic murmur heard best over the lower left sternal border. Tetralogy of Fallot (choice **E**) is characterized by the presence of a VSD, right ventricular hypertrophy, pulmonic stenosis, and overriding aorta. The murmur of tetralogy of Fallot is a long, systolic ejection murmur most audible at the midleft sternal border. In patients with pulmonic stenosis (choice **D**), there is a high-pitched systolic ejection murmur, most audible at the upper left sternal border, which transmits fairly well to the back. A systolic thrill may be present at the upper left sternal border and, rarely, in the suprasternal notch.

### 5 The answer is E *Surgery*

As a result of sustaining a spontaneous fracture of the neck of the femur, this patient is in hemorrhagic shock. Among the choices offered to account for this fracture, metastatic bone disease (choice **E**) is the most probable. Metastases in bone cause lytic lesions, thereby weakening the bone and possibly leading to a spontaneous fracture. The primary cancer may arise in any of several tissues, including breast, small-cell carcinoma of the lung, and follicular carcinoma of the thyroid. Lytic lesions are also found in multiple myeloma, which is the most common primary hematologic malignancy of bone, and in osteosarcoma, the most common primary cancer of bone. Nonmalignant diseases causing pathologic (spontaneous) fractures include bone cysts, Paget's disease of bone (in which the fractures are usually transverse and usually involve the femur or the tibia), osteogenesis imperfecta, and osteoporosis.

Chronic (not acute) osteomyelitis (choice **A**) results from acute hematogenous infection to the bone that may or may not have been treated adequately. The condition is usually quiescent for several months or even years before it flares up. The patient has fever, prostration, local inflammation, and a draining sinus. This patient had a furuncle on her thigh, not a draining sinus. Fractures are unusual in a setting of chronic osteomyelitis. Treatment is surgical, and cure is difficult. The goal is to remove the sequestrum (dead bone), which is a continual nidus for infection. Osteoporosis (choice **B**) is unlikely. Not withstanding the hot flushes that she has been experiencing recently, the patient is still premenopausal. Declining bone density in women usually commences shortly after menopause, but frank osteoporosis is rare before the age of 65. Colles' fracture, fracture of the proximal humerus, neck of the femur, and collapse of the vertebra are the most common fractures associated with osteoporosis. Only femoral neck fracture and vertebral collapse are not preceded by a history of fall. Stress fractures (choice **C**) are caused by repetitive excessive load on the bones. This can involve the second and third metatarsals (march fracture), which was initially noted in infantrymen during long marches, and femoral neck in the case of young soldiers who have to march for great distances carrying a full, heavily loaded backpack. Stress fractures can also involve the tibiae in runners, especially when they run over uneven surfaces. Physical examination usually reveals localized tenderness without deformity. A radiograph may not show the fracture, especially in the early stages. A bone scan using $^{99m}$Tc-labeled bisphosphonate will clinch the diagnosis, by demonstrating increased uptake at the site. Most stress fractures resolve with rest. Osteogenesis imperfecta (choice **D**), also known as brittle bone disease, presents itself in four forms, of varying severity. Type I is the most common form and is associated with a blue sclera 98% of the time (not blue irises, as in this woman); typically, fractures are not excessive and primarily occur prior to puberty. Type II manifests in utero or in infancy and is lethal. Type III is relatively rare; fractures abound, causing bone deformities such as scoliosis and deformed limbs and may result in dwarfism. Blue sclera is also a prominent symptom in types II and III. Type IV is similar to type I but much rarer and differs in that blue sclera are not seen. Both types I and IV are associated with childhood fractures after minimal trauma and are easily mistaken for child abuse, particularly type IV, in which blue sclera are not present. Although in both type I and IV fractures become less frequent after growth ceases, the bone structure remains less dense than normal, making then susceptible to fractures throughout life and to osteoporosis as the patients age. Types I and IV are autosomal dominant, and commonly, cases can be traced back several generations. In contrast, type II and III cases lack a family history and are either autosomal recessive conditions or new mutations.

### 6 The answer is E *Surgery*

This patient has a ruptured abdominal aortic aneurysm. The abdominal aorta is retroperitoneal. Rupture can be heralded by severe flank or back pain due to bleeding posteriorly into the retroperitoneal space. This is true in 80% of cases; however, in the remaining 20%, the aneurysm ruptures anteriorly into the peritoneal cavity. Hypotension due to blood loss and a pulsatile mass in the epigastrium are also found. Prior to rupture, patients may have a history of backache or a vague discomfort in the epigastric region. Some 95% of cases of abdominal aortic aneurysm are due to atherosclerosis (choice **E**). Other causes include Marfan syndrome, trauma, mycotic infection, and syphilis. Most aneurysms occur below the renal arteries, as the vasa vasorum are lacking here. Lack of inherent blood supply here leads to tissue hypoxia, atherosclerosis, and weakening of the aortic vessel wall. There may be associated atherosclerosis elsewhere, such as the iliacs, and coronaries.

Cystic medial degeneration (CMD, choice **A**) is involved in the pathogenesis of aortic dissections due to hypertension in elderly men or connective tissue disorders in younger individuals. CMD occurs in the middle and outer part of the aorta and is characterized by elastic tissue fragmentation and the presence of cleft-like spaces containing acid mucopolysaccharides. CMD also occurs in Ehlers-Danlos syndrome, in which there is a defect in collagen (choice **B**) and Marfan syndrome, in which there is a defect in fibrillin (choice **C**). Aortic dissections are the most common cause of death in these connective tissue disorders. An immunologic reaction (choice **D**) has been implicated in the pathogenesis of some cases of abdominal aortic aneurysms; however, it is rare.

### 7 The answer is C *Pediatrics*

Most 3-year-old children are toilet-trained, play interactive games, give their first and last names, and pedal a tricycle. At age 3 (choice **C**), most children should be able to copy a circle, and some will be able to copy a cross.

A 1-year-old child (choice **A**) would not be able to pedal a tricycle, give his first and last names, or copy a circle or a cross. At age 1, a child should be able to stand momentarily, say "dada" and "mama," and bang two cubes held in his hands. Although some 2-year-old children (choice **B**) may be able to accomplish the tasks noted in the scenario, they would not be able to hop on one foot. Most 4-year-old children (choice **D**) are able to dress without supervision, hop on one foot, and catch a bounced ball. A 5-year-old child (choice **E**) would be able to copy a triangle.

**8** **The answer is A** *Preventive Medicine and Public Health*

The perinatal mortality rate is calculated by adding the number of fetal deaths, i.e., stillbirths ($\geq$20 weeks' gestation), and the number of neonatal deaths (within first 28 days of life), then dividing that sum by the total number of births (including both live and still births):

$$\frac{(\text{Number of Fetal deaths} + \text{Number of Neonatal deaths})}{(\text{Total number of Live births} + \text{Total number of stillbirths})}$$

In the data presented, the perinatal rate is calculated as follows: 85 (stillbirths) + 15 (neonatal deaths) divided by the sum of 1,600 (live births) + 85 (stillbirths). This equals 100/1,685 (choice **A**).

Therefore, it is apparent that choices **B** (85/1,600), **C** (125/2,205), **D** (100/1,700), and **E** (59/2,205) are incorrect because these data sets do not represent the perinatal rate.

**9** **The answer is C** *Obstetrics and Gynecology*

A diagnostic cervical cone biopsy is performed only if the combination of Pap smear, colposcopy, and directed cervical biopsies cannot unequivocally rule out frankly invasive carcinoma. A cone biopsy would be in order if the cervical biopsy showed mild dysplasia (choice **C**), because the high-grade squamous intraepithelial lesion (HSIL) Pap smear suggests a more severe lesion than was identified on colposcopy.

No cone biopsy is indicated for intraepithelial neoplasia on biopsy with satisfactory colposcopy (choice **A**). Satisfactory colposcopy means the entire transformation zone (T-zone) is seen and no lesion or squamous epithelium enters the endocervical canal. A negative endocervical curettage (ECC) result with satisfactory colposcopy (choice **B**) means that the entire T-zone was seen and the ECC pathology report showed normal histologic findings. A cone biopsy is not needed if the cervical biopsy showed carcinoma in situ (choice **D**), because frankly invasive disease is ruled out. When frankly invasive carcinoma is found on cervical biopsy (choice **E**), further confirmation of invasive disease becomes superfluous.

**10** **The answer is B** *Obstetrics and Gynecology*

Infection with the human immunodeficiency virus (HIV) results in the development of the acquired immune deficiency syndrome (AIDS), which has been a recognized disease in the United States since 1981. All HIV-positive pregnant women, regardless of HIV RNA viral load and CD4 count, should be placed on triple therapy (including a protease inhibitor and Combivir) at 14 weeks and continued on it throughout pregnancy and labor. Mode of delivery is one of the most significant factors that affect maternal–neonatal transmission (choice **B**). Current recommendations are that HIV-positive women should be offered elective cesarean section at 38 weeks to minimize vertical HIV transmission. This is particularly important if the CD4 count is low and the HIV viral load is high. If the CD4 count is normal and the HIV viral load is undetectable, a cesarean may not confer much benefit to the neonate.

Pregnancy does not appear to accelerate progression of HIV to AIDS (choice **A**). Neonates can be infected from HIV-positive breastfeeding mothers (choice **C**). There is no current effective immunization for neonates (choice **D**), or for adults for that matter. Disease progression of HIV to AIDS in neonates and infants is more rapid than in adults (choice **E**).

**11** **The answer is E** *Psychiatry*

A person can be involuntarily hospitalized if he is a significant danger to himself or others. Possessing a gun and voicing suicidal intent (choice **E**) suggests such a danger.

Because self-neglect is not sufficient grounds for involuntary hospitalization unless the person is so gravely disabled that he is unable to provide for food, clothing, or shelter, and as a consequence, has an imminent and significant threat to life, neither living in a makeshift shelter (choice **A**) nor being disheveled and malnourished (choice **D**) can be legal reasons for keeping the man hospitalized against his will. Hallucinations (e.g., hearing voices [choice **C**]) or delusions (e.g., believing he or she is followed by central intelligence agency members [choice **B**]) are seen commonly in patients with schizophrenia but do not necessarily pose a significant danger to self or others or signify grave disability, as legally defined.

**12** **The answer is E** *Medicine*

This lady has Graves disease and the optometrist recognized signs of Graves' ophthalmopathy. Graves disease is a form of hyperthyroidism caused by an autoimmune reaction of unknown etiology. The core of treatment is to reduce the production of thyroid hormone by the gland. This can be done by antithyroid drugs, radioactive iodine treatment, or surgery. Usually, the first line of treatment is by drugs and in the United States either propylthiouracil (choice **E**) or methimazole is used. The problem with this lady's eyes also needed to be treated with surgery to relieve the pressure behind the eyes caused by the infiltrating exophthalmos, which causes the swollen, bulging eyes very often associated with Graves disease. It is thought that this exophthalmus is due to common antigens shared by the tissues behind the eye and the thyroid gland; as a result exophthalmus is an almost 100% specific symptom for Graves disease. It is estimated that the incidence of Graves disease is about 30–80 cases per 100,000 individuals, and it affects seven to eight females for every one male. Typically, the incidence peaks between the ages of 20–40 years. It is likely that this lady's primary health care provider did not think Graves disease because she was so far out side of the "typical" range. Had the disease not been discovered and treated it would have continued to ravage her body, possibly even leading to irreversible blindness and/or death.

A prescription of levothyroxine would be used to treat a case of hypothyroidism, not hyperthyroidism (choice **A** is incorrect). The most common cause of hypothyroidism in the United States is Hashimoto's thyroiditis; in adult women, the incidence is about 3.5 per 1,000 persons per year, and in men it is about 0.8 cases per 1,000 persons per year (but the incidence in both sexes is much higher in the Appalachian region). Like Graves disease, Hashimoto's thyroiditis is an autoimmune disease, but it causes hypothyroidism rather than hyperthyroidism; however, short intervals of hyperthyroidism may intervene, particularly at the initiation of the disease. It is usually diagnosed by the presence of signs and symptoms of hypothyroidism (such as weight gain, sluggishness, sensitivity to cold, and depression), and confirmed by measuring the thyroid-stimulating hormone (TSH) level and presence of autoantibodies against various thyroid antigens. Chronic Hashimoto's can also cause goiter. Interferons are a class of cytokines produced by many cells in response to double-stranded RNA. They may aid the immune response by inhibiting viral replication within infected cells; they may also activate natural killer cells and macrophages and facilitate antigen presentation to lymphocytes. Although interferons β 1a and β 1b have anti-autoimmune activity that has made them useful in treating multiple sclerosis they have no known function in treating Graves disease (choice **B** is incorrect). Watchful waiting is defiantly not an acceptable treatment for Graves disease; morbidity will only progress with time, perhaps even resulting in death (choice **C** is not correct). Zolpidem (choice **D**) is used to treat insomnia. Although it might be used to treat the insomnia associated with hyperthyroidism, it will not alleviate the underlying cause of her symptoms (choice **D** is incorrect).

**13** **The answer is A** *Medicine*

The triad of rapidly progressive dementia, myoclonus, and periodic complexes found on electroencephalogram (EEG) are pointers to Creutzfeldt-Jakob disease (CJD) (choice **A**). Magnetic resonance imaging (MRI) will show bilateral areas of increased signal intensity in the caudate and putamen in T2-weighted images. The disease is more common among butchers and farmers. This patient contracted it after a corneal transplant. CJD represents the most common of the prion (*prion* is short for *proteinaceous infectious particle*) diseases, also know as the transmissible spongiform encephalopathies; it is rapidly fatal. Prions are highly infectious protein particles that do not contain nucleic acids. They are extremely resistant to heat and formaldehyde. Brain biopsy is the gold standard for diagnosis. It reveals extensive vacuolation (spongiform change) within the neuropil between nerve cell bodies. Most cases of CJD are sporadic in which there is a mutation in the protease resistant protein (PrP) gene, leading to deposition of amyloid. PrP is a membrane-bound glycoprotein whose exact function is still unknown. CJD can be inherited as well.

Some cases of spongiform encephalopathies may be transmitted to humans by eating beef obtained from cows suffering from bovine spongiform encephalopathy (choice **B**), also known as "mad cow" disease. This also is a transmissible spongiform encephalopathy caused by prions. The clinical features are similar to CJD, and have been found in young individuals in Britain who consumed contaminated beef. There has been no reported case of "mad cow" disease contracted in the United States to date. Although an infected cow had wandered across the border from Canada, the beef did not make it into the U.S. market. Since this patient never left the United States, it makes him a highly unlikely candidate to contract this disease. Parkinson disease (choice **C**) is due to degeneration of neurons in the substantia nigra that synthesize dopamine, a neurotransmitter involved in voluntary muscle movement. Clinical findings include bradykinesia, cogwheel rigidity, postural instability, and resting tremors. Patients have a mask-like face, and a monotonous voice. Dementia is a late feature. Alzheimer disease (choice **D**) is the most common cause of dementia in patients older than 65 years of age. The disease is due to neuronal destruction by β-amyloid protein, which derives from amyloid precursor protein (APP). Dementia is gradual, involving impairment of memory, cognition, and thought process.

Patients show change in behavior and personality, and have difficulty with activities of daily living. Motor function is usually preserved. They often lose their way in their own home. Acetylcholinesterase inhibitors are used in the treatment of mild to moderate Alzheimer disease, together with adjunctive medications for other associated problems. Progressive multifocal leukoencephalopathy (PML) (choice **D**) is a subacute demyelinating disease, caused by a papovavirus. Destruction of oligodendrocytes leads to demyelination of the white matter. It is usually seen in immune-compromised patients, most commonly in those with human immunodeficiency virus (HIV). Seizures and focal neurologic deficits, such as hemiparesis, may be a feature.

### 14 The answer is B  *Surgery*

Roux-en-Y gastric bypass surgery removes most of the stomach, leaving only a small pouch, which is attached directly to the small intestine at the level of the jejunum, bypassing most of the stomach and the duodenum. This leaves patients vulnerable to nutritional deficiencies, since many vitamins and minerals are normally absorbed from these missing areas. To avoid deficiency states, all persons who have had gastric bypass surgery are told consume specific vitamin and mineral supplements. Studies have show that special supplements, in addition to a standard multivitamin-mineral pill are required to prevent deficiencies of iron and vitamin $B_{12}$. This patient did not take such supplements, and not too surprisingly, he demonstrated classic symptoms of $B_{12}$ (cobalamine) deficiency (choice **B** is correct). Even individuals who have not had bariatric surgery are at some risk for cobalamine deficiency because of the way it is absorbed from the gut. Initially, it must be separated from the foods to which it is usually bound; once free, it must then bind to the "intrinsic factor," a substance normally released from the parietal cells of the stomach; this normally occurs in the duodenum. This $B_{12}$ intrinsic factor complex is then absorbed in the ileum. The classic presentation of $B_{12}$ deficiency is pernicious anemia caused by a lack of intrinsic factor due to an autoimmune attack on the partial cells; similarly, in the Roux-en-Y process, the part of the stomach removed by the surgeon includes most of the partial cells; consequently, these patients will become $B_{12}$ deficient unless their diet is supplemented. Initially, it was thought this need be by intramuscular injections. However, more recently, it has been demonstrated that rather massive oral supplementation worked just as well. (The amount in a normal multivitamin pill is usually 2 mcg, but in the oral supplements used for post Roux-en-Y patients the amount used is 1,000 to 2,000 mcg). This is what this patient admits he did not take. In humans, only two reactions require a cobalamine cofactor. The first is a reaction catalyzed by homocysteine methyltransferase. When too little cobalamine is available to permit this reaction to occur, folate accumulates in the otherwise nonfunctional $N^5$-methyl form making the $N^5$-$N^{10}$-methylene and the $N^{10}$-formyl derivatives unavailable for synthesis of the nucleotides required for RNA and DNA metabolism. Consequently, in the absence of excess folate to form these derivatives, a vitamin $B_{12}$ deficiency causes a macrocytic (megaloblastic) anemia. However, if sufficient exogenous folate is available to form the $N^5$-$N^{10}$-methylene and the $N^{10}$-formyl derivatives, a vitamin $B_{12}$ deficiency does not cause an anemia. Since the multivitamin supplement used in the post Roux-en-Y gastric bypass surgery protocol supplies excess folate, this vitamin $B_{12}$ deficiency does not cause an anemia. The second reaction requiring cobalamine as a cofactor is methyl malonyl CoA mutase, a reaction required in a sequence in which fatty acids with an odd number of carbons can be converted into succinyl CoA. When this sequence is inhibited by a lack of vitamin $B_{12}$, odd-numbered fatty acids accumulate and are incorporated into the myelin sheet of nerves. This leads to demyelination and symptoms of peripheral neuropathy, such as those described for this patient. It may also cause sensory ataxia due to loss of proprioception initiated by dysfunction of the dorsal and lateral columns of the spinal cord; this leads to the stomping gait described. If not treated in time, it will also bring about malfunctions in various parts of the brain.

It may be that he also has an iron deficiency because a special iron supplement is also recommended for post-surgery patients. Since adult males require very little iron, this is most important for menstruating females; moreover, if he was iron deficient this would cause a microcytic anemia contributing to fatigue but not to the neurological problems this patient has (choice **A** is incorrect). Most post Roux-en-Y patients have higher serum folate levels after surgery than before surgery without use of a special supplements. Thus, it is unlikely that this patient suffered a folate deficiency (choice **C** is incorrect). Similarly, there is no reason to suspect either a zinc or copper deficiency (choices **D** and **E** are not correct).

### 15 The answer is D  *Psychiatry*

This man's behavior is most suggestive of transvestic fetishism (choice **D**), a paraphilia characterized by an obsession with cross-dressing for the purpose of sexual arousal.

Other paraphilias include exhibitionism (choice **A**), in which an individual exposes his genitals to others; frotteurism (choice **B**), in which an individual derives sexual pleasure by rubbing his genitals against an unsuspecting person; and voyeurism (choice **E**), in which a person secretly observes people dressing or engaging in sexual activity. Gender identity disorder (choice **C**) also involves wearing the clothes of the opposite sex, but it is not done for sexual pleasure. Individuals with gender identity disorder feel more comfortable with the opposite gender identity.

#### 16 The answer is B *Obstetrics and Gynecology*

The description of this young woman, in the beginning of her reproductive life, is characteristic of anovulation with unopposed estrogen. The expected finding would be a proliferative histologic picture; therefore, tubular endometrial glands with many mitoses (choice **B**) would be the correct finding in this case.

There will not be evidence of ovulation (serrated endometrial glands with inspissated secretions (choice **A**), since these findings are characteristic of secretory endometrium seen in the luteal phase of a normal cycle. Secretory changes are dependent on progesterone from a corpus luteum. Since she is not ovulating, there is no corpus luteum to produce progesterone. Changes consistent with endometrial carcinoma (back-to-back endometrial glands with prominent nuclei, hyperchromism, and loss of cellular polarity [choices **C** and **E**]) essentially are never seen in a pubertal girl. Even though this girl is experiencing the effects of unopposed estrogen, the progression to malignancy takes many years. Endometrial changes of pregnancy (decidual reaction forming around endometrial arterioles [choice **D**]) would not be expected with anovulation.

#### 17 The answer is D *Medicine*

This patient is suffering from cluster headaches, often striking young men in the nocturnal hours. Oxygen in a high concentration (choice **D**) is a vasoconstrictor that aborts cluster headaches.

Both nitroglycerin (choice **A**) and alcohol (choice **B**) are vasodilators and may worsen vascular headaches. Exercise (choice **C**) and a warm pack (choice **E**) may distract the sufferer, but do nothing to end the underlying cluster attacks.

#### 18 The answer is A *Obstetrics and Gynecology*

The cause of the vaginitis is *Trichomonas vaginalis*, as evidenced by the pruritic discharge and the highly motile protozoan. The elevated vaginal pH and frothy greenish discharge are frequent clinical findings with trichomoniasis. The agent of choice is metronidazole (choice **A**). Due to an Antabuse effect of this medication, she should be advised not to drink alcohol while taking it. She also needs to be informed this is a sexually transmitted disease and her sexual partners also need to be treated. Ninety percent of females are symptomatic, compared with only 50% of males.

Clotrimazole (choice **B**) and miconazole (choice **C**) are topical intravaginal antifungal agents used to treat vaginal yeast infections. Acyclovir (choice **D**) is an antiviral agent used in genital herpes management. Azithromycin (choice **E**) is an antibacterial macrolide antibiotic administered orally for the treatment of *Chlamydia*.

#### 19 The answer is E *Preventive Medicine and Public Health*

The range is the difference between the largest and smallest values; in this set it is $8 - 2 = $ **6**

The mean is equivalent to the average; that is: it is equal to the sum of all the numbers divided by the number of numbers. In this list that is: $7 + 5 + 8 + 2 + 8 / 5 = $ **6**

The median is the "middle" value in the list of numbers; i.e., it is the number equidistant in order from the lowest and highest value in a sequentially ordered set of numbers. The numbers in this question arranged sequentially are 2, 5, 7, 8, 8. The middle number is 7 because there are two numbers of lesser value and two numbers of greater value. Hence, the median is **7**. The mode, on the other hand is the most frequently occurring number, which in this set is **8**; it occurs twice. Therefore, the answer choice that correctly states the mean, median, and mode (numbers 6, 6, 7, and 8) is choice **E**.

Choices **A**, **B**, **C**, and **D** are wrong. They represent the wrong numbers and/or the proper numbers in the wrong order.

#### 20 The answer is C *Medicine*

This boy is in status epilepticus. The initial management *always* is to secure the airway (choice **C**) by clearing it and inserting an oropharyngeal airway. Ensuring that adequate ventilation (breathing) is occurring follows this, and circulation is checked thereafter—the ABCs of initial airway management.

Insertion of a tongue blade (choice **A**) in a convulsing patient does not contribute to airway management and may lacerate the tongue. A bolus of 50% dextrose (choice **B**) should be preceded by intravenous (IV) thiamine. Lorazepam followed by phenytoin (choice **D**) should be started only after IV thiamine and dextrose have been administered. In case lorazepam is unavailable, diazepam could be substituted. Lorazepam usually stops seizures. However, it should be followed by phenytoin or phosphenytoin infusion, as neither lorazepam nor diazepam alone will prevent their recurrence. If seizures continue, the patient should be intubated. Intravenous *pheno*barbital should be administered and followed by *pento*barbital for maintenance (choice **E**) (note pheno vs. pento).

### 21 The answer is E *Obstetrics and Gynecology*

The fetal presentation in this case is a frank breech (choice **E**). In frank breech, the thighs are flexed and the legs are extended. This is the only kind of breech in which vaginal delivery may be safely considered. Breech presentation occurs when the fetal buttocks or lower extremities present into the maternal pelvis, a finding in 3%–4% of deliveries. Breech presentation is more common in premature fetuses, and uterine and fetal anomalies. A major concern with vaginal delivery of fetuses in breech presentation is fetal head entrapment due to inadequate time to mold to the maternal pelvis. Trauma could result to the neck and arms with hasty delivery, and if the fetal head is hyperextended, cervical spine injury could result, with tragic consequences. For these reasons, many breech fetuses are delivered by cesarean section.

Transverse breech (choice **A**) is not a medical term, but transverse *lie* is. In complete breech (choice **B**), both thighs and knees are flexed. However, if one lower limb is extended at the hip and the knee joints instead, it is called a *footling breech*. On the other hand, in double-footling breech (choice **C**), both lower extremities are extended at the hip and the knee joints. Incomplete breech (choice **D**) occurs when one or both thighs are extended at the hip joint only and one or both knees are flexed and lie below the buttocks.

### 22 The answer is B *Pediatrics*

The patient in this question has trisomy 21, or Down syndrome, which is characterized by hypotonia, a simian crease, a short fifth finger, and upward and slanted palpebral fissures and epicanthic folds. These patients will also have differing degrees of mental and growth retardation. Duodenal atresia (choice **B**) is often associated with Down syndrome and appears in the first day of life as bilious vomiting after feedings without abdominal distention. Plain abdominal radiographs typically show the "double-bubble" sign, caused by a distended and gas-filled stomach and proximal duodenum. The initial treatment for patients with duodenal atresia is nasogastric or orogastric decompression and intravenous fluid replacement. The definitive treatment is duodenojejunostomy.

Pyloric stenosis (choice **A**) appears at 2–3 weeks of age with nonbilious vomiting. Bile-stained emesis may be seen in the later phase of intussusception (choice **C**); however, it is rare under 3 months of age. It is associated with colicky abdominal pain, a sausage-shaped mass, and currant-jelly stool. If a diaphragmatic hernia (choice **D**) presents at birth, the infant usually has a scaphoid abdomen and respiratory distress due to herniation of the abdominal contents into the chest that compresses the lungs. Bowel sounds can be auscultated in the chest, and the presence of abdominal contents in the thorax can be visualized on chest roentgenogram. A perforated viscus (choice **E**) will cause free air in the abdomen that is evident on plain abdominal radiographs as air under the diaphragm.

### 23 The answer is D *Medicine*

This patient most likely has had an infarction involving the posterolateral portion of the medulla oblongata as a result of blockage of the posterior inferior cerebellar artery (PICA) on the left side. The condition is also known as Wallenberg syndrome, which might also be caused by occlusion of the vertebral artery. The computerized tomography scan shows no evidence of hemorrhage, and therefore the diagnosis of ischemic infarction is appropriate. Since his condition has been present for less than 3 hours, it is prudent to use a thrombolytic agent (choice **D**) as the initial medication. In the thrombolytic system, plasminogen is activated into plasmin by tissue plasminogen activator (tPA); plasmin then further decreases fibrin into degraded peptides. Plasminogen activator must be administered within 3 hours of the onset of the acute event to be efficacious. It is contraindicated if the blood pressure is sustained above 185/110. No other antithrombotic treatment should be instituted for 24 hours.

Heparinization (choice **A**) followed by warfarin is appropriate in the management of a patient with a nonhemorrhagic stroke and would have been the choice had it been more than 3 hours after the onset of the acute event. Right or left carotid endarterectomy (choices **B** and **C**) are incorrect, because the problem involves the vertebral circulation. Antiplatelet agents, such as aspirin and clopidogrel (choice **E**), are not used in the initial management of infarctions. They have a role to play in the prevention of strokes.

### 24 The answer is C *Surgery*

This patient has sustained a pneumothorax in the left hemithorax secondary to trauma. A pneumothorax can occur spontaneously or secondary to trauma resulting from a blunt or penetrating injury. A pneumothorax is the presence of air trapped in the pleural space that is unavailable for gaseous exchange. Physical findings include hyperresonance to percussion (also known increased timbre) on the side of the problem (choice **C**).

The breath sounds are not increased on the left side (choice **A**) but are absent instead. Egophony (choice **B**) is usually heard in patients with a pleural effusion. It occurs rarely in patients with consolidation of the lung. It is a bronchial sound that is heard when the patient speaks during auscultation. The syllables have an odd nasal or bleating quality. The tonal change is due to compression of the lung and the air passages. The width of the intercostals will not be increased (choice **D**). Widened intercostal spaces are found in patients with chronic obstructive airway disease such as emphysema. Nor will mediastinal shift occur to the left (choice **E**). The shift in fact will occur to the right, especially if the pneumothorax is large or if a tension pneumothorax has occurred.

### 25 The answer is E *Medicine*

This patient has symptoms of digitalis toxicity in addition to cardiac failure. Digitalis toxicity leads to vomiting, increasing confusion, hallucinations, photophobia, yellow vision, and cardiac arrhythmias that could be potentially dangerous if left untreated, because supraventricular tachycardia (SVT) and atrioventricular (AV) block could supervene, or even worse, ventricular tachycardia and fibrillation. The presence of SVT and AV block signifies cardiotoxicity. Digitalis toxicity may be precipitated by hypokalemia, and therefore, the serum potassium level should be increased (choice **E**), maintaining it between 4.0 and 5.0 mmol/L. There is a strong possibility the patient is on a loop diuretic (such as furosemide), which restricts sodium and chloride reabsorption in the proximal part of the ascending loop of Henle, with resultant excretion of sodium, water, chloride, and potassium. Digitalis administration should be discontinued temporarily. The serum digitalis level does *not* correlate with digitalis toxicity.

Raising the serum sodium level will have no effect on the heart (choice **A**). Sodium has its primary effects on the brain and not the heart. Lowering serum magnesium levels (choice **C**) would aggravate the problem further, as one of the causes of digitalis toxicity is hypomagnesemia. Raising the serum calcium level (choice **D**) would be disastrous, as hypercalcemia promotes digitalis toxicity. Although hypomagnesemia could result from use of loop diuretics, this effect is less common than that of hypokalemia; therefore, raising the serum magnesium level (choice **B**) is not indicated. Other causes of digitalis toxicity include hypothyroidism, myocardial ischemia, advancing age, renal insufficiency, volume depletion, and concomitant use of drugs that delay elimination of digitalis, such as amiodarone, verapamil, β-blockers—such as carvedilol (which has been prescribed to this patient) and quinidine, a cinchona alkaloid that is used to treat cardiac arrhythmias. Although with coadministration of angiotensin-converting enzyme (ACE) inhibitors, such as enalapril, digitalis toxicity can potentially induce hyperkalemia, in the case presented, the electrocardiogram did not show evidence of hyperkalemia (peaked T waves); if it did, one would consider lowering the serum potassium level.

### 26 The answer is D *Surgery*

Fat necrosis is usually seen in stocky women with large pendulous breasts. Its importance lies in its ability to mimic breast carcinoma. A history of trauma (such as that from use of a seat belt) may or may not be present. Furthermore, a history of trauma alone is not diagnostic. Trauma on the other hand, may have drawn the attention of the patient to the lump, which is often painless. Fat necrosis usually presents as a nontender, irregular, firm breast lump with thickening of the overlying skin or retraction, giving it the classic *peau d'orange* appearance—and raising doubts about the diagnosis. The lump usually decreases in size with time. However, a residual cyst within the confines of the breast may linger on. The patient should be reassured and followed up in a few weeks (choice **D**). Although mammography may demonstrate nonspecific changes or mimic carcinoma, ultrasound will often prove useful in coming to a diagnosis. The diagnosis can be confirmed by core biopsy under ultrasound guidance, as was done in this case. Histologically, the lesion consists of lipid-laden macrophages, scar tissue, and chronic inflammatory cells. Since epithelial tissue is not involved, there is no potential for malignancy.

Excision of the mass (choice **A**) is not indicated, as the mass resolves over time. A repeat fine-needle biopsy (choice **B**) will not contribute to diagnosis in case of doubt. Should the need arise, an open biopsy would be in order. Repeating the mammography after a month (choice **C**) would not be helpful. Mastectomy (choice **E**) is totally uncalled for, and would constitute malpractice.

### 27 The answer is A  *Surgery*

The patient has acute glaucoma, which refers to a sudden increase in intraocular pressure, in which the tonometer pressures exceed 22 mm Hg (choice **A**); the normal range is between 8 and 21 mm Hg. There are two major types of glaucoma, acute and chronic. Acute, also known as closed-angle glaucoma is characterized clinically by sudden onset blurry vision, intense pain, and minimal photophobia. The patient may complain of seeing halos around light fixtures and is usually uniocular. Other findings include ciliary injection, a steamy-appearing cornea, and lack of discharge from the eye. The pupil is mid-dilated, fixed, and irregular. A shallow anterior chamber is noted on gonioscopy. Gonioscopy is useful in differentiating between open- and closed-angle glaucoma. The cup-to-disc ratio is greater than 0.6. The normal cup is one-third the size of the disc. Acute-angle closure glaucoma is less common than open-angle glaucoma. It is usually unilateral and occurs as the lens develops cataract, enlarging with age, pushing it forward into the ciliary body, narrowing the angle between the iris and the cornea, and eventually closing off the canal of Schlemm. This process is accentuated by inherited anatomic features that also cause farsightedness and by widening of the pupil in dim light, accounting for the transitory attacks noted by this patient. Dilating the pupil can also provoke this latter effect. An attack of closed-angle glaucoma is a medical emergency. Initial treatment is to lower the intraocular pressure with a β-blocker such as timolol; a carbonic anhydrase inhibitor, such as acetazolamide; and osmotic agents, such as oral isosorbide. One of the prostaglandin analogues, such as latanoprost, bimatoprost, or travoprost, is becoming increasing popular. In most cases, laser iridectomy is necessary. In this procedure, a full-thickness opening is created in the peripheral iris to allow the flow of aqueous from the posterior to the anterior chamber.

Chronic (open-angle) glaucoma is much more common and is an insidious disease with few clinical symptoms other than elevated intraocular pressure. There is a gradual progressive contraction of peripheral vision that may not be noticed at all. If left untreated, the chronic high pressure damages the optic nerve, resulting in a loss of peripheral vision that occurs so gradually that it may not be noticed until it is too late. Chronic glaucoma is a leading cause of blindness in the United States, where about 3% of the population older than 65 years is affected; this amounts to about 2 million individuals, of whom some 60,000 are legally blind. Open-angle glaucoma is eight times more common in African Americans than in other ethnicities. Other risk factors include diabetes mellitus and prolonged corticosteroid use. Intraocular pressure is lowered with medications already described for angle-closure glaucoma. Surgical intervention is carried out if medical therapy fails and consists of laser trabeculoplasty or filtering surgery.

Blood in the anterior chamber (choice **B**) is called a hyphema and is associated with acute visual loss. The most common cause is ocular trauma. The presence of a hyphema in a small child should always be considered to be secondary to child abuse until proved otherwise. African American children who present with hyphema should be screened for sickle cell disease or trait. Corneal abrasions (choice **C**) produce blurry vision, pain, moderate photophobia, watery discharge, mild to moderate conjunctival injection, a hazy cornea, a positive fluorescein stain, a normal or constricted pupil, a poor to normal pupillary light reflex, and normal intraocular pressure. Papilledema (choice **D**) refers to swelling of the optic disc due to increased intracranial pressure. Patients with papilledema present with venous stasis, prominent disc vessels, a swollen disc with blurred margins, and absence of the physiologic cup. Bloodless arterioles and a cherry-red fovea (choice **E**) characterize a central retinal artery occlusion.

### 28 The answer is E  *Medicine*

This patient has a lower motor neuron lesion (choice **E**) affecting cranial nerve VII—the facial nerve (CN VII) on the right side—and is also known as Bell's palsy. Facial palsy is the most common of the cranial neuropathies. Most cases are due to infection with herpes simplex virus and are not idiopathic, as was believed earlier. The facial nerve innervates the muscles of the face and the stapedius muscle in the ear and conveys taste fibers to the anterior two-thirds of the tongue, via the chorda tympani nerve. The roaring in the ear (hyperacusis) and lack of taste in the anterior portion of the tongue are due to involvement of the aforementioned innervation. The problem with speech is due to dysarthria, resulting from paralysis of the muscles around the mouth. The inability to close his eye can put his cornea, and indeed the eye, in danger. Hence, the eyelid should be taped shut or covered with an eye patch. The facial nerve also supplies the lacrimal gland; absence of tears could result in xerophthalmia (corneal drying) and attendant complications, hence artificial tears are necessary. Corticosteroids are helpful. The disorder usually resolves over time. Other causes of lower motor neuron facial paralysis include lesions in the brainstem, cerebellopontine angle, middle ear infection, multiple sclerosis, human immunodeficiency virus (HIV) infection, Lyme disease, parotid tumor tumors, diabetes mellitus, and trauma to the facial nerve.

An upper motor neuron (choice **A**) lesion of the facial nerve will spare the upper half of the face because of the bilateral innervation to that region. An upper motor neuron VII nerve paralysis is due to involvement of the contralateral motor neurons of the descending corticobulbar pathway or of the pathway used en route to the seventh cranial nerve nucleus in the pons. A brainstem glioma (choice **B**) is unlikely, given the sudden nature of the event, lack of symptoms such as headache, nausea and vomiting, and bulbar signs involving the lower cranial nerves. These patients could have ataxia as well. A left middle cerebral artery embolus (choice **C**) could very well occur given his history of atrial fibrillation. However, embolism involving the middle cerebral artery would be associated with headache, confusion, right hemiparesis or hemiplegia, and an upper motor neuron facial paralysis on the right as well. Hemorrhage into the internal capsule (choice **D**) could occur, given the history of hypertension in this patient. However, the patient would have severe headache, obtundation, and a dense right hemiplegia, together with a right upper motor neuron facial nerve paralysis.

### 29 The answer is D  *Medicine*

Rapid (but temporary) control of arrhythmia follows achievement of a therapeutic blood level of lidocaine. The temporary nature occurs because lidocaine rapidly redistributes from blood to other tissues (choice **D**). In this situation, the reappearance of the arrhythmia reflects the rapid distribution of lidocaine from the blood to highly perfused body tissues, resulting in a decrease in plasma concentration of the drug below therapeutic levels. A similar process, involving redistribution of thiopental from the brain to other highly perfused tissues, is responsible for termination of the anesthetic effects of the intravenous (IV) barbiturate.

Although the liver metabolizes lidocaine extensively, the elimination half-life of the drug is 1–2 hours (not 2 minutes [choice **C**]), which cannot account for such a rapid reappearance of the arrhythmia (choice **A**). While the blood levels following IV administration of lidocaine may be variable, this is due to redistribution processes and not to errors in laboratory determination of drug levels (choice **B**). There is no evidence that cardiac cells are capable of rapid (and reversible) changes in sensitivity to any antiarrhythmic drug (choice **E**). Conversely, the lidocaine level may be increased in patients taking cimetidine, and the dosage needs to be reduced in patients with congestive cardiac failure or liver disease.

### 30 The answer is C  *Preventive Medicine and Public Health*

Most recessive diseases (e.g., cystic fibrosis) will present in isolated individuals. When two carriers of a recessive disease have children, those children will have a 25% chance of expressing the disease (choice **C**).

Although new mutations (choice **A**) are a possibility, most often it will turn out that both parents are carriers. It is only in families with many siblings and/or cases with obvious consanguinity that recessive inheritance can be clearly identified on the basis of family relationships alone. As long as outbreeding predominates in a family, the chances of a recessive disease being expressed are remote, largely depending on the incidence in the general population. The recessive gene will be carried from generation to generation, only becoming evident when it shares an allelic site with a second mutated gene. That is, excluding a new mutation, there is zero chance of a recessive disease being expressed if a normal individual mates with a carrier. *Penetrance* is a term primarily used in conjunction with dominant disorders and is a measure of the chance of such a disorder not being expressed clinically (choice **B**). There is often variability in dominant disorders because dominant disease most often involves proteins having a structural function, as opposed to recessive disorders, which most often involve an enzyme. Thus, you can analogize a dominant genetic defect to a house in which every other normal 2 × 4 stud is replaced by a 1 × 2 stud. Externally, the two may be indistinguishable, until an environmental stress is applied. Currently, it is often easy to identify carriers by simple biochemical techniques. However, there is no simple physiologic method available permitting the identification of carriers of cystic fibrosis (choice **D**). Even analysis involving DNA fingerprinting (choice **E**) is complicated by the fact that more than 400 different mutations in the cystic fibrosis gene have been identified; that is, it is not caused by a unique mutation.

## 31 The answer is B *Medicine*

This patient has had a possible hemorrhagic stroke involving the right cerebral hemisphere. This is likely due to the history of treatment with warfarin. The initial investigation is a noncontrast computed tomography (CT) scan of the brain (choice **B**) to establish whether the problem was due to a hemorrhage or an infarct. If it were an infarct, management would include anticoagulants. On the other hand, administering anticoagulants to a patient who has a cerebral hemorrhage would be disastrous.

A magnetic resonance imaging (MRI) scan (choice **A**), although helpful, is less sensitive for acute bleeding, takes longer, and is less likely to be available on an emergent basis. The electroencephalogram (EEG) (choice **C**) would be expected to show focal slowing on the right; however, it cannot differentiate between an ischemic and a hemorrhagic stroke. Carotid duplex ultrasonography (choice **D**) would be useful to determine if the source of an embolus was a plaque within the carotid artery. Since 80% of emboli are cardiac in origin, an echocardiogram would be an appropriate initial investigation in such an event. Neither carotid duplex ultrasonography nor echocardiography can distinguish between cerebral ischemic and hemorrhagic stroke. They can only support the diagnosis of ischemic stroke based on CT scan findings in the brain. Finally, a spinal tap (choice **E**) is not helpful in differentiating an ischemic from a hemorrhagic stroke and places an anticoagulated patient at risk for a developing a spinal epidural hematoma with subsequent spinal cord compression. Worse still, if a spinal tap was inadvertently carried out in the presence of raised intracranial pressure, tonsillar herniation and death could ensue.

## 32 The answer is A *Obstetrics and Gynecology*

The group B β-hemolytic streptococcus (GBS) neonatal attack rate is only 1–2 cases per thousand women with a positive vaginal culture (choice **A**); most women with a positive vaginal culture will have uninfected infants. However, GBS still has the potential for significant adverse impact on the fetus, neonate, or both, because if neonatal sepsis does occur, the mortality rate approaches 50%. This is why screening for GBS is now recommended by the Centers for Disease Control and Prevention (CDC) for all women at 36 weeks' gestation, with intrapartum penicillin prophylaxis if culture positive.

Even though most infants born to women with a positive GBS culture are not infected, a negative culture does not rule out the presence of the organism at the time of delivery because most GBS carriers harbor the bacterium only intermittently or transiently (choice **B**). Treating carriers is ineffective for eradicating the organism (choice **C**). Up to 30% of women of reproductive age will have colonization with GBS; the organism is part of normal female genital tract flora (choice **D**). Current nonculture assay tests are specific but not very sensitive (choice **E**). The diagnostic modality of choice is a culture.

## 33 The answer is B *Pediatrics*

External otitis, or "swimmer's ear," is caused by excessive moisture in the ear canal, which causes the loss of protective cerumen leading to chronic irritation. However, cerumen impaction with trapping of water can also cause infection. The patient presents with ear pain that is worsened by manipulation of the pinna. The ear canal is erythematous and edematous. Otorrhea may be seen. *Pseudomonas aeruginosa* (choice **B**) is the most commonly isolated bacterium in external otitis. Other organisms include *Enterobacter aerogenes*, *Proteus mirabilis*, coagulase-negative staphylococci, *Klebsiella pneumoniae*, streptococci, *Staphylococcus aureus*, diphtheroids, and fungi.

Both *Haemophilus influenzae* (choice **A**) and *Moraxella catarrhalis* (choice **C**) cause otitis media, but not as often as *Streptococcus pneumoniae*. *Streptococcus agalactiae* (choice **D**) has been isolated from middle ear fluid in neonates with otitis media. However, both *S. agalactiae* and *Escherichia coli* (choice **E**) are leading causes of sepsis and meningitis in neonates.

## 34 The answer is D *Medicine*

Ventricular tachycardia (choice **D**) is defined as three or more beats of ventricular origin that occur in succession, at a rate in excess of 100/min, usually between 120 and 220/min. The rhythm may be regular or irregular. P waves may be present, with no fixed relationship to the QRS complexes, or absent, depending on the ventricular rate. The width of the QRS is 0.12 second or above, and the morphology is bizarre, with notching frequently present. This patient's ventricular rate is approximately 150/min, and the rhythm is slightly irregular. A burst of seven consecutive wide complexes follows a normal sinus rhythm and ends with a premature ventricular complex coupled to a sinus complex. The configuration of the premature complex is similar to that of the tachycardia complexes, so this configuration represents a ventricular tachycardia. When prompt therapy is indicated, lidocaine is the treatment of choice.

Premature atrial contractions (choice **A**) originate in the atria outside of the sinus node. The rhythm is irregular because ventricular activation may not occur (nonconduction), resulting in a pause in the cardiac rhythm. Atrial flutter (choice **B**) is a regular atrial rhythm that results from reentry at the atrial level. The atrial rate varies from 220 to 350/min, whereas the ventricular rate varies from 150 to 175/min, indicating atrioventricular (AV) conduction ratios ranging from 2:1 to 4:1. The atrial waves have a "sawtooth" or "picket fence" configuration. Paroxysmal (supraventricular) tachycardia (choice **C**) has a regular atrial rate of 160–220/min and a similar ventricular rate if the atrial rate is below 200/min (AV conduction ratio of 1:1). The atrial rhythm is usually regular. P waves are frequently difficult to identify; but when present, they may have different contours than sinus P waves. The P-R and QRS intervals are variable. The QRS complexes are of normal configuration. Carotid sinus massage or the Valsalva maneuver (patients hold their breath) is frequently used to convert paroxysmal tachycardia to normal sinus rhythm. Sinus tachycardia (choice **E**) is caused by an increased rate of discharge from the sinus node. The rate is regular and exceeds 100/min. Each QRS is preceded by an upright P wave in leads I and II, and a Vr.

### 35 The answer is D *Surgery*

Heparin blocks the intrinsic pathway of the coagulation cascade, and its activity can be measured by determining the activated partial thromboplastin time (aPTT) (choice **D**). The intrinsic system begins with the conversion of factor XII to an active enzyme called XIIa once it has come into contact with negatively charged surfaces. In addition to monitoring adequacy of heparinization, aPTT is used to monitor replacement therapy in hemophilia A and B. The therapeutic range for aPTT is 1.5–2.5 times the reference range.

The prothrombin time (PT) (choice **B**) blocks the extrinsic pathway (e.g., after oral anticoagulation). The extrinsic portion of the coagulation cascade is initiated by the interaction between factor VII and tissue factor. The PT is normal in patients who are on heparin alone, because heparin acts on the intrinsic pathway. Thrombin time (TT) (choice **A**) is used to screen for abnormalities of fibrinogen. It measures conversion of fibrinogen to fibrin by thrombin. This is accomplished by polymerization of fibrin polymers to a fibrin gel. TT does not measure fibrinolysis or stabilization of fibrin. The most common cause of prolongation of TT is heparin; however, prolongation can also occur in uremia and defects in fibrin (e.g., dysfibrinogenemia, hypofibrinogenemia). Thus, although heparin prolongs TT, it is not used as a test to monitor heparin therapy. The fact that the TT is not due to heparin can be determined by blocking its action with protamine sulfate or, even better, measuring the reptilase time. Reptilase time is most commonly used to determine the cause of prolonged TT. Reptilase is an enzyme obtained from the venom of a reptile, *Bothrops atrox*, which clots human fibrinogen. Prothrombin and proconvertin test (choice **C**), an assay of prothrombin (factor II) and proconvertin (factor VII), is actually a modified PT in which factor V and fibrinogen are added to it. Thus, the assay is sensitive to defects in factors II, VII, and X. It can be used to monitor oral anticoagulant therapy, not heparin therapy. The test is usually reported in terms of percentage of activity based on a series of normal plasmas diluted with normal saline. This test is no longer used, because it has no advantage over the PT or the international normalized ratio (INR). Furthermore, results from prothrombin and proconvertin tests cannot be converted to INR values. Bleeding time (choice **E**) measures the interaction between platelets and the vessel wall. Defects in platelets or a defect in the vessel wall will result in a prolonged bleeding time. It is the most commonly used test to measure in vivo platelet function. The most common cause for prolonged bleeding time is drug therapy, especially aspirin. Patients with von Willebrand disease also have prolonged bleeding time due to a deficiency or abnormality in von Willebrand's factor. Von Willebrand disease is the most common hereditary bleeding disorder.

### 36 The answer is A *Psychiatry*

Maintenance therapy after response to antidepressants should generally be continued at an effective dose for 6 months after initial response (choice **A**).

Quick relapse is more likely if antidepressants are tapered (choice **C**) or stopped earlier (choice **D**). Some studies suggest much longer treatment after recovery from a depressive episode (choice **B**) if the patient has a history of multiple relapses, but not for a single episode. Therapy should not be switched to fluoxetine (choice **E**) another selective serotonin reuptake inhibitor (SSRI), since sertraline has been effective and shows no untoward adverse effects.

**37 The answer is D** *Medicine*

This patient is in the early stages of metabolic syndrome and increases insulin resistance, which, when fully developed, is characterized by type 2 diabetes, dyslipidemia, hypertension, and obesity. Although only tested once, at this time, it is highly probable that he is in a prediabetic state, which is defined as having fasting plasma glucose levels between 100 and 126 mg/dL on two consecutive days. His fasting total cholesterol (TC) level is also in the borderline high range. (For TC, the normal value is defined as equal to or less than 200 mg/dL [5.2 mmol/L], borderline is between 200 and 240 mg/dL [5.2–6.2 mmol/L], and elevated as equal to, or greater than 240 mg/dL [6.2 mmol/L]. Whereas the new American Heart Association definitions for LDL levels are: optimal less than 100 mg/dL [2.5 mmol/L], near optimal 100–129 mg/dL [2.5–3.3 mmol/L], borderline high 130–159 mg/dL [3.4–4.0 mmol/L], high value 160–189 mg/dL [4.1–4.8 mmol/L], and very high 190 mg/dL [4.8 mmol/L] and above.) In addition, he is definitely hypertensive (systolic/diastolic values reported as mm Hg are defined as normal, <120/80; prehypertension, 120/80 to 139/89; stage 1 hypertension, 140/90 to 159/99; and stage 2 hypertension, ≥160/100). In summary, he is well on his way to becoming a full-blown diabetic, with a high blood glucose level as well as high LDL and total cholesterol levels, and also is liable soon to be a stage 2 hypertensive and a candidate for severe coronary artery disease (CAD). The primary driving force for these conditions is his obesity, created by his lifestyle. His body mass index (BMI) is 30.2 kg/m$^2$, calculated using the following formula: BMI = weight in kg divided by height in meters squared, where 1 kg = 2.2046 lb, and 1 m = 39.37 inches. A BMI between 25 and 29.9 kg/m$^2$ is defined as overweight, and 30 kg/m$^2$ or greater as obese. The first step in managing obesity in this patient is to get him off his couch and moving about. Taking his wife out dancing at least twice a week (choice **D**), while not a solution in itself, would be a step in the right direction, and it might be easier to persuade this obviously recalcitrant man to do this, which may also please his wife, than to initially recommend the more stringent dietary and exercise regimes that will be required. In the interim, it also may be possible to persuade him to return to treat his hypertension and incidentally better deal with his lifestyle issues, including the possibility of depression.

Gastroplasty (choice **A**) will cause him to lose weight. However, it requires surgery and has concomitant short- and long-term risks. As a consequence, it should be reserved only for the morbidly obese. Although short-term weight loss is enhanced by the prescription of an anorexic drug (choice **B**), patients taking such agents usually end up even heavier than before they started treatment because of a rebound effect. Management in this case clearly entails a lifestyle change, which may require long-term treatment and a great deal of patience. One would prescribe gemfibrozil (choice **C**) as a way to lower triglyceride levels only after they were acutely high and more conservative measures failed. A dietary supplement containing ephedra (choice **E**) would not be a wise move since several studies have shown that it can cause serious reactions including hypertension, which certainly would not be recommended in this case. Ephedra (also known as ma huang) contains the chemical ephedrine, which was used as an asthma medication until the 1980s, when it was taken off the market because of its dangerous effects on the heart and blood pressure. Tolbutamide is a first-generation sulfonylurea, an oral hypoglycemic agent. Not only are more effective agents available, but also tolbutamide, like all sulfonylureas, runs the risk of inducing hypoglycemia and promotes weight gain. Thus, the physician would not likely prescribe tolbutamide (choice **F**). Until recently, prediabetes would only be treated by lifestyle changes, diet, and exercise. However, it now is deemed acceptable to be more aggressive and prescribe an oral hypoglycemic agent. Metformin is often recommended because it neither causes hypoglycemia nor promotes weight gain.

**38 The answer is B** *Pediatrics*

Phenylketonuria (PKU) is caused by a deficiency in phenylalanine hydroxylase, which has a prevalence of 1 case per 11,000 births. The normal pathway is disrupted, so phenylalanine and other metabolites accumulate and cause brain damage. Clinically, affected infants are blond, with fair skin and blue eyes. A mild eczematous rash disappears with age. Vomiting can be confused with pyloric stenosis. Mental retardation is usually severe. The infants have a musty, mousey odor of phenylacetic acid. Screening is recommended after 72 hours of age and after feeding of proteins. Early institution of a diet low in phenylalanine is essential in preventing brain damage. Women who have PKU and want to have children should go on a low-phenylalanine diet before conception and throughout pregnancy to reduce the risk of spontaneous abortion and birth defects. The blood phenylalanine levels should be kept below 6 mg/dL throughout pregnancy (choice **B**).

Pregnant women with PKU and phenylalanine levels above 6 mg/dL (choices **C**, **D**, and **E**) have a higher risk of spontaneous abortions. Infants born to such mothers may have mental retardation, microcephaly, and/or a congenital heart anomaly. Blood levels of 1 mg/dL (choice **A**) are below the risk level but are not the highest safe level.

### 39 The answer is C *Surgery*

The patient has an acute arterial occlusion (choice **C**), which is associated with the six P's—**P**ain, **P**allor, **P**aresthesias, **P**aralysis, **P**oikilothermia, and **P**ulseless (absence of pulse). The most likely cause is an embolus, but trauma could also be responsible. In an embolic arterial occlusion, there is no antecedent history of claudication pain. Emboli can spring from a recent myocardial infarct, mitral stenosis, artificial heart valve, or an aortic aneurysm. The condition occurs suddenly. The limb is cold to touch, and loss of motor function generally ensues within hours after onset of pain. For this reason, embolic arterial occlusion is an emergency. The first loss of function is the inability to move the toes. (In the case of venous occlusion, on the other hand, motor function is not lost.) Heparinization followed by embolectomy and thrombectomy is the preferred treatment. The popliteal artery is the most susceptible vessel for occlusion because it is commonly affected by atherosclerosis and is a small-caliber artery.

Superficial thrombophlebitis (choice **A**) in the saphenous system of the legs presents with pain and tenderness along the course of the vessel. A herniated disk (choice **B**) would not be expected to involve the whole leg, nor would it present with the given symptom/sign complex. A history of back pain followed by pain going down the leg (radicular pain) would be usual. Findings would include hypesthesia along the lateral or inner aspect of the leg, depending on which intervertebral disk has herniated, and weakness of the plantar or dorsiflexors of the foot. Sciatic stretch sign would be positive, and the deep tendon jerks may or may not be affected, depending on the level of herniation. The pulses will be normal, and skin temperature would be normal. Deep venous insufficiency (choice **D**) is associated with superficial varicose veins and stasis dermatitis around the ankle. Hypovolemic shock (choice **E**) produces hypotension, generalized pallor, and cold, clammy skin.

### 40 The answer is C *Psychiatry*

The clinical course of cyclothymic disorder (graph **C**) is characterized by numerous periods of hypomanic symptoms and numerous periods of depressive symptoms. During none of these episodes do patients have full manic or depressive episodes. Cycling is often rapid.

### 41 The answer is B *Psychiatry*

The clinical course of bipolar II disorder (graph **B**) is characterized by depressive episodes and one or more hypomanic episodes.

### 42 The answer is D *Psychiatry*

Bipolar I disorder (graph **D**) includes both manic and depressive episodes

Graph **A** represents the clinical course of major depressive disorder, recurrent type. Graph **E** represents the clinical course of dysthymic disorder.

### 43 The answer is F *Medicine*

This unfortunate young woman contracted a genital herpes simplex infection (choice **F**). Presently, eight different DNA herpes virus strains are recognized, five of which bear the name herpes simplex virus (HSV); these are HSV1, HSV2, HSV6, HSV7, and HSV8. HSV 6 causes exanthema subitum (aka, roseola infantum or sixth disease) in infants, and in adults, is associated with immune-compromised conditions, such as acquired immune deficiency syndrome (AIDS). HSV 7 is a T-cell lymphotrophic virus, and HSV 8 is associated with Kaposi's sarcoma in AIDS patients. Both HSV 1 and 2 cause outbreaks of blisters and ulcers: HSV 1 primarily around the mouth and oral cavity, and HSV 2 primarily in the genital region. Both of these viruses are spread by physical contact, and both tend to retreat into sensory dorsal root ganglia, causing a remission of symptoms; these latent infections tend to flare up and cause symptoms to reappear at intervals, usually in times of stress. Such recurrences are usually milder, cause fewer lesions, and tend to heal faster than the initial ones. Transmission of the disease is most effective during such outbreaks, but viral shedding and infectivity can happen during asymptomatic periods. About 80% of the adult population contracted oral HSV 1 infections as children, and about 30% of these have observable recurrent symptoms, which generally are mild; however, occasionally optical or other complication will arise. Although oral infections with the HSV 2 virus are still uncommon, the prevalence has been increasing during the past few decades because of changing sexual behaviors. The prevalence of genital herpes has also been increasing, and at least 80% of these cases are due to infection by HSV 2. Nationwide, about 25% of females and 20% of males over the age of 12 are infected. It is hypothesized that more females are affected than males because the transmission from males to females is more efficient than from females to males. About half of the seropositive individuals show few or no symptoms but still may transmit the disease, and about 1 neonate in 3,500–5,000 births has an HSV 2 infection that was transmitted to the fetus during delivery; such infections can cause serious morbidity and even death of the newborn.

### 44 The answer is D *Medicine*

This hunter suffers from Rocky Mountain spotted fever, a disease caused by *Rickettsia rickettsii* (choice **D**) and transmitted to humans by the bite of an ixodid tick. Cases are most frequently reported during the mid-summer months when the ticks flourish, and although cases occur in almost all the contiguous states they are more common in the Carolinas and Oklahoma than in the Rocky Mountain States. Infected patients generally visit a physician when they first feel ill from nonspecific symptoms after an incubation period of 5–10 days. However, a diagnosis cannot generally be made until later signs and symptoms appear; knowledge of a tick bite is often the earliest factor leading to suspicion of the disease. Rocky Mountain spotted fever remains a serious and potentially life-threatening condition. Prior to the advent of antibiotics, the mortality rate was close to 30%, and still today, despite the availability of effective treatment, approximately 3% to 5% of individuals who become ill die from the infection. Survivors, particularly those recovering from severe, life-threatening disease, may have long-term complications including partial paralysis of the lower extremities, gangrene requiring amputations, hearing loss, loss of bowel or bladder control, movement disorders, and language disorders.

### 45 The answer is B *Medicine*

This young man contracted a case of mononucleosis caused by infection with Epstein-Barr virus (choice **B**). EBV is one of the eight known herpes viruses and is essentially ubiquitous in the American population. More than half the population is infected in infancy and early childhood, and by the age of 35–40 years, at least 95% of the population test serologically positive for EBV antibodies. Infection in childhood is usually symptomless and goes unnoticed, but infection in adolescents and young adults induces symptoms of mononucleosis 35%–50% of the time; however, even among diagnosed cases, a wide range of symptoms is expressed, the case described having most of them. More extreme problems involving the heart or central nervous system can arise, but these are extremely rare. Although symptoms almost always resolve within 2 months at most, EBV behaves like other herpes viruses in that it remains dormant only to resurface on occasion. The dormant EBV resides in the back of the throat and causes no symptoms on reactivation but makes the carrier infective. According to the Centers for Disease Control (CDC), the only mode of infection is by contact with saliva, leading to mononucleosis' nickname "the kissing disease"; however, clearly, there are other ways to catch this disease. EBV has long been a suspected cause of chronic fatigue syndrome, but this has never been proven and the contemporary consensus is that it most likely is not. EBV also has some sort of ill-defined relationship with several neoplasms, in particular with Burkitt's lymphoma and nasopharyngeal carcinoma; in fact Epstein and Barr first isolated it from Burkitt's lymphoma.

### 46 The answer is C *Medicine*

This lady had Brill-Zinsser disease, which is a recurrent form of epidemic typhus cause by infection with *Rickettsia prowazekii* (choice **C**). It may appear many years after an initial infection caused by feces from a human body louse: the louse's bite itches, the affected person scratches, and the rickettsial laden feces penetrate the skin. The symptoms of Brill-Zinsser disease are similar to those of a primary *R. prowazekii* infection but milder, and death almost never occurs. There are several different but related diseases that bear the name typhus. *Epidemic typhus* produces the most severe symptoms and is the classic disease that raises its ugly head whenever war, natural diasters, or other conditions arise that force humans together under crowded unsanitary conditions. Presently, it rarely occurs in the United States, except for a few cases annually spread by an unknown vector that passes the organism to humans from infected "flying squirrels," and in an attenuated form as Brill-Zinsser disease carried in immigrants exposed years earlier. Other forms of typhus in the United States are *murine typhus*, caused by infection with *Rickettsia typhi*, in which the rat flea is a vector, and *cat-flea typhus*, caused by infection with *Rickettsia felis*. Both have symptoms less severe than epidemic typhus and are endemic with low frequency in the United States. A third form of typhus is *scrub typhus*, an acute, febrile, infectious illness caused by *Orientia tsutsugamushi*; this organism was originally classified as a *Rickettsia* because, like the *Rickettsia*, it is an obligate intracellular gram-negative bacterium and it causes a rickettsial-like disease; because recent DNA studies have shown it to be genetically different from the Rickettsia, it has been reclassified. Humans are accidental hosts in this disease, which is essentially unknown outside of Asia.

### 47 The answer is A  *Medicine*

Varicella-zoster virus is one of the eight herpes viruses and is also known as herpes zoster virus. It causes chickenpox in children and shingles and postherpetic neuralgia in adults. The case describes shingles (choice **A** is correct). As an episode of chickenpox resolves, the virus retreats into the nerve cell bodies of the dorsal root, cranial nerve, or autonomic ganglion, where it lies dormant until the infected individual becomes immune-compromised in some way, such as by older age, disease, or immune-inhibiting drugs. In such persons, the virus becomes activated, migrates along the nerve axons to cause symptoms along the path of the nerve and perhaps its branches in the corresponding dermatome; these symptoms characterize the condition called shingles. Approximately half of patients with zoster or postherpetic neuralgia describe their pain as "horrible" or "excruciating," ranging in duration from a few minutes to constant on a daily or almost daily basis; in addition, ophthalmic or other complications can also occur. The antiviral oral drugs acyclovir, valacyclovir, or famciclovir administered within 72 hours after the first appearance of the rash can help to alleviate these symptoms. The rash usually heals within 2–4 weeks, but nerve pain sometimes lingers on for months or even years; the patient then has postherpetic neuralgia. The incidence rate for shingles for individuals older than 65 years has been estimated to be as high as 12 cases per 1,000 individuals annually. Persons who have not had chickenpox can get this disease by contacting the rash before it crusts. Individuals vaccinated against chickenpox apparently can develop shingles even though they never developed symptoms of chickenpox; however the symptoms associated with the shingles seem to be milder than if they were infected with the native virus; however, it should be cautioned that few data are available since the chickenpox vaccine introduced in 1995 was not available to those older individuals most susceptible to developing shingles. On May 25, 2006, the U.S. Food and Drug Administration licensed an anti-zoster vaccine that is now recommended for use in person's aged 60 or more. This vaccine losses efficacy in older patients but even if it does not prevent an attack of shingles it does reduce symptoms and the incidence of severe postherpetic neuralgia.

### 48 The answer is E  *Medicine*

Cytomegalovirus infection is very common. It is estimated that 50%–85% of the U.S. adult population had been infected with cytomegalovirus, a member of the herpes virus family, sometime during development, typically in early childhood. As a rule, such early infection causes few if any symptoms in young children. Older children, teens, and adults who become infected for the first time typically develop mononucleosis-like symptoms, including fatigue, muscle aches, headache, fever, and enlarged liver. Since mononucleosis has been ruled out as the cause of the symptoms in the patient described, it is very likely that her symptoms are caused by a recent cytomegalovirus infection (choice **E**). This virus can also lie dormant after an early infection only to become reactivated later in life if an infected person becomes immunocompromised.

### 49 The answer is J  *Psychiatry*

The symptoms are most suggestive of separation anxiety disorder (choice **J**), a condition characterized by fear of separation from caregivers. It can manifest itself as worry about separation, severe protest over separation, or severe anxiety after separation. Often, the presenting complaint involves marital problems caused by these behaviors. Behavioral therapies are often effective for the child. Treatment also involves parent education and therapy to resolve potential ambivalence about allowing the child more independence.

### 50 The answer is H  *Psychiatry*

The symptoms are most suggestive of social phobia (choice **H**), characterized by fear and avoidance of social situations. Individuals with this disorder tend to be solitary and reclusive. Their presenting complaint is often depression and loneliness. Treatment often includes cognitive-behavioral techniques such as assertiveness training in which social interactions are rehearsed.

## REMAINING INCORRECT CHOICES

Pervasive anxiety in many situations would suggest generalized anxiety disorder (choice **C**). Anxiety after severe emotional trauma, objects (e.g., animals), or situations (other than social situations), would suggest specific phobia (choice **I**). Other disorders associated with childhood behavioral problems are conduct disorder (choice **A**), in which major age-appropriate societal norms are violated, and oppositional defiant disorder (choice **E**), which is characterized by defiance of authority. Delirium (choice **B**), characterized by acute and severe cognitive disturbances, may be associated with anxiety.

Many disorders associated with anxiety are not limited to social situations. In panic disorder (choice **F**), attacks of anxiety occur without obvious triggers. Obsessive-compulsive disorder (choice **D**) is often associated with anxiety about the obsessive thoughts or anxiety when the compulsions are resisted.

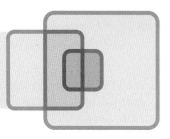

# test 3

# Questions

**Single Best Choice Directions:** *This section consists of numbered statements or questions followed by a list of potential answers; you are to select the ONE best answer.*

**1** A 48-year-old female type 2 diabetic with mild hypertension presents with a 6-week history of tiredness that has come on gradually; there even are days when she feels that there is no point in getting up in the morning. She has been turning up late for work, and her supervisor has "written her up" for tardiness. In addition, she states that her clothes have become tighter, that she has difficulty getting into her shoes, and that her voice seems hoarse. For the past few days, she also has noticed pain in the right wrist, especially when she uses the computer. She constantly fights with her husband, saying that the bedroom is cold at night, and insists on using several blankets. Her only medications are metformin for diabetes and hydrochlorothiazide for hypertension. Her vital signs are as follows: blood pressure, 130/90 mm Hg; pulse 60/min regular; respirations, 16/min; and a body temperature of 36.50°C (97.70°F). She has rather coarse features, her face and eyelids are puffy, and pretibial nonpitting edema is present. Examination of her neck reveals a diffuse nontender enlargement in the anterior region that moves with swallowing. No other abnormality is noted. Which of the following set of laboratory test values best supports the proper diagnosis?

| | Total Serum $T_4$ | Free Serum $T_4$ | Serum TSH |
|---|---|---|---|
| (A) | ↑ | Normal | Normal |
| (B) | ↑ | ↑ | ↓ |
| (C) | ↓ | Normal | Normal |
| (D) | ↓ | ↓ | ↑ |
| (E) | ↓ | ↓ | ↓ |

The arrow = direction of deviation from normal; $T_4$, thyroxine; $T_3$, triiodothyronine; TSH, thyroid-stimulating hormone.

**2** A 23-year-old woman, gravida 3, para 1, abortus 1, comes to the maternity unit examination room at 39 weeks' gestation by dates. Onset of prenatal care was at 10 weeks. Gestational age was confirmed by a 12-week sonogram. Her diabetes screening at 26 weeks' gestation was within normal limits. She reports uterine contractions that have been regular for the past 3 hours. On examination, you find that the contractions are 3 minutes apart, last 50 seconds each, and are firm to palpation. Her membranes ruptured 1 hour ago, and you note clear Nitrazine-positive fluid leaking from her vagina. Digital cervical examination reveals dilation of 5 cm, effacement of 100%, and the presenting vertex at 0 station. Which of the following criteria is most accurate for assessing whether she has entered the active phase of labor?

(A) Cervical effacement over 90%
(B) Contraction duration over 30 seconds
(C) Presenting fetal part is engaged
(D) Cervical dilation of at least 4 cm
(E) Ruptured membranes

**3** A physician sees a 7-year-old girl who has been referred to him by the school nurse, who informs him that the child often has cessation of speech in mid-conversation, accompanied by a blank stare and flickering of the eyelids. These symptoms last approximately 10 seconds before she resumes regular activity. The physician suspects that the child has a seizure disorder and asks the child to hyperventilate. During hyperventilation, the aforementioned symptoms appear. Which of the following electroencephalogram patterns is most characteristic of this disorder?

(A) Hypsarrhythmia
(B) Interictal slow-spike waves
(C) Centrotemporal spikes
(D) Three-per-second spike-and-wave pattern
(E) Four- to six-per-second spike-and-wave pattern

**4** A 44-year-old woman consulted her primary care physician because of a nagging feeling of fatigue, pain, and stiffness in both hands upon rising; the pain persisted for at least 1 hour after arising and was severe enough to make getting herself ready for the day's work difficult. The physician found that she had a low blood count, an elevated sedimentation rate, and an elevated C-reactive protein level, but x-rays of her hands were essentially normal. Feeling that she may have some sort of autoimmune condition, he referred her to a rheumatologist, who immediately had her haplotype determined and ran immunological tests for rheumatoid factor and an anticyclic citrullinated peptide antibody (ACPA) test, as well as testing for antinuclear antibodies (ANAs). Her haplotype serotype was HLA-DR4, and she tested positive for ANA and ACPA and negative for rheumatoid factor. Most likely, this lady suffered from which one of the following conditions?

(A) Systemic lupus erythematosus
(B) Multiple sclerosis
(C) Sjögren syndrome
(D) Diabetes mellitus type 1
(E) Rheumatoid arthritis

**5** A 38-year-old man was taken to an emergency facility after his car skidded on the freeway and struck a pillar. His vital signs were as follows: pulse, 88/min; respirations, 20/min; blood pressure, 100/70 mm Hg. Physical examination revealed nonprominent jugular neck veins, no indication of cyanosis, and symmetric breath sounds. A posterior–anterior chest x-ray film revealed a widened mediastinum. Which of the following choices is the most likely diagnosis?

(A) Ruptured aortic aneurysm
(B) Cardiac tamponade
(C) Dissection of the thoracic aorta
(D) Myocardial contusion
(E) Pulmonary contusion

**6** An executive was fired 2 years ago and experienced several months of depression. However, he seemed to regain his confidence spontaneously and now states that losing his job has been helpful, in that it gives him more time to spend with his family. Which of the following psychodynamic defenses is most strongly suggested by this statement?

(A) Splitting
(B) Compensation
(C) Displacement
(D) Rationalization
(E) Projection

**7** A 20-year-old woman who is a business major at a local university sees her physician because she has not had a period for the past 5 months. She knows she is not pregnant because she is not sexually active. She attained menarche at 12 years of age, but her menses always have been irregular. She also expressed concern about being at least 25 pounds overweight and volunteers that her roommate has recently lost weight and was diagnosed with hepatitis A, suggesting that maybe she could do so too. Physical examination revealed that she is 168 cm (66 in) tall and weighs 46 kg (102 lb). Her secondary sex characteristics are normal, but she appears thin and underweight. Her pelvic examination is normal. Findings of laboratory studies of serum prolactin, estradiol, and human chorionic gonadotropin (HCG) measurements are normal. Which of the following is the most likely diagnosis?

(A) Turner syndrome
(B) Hypogonadotropic hypogonadism
(C) Polycystic ovary syndrome
(D) Asherman syndrome
(E) Anorexia nervosa

**8** A man married a young woman who lost her vision at the age of 28 years. They had three children, two girls and one boy, all of whom started to become blind after the age of 20. All three of these children married sighted persons and had children. One daughter had two boys and a girl, all of whom became blind. The other daughter had a boy and girl; both of them lost their vision as well. The son had three boys and a girl, all of whom were sighted and had excellent vision as long as they lived. In the third generation, all the boys who remained sighted and those who lost their vision early married women who remained sighted until they died, and all their offspring also remained sighted well into old age. The daughter of the second-generation male who retained her sight married a normally sighted man, and their offspring could see throughout their lives as well. The second-generation women who became blind married men who retained their sight but their offspring of either sex lost their sight at an early age. Which of the following inheritance patterns is most likely to be present?

(A) Autosomal dominant
(B) Autosomal recessive
(C) Mitochondrial
(D) X-linked dominant
(E) X-linked recessive

**9** A 3-year-old child presents with recurrent right lower lobe pneumonia. His growth parameters are at the 25th percentile, and he is developmentally appropriate for his age. His past medical history is positive for an ear infection at 18 months of age and gastroenteritis at 2 years of age. He has completed two courses of antibiotic therapy with minimal if any improvement. Which of the following conditions is most likely responsible for this patient's disease?

(A) Primary B- or T-cell immunodeficiency disorder
(B) Cystic fibrosis
(C) Chédiak-Higashi syndrome
(D) Congenital lung abnormality
(E) Foreign body aspiration

**10** A 65-year-old male jumps off of a bus to catch a train. He immediately feels very severe pain in the front of the knee and hears a snap. He falls to the ground and is unable to rise. The emergency physician determines that the patient is a diabetic whose diabetes is controlled by oral hypoglycemics. He has no allergies and is not on any other medications. He exercises occasionally, and he is overweight. His vital signs are as follows: pulse, 86/min; respirations, 18/min; blood pressure, 150/97 mm Hg. His temperature is normal. The patient complains of pain in the right knee. Clinical examination reveals swelling and tenderness in the anterior aspect of the knee, and a sulcus is palpable proximal to the superior pole of the patella; no fragments can be moved. The patient is unable to extend the knee. Hemarthrosis is absent. Which of the following is the most likely diagnosis?

(A) Tear of the quadriceps expansion
(B) Tear of the anterior cruciate ligament
(C) Transverse fracture of the patella
(D) Tear of the posterior cruciate ligament
(E) Avulsion of the quadriceps tendon from the tibial tuberosity

**11** A 35-year-old woman, gravida 5, para 4, abortus 1, is seen for an annual examination and cervical cancer screening. Her four successful pregnancies all ended with term spontaneous vaginal deliveries of neonates weighing between 3,000 g (6 lb 10 oz) and 4,000 g (8 lb 13 oz). All children are alive and well. She had an uncomplicated elective laparoscopic tubal sterilization procedure performed 2 years ago under general anesthesia. Her 30-year-old sister also comes in for a routine annual examination. She has never been pregnant. She uses combination oral contraceptive pills for birth control. Which of the following physical examination findings of the cervix would be more typical of this 35-year-old woman than of her 30-year-old sister?

(A) Increased bluish hue
(B) Purulent discharge
(C) Retracted squamocolumnar junction
(D) Transverse-appearing external os
(E) Absence of scarring

**12** A 25-year old mother takes her 5-year-old child to see a pediatrician for a rash that started on her trunk and then spread to her face and extremities. According to the mother, the rash occurred in varying stages. It began with crops of small, red papules that progressed to teardrop vesicles on an erythematous base. These vesicles became cloudy, broke open, and then formed scabs. Which of the following is the most common complication of this infection in a normal host?

(A) Reye syndrome
(B) Pneumonia
(C) Thrombocytopenia
(D) Encephalitis
(E) Secondary bacterial skin infection

**13** A very anxious 25-year-old man complains of severe right lower quadrant pain. Physical examination reveals rebound tenderness, and laboratory results include leukocytosis. He experiences much subjective pain relief after normal saline solution is administered. Which of the following is most strongly suggested by this situation?

(A) The pain is psychogenic.
(B) He has a histrionic personality disorder.
(C) He was volume depleted.
(D) He has factitious disorder.
(E) He is responding to a placebo.

**14** A 57-year-old woman has had a rather remarkable history. She was born to a poor immigrant family and worked her way through college as a bartender in a small night club where patrons enjoyed a "good smoke" along with their drinks. After college, she went to law school, passed the bar, got a job in a good law firm, and became a partner within a decade. Moreover, she married and has two children. All her life she has been active and full of energy, but about 6 months ago she began to fatigue early; 2 or 3 months ago, she noticed a shortness of breath and a loss of appetite and of weight. Several weeks ago, she developed a dry cough, and last week, she spat up sputum with streaks of blood. As a nonsmoker, she though herself essentially immune to lung cancer; however, the blood in her sputum alarmed her and she consulted a pulmonologist. He took a history, gave her a general physical examination, and took chest x-rays followed by a computed tomography (CT) scan. He reported back to her that he had both bad and good news: "The bad news is that you have lung cancer; the good news is that the cancer is located in a defined area near the center of the lung but only in the left lobe and at the root of the bronchus; this means it seems not to have spread and is a relatively slow-growing variant; this provides hope it can be successfully treated." Which of the following lung cancer variants does this lady most likely have?

(A) Adenocarcinoma
(B) Squamous cell carcinoma
(C) Bronchoalveolar lung cancer
(D) Large-cell carcinoma
(E) Small- (oat) cell cancer

**15** A 28-year-old woman complains that her mother is selfish, undereducated, devious, and bereft of any redeeming qualities. On the other hand, she idealizes an aunt whom she describes as kind, sage, and the source of strength in her life. Which of the following defense mechanisms is this woman using?

(A) Projection
(B) Idealization
(C) Conversion
(D) Splitting
(E) Symbolization

**16** A 74-year old Caucasian man recently made an appointment to see his physician because he had difficulty in swallowing his pills. It took 2 weeks to get an appointment; by that time, his problem had progressed to the point where he was having problem with solids in general but no problem with liquids. In the past, he also had a longstanding history of gastroesophageal reflux disease (GERD), which was treated with omeprazole starting last year; however, he admits not taking his pills religiously. At present, he does not smoke, but he had started smoking at the age of 14 and quit some 10 years ago. He did drink, but primarily beer and only at social occasion. Which of the following conditions is the most likely diagnosis?

(A) Diffuse esophageal spasm
(B) Achalasia
(C) Esophageal stricture
(D) Esophageal ring (Schatzki ring)
(E) Esophageal carcinoma
(F) Zenker's diverticulum
(G) Esophageal varices

**17** A multicentered retrospective research study involving 362 women of childbearing age with pregestational diabetes mellitus investigated the relationship between mean blood glucose values and major fetal malformations. The purpose of the study was to estimate the relative risk of pregestational women with diabetes mellitus to have major fetal malformations during their pregnancy. The presence of malformation was confirmed by sonography and amniocentesis. Of the 362 women, 60 had mean plasma glucose values of 130 mg/dL or above, whereas 302 women had mean plasma glucose values below 130 mg/dL. The first group had ten cases of major fetal malformations in their pregnancies, whereas in the second group, only two had major fetal malformations in their pregnancies. Findings from the study are summarized in the table below:

| Major Fetal Malformation is: | Totals | Maternal Mean Plasma Glucose Values | |
|---|---|---|---|
| | | ≥130 mg/dL | <130 mg/dL |
| Present | 12 | 10 | 2 |
| Absent | 350 | 50 | 300 |
| Totals | 362 | 60 | 302 |

Which of the following equations represents the odds ratio for this study?

(A) $300 \div 50 = 6$
(B) $50 \div 10 = 5$
(C) $60 \div (2 + 10) = 5$
(D) $(300 \div 2) \div (60 \div 10) = 25$
(E) $(10 \div 2) \div (50 \div 300) = 30$

**18** While working for the U.S. embassy in Jordan, a 44-year-old female citizen of the United States, who would not agree to immunizations for religious reasons, met a 54-year-old male citizen of Jordan, and after a whirlwind courtship, married him. Four months after the marriage, she felt ill. She first tired readily, and then she came down with abdominal pain and nausea. Subsequently, she started vomiting, grew feverish, developed joint pain, and jaundice, and excreted a dark urine and clay-colored feces. At the time of their marriage, both of them had serological tests for hepatitis B (HB) as suggested by the Centers for Disease Control and Prevention (CDC) guidelines published on September 19, 2008 for natives and their sexual contacts who are planning to enter the United States from countries in which the prevalence of HB is 2% or greater. At that time, the female's serological pattern was represented by which of the following patterns? (In these choices: HB = hepatitis B virus, HBsAg = viral surface antigen, anti-HBs = antibodies to the surface antigen, c = viral core antigen; anti-HBc = antibodies to the core antigen, IgM = immunoglobin M.)

(A) HBsAg negative, anti-HBc negative, HBsAg anti-HBs negative

(B) HBsAg negative, anti-HBc positive, anti-HBs positive

(C) HBsAg negative, anti-HBc negative, anti-HBs positive

(D) HBsAg positive, anti-HBc positive, IgM anti-HBc positive, anti-HBs negative

(E) HBsAg positive, anti-HBc positive, IgM anti-HBc negative, anti-HBs negative

(F) HBsAg negative, anti-HBc positive, anti-HBs negative.

**19** A 6-month-old infant presents to the emergency department with his mother. The mother says that the patient was born via spontaneous vaginal delivery. He weighed 7 lb (3.2 kg) at birth and currently weighs 15 lb (6.8 kg). Immunizations are up to date. Upon physical examination, the patient is noted to have fever, intermittent inspiratory stridor, retraction of the intercostal muscles, and flaring of the nostrils. The mother states that the child has had an upper respiratory infection for the last 1–2 days. Which of the following diagnoses is most likely in this patient?

(A) Laryngotracheobronchitis (croup)

(B) Whooping cough

(C) Acute epiglottitis

(D) Bronchiolitis

(E) Acute bronchial asthma

**20** A 73-year-old man with Scandinavian ancestors was undergoing a routine physical examination when his physician noted a roundish spot about 6 mm (14 inch) in diameter that was slightly pinker than the remainder of the man's face. When he ran his finger across it, he also noted that was dry and rough. The patient informed him that something had been going on with that spot for a year or so; its appearance seemed to wax and wane, essentially disappearing once in a while but then returning, sometimes covered with white scales that then dropped off. When asked, the patient admitted that as a boy and a young man he spent countless hours at the beach body surfing and never used sunscreen. The physician cauterized the lesion with liquid nitrogen. Within 2 weeks the area became crusted, shrank, and fell off. Two weeks thereafter, the rough spot returned, and after a month, the patient developed an open sore at the same location that would not heal. The sore is most likely to be which one of the following?

(A) Actinic keratosis

(B) Basal cell carcinoma

(C) Squamous cell carcinoma

(D) Nodular melanoma

(E) Herpes infection

**21** A 62-year-old woman with a 35-year history of treatment with antipsychotic medications for schizophrenia complains of the insidious onset of peculiar writhing movements that she could not control. These include unintended lip smacking, contorted facial expressions, and movements of her tongue and fingers. Her psychotic manifestations had been well controlled for some time, and her physician had begun to taper her medication doses. Moreover, she had been fairly successful in reintegrating herself into a normal social milieu but found these movements so embarrassing that she started to withdraw again. Which of the following is most likely responsible?

(A) Akathisia

(B) Huntington disease

(C) Parkinsonism

(D) Tardive dyskinesia

(E) Wilson disease

**22** A 56-year old woman presents at a family physician's office complaining of a chronic cough. She says she has had a cough for about the past 10 years, but it usually has been only during a brief period after waking up, especially on cold damp mornings. She confides she also is prone to catch chest colds in the winter but recovers without any problem. However, for the past 6 months or so, the cough has gotten worse. It lasts well into midday or later, and she hacks so badly that she can hardly work. Her bosses at the fan manufacturing plant where she has worked for the past 25 years have threatened to fire her unless she can get her all too frequent times of coughing under control; she adds "he also is pissed off because I miss so many days of work since I have so many colds." She continues, "My coughing sometimes is dry but more often produces a thick snotty-like spit which sometimes contains pus." When prodded, she admits she had been smoking since she was a teenager, and that for the last 10–20 years she probably smoked about two packs a day; she adds, "since cigarettes have became so expensive she has tried to cut back but can't because that long puff feels so good."

On physical examination, her blood pressure was 165/85 mm Hg. Her pulse is 100 and regular. Her weight is 185 pounds (83.9 kg), height 5 feet, 6 inches (2.2 m), and her body mass index (BMI) is 29.9. She wheezes while talking. On auscultation, adventitious breath sounds are heard in all lobes. X-ray demonstrates significant bronchial wall thickening and increased markings at the base of both lungs. Which is the most likely diagnosis in this patient?

(A) Emphysema
(B) Allergic bronchitis
(C) Asthma
(D) Chronic bronchitis
(E) Smoker's cough

**23** Potterville, USA, population 200,000, has an annual rate of 15 new cases of acute leukemia. A leading pharmaceutical company decided to try an experimental medication for the treatment of the disease. Patients with confirmed acute leukemia were selected from this population. Of the 300 known patients with cases of leukemia, 200 were female and 100 were male; all patients had received treatments earlier with established therapies. The treatment trial was double-blinded. The new treatment was received by 150 patients, whereas 130 received a placebo. Twenty patients dropped out of the study due to noncompliance or nonacceptance. The trial clearly showed that the new treatment extended the life span of the patients with the disease and increased the length of remission. It did not, however, cure the disease. From this study, one could conclude that treatment with this new drug caused which of the following?

(A) Increased incidence of acute leukemia
(B) Increased prevalence of acute leukemia
(C) Decreased incidence of acute leukemia
(D) Decreased prevalence of acute leukemia
(E) Decrease in both the incidence and prevalence of acute leukemia

**24** A first-year pediatric resident is called to the nursery to examine an infant who had a cyanotic and choking episode associated with feeding. The infant was born full term, weighed 3.5 kg (7 lb 14 oz), and no complications occurred during delivery. The mother had no prenatal care but denies use of alcohol, illicit drugs, or tobacco. She also denies any sexually transmitted disease. Physical examination of the infant reveals excessive oral secretions. These oral secretions improve with suctioning of the mouth and pharynx, but recur after a short time. The resident suspects tracheoesophageal fistula. Which of the following additional findings would support her suspicion?

(A) Cyanosis that occurs at rest but is relieved by crying
(B) A history of oligohydramnios during pregnancy
(C) The ability to pass a catheter into the stomach
(D) A stomach filled with air
(E) An associated renal anomaly

**25** A 76-year-old man consulted his primary care physician for his quarterly check up for diabetes and general health assessment. He was diagnosed with type 2 diabetes about 25 years earlier, and his diabetes is presently being treated with 1,000 mg metformin POS b.i.d., nateglinide 60 mg AC, pioglitazone 20 mg QD; his hypertension is being treated with hydrochlorothiazide, 12.5 mg QD, acebutolol 200 mg b.i.d., enalapril 20 mg b.i.d., doxazosin mesylate 2 mg b.i.d., amlodipine besylate 5 mg QD, and clonidine 0.3 mg t.i.d.; for hypercholesterolemia, atorvastatin 10 mg QD; and for hypothyroidism, levothyroxine 0.1 mg QD. In addition, he takes 400 mg of over-the-counter (OTC) ibuprofen for ostearthritis and 200 mcg OTC glucose tolerance factor. As part of this quarterly check-up, his physician also ordered some laboratory work. The results of his physical examination and laboratory analysis are summarized in the following table.

| Measurement | Value | Units | Normal or Desirable Range |
|---|---|---|---|
| Height | 66 | Inches | N/A |
| Weight | 142 | Pounds | N/A |
| Body mass index | 22.9 | $Kg/m^2$ | <29 |
| Blood pressure | 118/75 | mm Hg | <120/<80 |
| Glycosylated hemoglobin (HbA1c) | 6.0 | Percent | 4.3–5.9 = normal <7 desired |
| $Na^+$ | 139 | mmol/L | 135–147 |
| $K^+$ | 4.8 | mmol/L | 3.5–5.5 |
| $Cl^-$ | 102 | mmol/L | 96–108 |
| $CO_2$ | 28 | mmol/L | 22–29 |
| Anion gap | 11 | mmol/L | 5–14 |
| Fasting glucose | 121 | mg/dL | 65–99 |
| Calcium | 10.4 | mg/dL | 8.5–10.4 |
| Blood urea nitrogen (BUN) | 36 | mmol/L | 9–23 |
| Serum creatinine | 1.41 | mg/dL | 0.50–1.20 |
| Urea/Creatinine | 25.5 | Ratio | 10–22 |
| Osmolarity calculated | 288 | milliosmolar /kg | 268–292 |
| SGOT/AST[a] | 28 | Units/Liter (U/L) | 0–44 |
| GPT/ALT[a] | 26 | U/L | 0–44 |
| Alkaline phosphatase | 75 | U/L | 40–129 |
| Total protein | 7.9 | gm/dL | 6.3–8.3 |
| Albumin (A) | 4.5 | gm/dL | 3.6–5.0 |
| Total bilirubin | 0.7 | mg/dL | 0.2–1.2 |
| Conjugated bilirubin | 0.1 | mg/dL | 0.0–0.3 |
| Globulin (G) | 2.6 | gm/dL | 2.4–4.4 |
| A/G ratio | 1.7 | Ratio | 0.7–2.5 |
| Total cholesterol | 154 | mg/dL | >199 |
| Triglycerides | 90 | mg/dL | >149 |
| High-density lipoprotein (HDL) | 45 | mg/dL | <40 |
| Total cholesterol/HDL | 3.4 | Ratio | >6 |
| Low-density lipoprotein (LDL) calculated | 90 | mg/dL | <99 |
| Very-low-density lipoprotein (VLDL) calculated | 25 | mg/dL | <30 |

[a]SGOT = Serum glutamic oxaloacetic transaminase; AST, aspartate aminotransferase; GPT, glutamate pyruvate transaminase; ALT, alanine aminotransferase.

Which of the following drugs that he takes has recently been shown most likely to account for the abnormal values found?

(A) Pioglitazone
(B) Hydrochlorothiazide
(C) Ibuprofen
(D) Levothyroxine
(E) Glucose tolerance factor.

**26** An 18-year-old woman, gravida 1, para 0, underwent spontaneous vaginal delivery 10 minutes ago. She gave birth to a 4,030 g (8 lb 14 oz) male neonate with 1- and 5-minute Apgar scores of 8 and 9. Her prenatal course was uncomplicated, and labor began spontaneously. Pain relief in labor was achieved by continuous epidural analgesia. Monitoring of the fetal heart rate and uterine contractions was by external cardiotocography. The second stage of labor lasted 90 minutes. She did not receive an episiotomy. You note only minimal first-degree vaginal lacerations. The umbilical cord begins to lengthen, and you observe a gush of blood from the vagina. Which of the following is the most likely cause of these events?

(A) Rapidly falling estrogen levels in maternal circulation
(B) Avulsion of anchoring villi by contracting myometrium
(C) Falling levels of circulating, placentally produced prolactin
(D) A gradual decrease in $P_{CO_2}$ in the umbilical vein
(E) A progesterone-mediated decrease in gap junctions

**27** An apparently healthy, athletically inclined, 5-foot 3-inch, 104 pound 16-year-old girl was given a casual nonfasting serum glucose test; the resulting value was 250 mg/dL. Concerned, the pediatrician ordered determination of fasting serum glucose levels on 2 consecutive days; the values obtained were 135 mg/dL, and 130 mg/dL. On the basis of these values, plus the fact she was slightly underweight, the pediatrician concluded she had type 1 diabetes mellitis and started her on insulin therapy. Two years later, she became a patient of her mother's physician, who had been treating the mother for type 1 diabetes, a condition she apparently developed while carrying the daughter at the age of 17. Somewhat suspicious of the fact that a mother and daughter both developed type 1 diabetes as teenagers, she sent away to a commercial laboratory for a specific genetic test. The result of this test made the physician change the diagnosis and mode of treatment for both mother and daughter. Most likely, the gene tested for was which one of the following?

(A) The hepatocyte nuclear factor 4α (HNF4α) gene on chromosome 20
(B) The GCK gene for glucokinase on chromosome 7
(C) The hepatocyte nuclear factor 1α (HNF1α) gene on chromosome 12
(D) The gene coding for insulin promoter factor-1 (IPF1) homeobox on chromosome 13
(E) Hepatocyte nuclear factor 1β (HNF1β)
(F) The neurogenic differentiation factor 1 gene located on chromosome 2

**28** A 22-year-old woman consulted a physician because she had been feeling poorly. She informed the physician that she is extremely tired despite going to bed early and sleeping well. This first became a problem almost a year ago, and more recently she also noted she became extremely weak after exerting herself physically or even after eating a carbohydrate-rich meal. Additionally, she was thirsty all the time, even though she also craved extra salt; understandably, she also needed to urinate excessively, even at night, thus interrupting her sleep. In response to the doctor's questions, she also revealed that these spells of weakness involved all four limbs and were worse in and around her upper arms and shoulders, as well as in her hip muscles. This made walking almost impossible, while her weak arms caused her to drop and break things. She added that she also has been getting severe cramps and painful spasms in these muscles. In addition, she thought that she has more joint stiffness, some degree of numbness in her hands and feet, and sometimes she felt dizzy upon arising. She had no history of nausea, vomiting, or other gastrointestinal problems. She added that she does not smoke, only drinks alcohol at a few social occasions, and is not taking any prescription or over-the-counter drugs; no person in her family that she was aware of had similar problems; however, her parents are first cousins. A "weakness attack" was induced by making her lift weights while marching in place and then having her rest. During the ensuing attack, the muscles in all four limbs became flaccid and there were associated depressed tendon jerks. The muscles of her eyes, face, tongue, pharynx, larynx, diaphragm, and sphincters were not involved. Her blood pressure remained within the high normal limit. Laboratory studies showed her serum glucose was 132 mg/dL, sodium, 140 mmol/L (normal 136–145), serum calcium 2.5 mmol/L (normal 2.2–2.6), serum potassium ion value was 1.6 mmol/L (normal 3.5–5.0), serum magnesium ion level was 0.5 mmol/L (normal 0.8–1.2), and serum chloride ion value was 94 mmol/L (normal 98–106 mmol/L); the abnormal levels persisted even between the attacks. She also had metabolic alkalosis with a bicarbonate ion level of 33 mmol/L (normal 22–30 mmol/L) and a blood pH of 7.48 (normal 7.35–7.45). A 24-hour urine analysis revealed alkaline urine with higher than normal amounts of potassium ion, 285 mmol/24h (normal 25–125 mmol/24h); chloride ion, 625 mmol/24h (normal 110–250 mmol/24h); and magnesium ion, 50 mmol/24h (normal 2–5 mmol/24h). On the other hand, the urinary calcium ion was lower than normal (1.5 mmol/24h, normal 2.5–7.5/24 hr). Thyroid function tests (T3, T4, and TSH) were normal. Which of the following does this lady most likely have?

(A) Thiazide diuretic toxicity
(B) Bartter syndrome
(C) Dent syndrome
(D) Andersen-Tawil syndrome
(E) Gitelman syndrome

29 An African American couple, with no known family history of sickle cell disease, wants to know the probability that their child will have sickle cell disease. To obtain a more precise assessment, a hydrolysate of their red blood cells (RBCs) is subjected to electrophoresis. The man has no hemoglobin S (HbS), but the woman has an obvious HbS band. Given that the carrier rate among African Americans is approximately 8%, or 1 in 12, the likelihood that their child will have sickle cell disease would most likely be:

(A) 0
(B) 1/4
(C) 1/144
(D) 1/576
(E) 1/1,936

30 A 22-year-old woman, gravida 2, para 1, presents for a routine prenatal visit. She is 42 and 1/2 weeks' gestation by dates, 170 cm (67 in) tall, and weighs 67 kg (147 lb). During her pregnancy, she has had a total weight gain of 19 kg (43 lb). This was a planned pregnancy that was complicated in the first trimester by severe nausea and vomiting that ended by 15 weeks' gestation. She required intravenous hydration and antiemetic medications. She has a positive history of chronic hypertension treated with methyldopa. She has had five sonograms performed during her pregnancy, at 10, 20, 25, 30, and 40 weeks' gestation. Which of the following five sonograms will have provided the most accurate estimate of the duration of pregnancy?

(A) 10 weeks
(B) 20 weeks
(C) 25 weeks
(D) 30 weeks
(E) 40 weeks

31 A 5-month-old nonimmunized child presents with a 2-week history of paroxysmal coughing, low-grade fever, posttussive emesis, and a viscid nasal discharge. Physical examination reveals bilateral otitis media and conjunctival hemorrhages. Scattered inspiratory rales are present bilaterally. The complete blood count (CBC) shows a white blood cell (WBC) count of 45,000 cells/mm³, 95% of which represent lymphocytes. Which of the following is the most likely diagnosis?

(A) Acute lymphoblastic leukemia
(B) *Chlamydia trachomatis* pneumonia
(C) Whooping cough
(D) Bronchiolitis
(E) Respiratory syncytial viral pneumonitis

32 A 2-year-old child presents to the physician's office with her mother. The mother states that, for the past few days, the child has had a low-grade fever, upper respiratory tract symptoms, and has been tugging at her right ear. An examination of the right ear with the pneumatic otoscope reveals a hyperemic, opaque, bulging tympanic membrane with poor mobility. The patient attends daycare three times a week. There has been no recent travel, and no one else is ill in the household. Which of the following organisms is the most likely causative pathogen?

(A) *Haemophilus influenzae*
(B) *Staphylococcus aureus*
(C) *Moraxella catarrhalis*
(D) *Streptococcus pneumoniae*
(E) Respiratory syncytial virus

33 A 24-year-old male football player fell on his outstretched hand while running with the ball, hoping to make a touchdown. He was writhing in pain and had to be taken to the emergency room of a local hospital. The patient complained of severe pain in his right arm. His vital signs were: blood pressure, 140/80; pulse, 98/min regular; temperature 37°C (98.6°F); and respirations 22/min and regular. The right arm was swollen and angulated in the midarm area. It was tender to touch, and movement was painful. The humeral shaft appeared to be fractured. Capillary circulation in the nail beds was normal. However, there was clinical evidence of nerve damage. The arm was splinted, and the patient was given narcotic analgesia to minimize the pain. An x-ray film of the arm confirmed fracture of the humeral shaft, with some angular displacement. Which of the following is the nerve injury associated with this fracture?

(A) Axillary nerve
(B) Median nerve
(C) Ulnar nerve
(D) Radial nerve
(E) Brachial plexus

34 A 16-year-old woman, gravida 1, para 0, presents to the outpatient office for a routine prenatal visit at 34 weeks' gestation. Her blood pressure (BP) is 150/95 mm Hg and remains elevated after 10 minutes of rest in the left-lateral position. Urine dipstick testing reveals 1+ glucose and 2+ albumin. She denies vaginal bleeding, leakage of vaginal fluid, headache, epigastric pain, or visual disturbances. Her BP on her initial prenatal visit at 14 weeks' gestation was 120/75 mm Hg. An obstetric sonogram obtained at 18 weeks' gestation confirmed her dates and showed

normal fetal anatomy. Her maternal grandfather has adult-onset diabetes. Her mother and maternal grandmother both have chronic hypertension. Which of the following is the most likely explanation for the findings in this patient?

(A) Blunted angiotensin response
(B) Elevated β-endorphin level
(C) Acute diffuse vasoconstriction
(D) Primary renal disease
(E) Chronic hypertension

**35** A 4-year-old child presents with a temperature of 40°C (104°F), which she has had for the past 4 days. Her primary care physician had seen her on the first and third day of fever. He was unable to ascertain the source of the fever. However, he had assured the mother that the fever would go away spontaneously. The mother is very concerned about the fever and brings the child to you for a second opinion. On physical examination, the patient is noted to have conjunctivitis, an erythematous rash, cervical adenopathy, and swollen hands and feet. Laboratory findings include an absolute neutrophilic leukocytosis, left shift, normal platelets, and an elevated erythrocyte sedimentation rate (ESR). Which of the following is the most likely diagnosis?

(A) Scarlet fever
(B) Acute rheumatic fever
(C) Juvenile rheumatoid arthritis
(D) Toxic shock syndrome
(E) Kawasaki syndrome

**36** A 15-year-old boy presents to his family physician with a history of dysuria, fever, and urethral discharge of 3 days' duration. He confesses to having sex with an older girl a few days earlier. Physical examination reveals a well-nourished boy with no pallor. His blood pressure is 110/76 mm Hg, his pulse 79/min regular, his respirations 18/min, and he has an oral temperature of 100°F (37.7°C). A yellowish white discharge is noted through the urethra, and he has bilateral tender inguinal lymphadenopathy. Prior to treating this patient, the physician should:

(A) Obtain parental consent.
(B) Counsel him on safe sexual practices.
(C) Notify state health authorities.
(D) Notify his sexual partner.
(E) Notify his parents after treating him.

**37** While riding his bicycle, a 9-year-old boy loses control and falls. During the process, his abdomen strikes the handlebar. His parents bring him to the emergency department because he has vague midabdominal pain and some bruising of the anterior abdominal wall. His vital signs are stable, and he has no other visible injuries. Which of the following is the most likely diagnosis?

(A) Ruptured spleen
(B) Ruptured liver
(C) Ruptured pancreas
(D) Hematoma in the rectus muscle
(E) Ruptured duodenum

**38** A 77-year-old man fractured his femur and was undergoing surgery to insert a rod to facilitate healing. After the fracture, the distal portion of the femur was pulled up toward the hip by the action of his muscles; this caused a lot of bleeding, fortunately, the femoral artery was not punctured. Now, during the surgery itself, more bleeding occurred, and it was decided to transfuse him with two units of blood. About 90 minutes after the start of the transfusion, it was noted that the patient developed chills; a quick check of his temperature showed it rose by 1.5°C from a presurgical value of 37.8°C. Which of the following reactions is most likely occurring?

(A) A hemolytic transfusion reaction
(B) A nonhemolytic febrile reaction
(C) A delayed hemolytic transfusion reaction
(D) An allergic reaction
(E) A reaction due to volume overload
(F) An acute lung injury
(G) A reaction caused by increased oxygen affinity

**39** Four hours ago, a 28-year-old woman, gravida 1, para 0, at 38 weeks' gestation was admitted to the labor and delivery suite. On admission, she had regular uterine contractions occurring every 2–3 minutes, a dilation of 4 cm on cervical examination, effacement of 80%, and blood pressure of 115/75 mm Hg. The fetus is in longitudinal lie and cephalic presentation with an estimated weight of 3,500 g (7 lb 11 oz) by abdominal palpation. Her prenatal course was characterized by first-trimester bleeding that spontaneously resolved. Her blood pressure (BP) has gradually increased over the past 4 hours; it is now sustained at 150/95 mm Hg. Her patella deep tendon reflexes are brisk, but she has no clonus. A urine dipstick test shows 2+ albumin. Administration of which of the following agents is indicated as the next step in management?

(A) Phenobarbital
(B) Diazepam
(C) Magnesium sulfate
(D) Diphenylhydantoin
(E) Magnesium gluconate

*Directions for Matching Questions (40 through 50): Each set of matching questions is preceded by a list of 4 to 26 lettered options followed by a brief explanation of the required task and then by a series of numbered statements. For each lettered statement you are to select ONE lettered option that best fulfills the task as it relates to that statement. Remember that each of the listed options might be correctly selected once, more than once, or not at all.*

## Questions 40–42

(A) Photophobia

(B) Raccoon sign

(C) Lucid interval

(D) Optic nerve atrophy

(E) Enlarged sella

(F) Cavernous sinus thrombosis

*For each of the conditions depicted below, select the ONE most likely finding described above.*

**40** A 28-year-old motorcyclist collided with an automobile and was thrown off. His helmet was not secured properly and came off during the event. He sustained a linear fracture to the left temporal bone.

**41** A 26-year-old college student was in an automobile accident. She sustained a fracture to the base of the skull.

**42** A 75-year-old man was brought to the hospital by his daughter. She stated that he fell and hit his head several weeks ago. Since that time, he has had a dull headache, has become uncharacteristically aggressive, and has been unable to concentrate.

## Questions 43–48

(A) *Staphylococcus aureus*

(B) *Staphylococcus saprophyticus*

(C) *Bacillus anthracis*

(D) *Bacillus cereus*

(E) *Clostridium perfringens*

(F) *Clostridium tetani*

(G) *Clostridium botulinum*

(H) *Corynebacterium diphtheriae*

(I) *Listeria monocytogenes*

(J) *Actinomyces israelii*

**43** A 23-year-old woman 7 months pregnant develops a fatigue, a general feeling of malaise, mild fever, and muscle aches. However, she gets over it in a few days and attributes it to a mild flu. Five weeks later, she gives birth to a 3-week premature baby boy. The neonate is listless, jaundiced, feverish, has a full body rash and difficulty with breathing. Despite all efforts, the baby dies 12 hours later.

**44** A high school cafeteria prepares a meat stew and sets up to serve it. However, a fire drill is called before the students have a chance to eat it and the stew slowly cools down. An hour later, after the drill, the cook reheats the stew and serves it. That night, many of the students get severe stomach cramps and diarrhea.

**45** One evening, a 6-month-old baby girl was given several teaspoons of honey to help induce her to swallow some bitter-tasting medicine prescribed by her pediatrician. The next morning, she was found to be lethargic, unwilling to eat and constipated, and to suffer from placid muscle paralysis.

**46** A 16-year-old girl had a date to go on a picnic with her dream man, the 18-year-old captain of her high school's football team. Wishing to impress him, she prepared food to take along, consisting of a potato salad and ham sandwiches. Being somewhat naïve, she did not wash her hands or the potatoes before preparing the meal and although she did refrigerate the finished product, it rode in a warm car and then stood on the picnic table for about 2 hours before they ate. Forty-five minute after gulping down the food, the boyfriend had severe stomach cramps, followed by nausea, vomiting, and then diarrhea. The girl, who ate less and more slowly, only had cramps and nausea.

**47** A postal worker noted a white powder leaking from an envelope. Curious, he lifted it up to examine it further. He noted it did not have sufficient postage, so he returned it to the sender. A week later, he developed what he felt was the first sign of a cold. Shortly thereafter, he developed a fever with chills and night sweats and then a cough, shortness of breath, fatigue, and muscle aches. By the time he saw a physician, he also had a sore throat, enlarged lymph nodes, vomiting, and diarrhea, and painless raised bumps appeared on his arms, hands, and face. The physician who first saw him immediately suspected his problem and gave him ciprofloxacin IV. Despite the treatment, the bumps evolved into ulcers with black areas in the center and his respiratory problems worsened. He died the following day.

**48** A young man from Latvia joins a family in the United States who belong to a small isolated sect that believes vaccinations defile children. About 2 weeks after this man joins the family, his 5-year-old cousin develops a fever of 101°F (38.3°C) and chills. The child also has a sore throat, headache, hoarseness, wheezing, and a cough. The child has greater and greater difficulty in breathing, and his neck swells, inducing a bull-necked appearance. Even though it was against the sect's beliefs, the child's parents finally take him to an emergency medical facility. The physician on duty there notes the child has a grayish, thick, leathery membrane covering his tonsils, soft palate, nasopalatal area, and uvula.

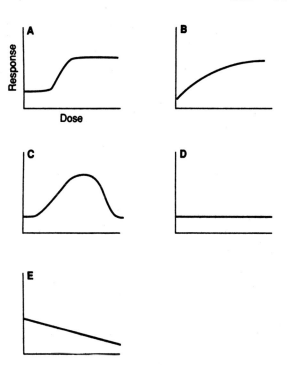

## Questions 49 and 50

The dose/response curves illustrated above represent the changes in therapeutic response for different medication doses. The ordinate (the vertical axis) represents increasing therapeutic response; the abscissa (the horizontal axis) represents increasing medication dose. Match each drug listed below with the proper graph.

**49** Nortriptyline

**50** Lithium

# Answer Key

| | | | | | | | | | |
|---|---|---|---|---|---|---|---|---|---|
| **1** | D | **11** | D | **21** | D | **31** | C | **41** | B |
| **2** | D | **12** | E | **22** | D | **32** | D | **42** | A |
| **3** | D | **13** | E | **23** | B | **33** | D | **43** | I |
| **4** | E | **14** | B | **24** | D | **34** | C | **44** | E |
| **5** | C | **15** | D | **25** | C | **35** | E | **45** | G |
| **6** | D | **16** | E | **26** | B | **36** | B | **46** | A |
| **7** | E | **17** | E | **27** | C | **37** | E | **47** | C |
| **8** | C | **18** | A | **28** | E | **38** | B | **48** | H |
| **9** | E | **19** | A | **29** | A | **39** | C | **49** | C |
| **10** | D | **20** | C | **30** | A | **40** | C | **50** | A |

# Answers and Explanations

**1** **The answer is D** *Medicine*

The clinical vignette describes a patient with hypothyroidism. This diagnosis is confirmed by the laboratory test profile of decreased total $T_4$, decreased free $T_4$, and increased thyroid-stimulating hormone (TSH) levels (choice **D**). The TSH value is the most sensitive test for diagnosing primary hypothyroidism, because it is increased even when the serum $T_4$ is only on the low side of normal, indicating a gland that is on the verge of failing. The presence of a smooth, nontender thyroid gland is a typical finding in Hashimoto's thyroiditis, the most common cause of hypothyroidism in the United States in patients older than 6 years of age. Initially, these patients have hyperthyroidism due to leakage of $T_3$ and $T_4$ from the cells; after that phase, hypothyroidism sets in. Antibodies to thyroglobulin (TG) and thyroid microsomes are found in the plasma of patients with Hashimoto's thyroiditis, indicating that autoimmunity plays a prominent role in causing the disease. Additional clinical features of hypothyroidism include macroglossia, congestive cardiomyopathy, depression, constipation, slow mentation, menstrual irregularities, and proximal muscle weakness. Elevated serum creatinine kinase should alert one to muscle problems. Levothyroxine is the treatment of choice, with a goal of bringing serum TSH into the normal range.

An analytic pattern of increased total $T_4$, normal free $T_4$, and normal TSH values typically is obtained from a person with an increase in TG levels (choice **A**); for example, a woman taking oral contraceptives. Increased total $T_4$, increased free $T_4$, and decreased TSH levels (choice **B**) represent data that might be presented by a patient with hyperthyroidism, most commonly due to Graves disease. A decreased total $T_4$, normal free $T_4$, and normal TSH values (choice **C**) is a pattern that would be obtained from a person with a decrease in TG levels; for example, an athlete taking anabolic steroids. A decrease in total $T_4$, decrease in free $T_4$, and decrease in TSH values (choice **E**) is characteristic of a patient with a problem in either the anterior pituitary (secondary hypothyroidism) or the hypothalamus (tertiary hypothyroidism), with decreased release of thyrotropin-releasing hormone (TRH).

**2** **The answer is D** *Obstetrics and Gynecology*

The determination of the stage of labor is important because the normal progress expected varies by which stage and phase of labor the patient is in. The first stage of labor (from onset of true labor to complete cervical dilation) has two phases: a latent phase, during which cervical effacement and early dilation occur, and an active phase, during which more rapid cervical dilation occurs. Cervical dilation of at least 4 cm (choice **D**) marks the active phase.

Cervical effacement over 90% (choice **A**), and contraction duration over 30 seconds (choice **B**) are frequently noted in active labor but can also occur in early labor. Engagement of the fetal presenting part (choice **C**) and membrane rupture (choice **E**) are not essential for active labor diagnosis.

**3** **The answer is D** *Pediatrics*

Absence, or petit mal, seizures cease as quickly as they commence. Motor activity stops abruptly, and patients develop a blank stare with fluttering of the eyelids. The seizures are brief (10–30 seconds), but may occur many times throughout the day. They end abruptly and have no postictal stage. Absence seizures can be triggered by hyperventilation. An electroencephalogram (EEG) shows a typical three-per-second spike-and-wave pattern (choice **D**).

Hypsarrhythmia (choice **A**) is seen on EEG in patients with infantile spasms. Interictal slow-spike waves on EEG (choice **B**) are seen with Lennox-Gastaut syndrome. Centrotemporal spikes (choice **C**) is the EEG finding diagnostic of benign partial epilepsy. A four- to six-per-second irregular spike-and-wave pattern (choice **E**) can be found on the EEG of a patient with juvenile myoclonic epilepsy (Janz syndrome).

**4** **The answer is E** *Medicine*

The lady has the early symptoms of rheumatoid arthritis (RA) (choice **E**). RA is an autoimmune inflammatory condition principally involving the synovial membranes of multiple joints, typically in a symmetrical bilateral fashion starting with the smaller joints on the hands. As the disease progresses, typically with periods of remission, it affects the feet and bigger joints, and causes malaise, weight loss, and fever. Although in this case the lady's symptoms and early laboratory studies are nonspecific, they are typical for some sort of inflammatory autoimmune condition. Moreover the HLA-DR4 haplotype serotype is strongly positively correlated with RA and a positive anticyclic citrullinated peptide (ACPA; also known as citrulline antibody, anti-citrulline antibody, anti-CCP, and cyclic citrullinated peptide antibody) test. This test measures a form of serum citrulline, and some investigators hypothesize that the conversion of arginine to citrulline plays a role in the autoimmune inflammatory process associated with RA. It has a specificity of about 95% for RA, although it does provide false-negative results about 33% of the time; in addition, it often is present in the earliest phases of the disease, even before clinical signs are clearly manifested. In contrast, the negative rheumatoid factor result does not rule out RA because it is frequently negative in early cases, even after the first year. ANA is a relatively nonspecific test for autoimmune and other inflammatory conditions; therefore, a positive test is compatible with RA but also other disease states. The prevalence of RA is about 1 case per 100 persons; females are affected three times more often than males, and the onset in most cases occurs between the ages of 25 and 50, peaking between the ages of 40 and 50 years. Recent treatments for RA have improved the lives of RA patents to a remarkable extent. Although the classic medications, corticosteroids and/or nonsteroidal anti-inflammatory drugs (including aspirin), are still employed to reduce pain and inflammation, so-called *disease-modifying antirheumatic drugs* (DMRDs) are now available and often prescribed early in the course of the disease to avoid disease progression to the point of causing irreversible damage. In addition, genetically engineered drugs called *biologics* have been developed that induce remissions in about two-third of cases. Unfortunately, these have to be administered by injection and are very expensive, thus they are often reserved for people in whom DMARDs are ineffective, or they are used to supplement DMARD treatments. Physical therapy is also an important adjunct used to help joint function.

All the incorrect choices also are autoimmune diseases. Systemic lupus erythematosus (SLE) (choice **A**) is a chronic inflammatory systemic disease that can affect any organ system. ANAs are present in the serum of most patients with active SLE, and antibodies to native double-stranded DNA are essentially diagnostic for this disease. A genetic component is also likely, since HLA-DR2 and HLA-DR3 human leukocyte antigens are more common than in the general population. SLE is erratic in its manifestations in that it follows a relapsing and remitting course. The prevalence in the United States is 6–35 per 100,000 people. The incidence is highest among women of childbearing age, and overall in adults, it is 10–15 times higher in women than in men. Cases of SLE vary from being relatively benign to being progressive and rapidly fatal. Prior to 1955, the 5-year survival was less than 5%, but now thanks to better medical care, the 10-year survival is about 90%. Nonetheless, 30% of SLE-related deaths occur before the age of 45 years. Multiple sclerosis (MS) (choice **B**) is a disease in which the immune system attacks the myelin sheets in the central nervous system, killing oligodendrocytes and causing demyelination. This may produce numerous physical and mental symptoms, depending on the nerves affected, and it often progresses to physical and cognitive disability. Disease onset usually occurs in young adults, and it is more common in women. It has a prevalence ranging between 2 and 150 per 100,000 depending on the country or specific population; it is more frequent among individuals of northern European descent. Although the condition is not curable, recently developed medications help mitigate symptoms; the type of medication used varies with the variant form of the disease. Sjögren syndrome (choice **C**) occurs when the immune system attacks and destroys moisture-producing organs, including the salivary and lacrimal glands and more rarely the lungs, kidneys, or gastrointestinal tract. It usually is characterized by dry eyes and mouth, and sometimes by enlargement of the parotid gland. More than 90% of individuals affected by Sjögren syndrome are women, and 90% of the time it is rheumatoid factor positive; it also may be associated with rheumatoid arthritis or other rheumatic diseases. Serum levels of ANA are also often elevated. Some people may experience only mild symptoms of dry eyes and mouth and are able to treat the disease symptomatically, while others have a more severe disease and must cope with blurred vision or recurrent oral infections and difficulties with swallowing and eating. Systemic problems can also occur including fatigue, joint pain, and even autoimmune tubulointerstitial nephritis leading to proteinuria, urinary concentrating defect, and distal renal tubular acidosis. Unlike diabetes mellitus type 2, type 1 (choice **D**) is a disease with an autoimmune component triggered by some still not clearly identified factor. Approximately 85% of patients have circulating islet cell antibodies, and the majority also has detectable anti-insulin antibodies before receiving insulin therapy. Most islet cell antibodies are directed against glutamic acid decarboxylase within pancreatic β cells. Some theorize that there is a virally induced etiology. The Coxsackie virus is commonly suggested, although the evidence is inconclusive. Since not everyone infected by this organism gets diabetes type 1, it also is suggested that, in addition, there is a genetic component; evidence for this is provided by the fact that up to 95% of patients with type 1 diabetes express human leukocyte antigen (HLA)-DR3 or HLA-DR4; in fact HLA-DQs are considered specific markers of type 1 DM susceptibility. Others claim cow's milk contains a triggering agent, which however never has been identified; this idea is derived from studies claiming a higher incidence among babies given cow's rather than breast milk after birth.

### 5 The answer is C *Surgery*

This patient most likely has traumatic dissection of the thoracic aorta (choice **C**) caused by a deceleration injury. Disruption of the aorta can occur at the root (the origin of the ligamentum arteriosum) or at the diaphragm. Prognosis is poor, with 85% of patients dying at the scene of the accident, and only 15% making it to the hospital. These patients have small tears or effective tamponading. The intima and media are fractured, leaving the adventitia intact. Blood collects subjacent to the adventitia, giving rise to a pseudoaneurysm, which is seen as a widened mediastinum on a posterior–anterior chest x-ray film. A widened mediastinum is the most consistent sign associated with traumatic disruption of the thoracic aorta and should immediately make one suspect this lesion. Approximately one-third of patients have no presenting clinical symptoms after traumatic disruption of the thoracic aorta.

Ruptured aortic aneurysm (choice **A**) is usually seen in the elderly. The most common cause for this condition is atherosclerosis. There may be a longstanding history of hypertension and associated coronary artery disease. A palpable pulsatile mass is present in the epigastric region. Unlike traumatic disruption of the thoracic aorta, this is a true aneurysm. Cardiac tamponade (choice **D**) most often follows blunt chest injury. It is associated with elevated venous pressure, hypotension, and muffled heart sounds. These three signs compose Beck's triad. Of these, hypotension is the most reliable symptom, because elevated venous pressure may not be seen in the presence of severe hypotension, and the heart sounds are not muffled on many occasions. Tachycardia is present, and the chest radiograph is noncontributory, as acute effusions are not discernible. Two-dimensional echocardiography is the best test to confirm the diagnosis. Treatment involves pericardiocentesis. Myocardial contusion (choice **D**) follows blunt chest trauma. It mainly involves the right ventricle. Patients may not have symptoms at initial presentation. Presence of a new right bundle branch block on electrocardiogram should point to the diagnosis. Radionuclide angiography is the most sensitive test to detect this condition. Pulmonary contusion (choice **E**) may also follow blunt chest trauma. Patients may appear remarkably fit. It is the most common cause of potentially lethal injury in the United States. Chest x-ray films may show a few patchy infiltrates that progress with time. Respiratory failure can develop rapidly. Therefore, one should have a high index of suspicion when confronted with a patient with vague symptoms after blunt chest injury.

### 6 The answer is D *Psychiatry*

Rationalization (choice **D**) refers to the distortion of reality, so that an act or event that actually is unpleasant seems to be desirable. This defense mechanism is often used when an individual cannot accept the implications of a particular outcome of events. The other defense mechanism choices do not apply as well to this patient.

Splitting (choice **A**) occurs when an individual psychologically separates positive qualities into one individual or group and negative qualities into another. Compensation (choice **B**) is an effort to use skills or competencies in one area to counterbalance self-perceived deficiencies in other areas. Displacement (choice **C**) occurs when the emotions associated with a psychologically unacceptable object, idea, or activity are transferred to another object or situation. Projection (choice **E**) is the attribution of uncomfortable internal feelings or thoughts, especially anger and guilt, to other individuals.

### 7 The answer is E *Obstetrics and Gynecology*

The patient's height/weight discordance, as well as her misconception concerning her weight, suggests anorexia nervosa (choice **E**) causing secondary amenorrhea.

Turner syndrome (choice **A**) is associated with primary amenorrhea, absence of secondary sexual development, and short stature due to aneuploidy (45, X); estradiol levels are low, but follicle-stimulating hormone (FSH) levels are high. Hypogonadotropic hypogonadism (choice **B**) is associated with absence of secondary sexual development due to hypothalamic-pituitary insufficiency; an example is Kallmann syndrome. Estradiol levels are low, and FSH levels are also low. Polycystic ovary syndrome (choice **C**) is associated with male pattern hair, infertility, and irregular menses. Estradiol and FSH levels are within normal limits, but luteinizing hormone (LH) level is increased. Asherman syndrome (choice **D**) is characterized by secondary amenorrhea, the result of intrauterine synechiae following overzealous curettage. Estradiol and FSH levels are within normal limits.

**8** **The answer is C** *Medicine*

In this pedigree, all affected females transmit a trait that causes early vision loss to offspring of both sexes. However, affected males and normal individuals of both sexes do not transmit loss of sight to their offspring. This non-Mendelian pattern of inheritance is characteristic of conditions caused by a mutation in a mitochondrial gene (choice **C**), due to the fact that only females transmit mitochondria to the ovum. This particular family has Leber's hereditary optic neuropathy. Individuals who inherit this condition suffer precipitous vision loss, usually in their 20s, due to optic nerve degeneration. In different families with Leber's hereditary optic neuropathy, 11 different missense mutations in three different mitochondrial genes encoding respiratory chain subunits have been described. Although the ultimate phenotype, loss of vision, remains consistent, the rate of vision loss and the age of onset vary considerably, even among members of the same family. Such variability in the phenotypic expression of conditions transmitted by mitochondrial mutations is characteristic of these conditions and is called *heteroplasmy*. It occurs because each cell carries multiple mitochondria, of which on average only half will be affected, but transmission of mitochondria with normal and mutated genes will occur in a random manner. Because mitochondrial-DNA (mtDNA)-encoded proteins are primarily associated with electron transport and adenosine triphosphate (ATP) synthesis, tissues that depend upon the electron transport system are affected most.

In an autosomal dominant disorder (choice **A**), either an affected male or female may transmit the mutant gene to a child of either sex, and the mutant trait will be expressed.

In an autosomal recessive disorder (choice **B**), both parents must transmit a mutant gene to the gamete for the trait to be expressed. An offspring of either sex who inherits one mutant gene from either parent will be a carrier.

In an X-linked dominant disorder (choice **D**), affected males will carry only one X chromosome, which will bear the mutated gene; this X chromosome will be transmitted to his daughters, in whom the trait is expressed since it is dominant. However, characteristically, the disease is more severe in hemizygous affected males than in heterozygous affected females. Since his sons only will inherit his Y chromosomes, they will not be affected, nor will they be carriers. Affected females almost certainly will have one X chromosome with the normal gene and one with the mutated gene; thus, they transmit the mutant gene to 50% of their daughters and to 50% of their sons. Since the trait is dominant, the mother as well as offspring of both sexes who inherit the affected chromosome will express the trait.

In an X-linked recessive disorder (choice **E**), males carrying an X chromosome with a mutated gene will express the trait since they only have one X chromosome; females carrying an X chromosome on the other hand will be carriers but will not expresses the trait since the recessive trait will not be expressed in the presence of an X chromosome carrying the normal gene. Sons of affected males will be neither carriers nor affected because they inherit a Y, not an X chromosome; however, 100% of the daughters will be carriers because they will receive the affected X chromosome from their father and a normal one from their mother. Fifty percent of the daughters of women who are carriers will become carriers themselves, since there is a 50% chance they will inherit the affected X chromosome. Although there is also a 50% chance that her son will inherit an X chromosome bearing the mutated gene, those who do will express the disease because that will be their only X chromosome.

**9** **The answer is E** *Pediatrics*

Foreign body aspiration (choice **E**) is the most common cause of recurrent pneumonia in an otherwise healthy 3-year-old child. Because of the lung's anatomy, right side aspiration is more common. When a child presents with pneumonia, a history of choking can often be elicited.

Immunodeficiency disorders (choice **A**) are characterized by recurrent infections, usually by opportunistic organisms, and failure to thrive. Cystic fibrosis (choice **B**) similarly results in failure to thrive, and malabsorption and clubbing are often seen. In cystic fibrosis, common organisms responsible for pneumonia are *Staphylococcus aureus*, *Pseudomonas aeruginosa*, and *Haemophilus influenzae*. In addition, *Burkholderia* *cepacia* is an organism that is increasing in frequency in patients with cystic fibrosis and may be associated with rapid pulmonary deterioration and death. Chédiak-Higashi syndrome (choice **C**) is autosomal recessive and is associated with giant granules in neutrophils and recurrent infections of the skin, mucous membranes, and the respiratory tract. Moreover, the fact that the patient is healthy indicates that this is not Chédiak-Higashi syndrome, in which albinism is a key to diagnosis. Congenital lung abnormalities (choice **D**) generally present at a much earlier stage.

### 10 The answer is D *Surgery*

This patient has a tear of the quadriceps expansion (choice **A**), which may result from direct or indirect injury. It can occur within the muscle, at the tendon-muscular junction, within the tendon itself, or at the tendo-osseous junction (most common in the elderly). Tears of the quadriceps expansion are most common in older individuals who are overweight and in poor physical condition. The usual history is of missing a step and tripping while descending a staircase or suddenly jumping down from a height. Patients complain of severe pain, often feel or hear a snap, and fall to the ground. Physical examination reveals swelling and tenderness at the site of the tear, and a sulcus or gap is felt at the site of separation, especially if the tear is complete. If the tear is partial, the patient has difficulty extending the knee; if the tear is complete, the patient cannot extend the knee. Tears of the quadriceps expansion can also occur in athletes and young individuals. In athletes, the tears are most often at the insertion of the tendon into the tibial tubercle.

Tears of the posterior cruciate ligament (choice **D**) usually occur because of hyperextension and are associated with a positive sag sign. They are not associated with inability to straight-leg raise, swelling of the anterior aspect of the knee, or a gap between the fibers of the quadriceps expansion or tendon. Although it is true that a snapping sound is heard in tears of the anterior cruciate ligament (choice **B**), there is hemarthrosis and a positive Lachman's test result. The inability to straight-leg raise, a gap felt at the site of the tear, and swelling confined to the anterior aspect of the knee are not features of this condition. Transverse fracture of the patella (choice **C**) is the main differential diagnosis. Fractures of the patella can result from direct or indirect trauma. In older individuals who are obese and in poor physical shape, an indirect injury resulting from tripping down stairs, jumping from a height, or even forcefully squatting can result in fracture of the patella. The patient complains of severe pain and falls to the ground. Difficulty in straight-leg raise, swelling over the knee, and hemarthrosis are seen. A gap can be felt in the patella, and the fragments can be moved, which distinguishes it from a pure tear of the quadriceps expansion. Avulsion of the quadriceps tendon from the tibial tuberosity (choice **E**) usually occurs in a younger individual. In teenagers, the epiphysis is weaker than the tendon, and it can be sheared off from its moorings. The gap is felt below the inferior pole of the patella. In the case presented, the gap is felt above the superior pole of the patella.

### 11 The answer is D *Obstetrics and Gynecology*

On physical examination, the astute observer can identify the irreversible changes that pregnancy brings to the female body, especially in the reproductive tract. A transverse-appearing external os (choice **D**) is more typical of a multiparous than a nulliparous cervix. This is sometimes described as a "fish-mouth"–shaped cervical os.

Increased bluish hue (choice **A**) is true of pregnancy (Chadwick sign) because of the increased vascularity of the cervix but is unrelated to parity. Purulent discharge (choice **B**) is characteristic of cervicitis but is unrelated to parity. A retracted squamocolumnar junction (choice **C**) is found in postmenopausal women but is unrelated to parity. Absence of scarring (choice **E**) is a characteristic of nulliparous, not multiparous, women.

### 12 The answer is E *Pediatrics*

The patient has a presentation that is most consistent with varicella (chickenpox). The most common complication of varicella is secondary bacterial infection of skin lesions (choice **E**).

The association of Reye syndrome (choice **A**) with varicella has become rare since salicylates are no longer prescribed as antipyretics for children. Pneumonia (choice **B**) is more common in adolescents and adults than in children. Thrombocytopenia (choice **C**) can result in hemorrhages of skin and mucous membranes and may be associated with transient petechiae. Hemorrhagic vesicles can be seen. Encephalitis (choice **D**) is the most common central nervous system (CNS) complication of varicella but is far less common than secondary bacterial infection of skin lesions.

**13 The answer is E** *Psychiatry*

Normal saline solution is unlikely to have corrected the patient's underlying pathology. However, it is common for patients to respond to the placebo effect (choice **E**) inherent in many medical interventions.

Such responses do not suggest that pain or discomfort is psychogenic (choice **A**), exaggerated as in a histrionic personality disorder (choice **B**), or factitious (choice **D**). The response does not suggest that the patient was volume depleted (choice **C**).

**14 The answer is B** *Medicine*

Lung cancer is the second most common cancer in both sexes, following prostate cancer in men and breast cancer in women. However, it is by far the leading cause of cancer death among both men and women. It is estimated that in 2008 there were 215,020 new cases resulting in 161,840 deaths from lung cancer, these will account for around 29% of all cancer deaths. More people will die from lung cancer than from colon, breast, and prostate cancers combined. Typically, lung cancer is divided into two major categories, small-cell and non-small cell. This is because small-cell cancers grow rapidly, metastasize readily, and are scattered throughout the lung, making them essentially impossible to treat by surgery or radiation. On the other hand, before they mature and spread, non-small cell cancers tend to remain concentrated in a localized area, making surgical or radiation treatment a possibility. Among the non-small cell lung cancers are adenocarcinomas, squamous cell carcinomas, bronchoalveolar lung cancers, and large-cell carcinomas. Squamous cell carcinomas are generally located in a defined area near the center of the lung, either on a bronchial branch or on a nearby major lobe; this matches the description of the cancer the case above (choice **B**). These cells are situated near the terminus of the bronchi; consequently, they are particularly susceptible to airborne irritants and carcinogens and cancers in this area are typically caused by smoking tobacco products. However, carcinogens do not have to be smoked in order to be breathed in, as for instance is the case of second-hand smoke, which likely happened to this lady while she worked as a bartender. Typically, the progression from early injury is one that takes years to achieve; cells progress from normal, to hyperplasia, through metaplasia and dysplasia, finally into a true neoplastic state, a carcinoma. In this lady, the original exposure caused a mutation, and the progression may well have been promoted over the years by further exposure, likely during conferences, etc. Prior to the popularity of filter-tipped cigarettes, squamous cancers were the most common type of lung cancer, and they still constitute 25%–30% of all lung cancers. If caught in time, as it appears it may have been in the case described, squamous cell carcinomas are possibly treatable by surgery and/or radiation; however, they will grow and form bronchial cavities and thus become inoperable. It is the cancer type most often associated with hypercalcemia.

Adenocarcinoma (choice **A**) usually occurs in a peripheral location in the lung and has become the most common form of non-small cell carcinoma in the United States, accounting for 35%–40% of all lung cancers. When contained, it tends to respond better than other lung cancers to surgical removal. This type of cancer is the most frequent form found in nonsmokers, but the relatively recent increase in its incidence is primarily due to smokers of low-tar filter-tipped cigarettes. Apparently, microscopic fragments from the filters imbedded with carcinogen from the cigarette are responsible for this cancer variant, which also is responsible for the rapid increase of this cancer among women and in individuals younger than 45. Bronchioloalveolar carcinoma (choice **C**) is a distinctive subtype of typical adenocarcinoma of the lung. A National Institute of Cancer survey found it differs from the typical adenocarcinoma in that it has a significantly higher 5-year survival rate among patients in all stages of the disease. Moreover, as compared to typical adenocarcinoma, bronchioalveolar carcinoma has a higher incidence of metastases within the lung but fewer to the brain. Bronchioloalveolar carcinoma also has been diagnosed with increasing frequency over the past few decades and now account for 3%–4% of cases of non-small cell lung cancer; according to estimates, some 5,000–7,000 new cases are diagnosed annually in the United States. A characteristic finding in persons with advanced disease is voluminous watery sputum. Large-cell carcinoma (choice **D**) cells are unusually large when seen under the microscope. In a chest x-ray, they usually appear in the central portion of the lung. They tend to be accompanied by extensive bleeding and tissue damage and to be undifferentiated, without the specific architecture found in other types of cancer cells. They grow quickly and metastasize at an earlier stage than other forms of non-small cell lung cancers. They also tend to induce paraneoplastic phenomena, including secretion of a hormone-like substance that causes gynecomastia in males. Small- (oat) cell cancers (choice **E**) differ from the non-small cell carcinomas in that the are more aggressive, grow rapidly, metastasize to distant sites earlier, and are more frequently associated with distinct paraneoplastic syndromes. Except in rare situations, surgery plays no role in their treatment; however, they are very sensitive to chemotherapy or radiation.

### 15 The answer is D *Psychiatry*

Splitting (choice **D**) is described as the psychologic separation of all good qualities into one individual and all bad qualities into another. This separation occurs when an individual cannot tolerate ambivalent feelings toward a particular individual. Children and persons with borderline personality disorder often manifest evidence of splitting.

Projection (choice **A**) refers to the attribution of one's feelings or beliefs to another. Idealization (choice **B**) refers to the exaggeration of an individual's qualities by an admirer. Conversion (choice **C**) refers to the transformation of psychologic stressors into physical complaints. Symbolization (choice **E**) refers to the selection of a particular object or event to represent other meanings.

### 16 The answer is E *Surgery*

The factors pointing toward esophageal carcinoma (choice **E**) include a dysphagia that is rapidly progressing, a long history of acid reflux disease that apparently is not being adequately treated, and a male over the age of 65 years; the diagnosis will of course need be confirmed by endoscopy with biopsy. The incidence of esophageal cancer in the United States is about three to six cases per 100,000 individuals; it is more common after the sixth decade, and is over seven times more prevalent in males than in females. In September 2008, the American Cancer Society estimated that during 2008 there will be 16,470 new cases of esophageal cancer in the United States (78.7% of these will be in males), and overall, 87% will die from the disease. Almost all esophageal cancers are either squamous cell or adenocarcinomas, and although squamous cell cancers are more common in African Americans, adenocarcinomas are more common in Caucasians. Historically, squamous cell carcinoma was the more common form, accounting for 95% of the cases in the United States as recently as the mid-twentieth century. However, during the past few decades, the trend has been for the proportion of adenocarcinomas to increase and squamous cell carcinomas to decrease, and by the mid-1990s, each accounted for about 50% of the cases. Worldwide, squamous cell carcinomas still predominate and account for some 95% of cases in most developing countries. The squamous cell carcinomas are induced by exposure of the nonkeratinizing stratified epithelial squamous cells that line the esophagus to carcinogens. In the United States, the primary source of such carcinogens is tobacco smoke, and the decline in squamous cell carcinomas is likely linked to the decrease in the number of smokers. Other risk factors for squamous cell carcinoma include heavy alcohol consumption, nitrosamine and other nitrosyl compounds found in smoked and pickled foods, and a host of irritants that might be ingested. Most squamous cell carcinomas are found distributed about the middle of the esophagus. In contrast, the adenocarcinomas are primarily found in the lower portion of the esophagus and are the end product of a series of transformations started by chronic exposure to gastric acid regurgitated as the result of GERD. The acid first inflames the stratified squamous epithelial cells, which then undergo metaplasia and eventually transformation into specialized epithelial cells called Barrett's epithelium. These Barrett's epithelial cells then undergo further transformation with the ultimate possibility of becoming an adenocarcinoma; about 10% of persons with Barrett's epithelia will develop an adenocarcinoma. The earliest symptom of either type of esophageal cancer is a mild dysphagia that is apt to be ignored. Consequently, by the time of diagnosis, the cancer is liable to have penetrated the esophageal wall—which is relatively thin, being composed of only two tissue layers—and has metastasized primarily via the lymphatics to nearby vital organs. The overall 5-year survival rate for both types of esophageal cancer is near 20%, still miserable but much better than the 5% of only a decade ago.

All the distractors represent different causes of dysphagia. Diffuse esophageal spasm (choice **A**; also known as "nutcracker esophageus") produces dysphagia and chest pain that is often relieved with nitroglycerine. It is characterized by uncoordinated spasms that occur after a swallow. A barium study will reveal a "corkscrew" esophageus. It is treated with bougienage, calcium channel blockers, or nitrates. Achalasia (choice **B**) is caused by incoordination of the esophageal peristaltic muscles and the failure of the lower esophageal sphincter (LES) to relax due to a lack of inhibitory input from nonadrenergic, noncholinergic, ganglionic cells. It is also associated with dysphagia for solids and liquids, but it is a rare disorder, with an incidence in the United States of about 1 per 100,000 and unlike esophageal cancer does not primarily affect older males and is not progressive. The proximal esophagus is dilated and aperistaltic. In 20%–25% of patients it is treated with pneumatic dilatation, drugs that decrease the LES's tone (e.g., nifedipine), or surgery (esophagocardiomyotomy). An esophageal stricture (choice **C**) is a narrowing of the esophageal lumen that inhibits the passage of foods. It usually is caused by scarring, most often by gastric juice due to chronic GERD at the distal end; however, stricture formation also can occur in response to other types of trauma, including swallowing caustic solutions, chronic swallowing of pills without water, or residual scarring after surgery. The usual treatment is dilation. A Schatzki ring (choice **D**) is usually characterized by an intermittent, nonprogressive dysphagia for solid foods that occurs while consuming a heavy meal with meat that was "wolfed down"; hence the pseudonym the "steakhouse syndrome." Sometimes the meal is regurgitated, relieving the block, and eating can be resumed. There is no known etiology but such a ring has been observed in 6%–15% of older patients undergoing a barium swallow. Despite their common occurrence, only 0.5% of those with rings have significant symptoms. The presence and severity of symptoms correlate with the diameter of the ring's lumen. Radiographic barium swallow or endoscopy is used to confirm the diagnosis, and if deemed advisable, the ring can be ruptured by dilatation. Zenker's diverticulum (choice **F**) is the most common acquired diverticulum of the esophagus and is treated by surgery. Because of stagnant food collected in the pouch, the patient has halitosis. Esophageal varices (choice **G**) are caused by portal hypertension.

### 17 The answer is E *Preventive Medicine and Public Health*

The odds ratio is a method of estimating relative risk in case-control studies:

$$\text{Odds Ratio} = \frac{\text{Odds of exposure among the diseased group}}{\text{Odds of exposure among the disease-free group}}$$

Using the data from the table, the numerator is $(10 \div 2)$ and the denominator is $(50 \div 300)$. Thus (choice **E**) $(10 \div 2) \div (50 \div 300) = 30$

Choices **A**, $300 \div 50 = 6$; **B**, $50 \div 10 = 5$; **C**, $60 \div (2 + 10) = 5$; and **D**, $(300 \div 2) \div (60 \div 10) = 25$ are incorrect.

### 18 The answer is A *Medicine*

The pattern HBsAg negative, anti-HBc negative, HBsAg anti-HBs negative is that for a susceptible person; there is no surface antigen in the serum, nor is there anti–surface or anti–core antibody the serum. This must be the pattern that this lady demonstrated at the time of her marriage because 4 months later, she demonstrated symptoms of acute hepatitis B (HB) (choice **A** is correct).

HBsAg negative, anti-HBc positive, anti-HBs positive (choice **B**) represents natural immunity because there is no surface antigen (no infection) but there is antibody against both the core and surface antigens; thus, the person having this pattern must have been exposed to HBV and recovered. HBsAg negative, anti-HBc negative, anti-HBs positive (choice **C**) is the pattern you would expect from a person made immune by vaccination; again, there is no infection, but this time, the anti-HBc reaction is negative, meaning the person did not see the intact virus. (The anti-HBc reaction appears at the onset of symptoms in acute hepatitis B and persists for life. Therefore, the presence of anti-HBc antibodies indicates previous or ongoing infection with hepatitis B virus but does not define a time frame; conversely, the absence of such antibodies means there has been no infection.) But the anti-HBs reaction is positive because this is the antigen used to vaccinate against HB. The pattern HBsAg positive, anti-HBc positive, IgM anti-HBc positive, and anti-HBs negative (choice **D**) is the one shown by an acutely infected person; the surface antigen is positive, meaning the virus is thriving; type M antibody has been made against the core antigen, indicating that the infected person has just begun (within the past 6 months) to mount an immune defense; moreover, no antibody has yet been made against the surface antigen. HBsAg positive, anti-HBc positive, IgM anti-HBc negative, anti-HBs negative (choice **E**) shows chronic infection; surface antigen is positive, but antibodies against it are not present whereas core antibodies are. The absence of IgM anti-HBc antibodies means this is not a new infection. Choice **F**, HBsAg negative, anti-HBc positive, and anti-HBs negative most likely indicates a resolved infection. There is no active infection (it is HBsAg and anti-HBs negative), but the core antibody is positive (there had been an active infection). However, less likely possibilities, still worthy of consideration are that it could be a false-positive anti-HBc test, in which case the person is susceptible; or a low-level chronic infection; or an acute infection still in the process of being resolved.

HB is a liver disease transmitted by exposure of a person who never has had the disease or never been vaccinated against it with blood, semen, or another body fluid from an infected person. Some infected people develop an acute short-term illness, whereas others develop a chronic long-term illness. Up to 1.4 million people in the United States and 350 million people worldwide may have chronic HB. Most are unaware of their infection, since they may have no symptoms. As a result, they can spread the disease to others, including people they live with, sexual partners, and for women, their newborns. Consequently, testing is now recommended by the U.S. Centers for Disease Control (CDC) for the following groups of persons: those born in geographic regions with HBsAg prevalence of $\geq 2\%$; U.S.-born persons not vaccinated as infants whose parents were born in geographic regions with HBsAg prevalence of $\geq 8\%$; injection-drug users; men who have sex with men; persons with elevated liver enzyme activities of unknown etiology; persons who require immunosuppressive therapy; pregnant women; infants born to HBsAg-positive mothers; household contacts and sex partners of HBV-infected persons; individuals who are exposed to blood or body fluid from infected persons (e.g., needlestick injury to a health care worker); and persons infected with human immunodeficiency virus (HIV). Most adults will recover spontaneously from an acute HBV infection. Unfortunately, that is not true for babies, who generally acquire a chronic infection. Infections are defined as being acute during the first 6 months following infection. A positive test after 6 months means the person has a chronic infection that can last a lifetime. Most individuals with chronic HB live long healthy lives, provided they are careful and avoid alcohol and drugs or foods that might stress the liver; however, they can infect others, so all close household contacts and sexual partners should be vaccinated. During the past couple of decades, drugs have been developed that slow down the progression of the disease (but do not cure it); this has helped make the optimistic outcome described possible. Presently there are seven U.S. Food and Drug Administration (FDA) drugs approved to treat HB. They are α-interferon, pegylated interferon, lamivudine, dipivoxil adefovir, telbivudine, tenofovir, and entecavir.

## 19 The answer is A *Pediatrics*

Croup, also known as laryngotracheobronchitis (choice **A**), is most commonly observed in infants between 6 months and 3 years of age. Caused primarily by parainfluenza virus, it typically presents with prodromal symptoms of an upper respiratory infection. The child then develops fever and a brassy, barking, seal-like cough, with intermittent inspiratory stridor. Acute respiratory distress can develop. The diagnosis of croup in a child older than 3 years should prompt suspicion of an underlying anatomic abnormality.

Pertussis (choice **B**) usually occurs in unimmunized infants and is usually preceded by a prodromal catarrhal stage with conjunctivitis. Spasms of coughing end with an inspiratory whoop. In younger infants, the whoop is not present, and the signs are more subtle (e.g., apnea and cyanosis). Acute epiglottitis (choice **C**) is a rare disease among children in the United States because of the *Haemophilus influenzae* B vaccine. However, occasional cases of epiglottitis from *H. influenzae* B may occur in unimmunized children, and there are also some cases of epiglottitis caused by group A streptococci. In a previous age of greater prevalence of epiglottitis, the peak incidence was commonly seen in the 3- to 7-year-old age group; however, infants and adults with epiglottitis have been well described. Drooling is usually present, but the barking cough is absent. Bronchiolitis (choice **D**) and asthma (choice **E**) can present with retractions of the intercostal muscles and nasal flaring, but wheezing is usually present.

## 20 The answer is C *Surgery*

The hallmark of a squamous cell carcinoma (choice **C**) is an open sore that won't heal. It is the second most prevalent form of skin cancer, with a yearly incidence in the United States of about 200,000 cases per year. Most occur in elderly subjects on areas exposed to the sun and are more prevalent in light-skinned individuals with an early history of time spent outdoors as a youth. Most of them are slow growing but if left untreated, will eventually penetrate the dermis and invade underlying tissue. A small fraction may become malignant. As a rule, squamous cell carcinomas of the lip are most dangerous; these are most commonly found among habitual pipe smokers.

Actinic keratosis (choice **A**) is a reddening and roughening of the skin found in sun-exposed areas, most commonly in light-skinned elders. It may present as a single spot, as in the case described, or it may be spread over a wider area, giving the affected person a blotchy appearance. Some 15% will transform into a cancer, almost always a squamous cell carcinoma, as in the case described. A basal cell carcinoma (choice **B**) is the most common of all the skin cancers. It has been estimated that some 800,000 Americans are affected at any given time. It too appears to be sun induced and is most commonly found on the exposed areas of skin in lightly pigmented persons. They have several modes of presentation, the most common one being a shiny, pearly, translucent nodule. Basal cells carcinomas arise from the basal cells of the epidermis and almost never metastasize. A nodular melanoma (choice **D**) is the most aggressive of all the melanomas. It generally is first recognized as a pigmented, usually dark brown or black, bump or node. Unlike most melanomas, it does not initially spread superficially but rapidly grows into deeper tissues, infiltrating the subcutaneous lymphatics and metastasizing to the nodes. The prognosis is understandably poor. Contrary to common opinion, nodular and other melanomas (with the exception of lentigo melanoma) are not usually induced by exposure to the sun, and more melanomas are found on the trunk or limbs than on the face or other exposed areas. A herpes infection (choice **E**) may exist as an open sore but rarely as an isolated lesion and is never preceded by a rough, pinkish lesion.

**21** **The answer is D** *Psychiatry*

Tardive dyskinesia (choice **D**) emerges in a substantial number of patients who have had long-term treatment with antipsychotics. This dyskinesia consists of choreoathetoid movements that are often first evident in the fingers and tongue, but later become more generalized, extending to the face, then to the limbs, and eventually even to the trunk in the most severe cases. Unfortunately, the symptoms do not necessarily reverse themselves when the drug is withdrawn and are difficult to treat, often creating untenable embarrassment for an indefinite period. It is not clear whether long-term use of newer antipsychotic medications is less likely to cause tardive dyskinesia. Clozapine is the only antipsychotic medication that is not associated with the condition.

Akathisia (choice **A**) also is sometimes drug induced; it is characterized by motor restlessness caused by painful feelings of inner tension and anxiety. It too is often induced by antipsychotic medications. Huntington disease (choice **B**) is also characterized by choreoathetoid movements, but also by increasingly severe behavioral and cognitive problems, and eventually dementia. It is inherited as an autosomal dominant trait due to a repeat expansion of a CAG trinucleotide sequence at the beginning of the Huntington gene sequence. Normal individuals have 11 to 34 CAG repeats; Huntington disease–afflicted individuals have 37 to 121; the longer the sequence, the earlier the onset of symptoms. Moreover, the number of repeats increases as the affected gene is passed on from generation to generation. Parkinsonism (choice **C**) (aka pseudo-Parkinson disease) is a catchall phrase used to describe disease conditions that mimic classical idiopathic Parkinson disease by presenting with tremor, bradykinesia, rigidity, and postural instability or impaired postural reflexes; as is true with Parkinson disease, these dyskinetic traits result from striatal dopamine deficiencies. There is a very rare X-linked recessive type almost exclusively found among young Filipino men, but nonidiopathic parkinsonism is more often drug induced, commonly by neuroleptics. Wilson disease (choice **E**) can also present with a dyskinesis mimicking parkinsonism, but is an autosomal recessive condition affecting copper metabolism and usually has an early onset.

**22** **The answer is D** *Medicine*

Chronic bronchitis is a recurrent problem defined by coughing up an abnormal quantity of viscous mucus nearly every day for at least 3 months of the year for two or more consecutive years, clearly this lady meets this definition (choice **D**). In chronic bronchitis, the mucociliary response that normally clears bacteria and mucus from the bronchia is inhibited by damage to the endothelium caused by pollutants, primarily those caused by cigarette smoke. The inability to clear bacteria efficiently makes these persons vulnerable to catching colds, as described for the case described. The inflamed endothelium, combined with loss of supporting alveolar attachments, allows airway walls to deform and narrow the airway lumen; this, plus the excess phlegm, obstructs the bronchia, causing the obstructive component of chronic bronchitis. The body responds by decreasing ventilation and increasing cardiac output, resulting in a rapid circulation of hypo-oxygenated blood. This produces hypoxia and eventually polycythemia, hypercapnia, and respiratory acidosis; these effects in turn cause pulmonary artery vasoconstriction, cor pulmonale, and signs of right heart failure. The difficulty these patients have in exhaling caused by the blockage of the bronchia tends to make these patients purse their lips, and the hypoxia makes the lips take on a blueish tinge. Consequently, persons with long-term chronic bronchitis are called "blue bloaters."

Emphysema (choice **A**) is defined as an abnormal, permanent enlargement of the air spaces distal to the terminal bronchioles accompanied by destruction of their walls without obvious fibrosis. It is believed that noxious irritants found in cigarette smoke (and less often to other pollutants) activate polymorphonuclear leukocytes and macrophages, which release human leukocyte elastase and other proteases; these eventually overwhelm the antiproteases of the lung, resulting in tissue destruction. As the alveolar septae and the pulmonary capillary bed are eroded, the ability to oxygenate circulating blood is diminished; the body compensates for these events by reducing cardiac output and hyperventilating. This results in a limited blood flow through a fairly well oxygenated lung. Because of low cardiac output and the collapse of the alveoli, the rest of the body suffers from tissue hypoxia and generalized cachexia. Eventually, these patients develop muscle wasting and weight loss and can be recognized as "pink puffers."

Both chronic bronchitis and emphysema lead to chronic obstructive pulmonary disease (COPD), an irreversible chronic disease state caused by obstructive air flow. The prevalence of COPD in the United States has been estimated to be between 8%–17% for men and 10%–19% for women (the prevalence rates increased in women by 30% in the last decade); COPD is also the fourth leading cause of death in the United States. Although most cases display characteristics of both chronic bronchitis and emphysema, it has been estimated that chronic bronchitis predominates in 85%–88% of the cases.

Acute bronchitis (choice **B**) refers to short-term inflammations of the tracheobronchial tree caused by infections, allergens, or irritants. Although found in all age groups, bronchitis is diagnosed most frequently in children younger than 5 years. In asthma (choice **C**), the airways narrow as they become inflamed, constrict, and produce excess mucus in response to a triggering stimulant such as an allergen, an irritant, temperature changes, exertion, or emotional stress. These responses of the airways cause symptoms such as wheezing, shortness of breath, chest tightness, and coughing. Between episodes, patients usually feel well but they may develop shortness of breath more rapidly while exercising and retain it longer after exercise than the nonasthmatic individual. Symptoms of asthma range from mild to life-threatening but most often can be controlled by use of bronchodilators, oral drugs, and/or environmental changes. Asthma can be mistakenly diagnosed as acute bronchitis if the patient has no prior history of asthma. In one study, one-third of patients who had been determined to have recurrent bouts of acute bronchitis were eventually identified as having asthma. Smoker's cough (choice **E**) typically is an early morning cough demonstrated by most smokers. Nonsmokers clear harmful substances from their lungs via the action of cilia, which beat outward, thereby sweeping the bronchi clean. Smokers, however, both accumulate more toxic materials in their lungs than do nonsmokers and also cigarette smoke poisons the action of the cilia. Consequently, during the day, these toxic, irritating substances accumulate in smoker's lungs. However, during the night, during which the smoker usually refrains from smoking, some cilia recover and begin working again and after waking up, the smoker coughs, trying to clear away the poisons that built up the previous day. Unfortunately, prolonged smoking leads to the permanent destruction of the cilia and chronic bronchitis.

### 23 The answer is B *Preventive Medicine and Public Health*

The study clearly demonstrated an extension in the lifespan of patients with acute leukemia. Thus, there will be a larger number of patients with active leukemia at any given point in time. In other words, the *prevalence* will increase (choice **B**).

There is no evidence that the drug influences the rate at which new cases of acute leukemia occur, which is the definition of incidence. Thus, it cannot be said that the incidence either increases (choice **A**) or decreases (choice **C**). Based on the aforementioned explanation, it is apparent that the other choices, namely, **D** and **E**, are incorrect.

### 24 The answer is D *Pediatrics*

Esophageal atresia is an esophageal malformation causing upper intestinal obstruction. In approximately 85% of cases, a fistula between the trachea and distal esophagus is present, usually allowing air to enter the abdomen (choice **D**).

Cyanosis that occurs at rest but is relieved by crying (choice **A**) is characteristic of choanal atresia, which is diagnosed by the inability to pass a catheter through each nares into the nasopharynx. There is an association with polyhydramnios during pregnancy, not oligohydramnios (choice **B**). Often, a catheter used at birth for resuscitation cannot be inserted into the stomach; there is an inability not an ability to pass a catheter into the stomach (choice **C**). Approximately 50% of infants with esophageal atresia have associated anomalies, the most common being cardiac anomalies, not renal (choice **E**).

### 25 The answer is C *Medicine*

The higher-than-normal values for serum creatinine and blood urea nitrogen (BUN) levels could indicate decreased glomerular filtration rate and kidney damage. Moreover, diabetic nephropathy is a common complication of diabetes, but it is not inevitable; the prevalence of microalbuminuria (an early symptom of developing renal failure) among long-term diabetics is about 25%. So, although it is possible that this person's high creatinine and BUN levels are due to his diabetes, there is no evidence indicating this is actually true and the question itself is focused on one of the many drugs he is taking. Moreover, analgesic nephropathy is a well-known medical phenomenon often involving ibuprofen, one of the drugs this patient has been taking (choice **C**). A recent (1/28/08) *New Times* article succinctly describes the possible toxic role of ibuprofen: "Ibuprofen relieves pain by interfering with the body's production of prostaglandin, a substance involved in inflammation. But at the same time, the drug constricts blood flow. Normally, the change poses little risk if used for a short period. But for those whose blood flow to the kidneys is already reduced by kidney, heart or liver damage, flu, or aging, ibuprofen could lead to acute kidney failure." A Johns Hopkins study gave 12 women 800 mg ibuprofen 3 times a day; after 8 days, three of these women developed kidney failure. The symptoms of kidney failure reversed after the drug was withdrawn, and after recovery, these women were given 400 mg three times a day; two of these three developed acute renal failure once again. The nine women who did not go into kidney failure after 8 days were continued on the 800 mg until the 11th day, when the experiment was stopped after these women showed changes in renal function, although they did not go into renal failure. These and other studies clearly demonstrated that high doses of ibuprofen can be toxic to some individuals, causing acute renal failure. There are also anecdotal reports of low doses causing renal failure when administered for longer periods of time. Whether this induces chronic irreversible renal failure is not clear, but these reports clearly indicate that ibuprofen and other analgesics should be used with caution in patients whose kidney functions might be compromised with conditions such as diabetes.

Pioglitazone (choice **A**) and rosiglitazone are thiazolidinediones (aka, glitazones), antidiabetic drugs used to treat type 2 diabetes. Their primary mode of action is to activate insulin receptors on insulin-sensitive cells, but they also reduce liver gluconeogenesis and may also decrease triglyceride levels and increase the concentration of high-density lipoprotein cholesterol. The first thiazolidinedione approved was troglitazone, which had to be withdrawn from the market because of hepatic-toxicity. Although neither pioglitazone nor rosiglitazone seem to cause liver toxicity, both have been required by the U.S. Food and Drug Administration (FDA) to add a black-box warnings about heart failure risk for diabetics, and in 2008, the American Diabetes Association and the European Association for the Study of Diabetes advised that the use of rosiglitazone (Avandia) may promote weight gain and edema, as well as heart failure. In addition, a May 2009 report in the *American Journal of Ophthalmology* indicates that these drugs also stimulate the development of macular degeneration in as many as 60% of diabetic patients. In September 2010 the FDA began a review of pioglitazone because of its possible promotion of bladder cancer and in November of 2010 they restricted used of rosiglitazone to patients with type 2 diabetes that cannot be controlled by another medication. However, of direct pertinence to this question, neither thiazolidinedione has been reported to cause kidney problems. Hydrochlorothiazide (choice **B**) is a diuretic that works by blocking salt and fluid reabsorption in the kidneys, thereby increasing urine output, which in turn decreases resistance to systolic blood pressure. Consequently, it has been used to treat hypertension and edema caused by many conditions, including kidney failure; however, it has not been accused of being a kidney toxin. Although overdoses of levothyroxine or ingestion by children can cause thyroid storm, this artificial thyroid hormone is not a known kidney toxin (choice **D**). Glucose tolerance factor (choice **E**) has not been found to be toxic in doses commonly employed.

### 26 The answer is B *Obstetrics and Gynecology*

This woman is in the third stage of labor, which starts with delivery of the infant and ends with delivery of the placenta. The upper limit of normal for duration of the third stage of labor is 30 minutes. The factor that contributes most to the mechanism of the third stage of labor is avulsion of anchoring villi by contracting myometrium (choice **B**).

It is true that the estrogen level falls after delivery of the placenta, providing the hormonal stimulus for breast engorgement, but this decrease does not contribute to the third stage of labor (choice **A**). The levels of prolactin and umbilical vein $P_{CO_2}$ are not involved in placental separation (choices **C** and **D**). A progesterone-mediated decrease in gap junctions is not relevant to the third stage of labor or placental separation (choice **E**).

### 27 The answer is C *Medicine*

Maturity-onset diabetes of the young (MODY) describes a group of monogenetic forms of diabetes inherited in an autosomal dominant fashion. Although not nearly as common as classical type 1 or type 2 diabetes mellitus, MODY diabetes is not rare; the six best characterized forms collectively account for as many as 5% of all cases of diabetes, and according to the Centers for Disease Control and Prevention (CDC) June 24, 2008 press release, 24 million Americans suffer from diabetes mellitus, thus the 5% of diabetics diagnosed with MODY amount to 1.2 million individuals; moreover, patients with MODY are often overlooked and misdiagnosed. In addition to the six well-documented types of MODY, there are several addition rare, less well characterized forms. As many as 70% of all reported cases of MODYs are MODY 3; this is also the form that is most easily confused with type 1 diabetes, as in the cases described in the above vignette. MODY 3 type diabetes is caused by a mutation in the HNF1alpha gene located on chromosome 12 (choice **C**). This gene plays an important role in the differentiation of pancreatic β cells, and several different mutations in this gene share the common clinical effect of causing MODY 3 diabetes by diminishing β-cell function. Typically, mutations in this gene induce symptoms of diabetes before the age of 25, and not uncommonly, these patients were first diagnosed as having type 1 diabetes and were being treated with insulin. Once properly diagnosed, treatment can be switched to oral antidiabetic agents with excellent results for years. This switch in treatment is not a trivial difference from the patient's point of view, saving him or her much money and the many complications of using insulin properly.

MODY 1 is caused by a mutation in the HNF4A gene on chromosome 20 (choice A). The gene product of the HNF4A gene is transcriptional factor 14 (TCF14) (also known as HNF4-α), which helps regulate the HNF1α transcriptional factor, coded for by the HNF1&α gene mentioned above. Thus, mutations in HNF4A also affect development of pancreatic β cells. In MODY 1, the β cells usually produce enough insulin to avoid a diagnosis of diabetes until the affected individual reaches adulthood, but usually is still diagnosed with diabetes before middle age. These patients are often diagnosed as early-onset type 2 patients. MODY 2 is caused by one of several different mutations on the GCK gene for glucokinase on chromosome 7 (choice **B**). In addition to its catalytic function, glucokinase also triggers insulin release from the pancreatic β cells when circulating glucose levels surpass about 90 mg/dL (5 mM). The mutations causing MODY 2 result in a glucokinase that is less efficient in producing this effect. Consequently, the otherwise normal β cells do not secrete sufficient insulin until the circulating glucose concentration exceeds 126 mg/dL (7 mM) and patients have a chronic, usually asymptomatic, hyperglycemia that often is only discovered by chance, most often in women during pregnancy screening. MODY 4 is caused by a mutation on the gene coding the IPF1 homeobox on chromosome 13 (choice **D**); IPF1 is a transcription factor required for pancreatic development. This disease was discovered in a family in which a homozygous child was born without a pancreas. Various heterozygous relatives were studied and were found to have mild hyperglycemia or diabetes; these all could be controlled with either diet or oral antidiabetics. MODY 5 is due to a mutation in HNF1β (choice **E**). This very rare mutation causes pancreatic atrophy and renal disease. The pancreatic atrophy is responsible for varying degrees of insulin insufficiency and can induce diabetes that may develop in early infancy or much later during adulthood. The kidney manifestations are often more severe than those relating to glucose hemostasis, and MODY 5 is often discovered during the workup for kidney disease. Patients may also have various malfunctions of the reproductive system. MODY 6 is produced by mutations in the neurogenic differentiation factor 1 gene located on chromosome 2 (choice **F**). To date, only three kindreds with mutations causing MODY6 have been identified. In these kindreds, most family members first developed diabetes after the age 40; consequently, other than family history, their symptoms are essentially typical of type 2 diabetes.

**28** **The answer is E** *Medicine*

Gitelman syndrome (choice **E**) is a disease of the kidney's distal convoluted tubule that results in the loss of magnesium, sodium, potassium, and chloride ions into the urine. Most cases are either isolated or inherited in an autosomal recessive fashion, although there is at least one reported family in which the disease was reported to be inherited in an autosomal dominant manner. The most common cause of Gitelman syndrome is a mutation in *SLC12 A3* gene, although a few cases have been attributed to aberrations in *CLCKKB*. Several different mutations have been described in *SLC12 A3* gene; this may account for differences in symptoms reported in various families. Most cases are relatively benign but some are more severe. The product of *SLC12 A3* gene functions in the distal convoluted tubule as part of the thiazide-sensitive NaCl co-transporter, and homozygous loss of function mutations in this protein induces a hypocalciuria, but there is excess urinary loss of sodium, potassium, and magnesium ions. Hydrogen ion is retained, causing an alkaline urine. These changes are reflected by low circulating levels of potassium and magnesium ions, which are responsible for the symptoms of fatigue, muscle weakness, spasms, and pain. As a rule, the disease is not recognized until adolescence and often not until middle or even old age. A high-carbohydrate meal precipitates an attack because increased levels of glucose increases insulin levels, and the resultant increase in glucose utilization lowers circulating potassium ion levels. Treatment usually consists of replacement of potassium and magnesium ion. Some investigators also recommend an antiprostaglandin such as oral indomethacin, which was found to assist in returning potassium ion levels to normal in at least one case.

In so much as thiazide diuretics act on the same NaCl co-transporter as affected in Gitelman syndrome, it is not surprising that thiazide diuretic toxicity produces effects similar to Gitelman syndrome. However, in the case presented here, the patient states she does not take medication, consequently choice **A** is not correct. Bartter syndrome (choice **B**) refers to a group of autosomal recessive conditions, all of which, like Gitelman syndrome, cause the loss of excess potassium and magnesium ions into the urine. At one time, Gitelman syndrome was thought of as a mild form of Bartter. However, they clearly are distinct entities. Bartter syndrome usually makes its presence know in neonates or early antenatals and essentially always before the age of 6 years; in contrast, Gitelman strikes adults. Urinary excretion of magnesium is high in Gitelman syndrome and within the reference range in Bartter syndrome; conversely urinary calcium ion levels are high in Bartter syndrome and low or within the reference range in Gitelman syndrome. The final clinching difference is that different genes are involved. Recent genetic analyses have shown that there are five Bartter syndrome variants, as summarized in the following table.

| Bartter Type | Gene | Affected Site | Age of Affect |
|---|---|---|---|
| Type I | *SLC12A1* | The Na-K-2Cl transporter in the distal convoluted tubule | Neonatal |
| Type II | *ROMK1* | Apical potassium channel | Neonatal |
| Type III | *CLCNKB* | Basal chloride channel in the thick ascending limb of Henle | Classic antenatal |
| Type IV | *BSND* | In barttin[a], a subunit protein of the basal chloride channel in the thick ascending limb of Henle | Neonatal with deafness |
| Type V | *CLCNKA* | In barttin, a subunit protein of the basal chloride channel in the thick ascending limb of Henle | Neonatal with deafness |

[a]Barttin is required for potassium-chloride membrane currents and is located in the inner ear as well as in the kidney.

Dent syndrome (choice **C**) is a rare X-linked recessive disorder sometimes called *idiopathic hypercalcuria*. It is caused by mutations in the renal chloride channel CLCN5, and it causes low-molecular-weight protein-uria, hypercalciuria, aminoaciduria, and hypophosphatemia. Affected males will usually show symptoms in early adulthood, including tubular proteinuria, hypercalcuria, calcium nephrolithiasis, nephrocalcinosis and hypophosphatemic rickets; a significant percentage will have end-stage renal failure before the age of 50. Because of these properties, it is one of the several diseases that cause Fanconi syndrome. Andersen-Tawil syndrome (choice **D**) is an autosomal dominant disease characterized by a triad of symptoms: (1) episodic flaccid muscle weakness (i.e., periodic paralysis typified by weakness that occurs spontaneously following prolonged rest or after rest following exertion); (2) ventricular arrhythmias with a prolonged QT interval; and (3) physical anomalies that may include low-set ears, eyes set far apart, small mandible, fifth-digit clin-odactyly, syndactyly, short stature, scoliosis, and mild learning disability. Most commonly, serum potassium levels are reduced during periods of weakness. The disease is caused by mutations in *KCNJ2*, which codes for the inward rectifier potassium channel 2, known as Kir 2.1, which is involved in setting and stabilizing rest-ing membrane potentials and is primarily expressed in skeletal muscle, heart, and brain. Phosphatidylinositol 4, 5 bisphosphate ($PIP_2$) is an important regulator of Kir2.1 and many *KCNJ2* mutations alter $PIP_2$ binding.

**29** **The answer is A** *Preventive Medicine and Public Health*

Patients with sickle cell disease are homozygous for HbS. Because in the case described only one potential parent has the HbS allele, the only way their child could inherit two HbS genes is if one of the father's nor-mal hemoglobin (Hb) genes underwent a new mutation in a sperm cell, an extremely unlikely event. Therefore, their child does not have a reasonable chance of inheriting the disease (choice **A**). However, there is a 1:4 chance that their child would be a carrier. Such heterozygous carriers may have mild symptoms and are said to have the *sickle cell trait*.

The probability that two heterozygous carriers of the trait will have a child with the disease is 1:4 (choice **B**); that is, 25% of their children will have the disease; whereas 50% will have the trait and another 25% will be normal. Assuming there is no knowledge of family histories or Hb patterns, choice **C** (1/144) represents the probability that two carriers will meet. That is, the carrier rate among African Americans is approximately 1 in 12 and $1/12 \times 1/12$ equals 1/144. Choice **D** (1/576) corresponds to the likelihood of a child having the disease if two African Americans having no knowledge of family histories or Hb patterns had children. As indicated in choice **C**, the random chance of two African American heterozygotes meeting is 1/144. Since only 25% of their children will have the disease (see choice **B** above), those having the disease will equal $1/144 \times 1/4$, or 1/576. Choice **E** is not a sensible representation of the probability of a child inheriting sickle cell anemia.

**30** **The answer is A** *Obstetrics and Gynecology*

Determination of gestational age is of crucial importance. The last menstrual period, obtained from patient history, albeit subjective, can be very useful in identifying the number of pregnancy weeks, if it is reliable. An objective parameter for estimating the duration of pregnancy is ultrasonic measurement of fetal size. The ear-lier in pregnancy that the sonogram is performed, the more accurate it is, because the proportionate change in fetal growth from week to week is greater earlier in the pregnancy than it is later. As pregnancy progress-es, the accuracy of gestational age estimation from sonographic measurement of fetal size is progressively less. Therefore, sonograms performed at 20 (choice **B**), 25 (choice **C**), 30 (choice **D**), and 40 (choice **E**) weeks' gestation would not be as precise as a sonogram performed at 10 weeks' gestation (choice **A**).

**31** **The answer is C** *Pediatrics*

Pertussis (whooping cough; choice **C**) is an extremely contagious respiratory disease caused by *Bordetella pertussis*. Neither natural disease nor vaccination can provide lifelong immunity against the disease. In the United States, infants have the highest morbidity associated with pertussis; however, the majority of reported cases (67%) now occur in adolescents or adults. After a 1-week incubation period, children present with three successive stages of the disease. The catarrhal stage consists of symptoms of an upper respiratory infection, thick nasal discharge, and conjunctivitis. The paroxysmal stage is characterized by spasms of forceful coughing ending in an inspiratory whoop. The cough is strong enough to force vomiting; and facial redness and cyanosis are frequently observed. Often, there is no whoop in infants, but apnea may be manifested. In the convalescent stage, the cough and vomiting gradually subside. Cough can persist for several months. Petechiae and conjunctival hemorrhages are seen. Otitis media is a common complication. Complete blood count (CBC) usually shows leukocytosis, predominantly lymphocytes toward the end of the catarrhal stage and during the paroxysmal stage.

The diagnosis of acute lymphoblastic leukemia (choice **A**) would be suggested by the presence of blast cells on a peripheral blood smear. Patients with *Chlamydia trachomatis* pneumonia (choice **B**) have cough, tachypnea, and lack of fever. Eosinophilia ($>400$ cells/mm$^3$) may be present. Patients with bronchiolitis (choice **D**) usually have a normal white blood cell (WBC) count and differential count. The peripheral WBC count of patients with respiratory syncytial viral pneumonitis (choice **E**) tends to be normal or elevated, and the differential count may be normal with a neutrophilic or mononuclear prevalence.

**32** **The answer is D** *Pediatrics*

The presentation of this patient is most consistent with the diagnosis of acute otitis media. The most common causes of acute otitis media are *Streptococcus pneumoniae* (choice **D**), found in approximately 40% of cases; *Haemophilus influenzae* (choice **A**) was found in approximately 25%–30% prior to the advent of a vaccine; and *Moraxella catarrhalis* (choice **C**), in approximately 15%; whereas *Staphylococcus aureus* (choice **B**), group A *Streptococcus*, and gram-negative organisms (e.g., *Pseudomonas aeruginosa*) are less common causes of acute otitis media, and together account for approximately 5% of cases. Respiratory syncytial virus (RSV) (choice **E**) and other respiratory viruses are also associated with acute otitis media. However, even though otitis media can be a sequela of bronchiolitis caused by RSV, rarely, if ever, is the aspirate from the middle ear solely positive for RSV. These children usually have a bacterial pathogen isolated in their aspirate. It remains to be discovered whether viruses alone can cause acute otitis media or if their presence only enhances the chances for bacterial invasion.

**33** **The answer is D** *Surgery*

Fractures of the shaft of the humerus involve the radial nerve (choice **D**), which winds around its posterior aspect, in the radial groove. As a result, a wrist drop may be present.

Dislocations of the shoulder or fractures involving the surgical neck of the humerus may be associated with trauma to the axillary nerve (choice **A**). In such an event, sensations over the lateral aspect of the shoulder will be impaired. The median nerve (choice **B**) may be traumatized in supracondylar fractures of the humerus. The brachial artery may be compressed as well. The ulnar nerve (choice **C**) can be injured after posterior dislocation of the elbow. The brachial plexus (choice **E**) is not injured in fractures of the upper extremities. Acute lateral flexion of the neck (e.g., after a fall) can damage the lower cord of the brachial plexus.

**34** **The answer is C** *Obstetrics and Gynecology*

The case presentation describes the findings in a patient with preeclampsia associated with acute diffuse vasoconstriction (choice **C**), which typically occurs in primigravidas during the last trimester of pregnancy. This entity is characterized by sustained hypertension (with blood pressure $\geq 140/90$) along with significant proteinuria (1–2+ on dipstick testing or $\geq 300$ mg on a 24-hour urine collection).

Preeclampsia is characterized by an enhanced angiotensin response rather than a blunted one (choice **A**), which is the normal physiologic response with pregnancy. This condition is usually unrelated to elevated β-endorphin level (choice **B**), which is a frequent physiologic stress response to the pain of labor. The history provided is not characteristic of primary renal disease (choice **D**) or chronic hypertension (choice **E**), which is diagnosed if the hypertension either was present prior to the pregnancy or had its onset prior to 20 weeks' gestation.

**35** **The answer is E** *Pediatrics*

Kawasaki syndrome (mucocutaneous lymph node syndrome [MLNS]) is a febrile vasculitis that affects all blood vessels but primarily affects the medium-sized arteries, with predilection for the coronary arteries. Criteria for diagnosis are unexplained fever of 5 days' duration and four of the following five conditions: bilateral nonpurulent conjunctivitis, changes of the mucosa of the oropharynx (dry, cracked lips; strawberry tongue), changes of the peripheral extremities (edema, erythema), a polymorphous rash, and cervical lymphadenopathy. Desquamation of the palms and soles is a late finding, usually appearing during the second or third week of the disease. Many experts believe that, in the presence of classic features, the diagnosis can be made before 5 days of fever. Kawasaki syndrome (choice **E**) occurs generally in children under 5 years of age. Thrombocytosis appears in the second or third week. Leukocytosis, elevated C-reactive protein, and elevated erythrocyte sedimentation rate (ESR) are common laboratory findings.

Scarlet fever (choice **A**) causes a strawberry tongue, maculopapular rash, Pastia's lines, and circumoral pallor. Acute rheumatic fever (choice **B**) is diagnosed using the Jones criteria. The Jones criteria consist of major and minor manifestations. Major criteria include carditis, polyarthritis, erythema marginatum, and subcutaneous nodules. Minor criteria include arthralgia, fever, elevated erythrocyte sedimentation rate (ESR), and C-reactive protein, as well as a prolonged PR interval. Two major criteria, or one major and two minor criteria, plus evidence of a preceding group A streptococcal infection indicate a high probability of rheumatic fever. Juvenile rheumatoid arthritis (choice **C**) includes findings of lymphadenopathy, hepatosplenomegaly, and an evanescent salmon-colored rash. Many features of toxic shock syndrome (TSS) (choice **D**), a multisystem disease, resemble those of Kawasaki disease. Both include findings of strawberry tongue, conjunctival hyperemia, and an erythematous macular rash. However, in TSS other abnormalities such as hypotension, vomiting, diffuse myalgia, azotemia, and shock help to differentiate the two.

**36** **The answer is B** *Preventive Medicine and Public Health*

Good medical practice would include counseling the patient about prevention (choice **B**).

Although parents must usually grant consent for medical procedures involving minor children, neither consent nor notifying them is necessary when they demonstrate drug or alcohol dependence, have emergencies, require medical care in pregnancy, or, as in this case, have sexually transmitted disease (choice **A**). In this case, it is not necessary to notify state health authorities (choice **C**) or his sexual partner (choice **D**), nor is it required to notify his parents after treating him (choice **E**).

**37** **The answer is E** *Surgery*

The presentation of this patient is classic for rupture of the duodenum (choice **E**). Patients have vague symptoms because the duodenum is retroperitoneal. If left untreated, mortality is almost 100%. The best way to diagnose it is to maintain a high index of suspicion and conduct repeated physical examinations. Serum amylase is often elevated but is not diagnostic. X-ray films of the abdomen reveal retroperitoneal air, which is the sine qua non of duodenal rupture. Duodenal rupture in children could also result from the use of the lap belt without shoulder support in motor vehicles. This results from acute hyperflexion of the thoracolumbar spine, which crushes the duodenum. Drivers of motor vehicles can also sustain duodenal rupture as a result of compression against the steering wheel. This possibility is greatly reduced by an air bag.

This patient does not have a ruptured spleen (choice **A**) or a ruptured liver (choice **B**), because his vital signs are stable. Moreover, neither condition is associated with midabdominal pain. Rather, pain is in the left or right upper quadrant, respectively, and there may be associated fractures of the lower ribs. A diagnostic peritoneal lavage is positive for hemorrhage, and a computed tomography (CT) scan confirms the diagnosis. Rupture of the pancreas (choice **C**) usually follows blunt trauma. Although this diagnosis is a possibility, the duodenum more usually ruptures in injuries like the one described in the scenario. Pancreatic rupture is associated with hypovolemic shock due to tear of the gastroduodenal artery. The common bile duct may be avulsed as well. Serum amylase is raised, but this alone does not confirm the diagnosis. However, a persistently elevated serum amylase suggests this possibility. The diagnosis is best established by maintaining a high index of suspicion. A CT scan confirms the diagnosis. Hematoma of the rectus muscle (choice **D**) is a benign condition. The pain is confined to the region of injury and is not vaguely defined. Pain increases with contraction of the abdominal muscles. A localized mass may be present. The diagnosis is clinical, and treatment is supportive.

**38** **The answer is B** *Medicine*

In the United States, a nonhemolytic febrile reaction happens during 3%–4% of transfusions, making it the most common type of transfusion reaction and thus the most likely reaction to have occurred in the case described (choice **B**). It is thought that the most likely cause of this reaction is the presence of antibodies against white blood cell human leucocyte antigen (HLA) in the donor blood. Another possibility is the release of cytokines from white cells during storage; however, this is most likely to happen in stored platelet preparations. Nonhemolytic febrile reactions occur most frequently in patients who have had blood transfusions before or in multiparous women. Such febrile reactions are successfully treated with acetaminophen, and some hospitals routinely give patients acetaminophen prophylactically prior to surgery and/or use prestorage leukocyte-reduced blood components, at least for high-risk patients. Once fever is noted, the transfusion must be terminated and the blood rechecked to make sure that it truly is the proper type for the patient and the blood pack in question is destroyed. This is an expensive interruption, making it worth while to take such measures to avoid it when practical.

A hemolytic transfusion reaction (choice **A**) is the most dangerous type of reaction and approximately 20 patients die each year because of it; it occurs in about 1 in 40,000 transfusions. ABO incompatibility is most common, although antibodies against Rh or other blood group antigens do occur. Most common causes are: mislabeling of the recipient's pretransfer sample, giving the wrong blood to a patient with the same name, or not checking the patient's blood bank identification tag with the identification number on the unit; a laboratory error in identifying the proper blood type very rarely occurs. The severity of the reaction depends upon the degree of incompatibility, the transfusion rate, the amount of blood product given, and the health of the recipient. Most often, the onset of symptoms is within an hour of initiation of the transfusion, but it can be delayed. If the patient is under general anesthesia, the only symptoms of the reaction may be hypotension, profuse bleeding from incision sites and mucous membranes caused by disseminated intervascular coagulation, and/or a dark urine caused by hemoglobinuria. If a hemolytic transfusion reaction is suspected, the transfusion must be stopped, the sample and patient identification rechecked, and supportive treatment begun. The initial goal of treatment is to maintain blood pressure and renal blood flow with IV isotonic saline and furosemide. A delayed hemolytic transfusion reaction (choice **C**) may occur if the patient has been exposed to an antibody level so low that it gave a negative pretransfusion test. In this case, the reaction may occur as late as 1–4 weeks after the transfusion. Usually, the reaction is not very severe, often limited to the transfused erythrocytes causing a drop in the hematocrit. If a more severe reaction does occur, it should be treated as if it were a hemolytic transfusion reaction. An allergic reaction (choice **D**) to an allergen in the donor blood is not uncommon. Usually, the reaction is mild with urticaria, edema, and maybe dizziness during or immediately after the transfusion. An anaphylaxis reaction is rare, most often occurring in IgA-deficient recipients. In the case of an anaphylactic reaction, transfusion should be stopped immediately and the reaction treated. Patients with IgA deficiency should be transfused with blood from an IgA-deficient donor. A reaction due to volume overload (choice **E**) might be induced in susceptible patients by the high osmotic load of blood products in the transfusion, which draws water into the intravascular space. To reduce this possibility, red blood cells should be infused slowly. Susceptible patients include those with renal insufficiency or cardiac problems. The patient should be observed carefully, and if signs of problems arise, the transfusion should be stopped and the patient treated; typical treatment is with a diuretic. An acute lung injury (choice **F**) may be caused by anti-HLA or anti-granulocyte antibodies in the donor plasma that agglutinate and degranulate recipient granulocytes in the recipient's lung. Such a reaction occurs in 1 case per 5,000 to 10,000 transfusions. Although many cases are mild, the reaction may cause severe acute respiratory symptoms, even death, making this the second most common cause of transfusion-related death following ABO incompatibility. In nonfatal cases, supportive therapy leads to complete recovery, but even mild incidents should be reported. Blood stored for more than 7 days has a marked decrease in the red cell 2, 3-diphosphoglylcate (DPG) level, and after 10 days, the DPG level is essentially nil. This absence enhances the affinity of hemoglobin for oxygen (choice **G**), slowing the release of oxygen to the tissues of a recipient. Such an effect can be significant in infants, sickle cell patients, and patients suffering a stroke or acute chest symptoms.

**39** **The answer is C** *Obstetrics and Gynecology*

This patient meets two criteria for mild preeclampsia: sustained blood pressure elevation ($\geq$140/90) developing after 20 weeks' gestation, along with significant proteinuria. At term, the goal of management with mild preeclampsia is prompt delivery, so induction of labor is appropriate. Patients with preeclampsia, however, are also at risk for progressing to eclampsia, which is characterized by generalized seizures. Prevention of seizures is a crucial aspect of the care of any woman with a hypertensive disorder of pregnancy. In the United States, magnesium sulfate (choice **C**) is the most commonly used preventive agent for this condition.

Phenobarbital (choice **A**), diazepam (choice **B**), and diphenylhydantoin (choice **D**) are standard anticonvulsant medications, but are not used primarily for seizure prophylaxis in preeclampsia. Randomized, controlled head-to-head studies show that magnesium sulfate is superior to these standard anticonvulsants in prevention as well as treatment of eclamptic seizures. Magnesium gluconate (choice **E**) has no anticonvulsant activity.

### 40 The answer is C   *Surgery*

This patient has sustained an epidural hematoma, which usually results from tear of the middle meningeal artery, which enters the middle cranial fossa through the foramen spinosum. Fracture of the thin temporal bone across the groove of the middle meningeal artery results in it tearing. As a consequence, the dura is stripped from the inner table of the skull, forming an expanding mass. Failure to intervene results in herniation of the uncus of the temporal lobe, pressure on the brainstem, and death. Fractures of the occipital bone tear the venous sinuses, resulting in a venous epidural hematoma. Most patients with epidural hematoma have a lucid interval (choice **C**), which is a hallmark of the condition. The initial period of coma is followed by recovery and then coma again. The pupil on the side of the lesion begins to dilate, and inequality of the pupils (anisocoria) is noted. Hyperventilation should be instituted early to decrease intracranial pressure. A computed tomography (CT) scan shows a bright-white, lens-shaped (lentiform) mass on the side of the hematoma, which represents blood that has collected between the inner table of the skull and the dura. A burr hole is made at the pterion to evacuate the hematoma. A lumbar puncture is contraindicated because it will induce herniation and death.

### 41 The answer is B   *Surgery*

This patient has sustained a basal skull fracture involving the anterior cranial fossa. The fracture occurs across the cribriform plate of the ethmoid bone. Cerebrospinal fluid (CSF) leaks through the nose (CSF rhinorrhea) and may be unilateral or bilateral. Presence of glucose in the discharge is diagnostic of CSF as its source. A computed tomography (CT) scan locates the fracture and excludes presence of injury to the frontal lobe and other areas of the brain. Hyperventilation is essential to avoid raising intracranial pressure. In about 24 hours, the patient has circumorbital discoloration, which is known as a raccoon sign (choice **B**). Blood leaks into the subcutaneous tissues of the periorbital area. This resolves on its own without treatment. Meningitis can result because of transmission of pneumococci (which are resident flora in the nose) to the intracranial cavity. In such an event, a lumbar puncture can be done, provided there is no clinical evidence of raised intracranial pressure. Performing a spinal puncture in the presence of raised intracranial pressure is fraught with risk of herniation and death. In patients with fractures of the petrous temporal bone, CSF escapes through the external auditory meatus and is associated with discoloration behind the ear (Battle's sign).

### 42 The answer is A   *Surgery*

This patient has a chronic subdural hematoma, which results from tear of the bridging veins. Cortical atrophy in alcoholics and the elderly results in stretching of the bridging veins that connect the cortical veins with the sagittal sinus. This tenuous connection may be ruptured even after minor trauma. In 20% of cases, the hematoma is bilateral. Symptoms usually begin about 3 weeks after minor head injury and include dull headache, change in personality or mental status, lack of concentration, poor memory, and seizures. Unlike Alzheimer disease, this condition is associated with fluctuating symptoms. A computed tomography (CT) scan shows a dark lesion due to a collection of blood that contains methemoglobin. Raised intracranial pressure is relatively rare in these patients, because the blood occupies the space vacated by the shrinking brain; thus, hyperventilation is usually not required. A burr hole is required to evacuate the hematoma. Photophobia (choice **A**), retinal hemorrhages, and papilledema (rare) are features of this condition.

Optic nerve atrophy (choice **D**) results in visual loss that is almost proportional to the degree of atrophy that has occurred. It is a physical sign and not a diagnosis. The etiology could be primary or secondary. In primary optic atrophy, the disk is white, has a sharp margin, and the physiologic cup and lamina cribrosa are clearly visible. The blood vessels are normal. Primary optic atrophy occurs in tabes dorsalis, in pernicious anemia, and as a consequence of chronic raised intracranial pressure, or where the optic nerve is compressed. In secondary optic atrophy, the disc is pale, margins are indistinct; the optic cup and lamina cribrosa cannot be seen. White lines may be seen along the emerging vessels, as a result of perivascular lymph sheathing. Like primary optic atrophy, secondary atrophy can result from increased intracranial pressure secondary to brain tumors. An enlarged sella (choice **E**) could result from a tumor, such as a pituitary adenoma. These patients will complain of headache and have bitemporal hemianopsia on testing of the visual field. Cavernous sinus thrombosis (choice **F**) is a rare disease that results from infection that travels in a retrograde manner via the ophthalmic or facial vein to the cavernous sinus. The patient complains of headaches and difficulty in vision, especially diplopia due to paresis of cranial nerve VI, which lies within the sinus. Oculoparesis, conjunctival edema, and blindness could occur. This is a potentially fatal condition that should be treated early.

### 43 The answer is I *Medicine*

*Listeria monocytogenes* (choice **I**) is a small gram-positive rod that is extremely virulent. Ingestion of fewer than 1,000 bacteria can cause human illness (listerosis), with an incubation period of 3–70 days. Despite the fact that healthy children and adults rarely get infected in the United States, and when they do symptoms are relatively mild, some 2,500 persons get listerosis annually and about 500 die. In large part, this is because certain segments of the population are susceptible, including pregnant women, newborns, and immunocompromised individuals, such as those with acquired immune deficiency syndrome (AIDS), persons taking steroids, the elderly, and those with chronic illnesses including diabetics and persons with kidney disease or cancer. Pregnant women are about 20 times more liable to contract listerosis than the general population; when they do, they often suffer mild symptoms but the fetuses they carry are liable to suffer more serious symptoms. Infection during pregnancy may result in abortions, stillbirths, and neonatal deaths, as in the case described; it is the third most common cause of neonatal meningitis, and produces granulomatis infantisepticum in disseminated disease. The disease is commonly transmitted by eating contaminated foods, unpasteurized dairy foods in particular, although a recent epidemic was attributed to contaminated hot dogs. The potentially long incubation period makes it difficult to trace foodborne epidemics to their source. The treatment of choice is ampicillin.

### 44

*Clostridium perfringens* (choice **E**) is a gram-positive, anaerobic, spore and toxin-forming rod. It is ubiquitous in nature and is found in soils, decaying vegetation, spoiling foods, and the human intestinal tract. Because of its ubiquitous presence and anaerobic growth properties, it can cause infections in deep wounds; before abortions were legalized, such infections commonly caused septic endometritis and even death in women undergoing illegal abortions. Although all such infections are serious health problems, most illnesses caused by *C. perfringens* are due to food poisoning. The Centers for Disease Control and Prevention (CDC) has estimated that in the United States, there are some 10,000 annual cases of food poisoning induced by *C. perfringens*. In most cases, these are due to allowing cooked preparations of meat and poultry products to cool slowly before serving or refrigerating. This permits the small number of bacteria that survive the original cooking to multiple. After 8–16 hours of incubation, disease symptoms caused by the heat-resistant enterotoxins cause abdominal cramping and diarrhea. Except in the elderly or infirm, symptoms are generally self-limiting and last for about 24 hours. Serious complications are essentially limited to infections by the C-strain of *C. perfringens*, which produce the potently ulcerative β-toxin that causes enteritis necroticans, aka the "pig-bel syndrome." Deaths from this condition commonly occur due to infection and necrosis of the intestines and from resulting septicemia. However, infection with the C-strain is very rare in the United States.

### 45 The answer is (G) *Medicine*

*Clostridium botulinum* (choice **G**) is a gram-positive rod-shaped spore-forming obligate anaerobic bacterium that produces botulinum, a neurotoxin that, in infected individuals, generates botulism, a serious paralytic illness. There are seven types of botulism toxin designated by the letters A through G; all but type G cause human illness. Annually, an average of 145 cases of botulism are reported in the United States. Of these, 15% are foodborne, caused by eating toxin-containing foods, 20% are caused by toxin produced in a wound infected with the organism, and 65% are infant botulism, which occurs in infants who ingest spores that then germinate in their intestines and release toxin. These numbers have remained relatively constant for about five decades, except that wound botulism has increased somewhat because of increased use of black tar heroin. All of these can be fatal and are considered medical emergencies. Foodborne botulism most often occurs from eating low-acid home-canned products such as asparagus, green beans, beets, carrots, and corn. Symptoms generally begin 18–36 hours after eating a contaminated food, but they can occur as early as 6 hours or as late as 10 days. The classic symptoms of botulism include double vision, blurred vision, drooping eyelids, slurred speech, difficulty swallowing, dry mouth, and placid muscle paralysis. Infants with botulism appear lethargic, suck and feed poorly, are constipated, and have a weak cry and poor muscle tone (choice **G**). Honey is a known source of bacterial spores that produce *C. botulinum* bacteria. When ingested by infants less than 1 year old, the relative high stomach pH allows the spores to germinate and produce toxin that can cause infant botulism, which affects a baby's nervous system and may result in death, although most babies with infant botulism do recover. Nonetheless, infants under 12 months of age should never be fed honey. Whether adult or infant, all these are symptoms of the muscle paralysis caused by the bacterial toxin. If untreated, these symptoms may progress to cause paralysis of the arms, legs, trunk, and respiratory muscles, potentially leading to death. In fact, the toxin is so potent that it takes only about 75 nanograms to kill a person; assuming that an average person weighs approximately 75 kg; 500 grams would be enough to kill half of the entire human population. Despite this innate toxicity, during the past five decades, the death rate in infected persons has dropped from 50% percent to 3%–5%, in large part due to the development of tri- and heptavalent equine antitoxins. Moreover, the toxin has been tamed to such an extent that it is now used to treat strabismus, blepharospasm, and hemifacial spasm. It is also prepared as Botox, which is used cosmetically to iron out wrinkles and even to treat facial pain, migraines, and many other (often off-label) ailments.

### 46 The answer is A  *Medicine*

*Staphylococcus aureus* (choice **A**) is a gram-positive, facultative anaerobic coccus that appears in grape-like clusters when viewed through a microscope. It survives as a long-lived resilient commensal organism on about 25%–30% of the population, making routine hand-washing a critical factor in limiting the spread of the organism. In the case described, it is likely that the young lady seeded the food she was preparing with a few bacteria that multiplied when the food sat around prior to its consumption. As the organisms multiplied in the food, they produced rapidly acting enterotoxins; typically, *S. aureus* enterotoxins cause illness in 30 minutes to 6 hours after eating contaminated food. Patients typically experience several of the following: nausea, vomiting, stomach cramps, and diarrhea. The illness is usually mild, and most patients recover after 1–3 days. The best treatments for the vast majority of patients are rest, plenty of fluids, and medicines to calm their stomachs; however, since the toxin is not affected by antibiotics, antibiotics should not be prescribed. Highly susceptible patients, such as the young and the elderly, are more likely to have more severe illness perhaps requiring intravenous therapy and care in a hospital. Food poisoning is but one of the many diseases caused by *S. aureus*. It is responsible for a range of illnesses, from minor skin infections, such as pimples, impetigo (may also be caused by *Streptococcus pyogenes*), boils, cellulitis, folliculitis, furuncles, carbuncles, scalded skin syndrome in young children (caused by an exfoliative toxin with protease activity of that peels off the skin), abscesses, and septic arthritis, to life-threatening diseases such as pneumonia, meningitis, osteomyelitis, toxic shock syndrome (caused by a pyrogenic endotoxin produced by some strains), endocarditis, and septicemia. It is also one of the four most common causes of nosocomial infections, often causing postsurgical wound infections. Each year, approximately 500,000 patients in American hospitals contract a staphylococcal infection. Non–antibiotic resistant strains of *S. aureus* infections can be treated in about a month with any of several antibiotics. Unfortunately, antibiotic resistance has become an ever-expanding problem. In 1943, when Alexander Fleming discovered penicillin, *S. aureus* resistance was unknown; by 1960, about 80% of hospital isolates were penicillin-resistant because the bacteria had developed penicillinase (a β-lactamase). By that time, pharmaceutical companies had developed lactamase-resistant penicillins, the prototype being methicillin. However, during the 1990s, methicillin-resistant *S. aureus* (MSRA) had become increasingly common. Presently, first-line treatment for serious MRSA invasive infections is a glycopeptide antibiotic, either vancomycin or teicoplanin. Unfortunately, *S. aureus* strains resistant to the glycopeptides have recently been reported. These new evolutions of the MRSA bacterium have been dubbed vancomycin intermediate-resistant *Staphylococcus aureus* (VISA). Newer antibiotics that may be used if vancomycin no longer works include linezolid, quinupristin, dalfopristin, daptomycin, and tigecycline.

### 47 The answer is C  *Medicine*

*Bacillus anthracis* (choice **C**) is a gram-positive, spore-forming rod. It is the cause of anthrax, which can occur in three forms: cutaneous, inhalation (aka, pulmonary), and gastrointestinal. The naive postal worker described in the case inhaled anthrax spores and developed a case of inhalation anthrax. Symptoms as described in the case occur in two stages: stage one resembles a cold or flu, with fever, chills, sweating, fatigue, malaise, headache, cough, and chest pain. Stage two usually develops suddenly and includes higher fever, severe shortness of breath, and rapid dissemination of the organism throughout the rest of the body, causing cutaneous symptoms, shock, development of a necrotizing pneumonia, and often death. Five persons died from inhalation anthrax in 2001, when an unknown individual or organization mailed spores of highly refined pulverized, allegedly weaponized anthrax spores to at least 11 persons. This heightened public awareness, and ever since anthrax has been considered a potential bioterror weapon—and rightly so, because of it lethalness. The limited information available estimates the case-fatality rate for inhalation anthrax to be about 75%, even with all possible supportive care, including appropriate antibiotics. A vaccine with limited availability is available for high-risk patients. Fortunately, inhalation anthrax is very rare under ordinary conditions. Cutaneous anthrax is the most common form of anthrax infection, accounting for 90%–95% of all cases. It typically is transmitted to individuals with a cut or scratch who handle animal skins; typically, the animal's fur picked up spores that were lying dormant in the soil. The human infection starts as a raised itchy bump that develops into a vesicle and ulcer with a characteristic black necrotic area in the center. Consumption of contaminated meat causes gastrointestinal anthrax. It too is rare, although not as rare as inhalation anthrax. Symptoms include loss of appetite, vomiting, and fever, and are followed by abdominal pain, vomiting of blood, and severe diarrhea and death in 25%–60% of cases. All forms of anthrax are normally treated with ciprofloxacin.

**48** **The answer is H** *Medicine*

*Corynebacterium diphtheriae* (choice **H**) is an aerobic, nonencapsulated, nonmotile, gram-positive bacillus that causes diphtheria. New cases in the United States are almost nonexistent since the introduction and widespread use of the diphtheria vaccine. Cases are more common worldwide, however, and asymptomatic carriers can still transmit the disease to nonvaccinated individuals, as in the hypothetical case presented above. Classically, diphtheria presents as a respiratory tract infection within the first few days of the onset of illness. It is characterized by the formation of a dense, gray pseudomembrane composed of a mixture of dead cells, fibrin, red blood cells, white blood cells, and organisms. A combination of cervical adenopathy and swollen mucosa imparts a "bull's neck" appearance to the victims. The most frequent cause of death is suffocation following aspiration of the pseudomembrane. In the early 1900s, diphtheria was common in the United States. In 1920, there were about 150,000 cases and 13,000 deaths. As immunization became common, cases and deaths decreased. Between 2000 and 2004, there have only been five reported cases.

**REMAINING INCORRECT CHOICES**

*Actinomyces israelii* (**J**) is an anaerobic, gram-positive filamentous bacterium that is part of the normal flora in the tonsils and crevices around the teeth. Transmission in the oral region is via dental extractions or trauma to the teeth. It presents with a draining sinus in the jaw. The pus contains yellow sulfur granules, which contains the organism. Other infections caused by the pathogen include draining sinuses in the chest and abdomen, and endometritis associated with intrauterine devices (now uncommon). Treatment is with penicillin. *Clostridium tetani* (**F**) is a gram-positive rod that has spores in soil that gain entrance to individuals via closed wounds. Germination of spores is enhanced by the presence of necrosis and poor blood supply. Bacterial proliferation in the wound releases a neurotoxin, called tetanospasmin, which is carried intra-axonally (retrograde) to the central nervous system, where it binds to ganglioside receptors of spinal afferent fibers and inhibits the release of the inhibitory neurotransmitters glycine and γ-aminobenzoic acid within the spinal cord. This causes sustained motor stimulation of all voluntary muscles, eventually causing muscle stiffness starting in the jaw, inducing "lock jaw." Tetanus toxoid is given for active immunization. *Bacillus cereus* (**D**) is a gram-positive rod that produces preformed toxin that stimulates adenylate cyclase, causing gastroenteritis. It is transmitted via reheated fried rice or tacos with rice. The disease is self-limited and does not require antibiotic treatment. *Staphylococcus saprophyticus* (**B**) is coagulase negative and catalase positive. It accounts for 10%–20% of acute urinary tract infections in young, sexually active women. Since the pathogen is not a nitrate reducer and produces a neutrophil inflammatory reaction, the dipstick test for nitrite is negative and dipstick test for leukocyte esterase is positive. The treatment of choice is trimethoprim-sulfamethoxazole.

**49** **The answer is C** *Psychiatry*

Nortriptyline is a tricyclic antidepressant with a therapeutic window. Dosages that achieve a blood level of 50–100 ng/mL are associated with good patient response. Increasing the dosage diminishes the therapeutic response (graph **C**). This therapeutic window has not been demonstrated for other antidepressants, but may be present with risperidone, an atypical antidepressant that demonstrates greatest therapeutic response at doses of 4–6 mg daily.

**50** **The answer is A** *Psychiatry*

Lithium has a threshold for responses at a dosage that produces a blood level of approximately 1.0 mEq/L. Lower doses are ineffective. Higher doses do not appreciably increase the response (graph **A**), but are associated with more untoward effects.

Graph **B** represents a gradually increasing response with increasing dosage, as might be seen with many antipsychotic medications. Graph **D** represents a lack of response. Graph **E** represents an increasingly poor response to medication with increasing doses, usually associated with increasing adverse effects.

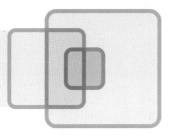

# test 4

# Questions

*Single Best Choice Directions: This section consists of numbered statements or questions followed by a list of potential answers; you are to select the ONE best answer.*

**1** A 4-day-old, 1,500-g (3 lb 5 oz) premature infant recovering from respiratory distress syndrome is noted to have bounding peripheral pulsations and a hyperactive precordium. A continuous machinery murmur is most audible at the left infraclavicular area. Left ventricle hypertrophy (LVH) is present on the electrocardiogram (ECG). The chest x-ray film shows slight enlargement of the heart and increased pulmonary venous markings. Which of the following is the most likely diagnosis?

(A) Ventricular septal defect (VSD)
(B) Atrial septal defect (ASD)
(C) Patent ductus arteriosus
(D) Pulmonic stenosis
(E) Tetralogy of Fallot

**2** A 48-year-old woman has been married for 8 years and desperately wants to have a child of her own before it is too late. She consults a new obstetrician for help because she has experienced multiple early second-trimester losses due to painless cervical dilation leading to expulsion of immature stillborn fetuses. She reports that she was exposed in utero to diethylstilbestrol (DES), explaining that when her mother was pregnant with her she experienced early pregnancy bleeding and, as a consequence, was treated with DES to prevent the pregnancy from being terminated. At this time, this patient is most likely to demonstrate which of the following conditions on physical examination?

(A) Cervical dysplasia
(B) Breast fibroadenoma
(C) Vaginal adenosis
(D) Müllerian agenesis
(E) Polycystic ovary syndrome

**3** A 20-year-old male college student is hospitalized after assaulting a girlfriend whom he accuses of using "radar" to place bizarre thoughts in his mind just after she broke off her relationship with him. He has been increasingly withdrawn and preoccupied over the last year but has no history of substance abuse or other physical problems. Mental status examination reveals an alert, anxious, and oriented male, with dysphoria, suspiciousness, constricted affect, mildly tangential thinking, bizarre ideation, and no memory impairment. Which of the following is the most likely specific diagnosis?

(A) Delirium
(B) Psychosis
(C) Depression
(D) Anxiety
(E) Mania
(F) Cocaine-induced psychosis
(G) Bipolar I disorder
(H) Schizophrenia
(I) Major depressive disorder with psychosis
(J) Shared psychotic disorder

**4** A 69-year-old man who has type 2 diabetes mellitus and lived in Bismarck, North Dakota, went fishing in nearby Long Lake with his 37-year-old son during late August. Although the fish weren't biting, the mosquitoes were, and in a few hours both men were bitten several times, so they only stayed briefly. Before they left, the son commented about the several dead crows they saw on their way back to the car. The following week, the older man developed a persistent headache followed a day later by loss of appetite, nausea, vomiting, muscle aches, rash on his trunk, and a fever. His condition did not improve during the following 2 days; in fact, his symptoms worsened. Consequently, his son, who felt fine, took him to the local ER. By that time, his fever had risen to 104.5°F (40.2°C), his aches and pains seemed to be worse, and he now also complained of a stiff neck. In addition, the admitting physician noted that he was confused and disoriented; he also had a parkinsonian-like tremor and a partial paralysis on his left side. Which virus among the following is the most likely cause of this gentleman's symptoms?

(A) LaCrosse encephalitis virus
(B) Eastern equine encephalitis virus
(C) West Nile virus
(D) Western equine encephalitis virus
(E) St. Louis encephalitis virus

**5** A 32-year-old anesthesiologist, married with two children and a successful hospital-based practice, is discovered by a colleague to be pilfering and using fentanyl. The colleague reports him to the hospital's physician well-being committee. The committee considers permitting him to stay on staff if he voluntarily enters a drug rehabilitation program that includes regular toxicological testing and submission of monitoring reports to the committee for 2 years. Which of the following statements about his case is most accurate?

(A) The physician well-being committee is required to report his fentanyl use to the state medical board.

(B) The committee can require him to submit regular toxicology reports.

(C) The prevalence of substance abuse among physicians is higher than in the general population.

(D) Treatment for substance abuse is more successful among physicians than in the general population.

(E) It is unethical for a physician to fail to report a colleague's impaired behavior to the state medical board.

**6** A 65-year-old man sees his primary care physician because of pain in his chest that he thinks might indicate heart trouble. He describes the pain as a burning sensation in his chest that radiates into the neck and his left arm. He also reports that he regurgitates a sour-tasting liquid that leaves a feeling of "pins and needles" in his throat and mouth. These symptoms are not aggravated by exercise but are by drinking coffee or chocolate, or by eating fatty foods. Results of a physical examination that included his heart sounds and an electrocardiogram (ECG) taken as part of an exercise tolerance test are unremarkable. An upper gastrointestinal barium x-ray study shows the presence of a hiatal hernia. Which of the following is the primary mechanism for this patient's complaints?

(A) Decreased acid production in the stomach

(B) Increased gastric emptying

(C) Decreased esophageal peristalsis

(D) Inappropriate relaxation of the lower esophageal sphincter (LES)

(E) Absence of ganglion cells in the myenteric plexus

**7** A 42-year-old woman complains of aching in the shoulder muscles, difficulty with climbing stairs, and difficulty with swallowing solids and liquids from her upper esophagus. Physical examination reveals atrophy of her shoulder and pelvic muscles. There is erythema over the bridge of her nose, with violaceous discoloration and edema of the upper eyelids.

Erythematous papules are noted over the proximal interphalangeal joints, metacarpophalangeal joints, elbows, and knees. An electromyogram (EMG) reveals low-amplitude polyphasic potentials, and laboratory testing reveals an increased creatine phosphokinase (CPK). Which of the following is the most likely diagnosis?

(A) Polymyalgia rheumatica

(B) Rheumatoid arthritis

(C) Polymyositis

(D) Dermatomyositis

(E) Systemic lupus erythematosus (SLE)

**8** A gravida 4, para 1, abortus 2, 31-year-old woman presents for prenatal care in the middle of her second trimester. She has a positive history of substance abuse preceding and during this pregnancy. Her first pregnancy ended with an emergency cesarean section delivery at 34 weeks' gestation because of significant painful vaginal bleeding associated with fetal bradycardia. On ultrasound examination, her singleton fetus is noted to have a limb reduction defect of the right lower extremity. Which of the following abused substances is most associated with this fetal anomaly?

(A) Tobacco

(B) Alcohol

(C) Narcotics

(D) Amphetamines

(E) Cocaine

**9** A 4-year-old girl fails to develop intelligible speech and simply repeats sentence fragments that she has heard. She spends hours sitting alone, facing a wall, and rocking back and forth. She shows little affection for others and sometimes bangs her head against the floor. Which of the following is the most likely cause for her symptoms?

(A) Childhood exposure to lead

(B) Childhood sexual abuse

(C) Emotionally distant parents

(D) Intrauterine rubella

(E) Maternal cocaine abuse during pregnancy

**10** A well-dressed but somewhat dishevel male presents at a walk-in clinic complaining of difficulty with breathing and a pain in his chest with a chronic cough. Upon providing a history, he says that he is a 31-year-old Harvard MBA graduate and admits that, although he is the CEO of a small business, he has been burning the candle at both ends for at least the past 5 years and has not taken care of his health. The attending physician notices his foul-smelling breath before anything else. The patient also indicates he has not been feeling well for a couple of weeks and is bothered by profound sweating, an inability to sleep, and has lost 5 pounds during the past month. Upon further questioning, he admits he has a drinking problem and more than occasionally drinks until he passes out. Upon examination, the doctor notices his teeth are in sad shape, and he has evidence of gingivitis. Additionally, his temperature was 37.5°C (99.5°F) and he has decreased breath sounds and crackles over the area where the pain was most intense; there is also egophony, and dullness to percussion in the presence of effusion. A chest x-ray was performed; it showed consolidation with a single cavity containing an air–fluid level in the posterior segment of the upper right lobes. Among the following choices, which represents the best next step in the treatment of this man?

(A) A prescription for oral metronidazole
(B) A prescription for oral clindamycin
(C) A prescription for oral vancomycin
(D) A prescription for oral penicillin G
(E) A prescription for oral isoniazid

**11** A 30-year-old woman, who is a nonsmoker, presents with bilateral puffiness and swelling of the fingers and joint pains. Cold exposure and stress cause episodes of blanching of the fingers. After turning white, these digits take on a blueish tint and then a red one. She is not on any medications, and her liver aminotransferase enzyme activities have always been stable and within the normal range. Her thyroid function tests are also normal. The mechanism for this patient's disease is most likely the result of which of the following?

(A) Vasospasm and thickening of the digital arteries
(B) Hyperviscosity due to cryoglobulins
(C) An immune complex vasculitis
(D) Thrombosis of the digital vessels
(E) An embolism to the digital vessels

**12** A 22-year-old woman with methamphetamine dependence intoxication is brought to the emergency department by the police in a state of extreme agitation. After a brief struggle, she is restrained and sedated. A cursory mental evaluation concludes that she probably has persecutory ideation. Physical examination finds hypertension and tachycardia. She is admitted to a medical psychiatric unit for observation and possible treatment. Which of the following statements about this patient is most accurate?

(A) Methylphenidate can be used to facilitate her detoxification from methamphetamine.
(B) Psychologic effects from withdrawal will likely be of short duration.
(C) She is likely to have additional serious psychiatric pathology.

(D) Simultaneous withdrawal from alcohol is unlikely.
(E) Use of antipsychotic medication during her withdrawal is likely to cause a severe toxic interaction with methamphetamine.

**13** A 20-year-old woman in her first pregnancy came to the maternity unit at 39 weeks' gestation after an uncomplicated pregnancy. She had spontaneous onset of labor and progressed normally through the first and second stages of labor. During the second stage of labor, the electronic fetal monitor tracing showed frequent prolonged variable decelerations of the fetal heart rate down to 90/min and lasting 45 seconds. She underwent an outlet forceps vaginal delivery of a 3,100-g (6 lb 13 oz) female neonate. One minute after birth, the infant is noted to have acral cyanosis and a weak respiratory effort at a rate of 30/min. The baby's heart rate is 105/min, and a systolic murmur is heard. She flexes all four extremities weakly but only after external stimulation. When the neonate's nose and mouth are suctioned, she shows no response. She keeps her eyes closed. Which of the following is her assigned Apgar score at 1 minute?

(A) 4
(B) 5
(C) 6
(D) 7
(E) 8

**14** An 85-year-old man is found wandering in a confused state in the middle of a busy thoroughfare. He is taken to the nearest emergency department, where the physician on duty determines he has a temperature of 102.6°F (39.2°C) as well as chills, a productive cough, and chest pain upon inspiration. His blood pressure is 98/68 mm Hg, his respiratory rate is 28/min (normal adult rate is 14–18/min), his respiration is labored, and he has pain upon inspiration. Physical examination shows a few bilateral rales and no other abnormality. His white cell count is 10,900/mm³ (normal range, 4.8–10.8 × 10³/μL) with a left shift. A chest x-ray film is ambiguous. His granddaughter is contacted, and she informs the hospital that her grandfather was self-reliant, had no observable memory problems, and still lived alone. However, earlier in the week, about 2 days ago, he had been complaining of nausea and loss of appetite. Which of the following is the most likely diagnosis?

(A) Alzheimer disease
(B) *Klebsiella pneumoniae* pneumonia
(C) Viral (atypical pneumonia) pneumonia
(D) *Streptococcus pneumoniae* pneumonia
(E) Primary tuberculosis
(F) Senile dementia due to chronic vascular disease

**15** Four years ago a 30-year-old heroin addict who habitually used shared needles when taking the drug intravenously (IV) tested positive for the human immunodeficiency virus (HIV) by the enzyme-linked immunosorbent assay (ELISA) and then by a Western blot test. He now presents to the physician on duty at a community clinic with fever, dyspnea, tachypnea, and peripheral cyanosis. A chest x-ray film reveals extensive "ground-glass" opacities in the lower zones of both lungs. The physician would expect which of the following?

(A) Organism response to amphotericin B
(B) Organism response to erythromycin
(C) Granulomas in the bone marrow
(D) Organism response to trimethoprim–sulfamethoxazole
(E) Gram's stain of sputum to be diagnostic

**16** A 33-year-old man presents as a new patient to a primary care physician. He tells the physician that he has had almost constant abdominal pain for at least the past month, and he lost his appetite and about 15 pounds during the past month; he also complains of being fatigued almost all the time. In addition, he has had frequent bouts of bloody diarrhea and the diarrhea and the concomitant need to wipe his bottom left his rectum sore. He adds that he had a similar sequence of events about 5 years previously, and at that time, his physician told him he had a nervous stomach. He adds that his younger brother seems to be having similar problems. The physician notes that he looks pale, and upon examination, she finds he has diffuse abdominal tenderness with the right lower quadrant being the most sensitive area. His temperature is 99.5°F (37.5°C), blood pressure 98/78 mm Hg, pulse 90 and regular; a complete blood count reveals that his serum hemoglobin value is 9.8 g/dL and a peripheral blood smear reveals a decreased mean corpuscular hemoglobin count (MCHC) and a decreased mean corpuscular volume (MCV). Among the following choices, which most likely represents the disease that this man suffers from?

(A) Crohn's disease
(B) Ulcerative colitis
(C) Irritable bowel syndrome
(D) Lactase deficiency
(E) Nervous stomach

**17** A 39-year-old woman consults a psychologist because she feels she needs help in dealing with her 62-year-old mother. She states that ever since her father died last year, her mother constantly nags her about finding a husband and producing grandchildren. The patient states that she has been living with another woman for the past 10 years in a stable, sexual relationship. The couple purchased a home several years ago, have separate and productive careers, travel widely, and do not want to raise children. Which of the following statements about this patient is most likely to be true?

(A) She has never had sex with a man.
(B) She would like to have a sex-change operation.
(C) She has never had children.
(D) She has abnormal estrogen levels.
(E) She has a history of satisfying interpersonal relationships.

**18** A 50-year-old man is hospitalized after experiencing racing thoughts, insomnia, increasing impulsivity, and grandiosity for 1 month. A 1-month trial of lithium with a blood level of 1.3 mEq/L fails to ameliorate his symptoms. Assuming no contraindications, which of the following is the most appropriate next medication to consider for long-term management of this patient?

(A) A trial of mirtazapine
(B) A trial of divalproex
(C) An increase in the dose of lithium
(D) Addition of clonazepam
(E) A trial of clozapine

**19** A 3-year-old child presents to the emergency department via ambulance with seizures followed by coma. The patient is initially stabilized, and diagnostic studies are obtained. The findings of the cerebrospinal fluid (CSF) include a total white blood cell (WBC) count of 250 cells/μL (normal, 0–5 cells/μL) with a predominance of lymphocytes and monocytes. The CSF glucose is 20 mg/dL (normal, 40–70 mg/dL), the total protein concentration is 50 mg/dL (normal, 15–45 mg/dL), and the chloride concentration is 105 mEq/L (normal, 118–132 mEq/L). Results of a Gram stain of spun-down CSF sediment are negative. A computed tomography (CT) scan with contrast shows enhancement at the base of the brain. Which of the following is the most likely diagnosis?

(A) Eastern equine encephalitis
(B) Subacute sclerosing panencephalitis
(C) Tuberculosis meningitis
(D) Cryptococcal meningitis
(E) Meningococcal meningitis

**20** A 27-year-old Irish Catholic woman gave birth to a 7-pound 5-ounce baby boy. The vaginal birthing was normal and everything seemed fine, but 26 days after the baby was born the mother began to have heavy vaginal bleeding. Her husband called 911, and an ambulance brought her to a nearby trauma facility. They managed to stop the bleeding, but she had lost so much blood that they gave her two units of replacement blood and admitted her into the hospital. There, the attending physician noticed she had many bruises on her legs, arms, and trunk, making him think abuse. But he took a careful history, starting with the questions: How did you get these bruises? Have you or any of your family ever had a bleeding problem before? She replied, "The bruises just appeared, but I always did bruise easily. As to bleeding problems I can't remember anything remarkable, except I used to have a bloody nose on a regular basis; so much so I sometimes missed school; the school nurse told me to stop picking my nose, even though I didn't think I did." The physician also asked: "How about your menses?" She replied, "No real problem, they occurred on a regular basis with minimal cramping, but I did lose a lot of blood. However, my family's doctor told me not to worry about it since my mother and grandmother also had heavy bleeding during their periods, thus it must simply be a familial trait." On the basis of this information, which of the following conditions does this lady most likely have?

(A) Hemophilia A
(B) Hemophilia B
(C) Hemophilia C
(D) Bernard-Soulier syndrome
(E) von Willebrand disease

**21** A 26-year-old woman frantically presents to her physician showing him that she lost patches of scalp hair at various places. She screams, "I cannot continue living looking like this!" She blames her hair dresser, saying she left her under the dryer too long when she got a permanent and that she must have cooked her scalp. She is thinking of bring a lawsuit. She also says she expects the physician to provide treatment and to tell her if a suit is justified. Which of the following choices represents the physician's best response? Tell her that:

(A) He can perform a hair transplant that will restore her hair within a few months but she doesn't have sufficient grounds for a suit.
(B) He can perform a hair transplant that will restore her hair within a few months and he will testify on her account if she sues.
(C) He feels confident that it is most likely that her hair will grow back spontaneously, but he has medication that may accelerate the process. However, there are no guarantees and he doesn't believe she has a case worth pursuing in court because the condition is an autoimmune reaction.
(D) He knows of several similar cases all caused by permanents and the end result always is complete baldness; so she should certainly sue.
(E) He recommends shaving her head so the bald spots are no longer discernible; he will be glad to testify in court as to the extent of her loss.

**22** A 32-year-old woman who is 40 weeks pregnant comes to the maternity unit in active labor. She states that she has painful genital blisters and ulcers, which she has experienced intermittently in the past. Pelvic examination reveals exquisitely tender vesicles and ulcers on her labia and vagina consistent with an active genital herpes infection. She is advised by the obstetrician that she should undergo a primary cesarean section delivery because of the increased risk of fetal infection via passage through an infected birth canal. She is mentally competent and tells the obstetrician that she refuses to have a cesarean section because her mother died during a surgical procedure. Although the doctor explains the risks of a vaginal delivery, she still refuses. The obstetrician should do which of the following?

(A) Allow a vaginal delivery
(B) Obtain a court order to perform the cesarean delivery
(C) Perform the cesarean section without her consent
(D) Obtain the consent of the husband to perform the cesarean delivery
(E) Refer her to another physician

**23** A 9-month-old child presents for well-child care. The patient's head circumference is noted to be two standard deviations above the norm. In addition, the child also has frontal bossing, translucent skin, and eyes that manifest a "setting sun" sign. A meningomyelocele is also evident on physical examination. A computed tomography (CT) scan of the head would show which of the following?

(A) Type I Chiari malformation
(B) Chronic subdural hematoma
(C) Shaken baby syndrome
(D) Protruding cerebellar tonsils
(E) Leptomeningeal cyst
(F) Epidural hematoma

**24** A 17-year-old boy was in his usual state of health until approximately 1 month ago when he developed a painful lump above his right knee. The patient says that he has fatigue and tells you that the leg pain awakens him from sleep. He also states that the leg pain is so bad that he has developed a limp that seems to be worsening. Physical examination reveals a hard, warm, tender mass. A radiograph of the right femur shows an "onion-skin" appearance at the location of the mass. Which of the following is the most likely diagnosis?

(A) Osteomyelitis
(B) Ewing's sarcoma
(C) Osteosarcoma
(D) Chondrosarcoma
(E) Eosinophilic granuloma

**25** A 66-year-old woman complains of fatigue, difficulty concentrating, constipation, headaches, and back pain. She says these symptoms have been present for several months. She has been living alone since her husband died 2 years ago, and she has few friends. She has no history of significant medical or psychiatric problems. Physical examination is unremarkable. Mental status examination reveals decreased psychomotor activity, intact memory and cognitive functions, and no evidence of psychosis. She denies feeling depressed or suicidal. Which of the following is the most likely diagnosis?

(A) Delusional disorder, somatic type

(B) Dementia

(C) Factitious disorder

(D) Hypochondriasis

(E) Major depressive disorder

**26** A 43-year-old woman, gravida 3, para 2, abortus 1, complains of increasingly worsening pain with menses along with progressively heavier menstrual blood loss. Pelvic examination reveals an asymmetrically enlarged uterus that felt soft and boggy. Results of a quantitative serum β-human chorionic gonadotropin (β-hCG) test were negative. Her symptoms were unresponsive to medical therapy. She underwent a total abdominal hysterectomy with complete resolution of her symptoms. Which of the following statements is correct about her condition?

(A) Endometrial glands are found within the myometrium.

(B) Age at diagnosis is usually in the early reproductive years.

(C) Surgical therapy is usually successful.

(D) Fertility is unimpaired.

(E) Diagnosis is made by pelvic examination.

**27** A group of junior college students were celebrating homecoming with a huge bonfire. In order to maintain the fire, they were savaging everything they could find. Two young men dragged in an old couch, which they broke up and threw on the fire. Rather than bursting into flame it smoldered and produced a black smoke that blew into the crowd. Immediately, the persons upon whom the smoke blew started coughing and choking, some complained of headaches and dizziness, two persons vomited, and one young lady collapsed. Onlookers quickly pulled her away from the smoke and because she didn't wake up called 911. The paramedics came within minutes and noted that she was breathing rapidly and her cheeks were unusually red; moreover, one claimed to detect the smell of burned almonds. Reacting quickly, the paramedics pull out a box labeled Cyanokit and started to administer a drug by IV drip. The primary antidote(s) in this kit is which of the following?

(A) Amyl nitrite, sodium nitrite, or 4-dimethylaminophenol (DMAP)

(B) Sodium thiosulfate

(C) Hydroxocobalamin

(D) Methylene blue

(E) Dicobalt edetate

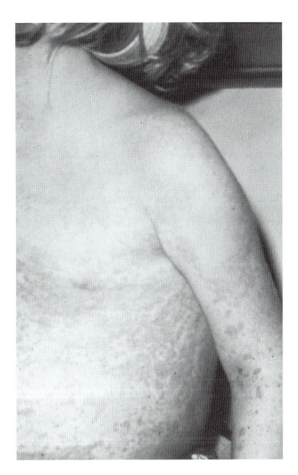

**28** A 3-year-old presents with a history of daily fever with temperature spikes of 39°C for the past 2 weeks. The parents state that the fever is followed by an evanescent rash over the trunk and extremities, as illustrated above. In addition, they say that the patient has arthritis-like pains. The patient also has hepatosplenomegaly, lymphadenopathy, and a pericardial effusion. The erythrocyte sedimentation rate (ESR) is elevated, and there is an absolute neutrophilic leukocytosis. Which of the following is the most likely diagnosis?

(A) Acute rheumatic fever
(B) Systemic lupus erythematosus (SLE)
(C) Juvenile rheumatoid arthritis (JRA)
(D) Lyme disease
(E) Ankylosing spondylitis

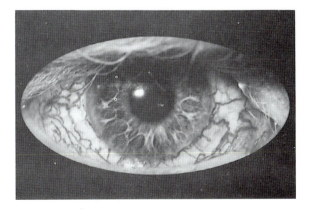

**29** A 3-year-old child with a long history of sinopulmonary disease is noted to have difficulty walking and dilated vessels in the conjunctiva and skin. In addition, the skin has lost its normal elasticity. Chest radiology reveals an absent thymic shadow. Pertinent laboratory data reveal elevated α-fetoprotein (AFP) levels, decreased serum immunoglobulin G (IgG) levels, and low IgA and IgE levels. Which of the following is the most likely diagnosis?

(A) Wiskott-Aldrich syndrome
(B) Ataxia-telangiectasia
(C) Rendu-Osler-Weber disease
(D) Friedreich's ataxia
(E) Cerebral palsy

**30** The N line heading from Coney Island to Ditmars Boulevard, Astoria in New York had to be terminated suddenly because some commuters complained of becoming ill. The driver reported this to the station at Avenue 36 and was advised to pull in. The station supervisor requested rapid-response teams of paramedical, law enforcement, and other personnel to be on hand. The press had somehow got wind of what was happening and rushed to the station in full force but were kept at a distance while law enforcement, paramedics, and other first responders took charge. Spectators were requested to leave the scene. The station was closed to all traffic. Announcements were made on radio and TV to commuters who may have transferred from the N line to other lines at several points including Atlantic Avenue-Pacific Street and at DeKalb avenue in Brooklyn; at Canal Street, Union Square, Herald Square, Times Square, and Lexington Avenue in Manhattan; and at Queensboro Plaza in Queens to go to the nearest emergency room to be examined, especially if they had developed symptoms. A large number of commuters were taken off the train, immediately triaged, and transported to various emergency departments, where physicians, nurses, and other responders were standing by. Hospital spokespersons were available to field questions from reporters. Symptoms that the patients had were variable. Some patients had severe pain in the eyes and copious tears. They were unable to keep their eyes open, and their eyes were red. Others complained of difficulty in breathing, chest pain, fatigue, excessive perspiration, fever, and muscle pain. Some of the patients who were admitted to the hospital developed pulmonary edema, respiratory failure, and then died due to multiorgan failure. Laboratory findings included marked leucocytosis (up to five times the normal value), metabolic acidosis, markedly elevated liver enzymes, hematuria, and abnormal renal function. The most likely agent that the commuters were exposed to was which of the following?

(A) Anthrax
(B) Phosgene
(C) Mustard gas
(D) Ricin
(E) Sarin

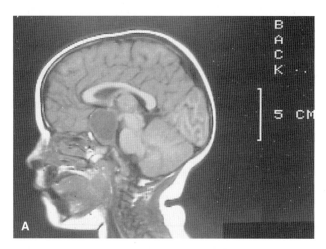
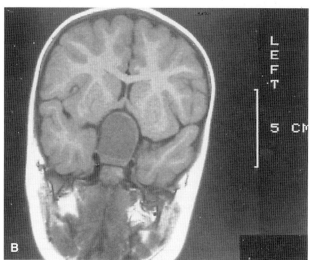

**31** A 59-year-old man works as an accountant in a high-rise office building in Manhattan. For many years, he habitually descended the 26 stories to the street at 10:30, noon, and 2:30 to smoke a cigarette and take a walk that lasted about a half hour during his lunch break. He figures walking is good for his health. However, starting about a month ago, he began to get pains in his calf that made walking difficult. These pains have become progressively worse, limiting his walks to just a few minutes before he had to find a place to sit and rest. He also found it hard to climb the stairs at home to go to bed; sometimes, he only managed three of four steps before he felt obliged to sit and rest. Worried, he consulted a physician who examined him and arrived at a tentative diagnosis. Which of the following choices best describes the first test the physician most likely preformed to verify this diagnosis?

(A) Peripheral Doppler ultrasound
(B) Peripheral angiography
(C) Computed tomography (CT) scan
(D) Ankle-brachial index (ABI) determination
(E) Magnetic resonance (MRI) scan

**32** A 3-year-old child with history of chronic headache is brought to the pediatrician by her mother. The mother states that the child had been in her usual state of health until 2 weeks ago, when she started to complain of a continuous headache. The mother states that she has given the patient over-the-counter medication for the headache but nothing seems to make the headache better. In fact, the mother thinks that perhaps the headache seems to be worse. On review of symptoms, the mother states that the patient has had to "pee" with increasing frequency. The physician notes that the child is short; the patient's height is below the 5th percentile for her

age. Although not very cooperative with the eye examination, the patient appears to have a bitemporal hemianopia. The physician orders a computed tomography (CT) scan of the head that shows a large suprasellar mass. (Figures A and B above.) Based on the history and physical examination, as well as on the result of the CT scan of the head, this patient most likely has which of the following?

(A) An astrocytoma of the third ventricle
(B) A pinealoma
(C) A craniopharyngioma
(D) Chromophobic adenoma
(E) Hand-Schüller-Christian disease

**33** A 28-year-old woman has a 15-year history of physical complaints, including chronic headaches, backaches, abdominal cramps, genital parenthesis, dizziness, nausea, and lack of energy. She abuses analgesics and benzodiazepines. Several relatives have histories of alcohol abuse and criminal behavior. Which of the following is the most likely diagnosis?

(A) Body dysmorphic disorder
(B) Delusional disorder, somatic type
(C) Factitious disorder
(D) Pain disorder
(E) Somatization disorder

**34** A 29-year-old man visits his family physician with a history of pain in his legs. He states that the pain occurs in the evening and even at night, which results in disturbed sleep. He has even tried waking up and walking around to try to get rid of the pain. At times, he feels a tingling sensation in the legs, as if something were crawling over them. Recently, he noticed a cramplike pain while he was driving, and he had to pull over. He had seen a psychiatrist recently and had been prescribed a neuroleptic medication. Based on the presentation, the most likely diagnosis to consider would be which of the following?

(A) Painful legs and moving toes syndrome
(B) Fibromyalgia
(C) Restless leg syndrome
(D) Cauda equina syndrome
(E) Akathisia

**35** A 19-year-old woman was given clindamycin prophylactically before undergoing breast augmentation surgery. Three days after the surgery, she started to feel badly. Initially, she felt lethargic, not wanting to get out of bed to go to work, but she did anyway. Her friends at work told her to go home, saying she looked sick. That night, she couldn't sleep because of acute abdominal pain and several bouts of a watery diarrhea. The following morning, she presented at the local emergency facility. The admitting physician noted she appeared haggard, with the sunken eyes and loose skin typical of dehydration; her temperature was 101.0°F (38.3°C), and she obviously was in great pain, with continuous abdominal cramping. She also continues to produce a watery, profuse, greenish, foul-smelling, liquid stool containing clumps of mucoid material. Her physician sent a stool sample to the laboratory with the expectation that the results would confirm his tentative diagnosis based upon the clinical observations already made. Unfortunately, he couldn't expect the results to become available for another 2–3 days. In the meantime, he started therapy, assuming his tentative diagnoses would be confirmed. Which of the following statements best describes the tentative diagnosis, the diagnostic test run on the stool sample, and the most likely treatment he started?

(A) *Staphylococcal enterocolitis* (*S. enterocolitis*) infection, Gram stain, and metronidazole
(B) *S. enterocolitis* infection, Gram stain, and administration of Imodium
(C) Pseudomembranous colitis, assay for *Clostridium difficile* (*C. difficile*) toxins, and administration of metronidazole
(D) Pseudomembranous colitis, assay for *C. difficile* toxins, and administration of loperamide
(E) Pseudomembranous colitis, assay for *C. difficile*, and administration of metronidazole
(F) Pseudomembranous colitis, assay for *C. difficile*, and administration of loperamide

**36** A 30-year-old man reports to his physician's office concerned about his well-being because his close friend recently had an acute myocardial infarction

(MI). The patient denies a history of chest pain, palpitations, shortness of breath, or swelling of the feet. He does not smoke or consume alcohol, and there is no family history of cardiac disease. His father died of carcinoma of the colon 5 years previously, at the age of 76, and his 74-year-old mother has diabetes, which is controlled with oral medication. Physical examination reveals a 173-cm (68-in) tall white male weighing 81 kg (180 lb), who is not in acute distress. His vital signs are as follows: pulse, 80/min (regular); respirations, 18/min; blood pressure, 128/80 mm Hg. Results of examination of the cardiovascular system and the rest of his physical examination are normal. The patient requests tests to exclude the possibility of him having coronary artery disease (CAD). Which of the following would be the most appropriate next step in the management of this patient?

(A) Order an immediate resting electrocardiogram (ECG) and, if the result is positive, perform an exercise ECG.
(B) Immediately order both a resting ECG and an exercise ECG.
(C) Schedule the patient for routine ECG screening.
(D) Explain to the patient that ECG screening is unnecessary in an asymptomatic patient.
(E) Order a total body computed tomography (CT) scan.

**37** A 55-year-old woman, gravida 4, para 4, comes to the outpatient office for a routine check-up and Pap smear. She underwent menopause 7 years ago, and initially she experienced hot flushes but they resolved within 2 years of menopause. She is not on any hormone therapy. Her cervical Pap smears since menopause have been read as negative for intraepithelial lesions or malignancy. She is 160 cm (63 in) tall and weighs 64 kg (141 lb). Which of the following endocrinologic profiles (**A** through **E**) (including follicle-stimulating hormone [FSH], gonadotropin-releasing hormone [GnRH], and sex hormone binding globulin [SHBG]) is most likely characteristic of this patient?

| | FSH | GnRH | Estrogen | SHBG |
|---|---|---|---|---|
| (A) | Increased | Decreased | Increased | Increased |
| (B) | Increased | Increased | Decreased | Decreased |
| (C) | Increased | Decreased | Decreased | Decreased |
| (D) | Decreased | Decreased | Decreased | Decreased |
| (E) | Increased | Increased | Increased | Increased |

**38** A 27-year-old primigravid woman presents for a prenatal visit at 32 weeks' gestation. She complains of a severe headache and epigastric pain for 24 hours. The headache is not relieved by acetaminophen. The epigastric pain is unrelieved by antacids. Her blood pressure (BP) today is 165/115 mm Hg. A urine dipstick test shows 3+ proteinuria. Her blood pressure on her first prenatal visit at 12 weeks' gestation was 120/70 mm Hg. She experienced severe nausea and vomiting during the first trimester, requiring antiemetic treatment, but her total pregnancy weight gain has been 22 pounds. She has taken thyroid replacement medication after undergoing iodine 131 ($^{131}$I) treatment for Graves disease 5 years ago. Which of the following medications would be indicated in the treatment of this patient?

(A) Phenytoin
(B) Magnesium sulfate
(C) Terbutaline
(D) Progesterone
(E) Indomethacin

**39** A pediatrician is called to attend a delivery of a 35-year-old primigravida. According to the patient and review of the medical record, the patient has had good prenatal care. And, except for the development of diabetes during the second trimester, the pregnancy has been uneventful. Cultures for sexually transmitted diseases are documented as negative. After many hours of labor the patient delivers an infant by spontaneous vaginal delivery with Apgar scores of 8 at 1 minute and 9 at 5 minutes. Birth weight is 4.5 kg (10 lb). Which of the following injuries is most likely to be found in this newborn?

(A) Cephalhematoma
(B) Facial nerve paralysis
(C) Intraventricular hemorrhage
(D) Brain contusion
(E) Fractured clavicle

**40** An 87-year-old man diagnosed with type 2 diabetes 27 years ago also has systolic hypertension and a body mass index (BMI) of 32. He presently is taking hydrochlorothiazide, atenolol, and amlodipine to control his systolic blood pressure, which when measured at home still averages about 167 mm Hg, and at the doctor's office, it ranges from 188 to 205 mm Hg. In addition, he also takes atorvastatin to help control his cholesterol level, which is now, with the help of this drug, at 125 mg/dL. In reviewing the results from a basic metabolic panel taken the previous week, his physician noted his serum creatinine level was 1.20 mg/dL (normal 0.70–1.30) and his blood urea nitrogen (BUN) 23 mg/dL (normal 9–23). After reviewing his history, the physician recommends starting enalapril to lower the patient's blood pressure. Three days after starting the enalapril, the patient checked himself into the emergency room (ER) complaining that he had hardly been able to urinate for the past 2 days. In addition, his arms and legs seemed to be swelling; he has abdominal pain, is unusually tired, and has problems concentrating. His serum creatinine level was now 1.80 mg/dL and his blood urea nitrogen (BUN) 36 mg/dL. Which of the following choices correctly describes the cause of this patient's symptoms?

(A) Vasodilation of the postglomerular efferent arterioles
(B) Vasoconstriction of the preglomerular arterioles
(C) Glomerulonephritis
(D) Acute interstitial nephritis
(E) A urethral stone

*Directions for Matching Questions (41 through 50): Each set of matching questions is preceded by a list of 4 to 26 lettered options followed by a brief explanation of the required task and then by a series of numbered statements. For each lettered statement you are to select ONE lettered option that best fulfills the task as it relates to that statement. Remember, each of the listed options might be correctly selected once, more than once, or not at all.*

## Questions 41–47

*For the following numbered descriptions of patients with orthopedic injuries, select the ONE lettered condition that is best associated with it from the list below.*

(A) Wrist drop may be present
(B) Fractured radius with dislocation of the radioulnar joint at the wrist
(C) Shoulder cannot externally rotate beyond neutral position
(D) Radial pulse should be felt during reduction
(E) Hypesthesia over the lateral aspect of the shoulder may be present
(F) Can be reduced by supination
(G) Fractured ulna with radial head dislocation

**41** A 28-year-old football player with anterior dislocation of the right shoulder.

**42** A 35-year-old man who presents with suspected posterior dislocation of the left shoulder.

**43** A 5-year-old child who was suddenly pulled by his right hand onto the curb by his mother.

**44** An 8-year-old boy who fell from a tree and landed on the back of his right elbow.

**45** A 30-year-old man who fell off a ladder and fractured the shaft of his right humerus.

**46** A 16-year-old boy with Monteggia's fracture.

**47** An 18-year-old man with Galeazzi's fracture.

## Questions 48–50

*The lettered values below represent percentage use of various substances by American high school seniors in 2004. Match the closest percentage use with the corresponding substance as described in questions 48–50.*

Percentage use
(A) 60.0
(B) 25.0
(C) 20.0
(D) 5.0
(E) 1.5

**48** Used anabolic steroids at least once during 2008

**49** Smoked tobacco at least once during the month of the survey

**50** Used some form of cocaine at least once during 2004

# Answer Key

| | | | | | | | | | |
|---|---|---|---|---|---|---|---|---|---|
| **1** C | | **11** A | | **21** C | | **31** D | | **41** E | |
| **2** C | | **12** C | | **22** A | | **32** C | | **42** C | |
| **3** H | | **13** B | | **23** D | | **33** E | | **43** F | |
| **4** C | | **14** D | | **24** B | | **34** C | | **44** D | |
| **5** D | | **15** D | | **25** E | | **35** C | | **45** A | |
| **6** D | | **16** A | | **26** A | | **36** D | | **46** G | |
| **7** D | | **17** E | | **27** C | | **37** B | | **47** B | |
| **8** E | | **18** B | | **28** C | | **38** B | | **48** E | |
| **9** D | | **19** C | | **29** B | | **39** E | | **49** B | |
| **10** B | | **20** E | | **30** D | | **40** A | | **50** D | |

# *Answers and Explanations*

**1** **The answer is C** *Pediatrics*

A patient with patent ductus arteriosus (choice **C**) has a continuous machinery murmur. Bounding pulses with hyperactive precordium also may be found on physical examination. Although the electrocardiogram (ECG) is usually not helpful, it may show left ventricular hypertrophy (LVH).

Patients with atrial septal defect (ASD) (choice **B**) have a widely split and fixed second heart sound. Patients with ventricular septal defect (VSD) (choice **A**) have a pansystolic murmur. Tetralogy of Fallot (choice **E**) is characterized by the presence of a VSD, right ventricular hypertrophy, pulmonic stenosis, and overriding aorta. The murmur of tetralogy of Fallot is a long, systolic ejection murmur most audible at the midleft sternal border. In patients with pulmonic stenosis (choice **D**), there is a high-pitched systolic ejection murmur, most audible at the upper left sternal border, that transmits fairly well to the back. A systolic thrill may be present at the upper left sternal border and, rarely, in the suprasternal notch.

**2** **The answer is C** *Obstetrics and Gynecology*

Diethylstilbestrol (DES) is a nonsteroidal estrogen that was used between 1940 and 1971 for treatment of threatened spontaneous abortion. Vaginal clear cell adenocarcinoma is the most serious consequence of prenatal DES exposure. However, numerous non-neoplastic uterine and vaginal anomalies also have been reported in women exposed to DES in utero, including cervical insufficiency, as is the case with this patient. Cervical insufficiency is treated with placement of a cervical cerclage at 14–16 weeks' gestation. Columnar epithelium is normally found only around the endocervical canal; in vaginal adenosis (choice **C**), the columnar epithelium extends onto the vaginal fornices. This condition is found in 4% of normal females, but 30% of women exposed to DES in utero have this condition. It is the most common physical finding observed during pelvic examination of DES-exposed women. During colposcopic examination, the immature metaplastic squamous epithelium of the cervix of these women resembles dysplasia, with a mosaic and punctate appearance. However, histologic examination demonstrates this epithelium is benign; it is not a true dysplasia, thus choice **A** is not correct.

The following conditions are not associated with prenatal DES exposure: Breast fibroadenoma (choice **B**), which is the most common breast tumor in young women; müllerian agenesis (choice **D**), which is characterized by absence of the oviducts, uterus, cervix, and proximal vagina; and polycystic ovary syndrome (choice **E**), a condition with bilaterally enlarged, smooth ovaries associated with anovulation, infertility, and hirsutism.

**3** **The answer is H** *Psychiatry*

The accusations represent bizarre delusions that indicate the presence of psychosis (choice **B**). Schizophrenia (choice **H**) is the most likely specific diagnosis. Key findings include a history of increasing pathology over the last year, deterioration of function, the presence of constricted affect, mildly tangential thinking, bizarre ideation, and social withdrawal.

The patient's normal awareness and lack of memory impairment make delirium (choice **A**) unlikely. Although the symptoms of dysphoria and anxiety (choice **D**) are present, they are readily explained by his psychosis, and there is little evidence to suggest that they represent primary mood pathology, such as depression (choice **C**) or mania (choice **E**). The lack of significant mood symptomatology makes bipolar I disorder (choice **G**) and major depressive disorder (choice **I**) less likely. The patient has no history of cocaine use (thus cocaine-induced psychosis [choice **F**] is not a likely diagnosis), and the girlfriend does not share the content of his delusions (i.e., shared psychotic disorder [choice **J**]).

**4** **The answer is C** *Medicine*

In the United States, West Nile virus (choice **C**) was first identified in New York State in 1999. Since then, the virus has infected humans in almost all 48 contiguous states. In 2007, 3,630 cases were reported in the United States, and North Dakota had one of the highest per capita rates of infection, about 5.8 cases per 10,000 residents. It is primarily spread to birds by the bite of a mosquito and then back to other mosquitos, some of which bite and infect humans. In the Old World, the *Culex pipiens* mosquitoes exist in two separate populations, one that bites birds and one that bites humans, but in North America many of these mosquitos are hybrids that bite both species; this probably accounts for the rapid spread of the virus in the United States. Only about 20% of infected humans develop symptoms; older individuals are more susceptible. Many infected individuals note no symptoms; others have relatively mild symptoms such as fever, headache, myalgia, swollen lymph nodes, and occasionally a skin rash on the trunk. However, a minority have serious symptoms; among the 3,630 case reported with symptoms in 2007, 1,217 (33.5%) developed encephalitis/meningitis and 124 (3.4%) died. In addition, a significant fraction of those who suffered neurological manifestation were left with some residual neurologic problems. The risk for developing encephalitis is greater among males who are over 70 years of age, particularly if they have type 2 diabetes or hypertension. A tentative diagnosis can be made based on the clinical symptoms, which can usually be confirmed serologically by the demonstration of specific IgG and IgM antibodies. The West Nile virus belongs to the Flavivirus genus and is a member of the Japanese encephalitis antigenic complex. False-positive serology results may occur with persons infected with or vaccinated for other flavivirus (e.g., St. Louis encephalitis, yellow fever, or dengue) or who were previously infected with the West Nile virus.

LaCrosse encephalitis virus (choice **A**) was first isolated in LaCrosse Wisconsin in 1963. It is quite rare and primarily affects children younger than 16. It is specifically transmitted by the *Aedes triseriatus* mosquito, and the intermediate hosts are small animalis such as chipmunks and squirrels. Consequently, the spread to humans is relatively rare (about 75 cases reported annually in the United States), and the range is very small (in recent years, most cases were confined to West Virginia). Eastern equine encephalitis virus (choice **B**) and the Western equine encephalitis virus (choice **D**) belong to the Togaviridae family. On average only five human cases of Eastern equine encephalitis occurs annually, almost entirely exclusively limited to Florida, Georgia, Massachusetts, and New Jersey. However, about 33% of persons who develop Eastern equine encephalitis die and half who survive are permanently impaired. In 1941, 3,336 human cases of Western equine encephalitis were reported. However, since that epidemic, the number of cases has dropped remarkably, and at present, cases average about 17 per year, mostly in California and none in North Dakota. The mortality rate of those with Western equine encephalitis is about 4%, primarily among the elderly. St. Louis encephalitis virus (choice **E**), like the West Nile virus, belongs to the Flavivirus family. St. Louis encephalitis is currently found throughout continental United States. It is named after the city of St. Louis, where the first cases were recognized in 1933. Prior to the onset of the West Nile invasion, it was regarded as the most prevalent mosquito-borne (as well as any other arthropod-borne) encephalitis in the United States. However, the incidence is not near as great as that of West Nile. The median rate of human infection has been reported as 35 cases per year in the United States (0.6 for North Dakota), with possible rates as high as 200 in epidemic years. The symptoms and outcomes are very similar as that for West Nile fever and encephalitis.

**5** **The answer is D** *Psychiatry*

Success rates for drug rehabilitation in physicians are higher than in the general population (choice **D**); at least in part, this is felt to result from the very high social and economic costs that continued abuse represents to those involved.

Physician well-being committees operate with confidentiality and are not required to arbitrarily report physician impairment to the state medical board or other agencies (choice **A**). Such committees cannot mandate treatment without a physician's consent, but may require treatment as a condition of withholding information about impairment from the state medical board (choice **B**). The prevalence of substance abuse among physicians is about the same as that of the general population (choice **C**). Although it is unethical for a physician to ignore impairment in a colleague, action may include report to a physician well-being committee in lieu of reporting to a state medical board (choice **E**).

**6** The answer is **D** *Medicine*

Although these symptoms clearly indicate that the patient has gastroesophageal reflux disease (GERD), it is always a wise move to rule out the possibility of cardioarterial disease (CAD), as was done by the exercise tolerance test. GERD is a chronic, recurrent disorder characterized by heartburn, belching, and epigastric pain. The primary mechanism is inappropriate relaxation of the LES (choice **D**). Agents that decrease LES pressure, such as chocolate, coffee, ethanol, fat, peppermint, anticholinergics, theophylline, diazepam, barbiturates, and calcium channel blockers, exacerbate GERD. About 1 in 10 nonpregnant adults complain about heartburn at least once a week, and prevalence of GERD increases with age, is found more commonly in older men than in older women, and is very common during pregnancy; approximately 1 in 4 pregnant women experience heartburn from acid reflux daily during pregnancy. This very high frequency is attributed to impaired LES competence coupled to increased abdominal pressure.

Secondary factors that predispose to GERD include hiatal hernia; acid concentration of the refluxate; delayed acid clearance, which is associated with low-amplitude peristalsis and recumbency; and decreased gastric emptying (not increased [choice **B**]), which aggravates reflux. The acid concentration of the refluxate is the most important factor in determining progression to reflux esophagitis. Complications associated with GERD are reflux esophagitis, stricture formation, and Barrett's esophagus. Barrett's esophagus is a premalignant condition characterized by glandular metaplasia of the distal esophagus. The risk of developing adenocarcinoma is 2%–10% in the United States, and distal adenocarcinoma of the esophagus has replaced squamous cell carcinoma of the esophagus as the most common esophageal cancer. GERD can also precipitate an asthmatic attack by reflux vagal stimulation or aspiration. Approximately 80% of adults with bronchial asthma have GERD. This percentage appears to be independent of bronchodilator therapy. Chronic aspiration is also linked to pulmonary fibrosis and bronchiectasis. Ambulatory monitoring of esophageal pH for 24 hours, the gold standard, can detect GERD and provide information relative to the potential for chronic aspiration of acid reflux. The treatment of GERD involves reducing gastroesophageal reflux, neutralizing the acid reflux, enhancing esophageal clearance, and protecting the esophageal mucosa from ulceration. Diet modification, weight loss, postural therapy (elevation of the head of the bed), restriction of alcohol, and cessation of smoking, along with pharmacologic treatment, are used in a stepwise approach reflecting patient response. A recommended progression of drugs includes antacids and alginic acid → histamine-2 ($H_2$) receptor antagonists at conventional doses → $H_2$ receptor antagonists at high doses, omeprazole, or prokinetic agents (metoclopramide) → antireflux surgery.

Absence of ganglion cells in the myenteric plexus (choice **E**) is the key finding in achalasia. Decreased peristalsis (choice **C**) is noted in both achalasia and systemic sclerosis. Decreased acid production in the stomach (choice **A**) is noted in pernicious anemia (destruction of the parietal cells) and *Helicobacter pylori*–induced atrophic gastritis involving the antrum and pylorus.

**7** The answer is **D** *Medicine*

The patient has dermatomyositis (DM) (choice **D**), which has some overlapping features with polymyositis (PM). Both disorders are a female-dominant type of myositis, with DM involving skin and muscle in adults and children, and PM involving only muscle in adults (choice **C**). Both disorders have muscle pain and atrophy, with the shoulders and pelvic muscles most commonly involved. The pelvic muscle weakness makes it difficult for patients to climb stairs. Dermatologic lesions associated with DM (not PM) include erythema over the bridge of the nose, with violaceous discoloration and edema of the upper eyelids; additionally, erythematous papular lesions may be noted over the dorsum of the proximal interphalangeal joints, knuckles, elbows, and knees. Dysphagia for solids and liquids is present, because of weakness of the striated muscle in the upper esophagus. Laboratory findings include a positive serum antinuclear antibody test result in 30% of cases. Anti Jo-1 and anti PM-1 antibodies are present in a small percentage of cases. The serum creatine kinase is increased, and muscle biopsies show a lymphocytic inflammatory reaction with destruction of muscle fibers. The treatment for DM and PM is chronic prednisone therapy. If patients fail to respond to steroid therapy, they may be placed on immunosuppressive agents such as azathioprine, cyclophosphamide, or methotrexate.

Polymyalgia rheumatica (choice **A**) may be associated with proximal muscle aching; however, serum creatine and the electromyogram (EMG) are normal. Likewise, rheumatoid arthritis (choice **B**) does not feature increased in serum creatine kinase or an abnormal EMG. Systemic lupus erythematosus (SLE) (choice **E**) could easily explain the "butterfly rash" but would not explain the myopathic features expressed in the EMG and the increased muscle enzymes.

**8** **The answer is E** *Obstetrics and Gynecology*

A frequent adverse effect associated with maternal prenatal use of many substances is intrauterine growth restriction (IUGR) and preterm delivery. However, of all the choices provided for this case, only cocaine (choice **E**) has clearly defined vascular disruption anomalies such as intestinal atresia, limb-reduction defects, and brain anomalies. It is also associated with abruptio placenta, which was the most likely cause of the problems that led to the 34-week emergency cesarean described in the scenario. Although the other choices have an adverse impact on pregnancy outcome, they do not cause limb-reduction defects.

Tobacco (choice **A**) is associated with IUGR, alcohol (choice **B**) is associated with fetal alcohol syndrome, and narcotics (choice **C**) and amphetamines (choice **D**) can lead to an addicted newborn.

**9** **The answer is D** *Psychiatry*

The symptoms are most suggestive of autistic disorder. Autistic disorder often presents with qualitative disturbances of interpersonal behavior, failure to develop normal communication, and a restricted range of interests. Abnormal behaviors, such as rocking and head banging, are common. There is a strong association between autistic disorder and intrauterine infections, most commonly rubella (choice **D**). Other prenatal and postnatal factors are also associated with subsequent autistic disorder, including encephalitis and errors of metabolism, such as tuberous sclerosis.

Psychosocial factors, such as emotionally distant parents (choice **C**) and childhood sexual abuse (choice **B**), are not causally associated with autistic disorder, although the resultant emotional pathology may mimic some autistic symptoms. Maternal cocaine abuse during pregnancy (choice **E**) and childhood lead exposure (choice **A**) have been associated with behavioral and attention disturbances in children, but not with autistic disorder.

**10** **The answer is B** *Medicine*

The chest x-ray showed a fluid-filled cavity characteristic of an abscess. Characteristically, this is due to a necrotizing lung infection that produced a pus-filled cavitary lesion. Such abscesses are generally caused by aspiration of oropharyngeal material by patients who are unconscious. The risk is increased in patients with gingivitis or poor oral hygiene. This patient has poor oral hygiene and confessed to bouts of unconsciousness under the influence of alcohol. The foul smell of his breathe suggests anaerobic bacteria are at least partially responsible for the infection. In the absence of additional data, the best course of treatment is a broad-spectrum antibiotic such as clindamycin (choice **B**). Had he been sicker and if available in a walk-in clinic, he would most likely been given clindamycin IV. In any case, he should be advised to either see his own physician, or to return within a week; unfortunately, walk-in clinics are not designed to provide continuous, coordinated, or comprehensive care.

Metronidazole (choice **A**) has activity against anaerobes and protozoa, but to be used in this situation it must be combined with an antibiotic such as penicillin to make sure the growth of aerobes is also inhibited. A prescription for oral vancomycin (choice **C**) would be used if infection by a methicillin-resistant *Staphylococcus aureus* (MSRA) organism were suspected; however, that is not the case, and it is best to reserve use of vancomycin for treatment of resistant bacteria, to minimize the development of vancomycin resistance. A prescription for oral penicillin G (choice **D**) would not effective because it would be degraded by the stomach's acidity; consequently, it always is administered parentally. Moreover, it would not be effective against gram-negative bacteria. A prescription for oral isoniazid (choice **E**) would be used to treat tuberculosis, which would be a very unlikely possibility in this patient.

**11** **The answer is A** *Medicine*

The patient has Raynaud's phenomenon, which most commonly affects women aged between 20 and 50 years. The phenomenon is marked by the changing color of the digits, as described for this patient. The blanching is due to a diminishing blood supply; the blue tint followed by a reddish color is caused by prolonged hypo-oxygenation, followed by flushing when the blood vessels open again. The phenomenon is commonly seen in association with various rheumatoid conditions, including scleroderma, rheumatoid arthritis, and systemic lupus erythematosus. In these conditions, the symptoms of Raynaud's phenomenon may precede the other symptoms of the underlying disease by years or even decades. This most notably occurs in sclerosis; it has been reported to be the presenting sign in 85% of the cases of systemic sclerosis and in 95% of the cases of localized scleroderma (aka, the CREST syndrome). Similar symptoms can be induced by other factors including hypothyroidism, carcinoid, frostbite, chronic use of vibrating tools, or a side effect of several medications, or the underlying factor(s) may be idiopathic. In idiopathic cases or those not involving generalized physical aberrations, in particular a rheumatoid disease, the multicoloration of the digits is often referred to as Raynaud disease rather than Raynaud's phenomenon. This question asks which choice most likely describes the underlying factor causing Raynaud's phenomenon in the patient described, and the data presented essentially eliminate most nonrheumatic causes of the phenomenon; in most, if not all, of the underlying rheumatoid conditions, the responsible factors playing critical roles responsible for initiating these changes are vasospasm and thickened digital vessels (choice **A**). Although these rheumatoid conditions are autoimmune diseases, immune complexes are not present in the vessels (choice **C**).

Two other systemic causes of Raynaud's phenomenon are thromboangiitis obliterans (Buerger disease), which is an inflammatory vasculitis producing thrombosis of the digital vessels (choice **D**) in male smokers (patient is female and a nonsmoker); and cryoglobulinemia, with proteins that precipitate in cold temperatures (choice **B**). The latter condition is commonly associated with chronic hepatitis C (not present in this patient, as demonstrated by her normal, stable liver transaminase levels). In addition to affecting the digits, in cold weather this condition also produces cyanosis of the nose and ears that reverses to normal when returning to a warm environment. Embolism to digital vessels in the hand is uncommon (choice **E**), and when it does occur, it is most commonly due to infective endocarditis or atrial fibrillation, neither of which is present in this patient.

## 12 The answer is C *Psychiatry*

Comorbidity for other severe mental disorders is greater than 50% in individuals with severe drug dependence. Mood disorders, anxiety disorders, and psychotic disorders are commonly present, any of which may cause additional serious psychiatric pathology (choice **C**).

Methylphenidate plays no role in methamphetamine detoxification (choice **A**). Psychologic effects from methamphetamine dependence, including mood and sleep disturbances, often continue for several weeks (choice **B**). Alcohol dependence is a common comorbid condition in individuals with methamphetamine dependence, and alcohol withdrawal may be seen during their hospitalization (choice **D**). Antipsychotic medications are often used to treat psychosis and agitation during methamphetamine withdrawal without an increased incidence of severe toxic interactions (choice **E**).

## 13 The answer is B *Obstetrics and Gynecology*

The Apgar score is a five-parameter clinical assessment of the newborn made shortly after birth. The score made at 1 minute indicates the degree of resuscitation that is needed, while the 5-minute score indicates the success of the resuscitation efforts. The five parameters used to assign a score are skin color, respiratory effort, heart rate, muscle tone, and reflex irritability. A score of 7 to 10 is excellent and requires no intervention. A score of 3 or less indicates that immediate life saving measures are needed. This infant will be assigned 1 point for pink body but blue extremities, 1 point for weak respiratory effort, 2 points for heart rate (because it is over 100/min), 1 point for muscle tone, and 0 for reflex irritability for a total score of 5 (choice **B**).

An Apgar score of 4 (choice **A**), 6 (choice **C**), 7 (choice **D**), or 8 (choice **E**) would be incorrect in this case.

## 14 The answer is D *Medicine*

The patient most likely has community-acquired bacterial pneumonia, as indicated by the abrupt onset of fever, chills, a productive cough, and chest pain upon inspiration. However, pneumonia in the elderly differs in some important ways from the classic findings of community-acquired bacterial pneumonia in younger adults. Commonly, the presenting symptoms are acute confusion with rapid breathing. Signs of consolidation, such as dullness to percussion, are also absent; rales are minimal; and x-ray studies can be difficult to interpret. Although present in the case described, chest pain, productive cough, and chills are not always present. The white cell count is not increased in 50% of cases or, as in this case, increased minimally; however, 95% of cases demonstrate a left shift. As in typical community-acquired bacterial pneumonia, *Streptococcus pneumoniae* (pneumococcus) (choice **D**) remains the most common cause.

*Klebsiella pneumoniae* pneumonia (choice **B**) is more commonly associated with alcoholics and nursing-home patients. Patients cough up mucoid-appearing sputum that is often tinged with blood. A Gram's stain of sputum shows fat, gram-negative rods with a capsule. The treatment of choice is the use of third-generation cephalosporins or fluoroquinolones. Viral pneumonias (atypical pneumonias) (choice **C**) are usually associated with a nonproductive cough and have an interstitial pattern on chest x-ray films rather than a consolidation. Primary tuberculosis (choice **E**) is rare in a 85-year-old otherwise healthy adult and occurs more frequently in children or immunocompromised patients. It involves the periphery of the lower part of the upper lobe or upper part of the lower lobe in the lungs. Alzheimer disease (choice **A**) and senile dementia due to chronic vascular disease (choice **F**) can be ruled out because of the sudden onset of symptoms.

### 15 The answer is D   *Medicine*

The patient has a *Pneumocystis carinii* pneumonitis with the characteristic radiographic findings of "ground glass" opacities in the lungs. Methenamine silver stains (not Gram's stain; choice **E**) of lung tissue or bronchoalveolar lavage specimens frequently demonstrate densely clustered cysts that resemble crushed ping-pong balls. Because the patient is human immunodeficiency virus (HIV) positive and has an opportunistic infection, the patient qualifies as having acquired immune deficiency syndrome (AIDS). *P. carinii* is the most common initial manifestation and cause of death in patients with AIDS. Once considered a protozoan, DNA analysis now shows that this organism is more closely related to a fungus; moreover, it cannot be cultured. Patients are generally susceptible to *P. carinii* infection when their CD4 helper T-cell count approaches 200 cells/mm$^3$ and infection is contracted in immunosuppressed patients by inhalation, producing an interstitial pneumonitis with extreme hypoxia. *P. carinii* predominantly affects the lungs, but it can also involve other head and neck organs, such as the thyroid or the skin. The treatment for *P. carinii* is trimethoprim–sulfamethoxazole (TMP-SMX; choice **D**) or pentamidine. Aerosolized pentamidine or low-dose sulfonamides are useful as prophylaxis against the infection. There is a 20% fatality rate with each infection; therefore, lifetime prophylaxis is needed. The infection does not respond to amphotericin B (choice **A**) or erythromycin (choice **B**). *P. carinii* is easily confused with *Histoplasma capsulatum*, but *Histoplasma* organisms are located in macrophages. Disseminated histoplasmosis could present with granulomas in the bone marrow (choice **C**). *P. carinii* does not produce granulomatous inflammation. Amphotericin B is the treatment of choice for histoplasmosis.

### 16 The answer is A   *Medicine*

Crohn's disease (choice **A**) is an inflammatory autoimmune condition with a significant genetic predilection; however, the course of the disease varies greatly from patient to patient. In many cases, attacks go into remission only to recur again years later; in other cases, the disease is consistent and persistent. The inflammation causes bowel cells to secrete large volumes of water with more salt than can be resorbed; consequently, it causes diarrhea. In mild cases, this may only be annoying but in severe cases patients may have dozens of bowel movements per day, interfering with daily activities and sleep. The inflammation also may cause thickening and scarring of the mucosa, which in turn causes cramping and pain. Again, the pain can vary from a minor annoyance to almost being intolerable. In addition, the inflammation can lead to ulceration and bleeding, which can induce a microcytic anemia, as in the case described, or less commonly it may interfere with vitamin B$_{12}$ absorption in the terminus of the ilium and induce pernicious anemia, a macrocytic event. The pain and cramping inhibits appetite, causing weight loss. In some cases, the ulceration can be so severe that fistulas are formed and organs adjacent to the colon become affected, causing a host of potential secondary problems. The inflammation is often localized in the ilium (about 50% of the time) or at the junction of the ilium and the colon (about 30% of the time), and in the body of the colon about 20% of the time, but it can occur at any place, varying from the mouth the rectum. In some patients, the affected area is a continuum, whereas in others it develops simultaneously in different areas, creating a patchwork effect. Ulceration can even happen outside the gastrointestinal system as, for example, in the mouth, skin, liver, joints, or eyes. What triggers the condition is unknown, but there appears to be a strong genetic component; approximately 20% of Crohn's disease patients have a first-degree relative who also is affected. The onset of the disease can start at any age but most typically appears between the ages of 15 and 35 years. It affects men and women to an equal extent, and Caucasians are at greater risk than other ethic groups.

Ulcerative colitis (choice **B**) is the other inflammatory gastrointestinal disease. Unlike Crohn's disease ulcerative colitis causes inflammation only in the colon or rectum, almost always only involves the superficial layer of the inner lining of the bowel, and the inflammation generally is diffuse and uniform rather than concentrated in some areas and pitted and nonhomogeneous. However, some relation must exist between the two diseases since having first-degree relatives with ulcerative colitis is a risk factor for developing Crohn disease. Irritable bowel syndrome (choice **C**) is not a disease per se but a description of a group of functional disturbances that may cause symptoms such as bloating, flatulence, diarrhea and/or constipation, and mucus in the feces. Unlike Crohn disease or ulcerative colitis, the syndrome very rarely causes inflammation or any type of tissue damage. Irritable bowel syndrome is very common; approximately 20% of adults in the United States have it. There is no know cause, but individuals may have heightened sensitivity to certain foods or to stress. It is more common in young adults, particularly in females. Lactase deficiency (choice **D**) is defined as too little of the intestinal enzyme lactase used to digest the lactose (milk sugar) found in the normal diet. By definition, all mammalian species drink milk at birth and therefore must produce sufficient amounts of lactase to thrive through infancy. However, as they age, most species develop an intolerance to lactose-containing foods (dairy products), and they lose the ability to synthesize sufficient lactase. This intolerance causes bloating and flatulence upon ingestion of diary products. Western Caucasian Europeans and their decendents are the major exceptions to the rule that lactase synthesis ceases with age. There isn't a specific diagnosis or a recognized disease called "nervous stomach" (choice **E**). Some doctors may use the term to generally describe symptoms of indigestion, bloating, or changes in bowel habits, especially after tests fail to reveal a specific cause.

## 17 The answer is E *Psychiatry*

The ability to maintain a stable relationship and a career over a significant period of time (at least 10 years) suggests that the individual has the general capacity to relate well to others; therefore, she has a history of satisfying interpersonal relationships (choice **E**).

Individuals with gender identity disorder seek sex-change surgery (choice **B**). Homosexual (lesbian) individuals, like this patient, are content with their biologic gender. There is some evidence for a genetic and prenatal hormonal basis for homosexuality, but in adulthood, homosexual individuals have normal sex hormone levels (choice **D**). Homosexual individuals often have experienced heterosexual sex (choice **A**), and many have had children (choice **C**).

## 18 The answer is B *Psychiatry*

This patient's condition is highly suggestive of bipolar I disorder that is not responsive to lithium treatment. This happens in at least 25% of cases. It would be unwise to increase the lithium dose (choice **C**) in this patient, because his level is already at the top of the therapeutic range. The medication of choice in such circumstances is divalproex (choice **B**), because some patients who do not respond to lithium will respond to it.

Mirtazapine (choice **A**) is a sedating antidepressant that would not be expected to control a manic episode. Clonazepam (choice **D**) no longer plays any first-line role in the treatment of bipolar I disorder. Newer antipsychotic medications may be useful in the acute and long-term treatment of bipolar I disorder, but clozapine (choice **E**) has untoward effects that make it a much less desirable choice for the long-term management of bipolar I disorder.

## 19 The answer is C *Pediatrics*

Tuberculosis meningitis (choice **C**) usually presents in recently infected individuals and is usually considered a disease of infants and children. The symptoms develop slowly in three stages. Stage 1 is a prodromal stage with nonspecific symptomatology. Seizures are common in stage 2; coma occurs in stage 3. A high index of suspicion is necessary for rapid diagnosis. A computed tomography (CT) scan of the head may show periventricular lucencies, edema, infarctions, and hydrocephalus. Cerebrospinal fluid (CSF) findings include an elevation in white blood cells (WBCs), usually from 250 to 500 cells/μL, predominantly lymphocytes. The CSF glucose is less than 40 mg/dL, or less than half the serum glucose found simultaneously. Protein concentration is normal or slightly high. Gram's stain is negative because the bacilli are acid-fast. CSF chloride is low.

Cryptococcal meningitis (choice **D**) is associated with elevated protein, hypoglycorrhachia, and mononuclear pleocytosis (rarely >300 cells/mm³). Children with subacute sclerosing panencephalitis (choice **B**) have CSF with normal white cell content (may show some plasma cells), normal or slightly elevated protein, and greatly increased γ-globulin. Eastern equine encephalitis (choice **A**) occurs more commonly in young infants, causing serious complications and fatalities. The spectrum and definitive diagnosis of meningococcal meningitis (choice **E**) are made by the isolation of the organism from the CSF.

## 20 The answer is E *Medicine*

Von Willebrand disease (choice **E**) is the most common of all the bleeding disorders; it affects both sexes equally, with a prevalence accounting for somewhat over 1% of the population. There are three major forms of the disease, types 1, 2, and 3, with four subsets of type 2: namely, 2A, 2B, 2M, and 2N. Patients with type 1 have less than the normal amount of von Willebrand's factor (vWF), patients with type 2 disease have aberrant forms of vWF, and patient's with type 3 disease have very little if any vWF. Types 1 and 2 are inherited as dominant traits; type 1 is the most common form, accounting for about 70% of case, and type 2A is the next most common form, making up about 17% of the cases. The type 3 disease is inherited as a recessive trait, is the most severe form, and is also not commonly encountered. During pregnancy, the levels of vWF normally rise throughout the third trimester and then decrease, normally to baseline about a mouth postpartum. However, in patients with von Willebrand disease, the decrease is exaggerated and levels of vWF decline even below the prepregnancy levels, which were already less than optimal. Consequently, as in the case described, a hemolytic crisis may take place some weeks after the birth (usually about a month). Recent National, Heart, Lung and Blood Institute (NHLBI) guidelines state that health care providers should remain in close contact with women with von Willebrand disease during this period. Although von Willebrand disease affects males and females to an equal extent, females more commonly become aware of otherwise borderline cases because of their menstrual periods. As in the case described, it is not uncommon for generations of women to have abnormally heavy menstrual flow, and while true that it runs in families, that does not make it normal. The function of vWF is to bind to other factors involved in coagulation and bring them to wound sites, thus permitting them to work together to inhibit bleeding. The basic vWF subunit is a 2,050 amino acid protein with specific domains for coagulation factor VIII, heparin, collagen, and platelet receptors and hence platelets. These monomers are N-glycosylated and converted into multimers in a process involving cysteine cross-linking at the C-terminus. These multimers are very large, containing up to 80 monomers, and only these larger forms of vWF are functional. Factor VIII is rapidly degraded when it is not bound to vWF, thus low circulating levels of vWF are accompanied by low levels of factor VIII. As mentioned, type 1 von Willebrand disease is due to reduced levels of functional vWF. Remember that, since this is a dominant condition, affected individuals all should have at least 50% of the normal levels of functional factor inherited from the normal parent. Variation in activity then depends upon residual activity remaining in the aberrant factor inherited from the other parent; thus, type 1 patients have half to near normal vWF levels and activity. In type 3 von Willebrand disease, a child inherits an aberrant factor from both parents; consequently, the type 2 diseases involve lack of functionality or hyperfunctionality in the factor that is synthesized.

Hemophilia A (choice **A**) and hemophilia B (choice **B**) are both sex-linked recessive conditions and consequently are rarely expressed in females; thus, they are clearly incorrect choices. Hemophilia A is the most common form, with a prevalence of about 1 case per 5,000 male births and results in a deficiency of blood coagulation factor VIII; hence, an alternate name, factor VIII deficiency. Patients may have cases that vary from severe to minor bleeding problems. Hemophilia B results in a deficiency of coagulation factor IX, and is also called factor IX deficiency or Christmas disease, after the first patient in whom the disease was described. It is less common than hemophilia A, with a prevalence of about 1 case per 25,000 male births. Hemophilia C (choice **C**) causes a deficiency of coagulation factor XI and affects members of both sexes. It is inherited in a recessive fashion and is quite rare, affecting about 1 person among 100,000 adults, almost only people of Ashkenazi or Iraqi Jewish decent, making it unlikely that this Irish Catholic lady suffers from this disease. Bernard-Soulier syndrome (choice **D**) is a very rare condition, with an incidence of about 1 case per 1 million individuals; it is characterized by a thrombocytopenia. The biochemical cause is decreased expression of the glycoprotein complex Ib/IX/V on the surface of platelets. This complex normally serves as a vWF receptor, and when it is deficient, platelet adhesion to wound sites is inhibited. In vitro, this can be demonstrated by the lack of aggregation of platelets in response to ristocetin, an antibiotic that normally induces platelets to aggregate. A deficient number of platelets at the wound site inhibits formation of the primary platelet plug and causes an increased tendency to bleed. The thrombocytopenia may be due to decreased platelet half life.

### 21 The answer is C *Medicine*

This lady has a case of alopecia areata. Alopecia is a general term for baldness; alopecia areata is a common type of specific hair loss that causes coin-sized areas of baldness, usually on the scalp, although it may occur any place on the face or trunk. It affects 1%–2% of the population, both males and females, most often teens or young adults, but may occur at any age. Hair generally grows back spontaneously, and it is thought to be an autoimmune reaction; thus, choice **C** is correct and permanents are not suspected as a cause (choice **D** is wrong). Person with this disorder sometimes have other autoimmune diseases, and there is a familial tendency to have the condition. As long as the loss is patchy and not all-inclusive, there is about an 80% chance it will grow back within a year. The early growth starts in the center of the bald patch; initially, it is fine and white, but with time, the hair usually regains its normal characteristics, although in older people it may not regain its color. The risk of not growing back is increased if there are large areas of hair loss, and in individuals with Down syndrome or eczema.

If the hair loss on the scalp is total, resulting in baldness, the condition is called alopecia areata totalis; if the loss is all over the body, it is called alopecia areata universalis. These are relatively uncommon conditions accounting for less than 1% of all alopecia areata cases and in these cases regrowth usually does not happen.

Alopecia areata usually does not lend itself to hair transplantation, thus choices **A** and **B** are incorrect. Some physicians would rather not treat alopecia areata, since odds are the hair will grow back spontaneously, but as it says in choice **C**, there are several treatments that may accelerate the rate of regrowth. Steroid creams, steroid injections or pills, dithranol treatment, and physical irritation all have been used and seem to jump-start hair growth, but often hair loss starts again once treatment stops. Steroids in particular may induce serious side effects. The least disruptive and probably the most effective treatment is minoxidil lotion. Shaving her head is a counterproductive response, and choice **E** is incorrect.

## 22 The answer is A *Obstetrics and Gynecology*

The physician should allow the patient to deliver her infant vaginally (choice **A**). Although the infant may contract herpes, the mother can refuse the cesarean section because competent adults have the right to refuse medical or surgical treatment. In this scenario, the fetus has no legal rights, the mother is the patient, and a court will not order a surgical procedure against the patient's will (choice **B**). Only the patient can consent to her own surgery. Although the risks of a cesarean are low, they can be major, including life-threatening. No one, including a husband (choice **D**), can consent to surgery for another person. Performing the cesarean without her consent (choice **C**) is legally considered "assault and battery" and is ethically not a viable option. The physician has the right to refuse treatment and to refer her to another physician; however, this will not solve the problem (choice **E**).

## 23 The answer is D *Pediatrics*

The symptoms described indicate that this patient has type II Arnold-Chiari malformation. In this condition, the hydrocephalus is a noncommunicating one. The fourth ventricle is elongated, there is kinking of the brainstem, and portions of the brainstem and cerebellum are displaced into the cervical spinal canal, causing obstruction of cerebrospinal fluid (CSF) flow. Skull films show a small posterior fossa and widened cervical canal (platybasia). Computed tomography or MRI will show hindbrain abnormalities and cerebellar tonsils protruding downward into the cervical canal (choice **D**). In noncommunicating hydrocephalus, the most frequent cause is aqueductal stenosis or the Arnold-Chiari malformation associated with meningomyelocele.

Type I Chiari malformation (choice **A**) is not associated with hydrocephalus and usually produces symptoms during adolescence or adult life. A leptomeningeal cyst (choice **E**) is a rare and late complication of a linear skull fracture and appears as an expanding pulsatile mass on the surface of the skull. Chronic subdural hematomas (choice **B**) are characterized by headache, personality change, and sudden loss of consciousness. Classically, patients with epidural hematoma (choice **F**) experience a brief period of unconsciousness followed by a variable lucid interval. As the hematoma expands, the patient has progressive loss of consciousness, headache, vomiting, and focal neurologic signs. Retinal hemorrhages would be seen in children who are victims of shaken-baby syndrome (choice **C**).

## 24 The answer is B *Pediatrics*

Ewing's sarcoma (choice **B**) is primarily a disease of adolescence but is far less common than osteosarcoma and is as likely to originate in almost any bone on the body. X-ray films are likely to show an "onion-peel," but this is not pathognomonic; the definitive diagnosis depends upon histologic examination, which will show small round cells. Primitive neuroectodermal tumors (pPNETs) show a histologic pattern similar to that of Ewing's sarcoma, respond similarly to chemotherapy, and both are characterized by a 11,12 chromosomal translocation. In spite of resection, chemotherapy, and irradiation, Ewing's sarcoma still has a 50% mortality rate.

Osteosarcoma (choice **C**) is the most common malignant bone tumor in children. The diagnosis of osteosarcoma may be suspected from good-quality radiographs. In advanced cases of osteosarcoma, possible findings include cortical destruction; sclerosis; a "sunburst" pattern of new periosteal bone formation; and calcified, soft-tissue extensions. Chondrosarcoma (choice **D**) is rare in children. It occurs most commonly in the pelvis. Metastasis is usually by local extension. Eosinophilic granuloma (choice **E**) presents as a painless or mildly painful swelling in the skull, long bones, ribs, pelvis, or vertebra. Radiographs show a lytic lesion with well-defined borders. Osteomyelitis (choice **A**) is an infection of the bone, with the femur and tibia most commonly affected. Radiographs are normal early in the course of osteomyelitis.

### 25 The answer is E  *Psychiatry*

This woman's symptoms are most suggestive of major depressive disorder (choice **E**). Depressive disorders may present as physical complaints, without subjective complaints of mood disturbance by the patient. This sort of clinical presentation is more common in patients who are stoic, are less able to introspect, and come from backgrounds in which emotional pathology is less acceptable. It is sometimes called "masked depression." Delusional disorder (choice **A**) is characterized by more improbable physical complaints. Dementia (choice **B**) presents with evidence of memory impairment and other cognitive deficits. In factitious disorder (choice **C**), symptoms are deliberately produced by the patient for the purpose of assuming the sick role. In hypochondriasis (choice **D**), a patient misinterprets minor physical complaints as evidence of more serious illness.

### 26 The answer is A  *Obstetrics and Gynecology*

The case scenario is characteristic of adenomyosis, a benign condition, in which endometrial glands and stroma are found within the myometrium (choice **A**). Adenomyosis usually develops in the later (not earlier [choice **B**]) reproductive years. Fertility may be impaired (choice **D**) if the site affected is in the region of the tubal ostia, a condition known as salpingitis isthmica nodosa. Although a physical examination finding of an enlarged, soft, boggy, tender, nonpregnant uterus may be suggestive of adenomyosis, the definitive diagnosis is based on histologic findings confirmed at the time of hysterectomy, not based on pelvic examination (choice **E**). A magnetic resonance imaging (MRI) study is strongly suggestive of adenomyosis if it demonstrates a symmetrically enlarged uterus. Surgical removal of the uterus is highly effective, not unsuccessful (choice **C**). The levonorgestrel-containing intrauterine contraceptive system (Mirena) is helpful in medical treatment of adenomyosis in some patients by decreasing menstrual blood flow.

### 27 The answer is C  *Medicine*

Cyanide is a deadly poison. It combines with ferric iron in the body, preventing oxygen from binding; this causes an increase in circulating $O_2$, thus imparting a pinkish to cherry red color to the skin. The most critical binding site is on mitochondrial cytochrome $a_3$, blocking the production of adenosine triphosphate (ATP). It is most commonly encountered as a solution containing a cyanide salt, such as NaCN or KCN, but the gas HCN is just as lethal. Annually, about 4,000 civilians die in the United States because of fires, and 60%–80% of these deaths are due to smoke inhalation. Traditionally, the treatment for smoke inhalation has been to pull the person into fresh air and administer 100% oxygen, on the assumption that the person is suffering from CO poisoning. However, recent studies have shown that at least as many deaths in home fires occur from HCN poisoning as from CO. Moreover, the proportion of cyanide-caused deaths will increase because of the increased use of synthetics containing nitrogen, as well as carbon in construction materials, clothing, and furniture, as for instance in polyurethane cushions and stuffings in couches. In 1994, France approved use of hydroxocobalamin (choice **C**) in the Cyanokit as the primary antidote to combat cyanide poisoning, and in 2007, the U.S. Centers for Disease Control and Prevention (CDC) also approved its use. Presently, the Cyanokit has been added to increasing numbers of emergency responder first-aid kits in the United States as a weapon to combat cyanide poisoning. The cyanide binds directly to the cobalt and no toxic by-products are produced. The major adverse effects are increased blood pressure, which maybe a welcome response since hypotension is a common symptom of cyanide poisoning, and reddish-colored urine that may persist for days.

Amyl nitrite, sodium nitrite, or 4-dimethylaminophenol (DMAP) (choice **A**) all are traditional antidotes for cyanide poisoning. They work by converting hemoglobin (ferrous iron) to methemoglobin (ferric iron), and since the concentrations of circulating hemoglobin are manyfold times greater than that of cytochrome $a_3$, the concept is that sufficient methemoglobin can be produced to draw the bound cyanide off of the cytochrome $a_3$. The disadvantages of these techniques are that there are no clear guidelines on how to estimate how much methemoglobin needs to be produced, and since this reduces the amount of functional circulating hemoglobin, it may be necessary to regenerate hemoglobin from the methemoglobin. Sodium thiosulfate (choice **B**) also is used as an antidote for cyanide poisoning. It acts as an endogenous sulfate donor, converting the poison cyanide to the innocuous thiocyanate. However, because the rate of this reaction is slow, thiosulfate is rarely used alone but is generally used after nitrite application. Methylene blue (choice **D**) is often used to correct over titration with a nitrate or DMAP; it converts methemoglobin back to hemoglobin. Dicobalt edetate (choice **E**) has also been used as an antidote for cyanide poisoning. It works by the same principle as hydroxocobalamin; however, it leaves residual free cobalt ions, which are toxic.

### 28 The answer is C *Pediatrics*

Juvenile rheumatoid arthritis (JRA) (choice **C**) is an autoimmune inflammatory disease that causes chronic synovitis as well as other extraarticular manifestations. This arthritis is divided into subgroups on the basis of presentation and laboratory findings. Systemic JRA occurs in approximately one-fifth of patients and is associated with high fevers, rash, hepatosplenomegaly, pleural and pericardial effusions, and anemia of chronic disease. The erythrocyte sedimentation rate (ESR) is elevated during active disease.

Acute rheumatic fever (choice **A**) can be differentiated from JRA by the evidence of carditis and its transient migratory arthritis. Systemic lupus erythematosus (SLE) (choice **B**) usually has milder joint manifestations and a characteristic malar rash. Lyme disease (choice **D**) should be considered in the differential diagnosis. A careful history and physical examination, searching for tick bites and characteristic rash of erythema chronicum migrans, should be performed. Ankylosing spondylitis (choice **E**) can be mistaken for JRA until spine involvement is seen. Its onset is later in life, and it is much more common in men.

### 29 The answer is B *Pediatrics*

Ataxia-telangiectasia (choice **B**) is an autosomal recessive disorder and the most common of the degenerative ataxias. The ataxia usually begins at approximately 2 years of age. It is progressive until full loss of ambulation occurs by adolescence. Telangiectasia (red spots on the skin due to dilated superficial blood vessels) is seen in the eyes, bridge of the nose, ears, and exposed surfaces of the extremities. The skin also loses elasticity. Sinopulmonary infections occur frequently, secondary to abnormal immune function. Low immunoglobulin A (IgA) and IgE levels are seen. The α-fetoprotein (AFP) level is elevated. Children with ataxia-telangiectasia have a much higher risk of developing lymphoreticular and brain tumors.

Wiskott-Aldrich syndrome (choice **A**) is an X-linked recessive syndrome that presents with atopic dermatitis, thrombocytopenic purpura, and an increased susceptibility to infection. Rendu-Osler-Weber disease (also known as hereditary hemorrhagic telangiectasia) (choice **C**) is characterized by angiomas of the skin, mucous membranes, gastrointestinal tract, and liver, as well as by pulmonary arteriovenous fistulas. Friedreich's ataxia (choice **D**) presents before 10 years of age with progressive ataxia, dysarthric speech, nystagmus, and skeletal abnormalities. Cerebral palsy (choice **E**) is a static encephalopathy that is a nonprogressive disorder of posture and movement. Cerebral palsy may be associated with mental retardation, epilepsy, and behavioral abnormalities.

### 30 The answer is D *Medicine*

Ricin is a waste product obtained while extracting castor oil from castor seeds. It is a toxic agent that inhibits protein synthesis in cells by inactivating the ribosome. It can enter the body via the cutaneous, gastrointestinal, or respiratory route. Ricin is not absorbed through intact skin, but when it comes into contact with mucosal surfaces, like the conjunctiva, it causes severe pain, blepharospasm, epiphora, and conjunctival injection. To penetrate the skin, ricin has been used in the form of bullets, which have been lethal. Following ingestion, symptoms appear after around 6 hours; these symptoms include vomiting, diarrhea, hematuria, fatigue, myalgia, hallucinations, and seizures; death can result. Following inhalation, symptoms can appear earlier. The patient complains of fever, excessive perspiration, fatigue, myalgia, cough, chest pain, and dyspnea. Pulmonary edema, cyanosis, and respiratory failure follow. In both cases, whether consumed by ingestion or inhalation, liver and renal failure ensues and death occurs from multiorgan failure within 2–3 days. There are no specific diagnostic tests to confirm exposure to ricin. Laboratory tests will show marked leucocytosis (up to five times normal values), elevated liver transaminases, hematuria, abnormal renal function, and metabolic acidosis. An immunofluorescence test using ricin antibody may be used to test samples from the environment for ricinine, an alkaloid present in castor bean. Some federal agencies, including post offices in the United States, have sensors that can detect the presence of ricin. Treatment is symptomatic and supportive. Eyes should be washed with copious amounts of water, IV fluids are administered to restore fluid lost through excessive perspiration and to prevent hypotension, oxygen is administered to maintain respiratory exchange, diuretics are given for pulmonary edema (confirmed on chest x-ray), and anticonvulsants are used to treat seizures. There is no vaccine against ricin. Differential diagnosis includes inhalation of phosgene or ingestion of poisonous mushrooms, arsenic, colchicines, and caustic agents. An important differential diagnosis is the inhalation or ingestion of staphylococcal enterotoxin B (SEB), a super antigen that stimulates cytokines that can cause widespread inflammation. The symptoms are similar to that of ricin and can be diagnosed by enzyme-linked immunosorbent assay (ELISA). The enterotoxin is secreted by *Staphylococcus aureus* and has been developed as a biological weapon. It is not lethal as an aerosol spray, but causes severe gastrointestinal symptoms, and victims are indisposed for up to 2 weeks. SEB can cause food poisoning or toxic shock syndrome in the general population. In addition to its possible use by terrorists, SEB is the most common cause of food poisoning and results from storing unrefrigerated food, especially milk, cheese, and meat, including those prepared in delis.

**Choice A** is incorrect. Anthrax is derived from *Bacillus anthracis*, a gram-positive, nonmotile, spore-forming bacterium. The spores gain access either through direct contact with the skin, ingestion, or inhalation, and then germinate. They lie dormant in the soil, and being hardy can survive for a long time in various environments, including clothing. Since spores can be grown in vitro, and *B. anthracis* produces a powerful lethal exotoxin, it can be, and has been, used as a biological weapon. Two strains of *B. anthracis* have been used in biological warfare; they are Ames and Vollum, of which the latter is more lethal. Anthrax is lethal because it has two components that play a role: a capsule and an exotoxin. The capsule prevents phagocytosis by neutrophils. This is achieved by disabling calmodulin, which is required to activate calcium ions, thus permitting neutrophils to phagocytose the bacterium. The exotoxin has three components: (a) a protective factor that enables the toxin to attach itself to the cell surface, permitting a (b) "lethal" and a (c) "edema" factor to enter the cell. The edema factor leads to leakage of vascular fluid into the tissue spaces, causing edema, or it attacks endothelial cells directly, ultimately causing hypotension. The lethal factor commands macrophages to produce tumor necrosis factor (TNF)α and interleukin 1, which attack tissues and cause septic shock. The symptoms will depend on the route of entry. When the inhaled spores enter the alveoli, they are captured by the macrophages and thereafter transported into the lymphatic system. Initially, patients have flu-like symptoms. Chest pain, cough, dyspnea, hemothorax, and hemorrhagic mediastinitis then result. Ingestion of anthrax will result in abdominal pain, hematemesis, and diarrhea. Contact with skin is the rarest form of the disease. The organism enters through a breach in the skin and a furuncle develops 2–5 days later. Thereafter, a black eschar forms in the center. The inhalational form of entry is the most lethal, and the preferred method for biological warfare. The diagnosis may be delayed because most patients assume they have the flu and do not seek immediate medical attention. Unfortunately, patients often present after the toxin has started to take effect. For the inhalational form of anthrax, the mortality rate is 97% despite treatment. In patients who have cutaneous lesions, diagnosis involves examining the fluid from the blister for spores and culture to reveal *B. anthracis*. For ingestional anthrax, examination of the blood, including culture for the bacteria is diagnostic. For inhalational anthrax, examination of blood, sputum culture, throat swab, and cerebrospinal fluid examination are diagnostic.

In inhalational anthrax, a chest x-ray will reveal classic widening of the mediastinum with clear lung fields. In some patients, a chest x-ray will reveal hemorrhagic pleural effusion as well. Treatment includes isolation, supportive measures, and intravenous antibiotics such as ciprofloxacin or doxycycline. Sometimes multiple drugs are required. Antibiotics are generally given for 2 months in those who survive. Although antibiotics kill the bacteria, they are ineffective against the toxin. Raxibacumab, a monoclonal antibody that specifically targets the enterotoxin is now available, and is used for treatment and prophylaxis. It prevents the binding of protective factor to the anthrax toxin receptor on the cell surface, thereby preventing the edema and lethal factors from gaining access to the cell and wreaking havoc. A vaccine is available; however, it does not afford immediate immunity. It takes several weeks to take effect and requires regular revaccination to maintain immunity. The vaccine is not available to the general population.

**Choice B** is incorrect. Phosgene is carbonic dichloride; it is a colorless gas that smells like freshly cut grass or hay, and is liquid below room temperature. It was used as a chemical weapon during World War I with great effect. Phosgene is a heavy gas and stays just above ground level; to allow better dispersion and diffusion, it is usually combined with chlorine. Phosgene is used in industry to produce pesticides and isocyanates from which certain plastics are made, and exposure to it is a known occupational hazard. Phosgene decomposes to hydrochloric acid and carbon monoxide in the presence of water, moisture, or steam. The effects of phosgene exposure do not occur until 48 hours have elapsed. Contact with skin result in features that resemble frost bite. Following inhalation, victims complain of burning in the eyes followed by blurry vision, burning in the throat, cough, dyspnea, nausea, and vomiting. In the lower airways, phosgene is converted into hydrochloric acid and chlorine, which then reacts with the sulfhydryl, ammonia, and hydroxyl groups in the proteins located at the alveolar interface. As a result, inflammation and pulmonary edema occurs. Oxygen–carbon dioxide exchange is compromised. Hypoxia and respiratory failure supervene, all in a matter of 2–6 hours following inhalation. An initial chest x-ray will be normal, but show evidence of pulmonary edema and bilateral interstitial infiltrates as the disease progresses. In those who survive, chronic bronchitis and emphysema can result. There are no specific diagnostic tests. Treatment involves taking off all contaminated clothing and washing the body with soap and water; eyes should be washed with water. Clothing, including contact lenses, used by the patient should be bagged and retained for examination. Patients should be observed for 48 hours in a hospital setting as symptoms generally begin thereafter. Treatment is supportive and includes intravenous fluids, oxygen, and ventilator support. There are no antidotes.

**Choice C is incorrect.** Mustard gas is a cytotoxic agent, dichlorodiethyl sulfide, belonging to the sulfur mustard family. It has the odor of mustard plants, hence the name, although it has been described by some as having a garlic-like odor and by others as odorless. It exists in three forms: liquid, powder, and gas. In pure form, it is colorless, but the form that is used as a chemical warfare agent is a brownish-yellow liquid. The gas is yellow in color and dissipates slowly. It was called "yellow fog" when it was used on soldiers during World War I. More recently, it was used during the Iraq–Iran conflict. The gas is used in warfare to induce ocular symptoms, thereby disabling the opponent's troops, and it can cause death as well. Sulfur mustard alkylates DNA, causing cellular injury and death. It is primarily a vesicant, meaning that it forms blisters on the skin and exposed mucus membranes. The epidermis is anchored to the dermis by laminin, a glycoprotein present in the basement membrane, and integrin, a transmembrane protein that promotes attachment of cells to extracellular matrix. Sulfur mustard suppresses the action of laminin and integrin, leading to separation of the epidermis from the dermis, thereby forming blisters. Symptoms usually develop anywhere from 6 to 24 hours after exposure and involve not only the skin, but the respiratory and gastrointestinal system as well. During the acute phase, patients complain of headache, nausea, smarting of the eyes, itching, blepharospasm, and photophobia; conjunctivitis and temporary blindness occurs, but in those who develop corneal ulceration, blindness can be permanent. Additional complaints include sore throat, a red face and neck, and palpitations due to tachycardia that can persist for months. Sulfur mustard penetrates clothing easily and is very soluble in fat; hence, penetration through skin is very rapid, leading to blister formation on both skin and exposed mucosal surfaces. Skin lesions usually occur in areas that are moist such as the axillae, perineum, and groin. They initially start as irritation that causes itching, followed by spots that progress to second- and third-degree burns with blister formation and excoriation of the skin. Blisters contain a yellowish fluid, which can be aspirated and tested for the presence of thio-diglycol, which confirms the diagnosis. Involvement of the respiratory system includes epistaxis, cough, hemoptysis, expectoration of purulent and necrotic material that has been sloughed off, dyspnea, and pulmonary edema. Involvement of the gastrointestinal system causes abdominal pain, vomiting, and diarrhea. Leucocytosis is present initially, followed by leucopenia even in the presence of infection. Anemia also occurs, and in some cases thrombocytopenia, suggesting bone marrow suppression. (The serendipitous finding of leucopenia led to the creation of mustine to treat leukemia, and thus began the era of chemotherapy.) Western Blot and immunofluorescence tests to confirm degradation of laminin and integrin using laminin antibody from animals exposed to sulfur mustard has been successful in animal experiments, and it is hoped that this test could be replicated for humans. Treatment includes washing the eyes with copious amounts of water, removal contaminated clothes, removal of the thick paste of mustard gas that is present on the skin, and immediately covering those area with anti-gas powder, which is a combination of calcium chloride and magnesium oxide. Thereafter, the patient should be washed with water and neutral soap. Blisters should be incised and drained, and a moist occlusive dressing with sulfadiazine cream should be applied. IV fluids, antibiotics, respiratory support, and analgesics should also be given as necessary. Burned areas usually heal within 4–6 weeks. Those who survive develop chronic respiratory problems such as chronic obstructive pulmonary disease (COPD), chronic bronchitis, bronchiectasis, asthma, and pulmonary fibrosis.

**Choice E is incorrect.** Sarin is an organophosphorus (OP) compound that is colorless and odorless and can change quickly from liquid to gas. It is a nerve gas that attacks the central nervous system and is 500 times more potent than cyanide. It was invented in Germany in 1939, but fortunately was not used for the extermination of prisoners of war, those deemed to be of inferior race, or those who opposed the Nazi regime—cyanide in the form of Zygon B was used instead. Sarin inhibits cholinesterase, so that acetylcholine continues to act on the postsynaptic receptor; it is fatal even in very low doses. Death can occur in less than a minute. Even a drop of Sarin on the skin can induce local perspiration and fasciculation. Initial symptoms include rhinorrhea, drooling, chest tightness, dyspnea, and miosis—all features of OP poisoning. Other symptoms include headache, confusion, blurred vision, ocular pain, lacrimation, tachycardia or bradycardia, variable blood pressure (hypotension or hypertension), nausea, vomiting, diarrhea, and diuresis. Seizures, coma, and death can result. Immediate intravenous administration of atropine, which blocks the action of acetylcholine at the muscarinic receptor, and pralidoxime 30 mg/kg body weight, is required. Diazepam can be used to treat seizures. Barbiturates should be avoided because of their anticholinesterase action. Other measures include washing the eyes if blurry vision is present, and if there has been contact with the skin, removal of all clothing and washing the body with water. Sarin was used during the Iraq–Iran war and in ethnic cleansing attacks against the Kurds. It has also been used by terrorists on a subway in Tokyo, Japan. Troops in danger of being attacked by sarin carry an autoinjector containing a combination of atropine 2 mg and obidoxime 110 mg.

## 31 The answer is D  *Medicine*

This man most likely has peripheral artery disease (PAD), sometimes called peripheral vacular disease (PVD), of the legs. The simplest and usually first diagnostic screening test is determination of the ankle-brachial index (ABI) (choice **D**). This is done by simply determining the brachial and ankle systolic blood pressures and then dividing the brachial pressure into the value for the pressure at the ankle. A ratio greater than 0.9 is considered normal; a ratio between 0.8 and 0.9 is consistent with mild PAD, between 0.5 and 0.8 moderate PAD, and less than 0.5 severe disease. If the ABI is abnormal, a test (or tests) to better determine the site and quantify the extent of the lesion causing the occlusion may also be run. These imaging tests are likely to be peripheral Doppler ultrasound (choice **A**), peripheral angiography (choice **B**), or a computed tomography (CT) scan (choice **C**) would be non-contributory. Although a magnetic resonance imaging (MRI) scan (choice **E**) will provide an accurate image of the interior of the artery, it is less likely to be used because of the cost. In the United States, it is estimated that 10%–25% of the population over the age of 55 years has discernible PAD. Risk factors include smoking, diabetes, high blood pressure, dyslipidemia, obesity, male, African American descent, age older than 55, or having any other known vascular disease. Additionally, since the cause of PAD is most likely arteriosclerosis, having PAD suggests that a person is at risk of having other arterial diseases, such as coronary arteriosclerosis. Moreover, thrombi may break off from the arteriosclerotic regions in the leg and travel to the heart or lungs. The first step in treatment is smoking cessation. Subsequent steps are bringing other risks factors, such as diabetes or hypertension, under control. Accomplishing this is likely to require specific medication in addition to lifestyle modification. Chelation therapy is a widely advertised alternative treatment; however, there is no sound evidence to support the use of this modality, which at the least can be expensive and on occasion dangerous. If such treatments are not beneficial, surgery (stents, bypass surgery and angioplasty, etc.) might be attempted. An unfortunate last resort most commonly utilized for diabetics is amputation.

## 32 The answer is C  *Pediatrics*

Craniopharyngioma (choice **C**) is the most common supratentorial tumor of children. About 90% of these tumors show calcifications on plain skull films or on computed tomography (CT) scanning. Many cases are originally discovered during an endocrine workup for short stature secondary to pituitary-hypothalamic involvement. Bitemporal field defects occur because of pressure or injury to the optic chiasm. The tumor can also compress the third ventricle, causing noncommunicating hydrocephalus. With prominent hydrocephalus, papilledema is evident. Polyuria from diabetes insipidus results from interruption of the supraoptic-hypophyseal tract. Treatment consists of surgical removal of the tumor and hormone replacement. In this patient, Figure A (the sagittal view) shows a large suprasellar mass, and Figure B (the coronal view) shows compression of the pituitary gland and a large suprasellar mass.

Astrocytoma of the third ventricle (choice **A**) commonly presents with symptoms of increased intracranial pressure (headache, nausea, vomiting, and hydrocephalus) and seizures. A pinealoma (choice **B**) presents with failure of upward gaze (Parinaud syndrome). Hand-Schüller-Christian disease (choice **E**) is a childhood histiocytosis. Presentation is variable, but skeletal involvement occurs in 80% of patients. Skin lesions, exophthalmos, and hepatosplenomegaly occur in 20% of these patients. Pituitary dysfunction may result in failure to thrive; however, calcifications are not seen on CT. Other central nervous system (CNS) symptoms are uncommon. Chromophobic adenomas (choice **D**) of the pituitary may also cause short stature and diabetes insipidus. Calcifications will not be present.

## 33 The answer is E  *Psychiatry*

The presentation is most suggestive of somatization disorder (choice **E**). Somatization disorder is characterized by a long history of physical complaints from multiple organ systems, commonly including general malaise, gastrointestinal symptoms, neurologic symptoms, and sexual symptoms. It almost always begins before 30 years of age, is often associated with analgesic and sedative-hypnotic abuse, and is more common in women.

In somatization disorder, the individual does not complain of an imagined physical deformity, as would be expected with body dysmorphic disorder (choice **A**). There is no evidence of the somatic delusions present in delusional disorder, somatic type (choice **B**). Also there is no suggestion that the complaints are intentionally produced or feigned, as in factitious disorder (choice **C**). Pain disorder (choice **D**) is diagnosed only when the predominant complaint is pain in the absence of complaints from other organ systems.

## 34 The answer is C *Medicine*

Restless leg syndrome (choice **C**) is a disorder of unknown etiology that affects both men and women equally. These patients complain of disagreeable sensations in the legs, cramplike pains, sometimes a crawling sensation, or even itching. These patients try to move their limbs to get rid of the pain, even getting up to walk or pace around. While the pain tends to disappear with movement, it returns during the resting phase. The pain can disturb sleep. It usually peaks by midnight and thereafter tends to improve by morning. The problem can occur during the day, either while being sedentary or while driving a car. It may be associated with iron deficiency anemia, diabetes, pregnancy, and chronic renal failure, especially in patients who are on dialysis. Some patient may go for months without symptoms. There are no clinical tests, and the diagnosis is based on a history of dysesthesia, motor restlessness, a desire to move the limbs, and worsening of symptoms at night or during periods of rest.

Painful legs and moving toes syndrome (choice **A**) does not occur at night and so does not induce insomnia. These patients complain of pain in the legs and feet, and involuntary writhing movements occur during this time. The pain does not get worse at the end of the day or during the night. Fibromyalgia (choice **B**) usually involves a large area of the body, including the axial skeleton. Symptoms generally occur throughout the day, and movement does not improve it. Cauda equina syndrome (choice **D**) is usually associated with low back pain, unilateral motor weakness, and sensory loss, and there may be loss of anal sphincter tone and problems with urination. Akathisia (choice **E**), an inner restlessness condition marked by an irresistible urge to move, is usually induced by medications such as phenothiazines or is a result of illness, such as Parkinson disease. These patients have restlessness that tends to affect the entire body, unlike restless leg syndrome, in which the problems are localized to the extremities. Symptoms occur less often at night, so insomnia is not a feature.

## 35 The answer is C *Medicine*

Pseudomembranous colitis is a condition in which the inner membrane of at least a segment of the colon becomes inflamed due to an infection that caused sloughing off of debris and white cells. These then tend to coat the colon, forming a pseudomembrane. The infection is caused by overgrowth of a minor endogenous organism, and it happens because most of the normal flora has been eliminated by an antibiotic. Most commonly, the overgrowing organism is *C. difficile*, which produces toxins that in turn cause gastritis leading to symptoms similar to those described in this case. Because the organism is difficult to grow, confirmation of *C. difficile* infection is generally done by assaying for its toxin B. Treatment is to remove *C. difficile* from the colitis, generally by using an antibiotic that will inhibit growth of anaerobes. Metronidazole is generally the first choice. Thus, in summary, the tentative diagnosis is pseudomembranous colitis, the diagnostic test run on the stool sample is assay for *C. difficile* toxin, and the most likely treatment is administration of metronidazole.

Choice **D** pseudomembranous colitis, assay for *C. difficile* toxins, and administration of loperamide is incorrect because provision of an antidiarrhea medicine most likely will be counterproductive because the net result will be to permit the *C. difficile* organism and its toxins to remain in the colon for a longer time. For the same reason, choices **B** and **F** will also not be correct. In addition, choices **E** and **F** are incorrect because *C. difficile* is difficult to assay for. Although at present *C. difficile* is the most common cause of infectious diarrhea, other organisms may also cause it; these include *C. perfringens* and *S. enterocolitis*. In fact, from about 1955 to 1970, *S. enterocolitis* was the most common cause of pseudomembranous colitis because *S. enterocolitis* strains were commonly methicillin resistant and gastroenteritis was generally treated with antibiotics that did not affect them. Thus, these antibiotics wiped out the normal intestinal flora, permitting *S. enterocolitis* to flourish. Starting around 1970, this situation was terminated with the introduction of antibiotics that inhibited growth of methicillin-resistant strains of *S. enterocolitis*. Unfortunately, *S. enterocolitis* species are starting to appear that are also resistant to some of these antibiotics and cases of pseudomembranous colitis caused by *S. enterocolitis* are being reported again, although not as commonly as by *C. difficile*. These cannot successfully be treated with metronidazole, thus making choice **A** wrong under any circumstance. Had vancomycin been used instead of metronidazole, choice **A** would have been correct.

**36** **The answer is D** *Preventive Medicine and Public Health*

There is insufficient evidence to recommend for or against screening middle-aged and older men and women for asymptomatic coronary artery disease (CAD) using resting, ambulatory, or exercise electrocardiograms (ECGs). Ischemic heart disease is the leading cause of death in the United States, accounting for approximately 500,000 deaths per year. It is estimated that approximately 1.5 million people have an acute myocardial infarction every year, and one-third will not survive the acute event. Nonetheless, routine ECG screening as part of the periodic health visit is not recommended for asymptomatic children, adolescents, or young adults (choice **D**). Therefore, in the case scenario, an ECG would be appropriate for a 30-year-old only if the patient had symptoms (e.g., chest pain) or a positive risk factor. Clinicians should emphasize proved measures for the primary prevention of CAD (e.g., reducing hypertension, lowering the blood cholesterol level) and counsel patients to avoid using tobacco, to consume a healthy diet, and to undertake regular aerobic physical activity.

Accordingly, choices **A**, **B**, and **C** are incorrect. Although total body computed tomography (CT) scans are the rage in some quarters, there is no evidence indicating that they should be recommended for screening for CAD (choice **E**).

**37** **The answer is B** *Obstetrics and Gynecology*

Menopause is characterized by absence of functional ovarian follicles resulting in estrogen levels that are decreased; therefore, choices **A** and **E** are incorrect. With the decline in estrogen levels, as well as loss of inhibin from the ovarian follicles, negative feedback to anterior pituitary gland is lost, resulting in increased follicle-stimulating hormone (FSH) levels; therefore, choice **D** is rejected. Choices **B** and **C** are identical except for the direction of gonadotropin-releasing hormone (GnRH). Because menopause is associated with increased GnRH levels, choice **C** is rejected, and choice **B** is found to be the only correct one. Estrogen levels move in the same direction as sex hormone-binding globulin (SHBG). With the normal fall in estrogen, we can expect SHBG to also be decreased.

**38** **The answer is B** *Obstetrics and Gynecology*

Hypertensive disorders of pregnancy are among the main causes of maternal mortality in the United States and require a sustained blood pressure (BP) above 140/90 for diagnosis. This patient's findings meet the criteria for severe preeclampsia. This includes the BP criteria (>160/110) and the proteinuria criteria of more than 3+ protein. In addition, the symptoms of persistent headache and epigastric pain support the concern regarding severe preeclampsia. The management priorities in this scenario are stabilization of the mother (by lowering her BP with hydralazine or labetalol to diastolic values between 90 and 100), prevention of seizures (using intravenous magnesium sulfate [choice **B**]), and then prompt delivery.

Phenytoin (choice **A**) is an anticonvulsant used in nonpregnant patients but is not appropriate in pregnant women. Terbutaline (choice **C**) and indomethacin (choice **E**) are tocolytics and would be contraindicated in this patient, who needs to be delivered. Progesterone (choice **D**) administration has been used for prevention of idiopathic preterm labor but has no demonstrable indication in severe preeclampsia.

**39** **The answer is E** *Pediatrics*

The clavicle is the most commonly fractured bone in infants during delivery (choice **E**). This fracture is more common in macrosomic newborns (e.g., infants of diabetic mothers). The newborn generally does not move the arm, giving an absent Moro reflex on the affected side. Crepitus is felt on palpation. Treatment is usually unnecessary, and the prognosis is good.

Cephalhematoma (choice **A**) is a hemorrhage confined within the area of the affected cranial bone. Cephalhematomas require no treatment, although phototherapy may be necessary to ameliorate hyperbilirubinemia. Facial nerve palsy (choice **B**) may result from pressure over the facial nerve in utero or from forceps during delivery. A patient with facial nerve palsy will have an eye that cannot be closed, an absent nasolabial fold, a corner of the mouth that droops, and a smooth forehead on the affected side. Prognosis depends on the extent of injury to the nerve. Intraventricular hemorrhage (choice **C**) is caused by rupture of the germinal blood vessels. Predisposing factors are prematurity, hypoxic injury, respiratory distress syndrome, reperfusion injury, and change in volume of cerebral circulation, compromised vascular integrity, hypervolemia (hypertension), and pneumothorax. The incidence of intraventricular hemorrhage increases with decreasing birth weight. Brain contusion (choice **D**) may be associated with a skull fracture.

**40** **The answer is A** *Medicine*

This man is suffering from acute renal failure (ARF) marked by oliguria and retention of nitrogenous wastes. Causes of ARF are customarily divided into three categories: prerenal, renal, and postrenal. Prerenal causes are those occurring in the blood supply leading up to the glomerulus, renal are due to events in the body of the kidney, and postrenal are due to obstructions in the urinary tract leaving the kidney. In the case described, the precipitating factor was the ingestion of enalapril. As a general rule, angiotensin-converting enzyme (ACE) inhibitors such as enalapril or of angiotensin II receptor blockers (ARBs) are beneficial and lower morbidity and mortality. However, they can trigger ARF because they inhibit the production or utilization of angiotensin II, which will cause vasodilation of the postglomerular efferent arterioles (choice **A**); the result is a decrease of glomerular pressure, which decrease the filtration rate and the production of urine, leading to acute renal failure. This usually only happens in persons whose vascular system is stressed in someway. The man's system in this case was stressed by old age, diabetes, and evidence of "inflexible" arteries as demonstrated by his resistant systolic hypertension.

Because the afferent preglomerular arterioles supply blood to the kidney, vasoconstriction of the preglomerular arterioles (choice **B**) also may cause prerenal ARF. Nonsteroid anti-inflammatory drugs (NSAIDs) may induce ARF via this mechanism because they inhibit cyclo-oxygenase (COX), and thus inhibit prostaglandin synthesis. Glomerulonephritis (choice **C**) rarely causes ARF, but it represents a type of renal ARF if it is quickly induced. It will be accompanied by systemic manifestations such as fever, rash, and arthritis. Acute interstitial nephritis (choice **D**) is another type of renal ARF. This condition often results from an allergic reaction to one of a host of drugs, including allopurinol, cephalosporins, cimetidine, ciprofloxacin, furosemide, NSAIDs, penicillins, phenytoin, rifampin, sulfonamides, and thiazide diuretics. Several diseases can also lead to development of acute interstitial nephritis. It again will be accompanied by a host of systemic manifestation. As indicated, obstruction of the outflow of urine from the kidney can also cause postrenal ARF. A urethral stone (choice **E**) is a cause easily visualized. Other causes include prostatic hypertrophy or cancer, catheters, and strictures.

**41** **The answer is E** *Surgery*

Anterior dislocation of the shoulder is more common than fracture. Joint stability has been sacrificed for mobility. Therefore, the shoulder joint has a shallow glenoid cavity with a small surface area, whereas the articular surface of the head of the humerus is disproportionately large. This permits one to move the arm to a great degree in several directions. The capsule of the shoulder joint is weak on its inferior aspect, and forced abduction leads to dislocation of the humeral head to a subglenoid and then a subcoracoid position. The subcoracoid position is the most common location for an anteriorly dislocated shoulder. Pull of the pectoralis major muscle attached to the upper end of the humerus results in displacement of the dislocated head to the subcoracoid position. Very rarely, the head is in the subclavicular position. Due to the proximity of the axillary nerve, it is most important to test for hypesthesia (choice **E**) over the lateral aspect of the shoulder, the presence of which signifies neural compression by the dislocated head. The musculocutaneous nerve is also in the vicinity, and hypesthesia over the lateral aspect of the forearm should also be excluded. Failure to document hypesthesia could result in a lawsuit. Unlike posterior dislocation, an anteriorly dislocated shoulder can be externally rotated. In fact, Kocher's method uses external rotation in reduction of shoulder dislocation.

**42** **The answer is C** *Surgery*

Posterior dislocations of the shoulder are rare and are usually caused by seizures. The posterior group of muscles attached to the humerus induces the dislocation during convulsions. Thus, a woman with eclampsia is more prone to a posterior dislocation of the shoulder than an anterior dislocation. The arm cannot be externally rotated beyond the neutral point (choice **C**). The problem can be missed on a standard x-ray, but a tangential view (transscapular view) will confirm the diagnosis.

**43** **The answer is F** *Surgery*

This patient has had a subluxation of the radial head. The radial head is ensconced within the annular ligament, which is still not fully mature. A sudden pull on the arm of a child (e.g., to prevent him from running onto the street) results in subluxation, in which the head of the radius slips inferiorly. There may be an associated partial tear of the annular ligament. This is not a dislocation of the head of the radius. Normally, no swelling is noted. The condition is reduced by supination of the forearm (choice **F**). The head relocates with a click. No immobilization is required. The child starts using the arm quite quickly. Recurrence is rare; however, after three recurrences, surgical repair is indicated.

**44 The answer is D** *Surgery*

This child has sustained a supracondylar fracture of the elbow. It usually results from a blow to the back of the lower end of the humerus, just above the medial and lateral condyles. These fractures may be associated with neurovascular trauma, most notably compression of the medial nerve and brachial artery. Normally, there is a great deal of swelling around the elbow. During reduction, the radial pulse should be felt constantly (choice **D**). If the pulse diminishes, the elbow should be extended to the position where the pulse returns to normal. Initially, the patient is kept immobilized in a Dunlop traction, in which the forearm and hand are kept elevated with countertraction while traction is maintained on the arm. Failure to ensure adequate circulation could lead to Volkmann's ischemic contracture, a disastrous complication. In the presence of an occult supracondylar fracture, a positive fat pad sign is noted, wherein the pad of fat normally present posterior to the capsule is pushed back further. Similarly, the pad of fat present anteriorly is pushed forward to form a triangular shape (a positive sail sign).

**45 The answer is A** *Surgery*

Patients who sustain fractures involving the shaft of the humerus can have concomitant injury to the radial nerve, which courses behind the shaft of the radius. In such an event, there may be an associated wrist drop (choice **A**). Sometimes, fractures of the humeral shaft may be associated with dislocation of the shoulder joint.

**46 The answer is G** *Surgery*

This patient has a Monteggia's fracture, in which the shaft of the ulna is fractured and the head of the radius is dislocated (choice **G**). In all cases of fractures, it is important to include the proximal and distal joint in the x-ray film so as not to miss associated joint injuries, as would occur in the case of a Monteggia's fracture.

**47 The answer is B** *Surgery*

This patient has sustained a Galeazzi's fracture, in which the shaft of the radius is fractured and the inferior radioulnar joint is dislocated (choice **B**). Just as in the case of a Monteggia's fracture, it is very important to include the proximal and distal joint while taking an x-ray film so as not to miss associated injuries.

**48 The answer is E** *Preventive Medicine and Public Health*

In a 2008 National Institute of Drug Abuse (NIDA) survey, 1.5% (choice **E**) of high school seniors reported use of anabolic steroids at least once. Although not addictive, use of anabolic steroids is a health hazard. Common side effects include severe acne and trembling; males may also undergo shrinking of the testicles and breast development, while females may grow facial hair, stop menstruating, and develop a deeper voice. Both sexes are also liable to irreversibly stunt their growth due to premature closure of their epiphyses. Prolonged use also increases the risk of developing jaundice, liver and/or kidney cancers, and hypertension.

**49 The answer is B** *Preventive Medicine and Public Health*

In 2004, 25% (choice **B**) of senior high school seniors reported that they used tobacco at least once during the previous 30-day period. This is a statistically insignificant increase from 2003, when 24% reported use. However, both values show an encouraging decline from 1997 data that reported 36.5% use in a comparable sample. Similar declines in use were also found in the lower grades. Another encouraging observation is that, over the same time period, high school students at all grades exhibited increased awareness of the health hazards associated with smoking. Despite these encouraging statistics among high school students, the next older bracket of adults studied in 2003 showed the heaviest use of tobacco products, 44.8%. It will be interesting to see if the apparent decline in use among high school students will carry forward into the future and be reflected by a significant decrease in use among young adults.

**50 The answer is D** *Preventive Medicine and Public Health*

Use of some form of cocaine during 2004 was reported by 5% (choice **D**) of 12th graders. There was a major increase in reported use between 1992 and 1999, from 3.2% to 6.2%, among this group of students. The rate then dropped to 5% in 2000 and has essentially remained steady since. Paradoxically, 12th graders also reported a perceived increase in availability of all forms of cocaine in 2004.

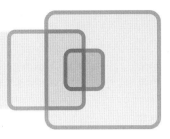

# test **5**

# *Questions*

***Single Best Choice Directions:*** *This section consists of numbered statements or questions followed by a list of potential answers; you are to select the ONE best answer.*

**1** A 68-year-old man presents at the emergency department because of such severe abdominal pain that he "just could not stand it any longer." He tells the triage nurse that he hadn't been feeling well for the past couple of months, primarily because he had been having abdominal pain about 30 minutes after eating and as a consequence lost almost 10 pounds, but last night he suddenly developed "a stomach ache from hell." He also has been vomiting and has had several episodes of bloody diarrhea. Upon physical examination, the physician notes hypotension and confirms the abdominal pain and notices abdominal distention. However, bowel sounds are absent, and there is no rebound tenderness present or other relevant findings upon abdominal examination. Laboratory data reveal an absolute neutrophilic leukocytosis and left shift plus lactic acidosis, and elevation of the serum amylase level. Which of the following is the most likely diagnosis?

(A) Acute ulcerative colitis
(B) Hemorrhagic pancreatitis
(C) Aortoenteric fistula
(D) Acute small bowel infarction
(E) Toxic megacolon

**2** Soon after birth, a term newborn is noted to be cyanotic with feeding. The infant was born to a 24-year-old primigravida who had excellent prenatal care. There is no history of tobacco, alcohol, or illicit drug use. Review of the mother's medical record shows that results of all diagnostic studies for sexually transmitted diseases have been negative. The delivery was uncomplicated. The infant weighed 6 lb 13 oz (3.1 kg), and Apgar scores at 1 and 5 minutes were 8 and 9, respectively. Examination of the newborn reveals that crying relieves the cyanosis. Which of the following is the most likely diagnosis?

(A) A tracheoesophageal fistula
(B) Bronchopulmonary dysplasia
(C) Respiratory distress syndrome
(D) Choanal atresia
(E) A patent ductus arteriosus

**3** A 54-year-old man presents to his physician for a physical examination. He is 5 ft 11 in tall and weighs 229 lb (body mass index [BMI] 33 kg/m²). His blood pressure is 165/80 mm Hg, pulse is 75/min and regular. Otherwise, results of his physical examination are unremarkable. He was asked to have a fasting blood sample taken for a lipid profile. The next week, the following data are reported: total cholesterol, 225 mg/dL; triglyceride level, 200 mg/dL; low-density lipoprotein, 145 mg/dL; and high-density lipoprotein, 40 mg/dL. Because his BMI defines him as being class I obese and because his total cholesterol is borderline high, the physician puts him on a diet and prescribes a cholesterol-lowering medication. Since starting the medication, the patient experienced problems with constipation and a bloating sensation that is relieved by increasing dietary fiber. Which of the following metabolic alterations is expected from the drug he is taking?

(A) Decreased activity of hydroxymethylglutaryl (HMG)-CoA reductase
(B) Decreased synthesis of triglyceride in hepatocytes
(C) Increased activity of capillary lipoprotein lipase
(D) Increased excretion of free cholesterol in feces
(E) Increased synthesis of hepatocyte low-density lipoprotein receptors

**4** A 62-year-old woman suffers a myocardial infarct (MI) while being examined in her physician's office. He attempts cardiopulmonary resuscitation, administers oxygen, and a bolus of epinephrine, all to no avail. The woman dies. Her family files a malpractice suit. For this claim to have merit, which of the following must the family prove about the doctor?

(A) He was improperly educated.
(B) He intended to cause the patient harm.
(C) He committed a crime.
(D) He overcharged the patient for the care given.
(E) He deviated from the established standard of care.

**5** A 48-year-old obese woman was admitted to the hospital with upper-right-quadrant pain and vomiting. She had no diarrhea or constipation. Clinical examination revealed tenderness in the right upper quadrant, and appropriate investigations demonstrated the presence of a stone in the common bile duct. Attempts to dislodge the stone endoscopically proved futile, so she underwent common bile duct exploration. Six days after surgery, she developed a temperature of 38°C (101°F). Which of the following is the most likely cause of her fever?

(A) Resorption of blood from the peritoneum
(B) Endotoxic shock
(C) Atelectasis
(D) A wound infection
(E) Renal failure

**6** A 6-month-old African American girl presents with low-grade fever and acute onset of painful swelling of the hands and feet. Radiographs taken at the onset of symptoms reveal soft-tissue swelling. A peripheral blood smear was made and is illustrated below. The findings described for this infant most likely correlate with which of the following events?

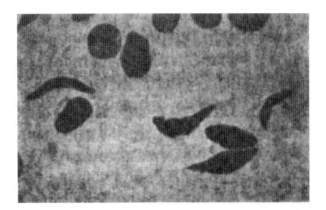

(A) A hemolytic crisis induced by an aberrant glucose-6-phosphate dehydrogenase (G6PD)
(B) Infection of the digital bones by *Salmonella*
(C) Replacement of fetal hemoglobin (Hb F) with Hb A
(D) A coxsackievirus infection
(E) Lymphedema of the hands and feet caused by the deletion of a chromosome

**7** A 3-year-old girl with autistic disorder has a buccal smear for chromosomal analysis. Her 14-year-old brother is retarded, with an unusually narrow face, a prominent forehead, large protruding ears, a prominent jaw, unusually large testes, and a high-pitched voice. The 55-year-old maternal grandfather of these children has had an inattention tremor for at least the past 5 years. With which of the following chromosomal abnormalities is the girl most likely afflicted?

(A) Cri du chat syndrome (deletion of short arm of chromosome 5)
(B) Fragile X syndrome
(C) Klinefelter syndrome (XXY)
(D) Down syndrome (trisomy 21)
(E) Turner syndrome (XO)

**8** A 42-year-old man complains of headaches when he wakes up in the morning. He reveals that has had these headaches for maybe as long as a year, but they have been occurring more often and are getting progressively worse. He also feels as though he is losing his strength and that he sometimes has trouble placing his feet where he wants to without looking down at the ground. The physician observes him to have an unusually prominent jaw with spaces between the teeth, and large hands and feet. By asking him to press against his arm, the physician confirms muscle weakness. Upon physical examination, his blood pressure was found to be 135/95 mm Hg, and his nonfasting blood glucose value was 195 mg/dL. Which of the following would be expected in this patient?

(A) Chest radiograph with normal-sized heart
(B) Normal-sized sella turcica
(C) Lack of suppression of glucose with an oral glucose challenge
(D) Decreased concentration of insulin-like growth factor-1
(E) Decreased serum growth hormone

**9** During a routine examination, a 65-year-old woman complains to her gynecologist that she has not been sleeping well for the past 5 or 6 months because of a sensation of pressure and burning in the middle of her chest. Further questioning reveals that she also feels the pressure and burning intermittently during the day; however, it is not induced by exercise and is relieved by antacids. The patient's blood pressure is 135/82 mm Hg, her pulse is 96/min and regular, and her temperature is 37.0°C (98.6°F). Her heart sounds are normal, and her lungs are clear. Palpation of her abdomen reveals no abnormalities. Which of the following is the most appropriate first step in the management of this patient?

(A) Refer her to a psychologist
(B) Prescribe cisapride
(C) Prescribe ranitidine, cimetidine, nizatidine, or famotidine
(D) Order an electrocardiogram (ECG)
(E) Prescribe antibiotics to eradicate gastric *Helicobacter pylori*
(F) Prescribe omeprazole, lansoprazole, rabeprazole, esomeprazole, or pantoprazole

**10** A 25-year-old man was thrown to the ground in a motorcycle accident. The paramedics transported him to the nearest emergency department. The physician on duty notes bruising about the orbit and blood in the external auditory meatus. Clear fluid exudes from his ear. The physician suspects that it is cerebrospinal fluid (CSF). Chemical analysis of the fluid compared with that of serum would be expected to show which of the following?

(A) A higher protein concentration than serum
(B) A higher chloride concentration than serum
(C) A higher glucose concentration than serum
(D) More white blood cells (WBCs) in the CSF than in the serum
(E) Absence of prealbumin on CSF electrophoresis

**11** You are reviewing the vaccine schedule with a group of nursing students. You explain that the measles-mumps-rubella vaccine (MMR) is a live attenuated vaccine that is generally given at 12–15 months, with a booster at 4–6 years. One of the students asks if there are any groups excluded from receiving the MMR vaccine. Your response is yes, all but one of the following groups should receive the MMR vaccine. Which one of the following groups should receive the vaccine?

(A) Pregnant women, persons with fever and upper respiratory infection, the immunocompromised, and those with allergy to neomycin causing contact dermatitis

(B) Pregnant women, patients with leukemia in remission, persons with moderate to severe fever, those with allergy to neomycin causing contact dermatitis
(C) Pregnant women, persons with no fever and upper respiratory infection, the immunocompromised, and those with allergy to neomycin causing contact dermatitis
(D) Pregnant women, patients positive for human immunodeficiency virus (HIV) not severely immunocompromised, persons with moderate to severe fever, and those with allergy to neomycin causing contact dermatitis
(E) Pregnant women, immunocompromised persons, persons with moderate to severe fever, and those with allergy to neomycin causing anaphylaxis

**12** A grossly underweight 52-year-old woman with chronic malnutrition is due to undergo major surgery. It is decided to start total parenteral nutrition (TPN) as part of the initial therapy. While introducing a central venous catheter into the right subclavian vein, the patient develops sudden dyspnea. Which of the following is the most likely diagnosis?

(A) Air embolism
(B) Pulmonary embolism
(C) Fat embolism
(D) Acute anxiety
(E) Pneumothorax

**13** A 56-year-old woman is taken to the emergency department with severe sunburn and dehydration. Her husband is in a similar condition. They explain that they have been living in their car in the desert for several weeks to elude a band of alien creatures disguised as humans. The husband has a history of one past psychiatric hospitalization 10 years ago with a diagnosis of delusional disorder. The wife has never been hospitalized. For the past 7 years, the couple has led an isolated existence, living in cheap motels for several months at a time before moving on. Mental status examination reveals a middle-aged woman who states that aliens have been pursuing her husband. Further questioning reveals that she has not actually seen the aliens herself, but that her husband frequently spots them. The woman's thought processes are otherwise logical, and there is no evidence of cognitive deficits. Which of the following is the most appropriate initial step in treatment for this woman?

(A) Behavioral psychotherapy
(B) Cognitive psychotherapy
(C) Conjoint psychotherapy
(D) Ziprasidone
(E) Separation from her husband

**14** A mother brings her 7-year-old son to an emergency clinic because he has been vomiting and has had diarrhea for the past 3 days. Upon taking a history, the attending physician determines that the emesis was nonbilious and nonbloody, and the diarrhea was nonbloody, loose, and watery. The patient states that he vomited more than ten times, and the number of times for his diarrhea are too numerous to count. He is in the second grade, and has had no ill contacts and no recent travel. There is no exposure to pets. On clinical examination, the physician determines that the patient is dehydrated with a loss of less than 5% of his total body water (TBW). Which of the following choices represents the next best step in management of this patient?

(A) Give the patient a bolus of 20 mL/kg of isotonic crystalloid over 20 minutes.

(B) Give the patient no less than 60 mL/kg of isotonic crystalloid to restore perfusion.

(C) Give the patient maintenance fluids of 5% dextrose and 0.45 N saline to replace the fluid deficit and to accommodate ongoing losses.

(D) Give the patient an antiemetic.

(E) Give the patient an antibiotic to treat the infectious process.

**15** A 42-year-old man with a 4-month history of increasing occupational and marital stress fails to return home from work at his usual hour of 6:00 PM, causing his spouse to file a missing persons report the next day. Based on a license plate and physical description, police find him in a bar in a neighboring metropolitan area during the following evening, alert, and sitting without a drink. He says that he lost his wallet, is unsure of who he is, and can't remember how he got there. Which of the following is the most likely diagnosis?

(A) Psychosis due to a general medical condition

(B) Conversion disorder

(C) Dissociative fugue

(D) Major depressive disorder

(E) Delirium

**16** A 23-year-old woman presents with crampy left-lower-quadrant pain, bloody diarrhea with mucus, and a history of tenesmus. Fecal culture reveals no contaminating organisms. The table below summarizes clinical findings.

| Symptom/Sign | Patient | Normal |
|---|---|---|
| Bowel movements | 5–6 per day | 3 per week to 2 per day |
| Pulse beats per minute | <85 | 95 |
| Hematocrit (percent) | 31 | 35–45 (young adult female) |
| Weight loss in last 3 months | 5% | 0% |
| Temperature (°F) | 100.0 | 98.6 |
| Erythrocyte sedimentation rate | 25 mm/h | <15 mm/h (female) |
| Albumin (g/dL) | 3.2 | 3.4–4.7 |

Which of the following is the most likely diagnosis?

(A) Ulcerative colitis

(B) Crohn disease

(C) An anal fissure

(D) Ischemic bowel disease

(E) Solitary ulcer syndrome

**17** A financially successful 65-year-old man, proud of the fact he could trace his ancestry to some of the early settlers in New Mexico and that all four of his children now had college degrees, made an appointment with his primary care physician for his Medicare B physical. The only complaint he had was that his knees ached from chronic arthritis resulting from an old injury he had while playing soccer in high school. After taking a history, getting his weight and height, checking his blood pressure, listening to his heart sounds, and giving him an electrocardiogram (ECG), the doctor told him everything seemed normal, but just to make sure he would order blood work (fasting), then ask him to come back so he could review everything in detail. The table summarizes the results of these tests.

| Measurement | Value | Units | Normal or Desirable Range |
|---|---|---|---|
| Height | 67 | Inches | N/A |
| Weight | 162 | Pounds | N/A |
| Blood pressure | 135/80 | Mm Hg | <120/<80 |
| Glycosylated hemoglobin (HbA1c) | 6.0 | Percent | 4.3–5.9 = normal <7 desired |
| $Na^+$ | 144 | mmol/L | 135–147 |
| $K^+$ | 3.9 | mmol/L | 3.5–5.5 |
| $Cl^-$ | 105 | mmol/L | 96–108 |
| $CO_2$ | 28 | mmol/L | 22–29 |
| Anion gap | 11 | mmol/L | 5–14 |
| Glucose | 119 | mg/dL | 65–99 |
| Blood urea nitrogen (BUN) | 21 | mg/dL | 8–23 |
| Calcium | 9.4 | mmol/L | 8.4–10.5 |
| Serum creatinine | 1.17 | mg/dL | 0.50–1.20 |
| BUN/Creatinine | 17.9 | Ratio | 10–22 |
| Osmolarity calculated | 290 | milliosmolar/kg | 268–292 |
| SGOT/AST[a] | 18 | Units/Liter (U/L) | 0–44 |
| GPT/ALT[a] | 16 | U/L | 0–44 |
| Alkaline phosphatase | 65 | U/L | 40–129 |
| Total protein | 6.9 | gm/dL | 6.3–8.3 |
| Albumin (A) | 4.4 | gm/dL | 3.6–5.0 |
| Total bilirubin | 0.5 | mg/dL | 0.2–1.2 |
| Conjugated bilirubin | 0.1 | mg/dL | 0.0–0.3 |
| Globulin (G) | 2.5 | gm/dL | 2.4–4.4 |
| A/G ratio | 1.8 | Ratio | 0.7–2.5 |
| Total cholesterol | 220 | mg/dL | >199 |
| Triglycerides | 150 | mg/dL | >149 |
| High-density lipoprotein (HDL) | 45 | mg/dL | <40 high risk >60 desirable |
| Low-density lipoprotein (LDL) | 145 | mg/dL | <100 optional; 130–159 borderline; >159 high |

[a]SGOT, serum glutamic oxaloacetic transaminase; AST, aspartate aminotransferase; GPT, glutamate pyruvate transaminase; ALT, alanine aminotransferase

Among the choices below the physician most likely might suggest which one of the following?

(A) A drug regime to treat his diabetes
(B) A drug regime to treat his hypertension
(C) A drug regime to treat his nephropathy
(D) A dietary regime to treat his diabetes and his hypertension
(E) A disease-modifying antirheumatic drug (DMARD) to treat his arthritis

18 A 72-year-old female is seen in the emergency department with a history of sudden, severe, colicky midabdominal pain and nausea and vomiting over the past 3 hours. During the examination, she throws up a bile-stained vomitus. Physical examination reveals generalized abdominal tenderness with diminished bowel sounds. Radiography of the abdomen shows a radiopaque mass in the distal small bowel on the right side, with dilated loops proximally. No free air is noted under the diaphragm, but air is present in the biliary tree. Which of the following is the most likely diagnosis?

(A) Lymphoma of the small bowel
(B) Acute pancreatitis
(C) Acute appendicitis with radiopaque fecalith
(D) Gallstone ileus
(E) Intussusception

19 For the past 6 months, a 55-year-old man with a 35-year history of smoking cigarettes has complained of persistent frontal headaches. For several days, he has had projectile vomiting and bilateral blurry vision. Physical examination shows bilateral papilledema. A magnetic resonance imaging (MRI) study shows a mass lesion involving the corpus callosum that has spread to both cerebral hemispheres. The patient dies a few days later of a transtentorial herniation. Which of the following underlying conditions is the most likely cause of the lesion?

(A) Cerebral infarction
(B) Glioblastoma multiforme
(C) Intracerebral hemorrhage
(D) Medulloblastoma
(E) Metastatic lung carcinoma

20 An article concerning the relative ability of a new drug to lower systolic blood pressure describes a study in which age- and ethnicity-matched male patients are divided into three groups. One group receives a well-recognized drug at a standard dose. The other two groups receive the new drug, but at different doses. At the end of 30 days, the systolic blood pressure of each group was determined, and the significance of the differences in the mean values was tested statistically. Which of the following statistical tests would provide the greatest confidence in the results?

(A) Student's *t*-test
(B) Analysis of variance
(C) Correlation coefficient
(D) Chi-squared test
(E) Logistic regression

21 Psychiatric consultation is requested for a 51-year-old woman on a surgical ward undergoing postoperative treatment for a mesenteric infarction. The consultation request notes "altered mental status; rule out delirium versus schizophrenia." Which one of the following combinations is more typical of schizophrenia than of delirium?

(A) Social withdrawal and a family history of psychopathology
(B) Memory impairment and waxing and waning of confusion within a period of hours
(C) Visual and auditory hallucinations
(D) A family history of schizophrenia and waxing and waning of confusion within a period of hours
(E) Social withdrawal and waxing and waning of confusion within a period of hours

22 An 18-year-old man enlisted in the Marines. He appeared to be in good physical shape, but his buddies sometimes remark about his unusual thirst, and he was annoyed by the fact that he often became so thirsty at night that he had to get up and drink a couple of glasses of water. Not surprisingly, he also had a need to urinate frequently. Since he acquired these traits around the age of 10, he did not regard them as being abnormal, just slightly annoying; his megathirst apparently started shortly after he fell from a tree and was knocked unconscious for a short time. He did fine during basic training until his unit went on a forced march during a hot August week. By the first night, he had emptied his canteen and suffered such a severe thirst that he actually woke up his sergeant begging for extra water. Luckily, his sergeant was a compassionate man and recognized something was truly wrong. In addition to his desperate pleading, he seemed too weak to stand straight at attention, looked and felt feverish, and his eyes appeared to have sunk deep into his forehead. Consequently, he was excused from the march and sent to the sickbay. Once there, his symptoms were recognized as dehydration, and he was given water and sent to the base hospital for further evaluation. The medics there quickly made a diagnosis and prescribed which of the following treatments?

(A) Metformin
(B) Foscarnet
(C) Desmopressin
(D) Increasing his daily water intake
(E) Demeclocycline

23 A 67-year-old woman presents to her doctor's office with a history of sudden severe backache. The patient states that she was working in the garden and tried to lift a sack of fertilizer when her "back gave out." She states that the pain was very intense, was stabbing in nature, and went across her abdomen, like a belt. She has a history of hypertension and diabetes mellitus and some urinary problems. Her vital signs are as follows: blood pressure, 130/100 mm Hg; pulse, 86/min, regular; respirations, 18/min; and temperature, 37°C (98.6°F). Physical examination reveals tenderness to deep palpation in the lower thoracic spine, paraspinal spasm, and a restricted straight-leg raise on both lower extremities. The deep tendon reflexes are normal in the knees, but are absent in both ankles. There are a few beats of clonus that were not sustained. She also has decreased touch in both legs below the knees. The most likely diagnosis is which of the following?

(A) Spinal cord tumor
(B) Epidural abscess
(C) Fractured vertebra
(D) Posterolateral lumbar disk herniation
(E) Central lumbar disk herniation

24 A young lactating mother is found to have a red, hot, painful, inflamed right breast consistent with mastitis. In addition, she has a temperature of 30.4°C (101.1°F), headache, and nausea. Her physician prescribes rest, antibiotics, plenty of fluids, and cold packs for the affected breast. The patient is concerned about breastfeeding. Which of the following is the best advice the physician can give the patient?

(A) Stop breastfeeding immediately because otherwise the baby might become infected.
(B) Stop breastfeeding immediately to prevent the possibility that the antibiotic will adversely affected the baby.
(C) Continue breastfeeding but only use the left breast.
(D) Continue breast-feeding using both breasts.
(E) Stop breastfeeding because commercial formulas are more nutritious.

**25** A 28-year-old woman who works as a computer analyst in a large company and does not exercise at all is concerned about the possibility of developing a myocardial infarction. This stems from the fact that her oldest brother, who is 42 years old, has already undergone coronary bypass surgery, and her mother died at 50 years of age after an acute myocardial infarction. She denies a history of chest pains, palpitations, or shortness of breath. The patient does not smoke, does not consume alcohol, and does not take any regular medication. Physical examination reveals an obese woman who is 163 cm (64 in) tall and weighs 112 kg (247 lb). Her vital signs reveal the following: heart rate, 92/min; respirations, 18/min; blood pressure, 125/90 mm Hg. A serum lipid panel yields the following values: total cholesterol, 250 mg/dL (normal, <200 mg/dL); high-density lipoprotein (HDL), 32 mg/dL (normal >60 mg/dL); low-density lipoprotein (LDL), 160 mg/dL (normal, <130 mg/dL), triglyceride (TG), 185 mg/dL (normal, <150 mg/dL), and very-low-density lipoprotein (VLDL), 260 mg/dL (normal <125 mg/dL). Based on this information, which of the following is the best step in the management of this patient?

(A) Start her immediately on 3-hydroxy-3-methyl-glutaryl-coenzyme A (HMG-CoA) reductase inhibitors.
(B) Start her on bile acid sequestrants and exercise.
(C) Commence a 6-month diet and exercise plan.
(D) Start her on the American Heart Association step 2 diet and exercise plan.
(E) Commence a combination of niacin, exercise, and diet.

**26** A 14-year-old girl complains bitterly that her mother intrudes into every aspect of her life and tries to control her. The mother admits that she closely monitors her daughter and sets many rules. The father has largely withdrawn from trying to control her behavior and is deeply involved in his work. The child has recently withdrawn from family interaction, refusing to speak to her parents or spend mealtimes with them. The mother has redoubled her efforts to maintain control. The cause of which one of the following disorders is most often ascribed to family dynamics similar to that described?

(A) Anorexia nervosa
(B) Dissociative identity disorder
(C) Narcissistic personality disorder
(D) Schizophrenia
(E) Separation anxiety disorder

**27** A 79-year-old man sees his family practice physician for a routine checkup concerning his diabetes. His physician tells him that he appears to be taking good care of himself; his HbAc1 level is only 6.2% and his lipid profile is acceptable, suggesting he is not at risk for a heart attack. He then adds that he thinks it would be wise for him to have a bone density test to see if he possibly has osteoporosis. The patient objects, saying he heard osteoporosis is a woman's disease, so why should he worry about it. Which of the following statements accurately reflects the truth about osteoporosis in men?

(A) Age-related osteoporosis in men is due to decreased ability to calcify bone matrix.
(B) Mortality rates after hip fractures are greater in women than in men.
(C) Loss of estrogen in aging men cannot be a factor that increases the risk of fractures.
(D) The prevalence of osteoporosis in men is about 20% that of women.
(E) The increase in rates of osteoporosis among aging men is primarily due to decreased ability to absorb vitamin D.

**28** A 23-year-old woman has tearing and moderate pain in her left eye. Her pupillary light reflex is normal. She recently was placed on topical corticosteroids for suspected allergic conjunctivitis. A Gram's stain and Giemsa stain are negative for organisms. A fluorescein stain of the eye exhibits a shallow ulcer with a dendritic appearance and irregular borders. Which of the following topical treatments would be most appropriate?

(A) Ketoconazole
(B) Trifluridine
(C) Phenylephrine
(D) Erythromycin
(E) Sulfacetamide

**29** While on a camping trip with his son in a remote location in Alaska a 69-year-old man accidently got a fish hook imbedded in the palm of his hand. They dug out the hook, washed the wound, and bandaged it. Apparently, they did not clean it out adequately because when they got back home a week later, it showed signs of infection. A doctor at the local ER cleaned it out thoroughly and gave him a shot of penicillin. The wound healed nicely but several weeks later, the man developed a mild fever, which persisted in the absence of any other symptoms. After a month, his temperature suddenly peaked and he developed excessive sweating, chills, fatigue, muscle and joint pains, night sweats, and painful lesions on the pads of the fingers. Which of the following is the most likely cause of this man's symptoms?

(A) Infection by *Staphylococcus aureus*
(B) Infection by *Streptococcus viridans*
(C) Infection by *Candida albicans*
(D) Infection by *Streptococcus bovis*
(E) Infection by *Clostridium septicum*

**30** A 64-year-old widow with substantial savings develops Alzheimer disease. She has a 36-year-old son who still lives at home and is anticipating receiving an ample inheritance. His mother is beginning to require around-the-clock supervision; consequently, the son starts to look into residential care options. He is appalled by the cost, but a friend tells him not to worry because at her age Medicaid will pick up the tab. Which of the following statements about her potential use of the federal Medicare or Medicaid program to finance her care is most accurate?

(A) Medicaid will not cover the cost of her medications.

(B) Medicaid will not pay for her residential care.

(C) She will become eligible for Medicaid only if she has contributed to the program through federal withholding of her wages.

(D) She will become eligible for Medicaid only upon turning 65.

(E) She will become eligible for Medicaid only if impoverished.

(F) In another year, Medicare will pay the cost of residential care.

**31** A 32-year-old man with a long history of substance abuse blames his parents for his inability to live without drugs. He insists that he obviously inherited his addictions from them. On this basis, he rejects any discussion about how changing the way he relates to others might decrease his drug cravings. While the man's conclusions about treatment may be wrong, for which of the following drugs is his surmise of heritability dependency best supported by clinical evidence?

(A) Opiate

(B) Cocaine

(C) Heroin

(D) Tobacco

(E) Benzodiazepine

(F) Alcohol

(G) Psychostimulant

**32** A girl is repeatedly sexually molested from age 7 through age 14 by her father, who warns her never to tell anyone or she will be killed. Although it seems hard to understand why she was not at least suspicious, the mother claims she never had an inkling that this type of deviant behavior was going on in her household. Which of the following has been most commonly suggested as a sequel to this situation?

(A) Dependent personality disorder

(B) Autistic disorder

(C) Dissociative identity disorder

(D) Hypochondriasis

(E) Major depressive disorder

**33** A 35-year-old fireman was badly burned when the roof of a house collapsed on him. He had second-degree burns involving 15% of his body surface and third-degree burns involving 20% of his body surface. He was rushed to the nearest emergency department and then transferred to a burn unit. A week later, he develops fever, and black patches are noted in the burn wounds. Biopsy and culture of one of the wound sites would most likely reveal which of the following organisms?

(A) *Staphylococcus aureus*

(B) *Pseudomonas aeruginosa*

(C) *Candida albicans*

(D) Group A streptococcus

(E) *Streptococcus pneumoniae*

**34** A 47-year-old man is described by coworkers as being intensely competitive, driven, hostile, distrustful, excitable, and anxious. The man complains of being tense, easily bored, and unhappy. Mental status examination reveals increased psychomotor activity with many quick shifts of posture, pressured speech, and irritability. According to psychosomatic theory, which of the following disorders is most likely to occur in such a person?

(A) Cancer

(B) Coronary artery disease

(C) Emphysema

(D) Migraine

(E) Peptic ulcer disease

**35** An internist at a major medical center received a letter from a physician located several states away. The letter said: "With your permission, I am asking a former patient of mine to see you. He is an 18-year-old man suffering from occipital bone syndrome. Physically, he has the pathognomonic bilateral exostosis of the skull and pili torti, extremely loose skin and joints, long neck, dysautonomia, and vascular tortuosity, as well as a somewhat unusual appearance including an abnormally long neck and face, with a high forehead and an arched palate. He also suffers from seizures, which are presently under control by medication. He has a very low normal IQ of 88. I am sure you will find his case interesting and his continued treatment challenging. If you accept him as your patient, I will send you his medical records." The patient described in this letter has an aberration in the metabolism of which one of the following trace elements?

(A) Zinc

(B) Selenium

(C) Chromium

(D) Copper

(E) Cobalt

(F) Manganese

**36** A 77-year-old man was brought to the local ER by his wife. She informed the admitting nurse that he had been suffering from what seemed to be a slight case of the flu, but instead of recovering he began to act somewhat weird—he was unable to find his keys or get his pants on correctly. He also complained of a severe headache, and just before getting in the car to come to the ER, he started to throw up. The triage nurse also noted that he had a temperature of 102.5°F (39.2°C), his left hand's grasp was very weak, and he appeared to have limited seizures in both arms; moreover, he seemed to drift in and out of consciousness. Upon physical examination, the presence of fever was confirmed, no evidence of nuchal rigidity was found, and both Kerning's and Brudzinsky's signs were absent; additionally, transient bouts of hemiparesis and both focal and generalized seizures were noted, and his movements were grossly uncoordinated. He also had ptosis, diplopia, and his left pupil was abnormally dilated. Papilledema was also noted in the optic disc of the same eye. The patient also drifted into unconsciousness for longer and longer periods of time. A computed tomographic (CT) scan and a lumbar puncture was performed to draw cerebral spinal fluid (CSF). The table below summarizes the results of the CSF analysis.

| Test | Normal | Result |
| --- | --- | --- |
| Color/turbidity | Colorless and clear | Pinkish and slightly turbid |
| Pressure | 8–15 mm Hg lying on a side 200–300 mm Hg sitting up | Normal |
| White blood cell count | 0–5 cells | 100 per mm³ |
| Cell differential | Mainly mono- nuclear lymphocytes | Mainly mono- nuclear lymphocytes |
| Protein | 15–45 mg/dL | 110 mg/dL |
| Glucose | 50–80 mg/dL | 35 mg/dL |

The CT results were ambiguous, but there was a suspicion of changes in the temporal lobe. Which of the following tests is most likely to yield a definitive diagnosis?

(A) Serologic analysis
(B) Increases in antibody levels
(C) Magnetic resonance imaging (MRI) studies
(D) Electroencephalography studies
(E) DNA analysis, using the polymerase chain reaction

**37** A 64-year-old man just completed his pre-Medicare physical and was in the process of getting an assessment from his physician. The physician informed him that basically he was in good health, but she would recommend a few things to him that would help preserve his health. First and foremost, she was glad to hear that he had given up smoking some 10 years earlier, but she felt he should modify his diet to one modeled on the so-called Mediterranean diet. She also recommended getting more exercise, at least a half hour per day at least 6 days a week. Finally, she recommended he take a baby aspirin (about 81 mg) before going to bed every night and either eating fatty fish two or three times a week or taking fish oil capsules daily. Which of the following choices best describes why aspirin and fish oil reduces the risk of heart problems?

(A) Aspirin covalently binds to the cyclo-oxygenase (COX) enzymes, and fish oil contains omega-3 fatty acids that are converted to series-3 prostaglandins.
(B) Aspirin covalently binds to the COX enzymes, and fish oil contains omega-3 fatty acids that are converted to arachidonic acid, the major precursor of the prostaglandins.
(C) Aspirin, the other nonsteroidal anti-inflammatory drugs, fish oil, and acetaminophen all block the COX enzymes.
(D) Aspirin noncovalently blocks the COX enzymes, and fish oil contains omega-3 fatty acids that are converted to series-2 prostaglandins.
(E) Aspirin noncovalently binds to the COX enzymes, and fish oil contains significant quantities of omega-3 fatty acids that are converted to series-1 prostaglandins.

**38** A poorly dressed 56-year-old lady enters an emergency department facility at a local hospital in an agitated manner saying she needs attention immediately because she just discovered she has colon cancer. The triage nurse calms her down a bit by asking her what makes her think that is true. She responds: "For the past week, each time I make number two, I get a sharp pain, and because the pain lasts for around a half hour after I wipe myself I know it must be coming from my insides. The worst was today when I saw bright red blood; I heard on the TV that blood when you go to the bathroom is a sign of cancer." The nurse tells her that there are also many other additional causes for blood in the stool. She finds that the lady is hypertensive but has not seen a physician since she was pregnant at the age of 18 years; the nurse then arranges for the woman to see one of the ER doctors. When the doctor sees the patient, he arranges for her to see a primary care physician but also recommends treatment. Which of the following choices is the most probable treatment recommended?

(A) Removal of a mass that may be protruding from the patient's anus

(B) Perform a sigmoidoscopy and during this procedure excise any polyps found

(C) Application of a local steroid cream twice daily, plus use of stool softeners and hot sitz baths

(D) Prescription of antihypertensive drugs and antibiotics

(E) Cautery by argon plasma coagulation applied via an endoscope

**39** A 47-year-old woman made an appointment to see her primary care physician because she thought she felt a small mass in her left breast. It was painless but seemed to be growing rapidly. The moment her primary care physician saw her, he arranged for her to have a mammogram and an open biopsy. The mammogram showed the mass to be round with smooth borders. By the time she had her biopsy, it had grown large enough to distort the shape of her breast. The gynecologist noted the mass to be firm, nontender, and mobile still with clearly defined boundaries. The overlying skin had become warm to the touch and appeared reddish, shiny, and translucent, causing the breast veins to become visible. The mass itself was about 6 cm in diameter. Which of the following choices most likely represents the proper diagnosis?

(A) Fibroadenoma

(B) Phyllodes tumor

(C) Invasive (also known as, infiltrating) ductal carcinoma

(D) Invasive (also known as, infiltrating) lobular carcinoma

(E) Inflammatory breast cancer

**40** A 23-year-old woman with an 18-year history of insulin-dependent diabetes is brought to the emergency department by her date, who became alarmed by her acute mental confusion and sudden-onset bizarre behavior. He explains that they spent the day at the beach, where she had been very active, playing volley ball and swimming, and that they missed lunch but were on their way to eat dinner when this sudden change in behavior occurred. He states over and over again that they had not been using drugs or drinking alcohol. The triage nurse notes perspiration, increased salivation, restlessness, and tachycardia. Which of the following is the most appropriate next step in the management of this patient?

(A) Order a complete blood count (CBC)

(B) Order an immediate blood glucose analysis

(C) Order serum electrolytes analysis

(D) Order an immediate drug screen

(E) Order arterial blood gases (ABGs) analysis

*Directions for Matching Questions (41 through 50): Each set of matching questions is preceded by a list of 4 to 26 lettered options followed by a brief explanation of the required task and then by a series of numbered statements. For each lettered statement, you are to select ONE lettered option that best fulfills the task as it relates to that statement. Remember that each of the listed options might be correctly selected once, more than once, or not at all.*

## 41–50 (Obstetrics and Gynecology)

(A) Ectopic pregnancy

(B) Vaginal foreign body

(C) Endometrial carcinoma

(D) Submucous leiomyoma

(E) Molar pregnancy

(F) Cervical carcinoma

(G) Simple hyperplasia without atypia

(H) Sarcoma botryoides

(I) Uterine adenomyosis

(J) Ovarian carcinoma

*For each of the numbered questions below (41 to 50), select the ONE lettered condition above to which it relates best.*

**41** A 3-year-old girl who has been experiencing vaginal bleeding is brought for evaluation by her worried mother. The girl's medical history is unremarkable, with normal physical growth and appropriate developmental landmarks. She has had all the recommended immunizations. On visual examination of the perineum, bleeding and multiple cystic masses resembling grapes are seen at the introitus.

**42** For the past 6 months, a 32-year-old multiparous woman has complained about intermittent vaginal bleeding between normal menstrual periods. The bleeding is painless and is not associated with cramping. She denies postcoital bleeding. Her last Pap smear, 6 months ago, was negative for dysplasia or malignancy. She underwent a tubal sterilization after her last pregnancy 3 years ago. Pelvic examination reveals normal external genitalia and vulva. Her vagina and cervix are without lesions. Her uterus is asymmetrically enlarged, about 8 week size, and nontender. Results of a qualitative urine β-human chorionic gonadotropin (β-hCG) test are negative.

**43** Starting over 9 months ago, a 39-year-old multiparous woman complains about having increasing heavy vaginal bleeding and pain with her menstrual periods. Two years ago, after workup for an abnormal Pap smear reported a low-grade squamous intraepithelial lesion (LSIL), she underwent cryotherapy for biopsy-confirmed cervical intraepithelial neoplasia grade I (CIN 1). Subsequent follow-up Pap smears have been negative. Her present pelvic examination is unremarkable except for a diffusely enlarged, globular, soft, tender uterus. Results of a qualitative urine β-human chorionic gonadotropin (β-hCG) test are negative.

**44** A 14-year-old girl complains of irregular, unpredictable heavy menstrual bleeding. She denies pain or cramping. Her first menstrual period was at age 13, and they have always been irregular, but the bleeding seems to be getting heavier. She has no chronic health problems and states she has never been sexually active. She appears well developed and well nourished, with normal female secondary sexual characteristics. Inspection shows normal female external genitalia. Results of a qualitative urine β-human chorionic gonadotropin (β-hCG) test are negative.

**45** A 39-year-old multiparous woman complains of intermittent vaginal bleeding between normal menstrual periods that has been going on for the past 4 months. The bleeding is painless and occurs after sexual intercourse. She has had three cesarean sections, along with a tubal sterilization with her last delivery. She has a 30 pack-year history of cigarette smoking. She is currently in a monogamous sexual relationship but has had multiple sexual partners in the past. She has not been regular in her annual examinations. Her last Pap smear was 5 years ago.

**46** A 6-year-old girl states that she has had vaginal bleeding for the past 3 days. She is brought to the office by her worried mother. The mother states that the child has no medical problems and is not on any medications. She denies headache or visual changes. General physical examination is consistent with a normal 6-year-old female without breast budding. External genitalia are unremarkable with no pubic hair.

**47** A 63-year-old nulligravid woman comes to the outpatient office complaining about intermittent painless vaginal bleeding. Her last menstrual period was 10 years ago. She is not on hormone therapy. She has never used oral contraceptives. She has struggled with obesity all her life. Her last Pap smear was a year ago and was negative for dysplasia or malignancy. Her pelvic examination is unremarkable without vulvar, vaginal, or cervical lesions. Her uterus is small, mobile, and nontender. No adnexal masses are palpable.

**48** A 21-year-old nulligravid woman complains that she has nonmenstrual vaginal bleeding and left-sided lower-abdominal pain. Her last menstrual period was 7 weeks ago. She is sexually active with multiple sexual partners. She uses barrier contraception irregularly and was treated with antibiotics 6 months ago for bilateral lower-abdominal pelvic pain. Her vital signs are stable. On pelvic examination, she has dark blood in the vagina with no active bleeding. Her uterus is slightly enlarged but nontender. She has left adnexal tenderness to palpation without an obvious mass.

**49** A pregnant 22-year-old Taiwanese woman presents at 15 weeks' gestation with vaginal bleeding and severe nausea and vomiting. She states she recently experienced vaginal passage of tissue that looked like grapes. Her uterine fundus is at her umbilicus and no fetal heart tones can be heard with a Doppler stethoscope. Ultrasonography of the uterus shows a "snow storm" image with no fetus or placenta.

**50** A 38-year-old woman presents with abdominal pain, spotting, and ascites.

# Answer Key

| | | | | | | | | | |
|---|---|---|---|---|---|---|---|---|---|
| **1** | D | **11** | E | **21** | A | **31** | F | **41** | H |
| **2** | D | **12** | E | **22** | C | **32** | C | **42** | D |
| **3** | E | **13** | E | **23** | C | **33** | B | **43** | I |
| **4** | E | **14** | A | **24** | D | **34** | B | **44** | G |
| **5** | D | **15** | C | **25** | C | **35** | D | **45** | F |
| **6** | C | **16** | A | **26** | A | **36** | E | **46** | B |
| **7** | B | **17** | D | **27** | D | **37** | A | **47** | C |
| **8** | C | **18** | D | **28** | B | **38** | C | **48** | A |
| **9** | D | **19** | B | **29** | A | **39** | B | **49** | E |
| **10** | B | **20** | B | **30** | E | **40** | B | **50** | J |

# Answers and Explanations

**1** **The answer is D** *Surgery*

Acute small bowel infarction (choice **D**) is indicated by the sudden onset of severe abdominal pain with vomiting and abdominal distention out of proportion with the physical findings, absent bowel sounds, a striking neutrophilic leukocytosis with left shift, lactic acidosis, hypotension, and increased serum amylase concentration of bowel origin. The increased serum amylase concentration is sometimes misinterpreted as representing acute hemorrhagic pancreatitis. Barium studies reveal "thumbprinting" of the mucosa due to submucosal hemorrhages and edema. Peritoneal signs (e.g., rebound tenderness) are generally late findings. These signs of acute infarction are often preceded by abdominal angina (also known as, mesenteric angina) 30 minutes after eating. Because of the pain, patients tend to have a fear of eating, and they lose weight. In 50% of cases, acute small bowel infarction occurs in elderly patients with atherosclerotic disease; usually, the pathogenesis relates to sudden occlusion of the superior mesenteric artery by thrombosis over an atherosclerotic plaque, less often to an embolism from the left heart (mitral valve disease, atrial fibrillation, or left ventricular mural thrombosis), and rarely from vasculitis. In about 25% of cases, nonocclusive infarction can occur from a low rate of blood flow, as in vasospasm or shock. Causes of vasospasm include ergot or cocaine poisoning and sympathomimetic drugs, such as digitalis. Shock can be induced by hypovolemia and hypotension, as may be caused by cardiac failure or loss of blood, as would occur with aortic aneurysm repair or dissections of the aorta (uncommon). The remaining 25% of cases of small bowel infarction may result from superior mesenteric vein occlusion related to hypercoagulable states, which could be associated with polycythemia rubra vera, oral contraceptives in females, malignancy, or one of the hereditary hypercoagulable states (e.g., antithrombin III deficiency, protein C and S deficiencies). Whatever the underlying mechanism, transmural, hemorrhagic infarctions damage the integrity of the mucosa, thus predisposing the bowel to secondary bacterial penetration and generalized peritonitis. The reestablishment of blood flow frequently results in further damage due to reavailability of oxygen, which may cause free radical formation. Treatment of the ischemic bowel must occur within 12 hours; otherwise, a 100% mortality rate can be expected. Surgery is always indicated if a grossly obvious hemorrhagic infarction has already occurred. Visible peristalsis is the best way to determine if the bowel is viable or dead. Embolectomy and intraarterial vasodilators are also used, depending on the cause of the ischemia.

The symptoms presented in this case are unlikely clinical presentations for acute ulcerative colitis (choice **A**); moreover, ulcerative colitis is most often seen in young adults. Although hemorrhagic pancreatitis (choice **B**) involves an elevated serum amylase concentration, it is not associated with diffuse abdominal pain and bloody diarrhea. An aortoenteric fistula (choice **C**) is usually a late complication of repair of an abdominal aortic aneurysm. Toxic megacolons (choice **E**) are associated with ulcerative colitis.

**2** **The answer is D** *Pediatrics*

Choanal atresia (choice **D**) should be suspected in any infant who develops cyanosis that occurs with feedings or at rest but is relieved by crying. The cyanosis occurs because newborns are obligate nose breathers, and this congenital anomaly consists of a unilateral or bilateral bony or membranous septum between the nose and the pharynx. Diagnosis is made by failure to pass a catheter through the nasal passages.

Tracheoesophageal fistula (choice **A**) is characterized by choking with feeding. An orogastric tube curls up and does not pass to the stomach. Bronchopulmonary dysplasia (choice **B**) is a complication of respiratory distress syndrome (choice **C**) and appears later in the infant's life. Cyanosis is not relieved by crying in either entity. A patent ductus arteriosus (choice **E**) is a left-to-right shunt and is not associated with cyanosis.

**3** **The answer is E** *Medicine*

The patient is most likely taking a bile acid-binding resin (e.g., cholestyramine) to lower his cholesterol level. These resins work by binding bile acids in the intestine to form an insoluble, nonabsorbable complex that is excreted in the feces along with the resin. This action reduces circulating cholesterol levels and causes a compensatory increase in the synthesis of hepatocyte low-density lipoprotein receptors (choice **E**) to more efficiently recover reduced levels of cholesterol from the blood. Recovered cholesterol is then converted to bile acids to replenish the bile acids that are lost in the stool. The most common complaints are constipation and bloating that are relieved by increasing fiber or mixing psyllium seed with the resin. Heartburn and diarrhea are occasionally reported. Problems may also arise from the resin forming complexes and promoting the excretion of other substances such as digitalis, folic acid, thiazides, and warfarin.

Normally, cholesterol is effectively reabsorbed from the intestine as part of the bile acids and is not excreted as the free compound. A bile acid-binding resin does not change this condition; however, now rather than being reabsorbed as an integral part of the bile acid, it is excreted as a component in a bile acid–bile acid-binding resin complex, not as free cholesterol; increased excretion of free cholesterol in feces (choice **D**) does not happen. The "statin" drugs (e.g., lovastatin) inhibit HMG-CoA reductase (choice **A**), the rate-limiting enzyme of cholesterol synthesis. This decreases the synthesis of cholesterol. Rare side effects of statin drugs include hepatic toxicity with an increase in transaminases, and a myopathy with an increase in creatine kinase; however, evidence suggests that the statins are also antiosteoporotic, an unexpected boon. Fibric acid derivatives (e.g., gemfibrozil) and nicotinic acid lower serum triglyceride (TG) levels. Fibric acid derivatives decrease hepatic TG synthesis (choice **B**) and also interfere with the formation of very-low-density lipoproteins (VLDLs) in the liver. Complications that might be associated with fibric acid derivatives include rash and myopathy, the latter sometimes causing rhabdomyolysis with marked elevation of creatine kinase and myoglobinuria. Nicotinic acid is also used in the treatment of hypertriglyceridemia (also hypercholesterolemia). The drug interferes with the formation of VLDL in the liver. Flushing is the major side effect of nicotinic acid and is diminished by taking a nonsteroidal anti-inflammatory drug 30 minutes before taking nicotinic acid. Flushing is not present in this patient. Fibric acid derivatives and nicotinic acid both activate capillary lipoprotein lipase (choice **C**), promoting increased delivery of fatty acids to the adipose.

### 4 The answer is E *Preventive Medicine and Public Health*

Malpractice is generally defined as deviation from the established standards of professional care (i.e., professional negligence). For a claim of malpractice, the patient must prove that the doctor was negligent by deviating from the established standard of care (choice **E**) and that this deviation caused injury (not necessarily deliberately). Additionally, the physician has to have a duty to the patient because of their professional relationship.

Neither the doctor's education (choice **A**) nor how much he charges the patient (choice **D**) is related to malpractice claims. Malpractice is a civil wrong (a tort), not a crime (choice **C**), and intent to cause harm does not have to be shown (choice **B**).

### 5 The answer is D *Surgery*

The patient most likely has a postoperative wound infection (choice **D**), which occurs in 2%–5% of patients who have had biliary tract surgery. The infections are usually the result of contamination of the wound either during or after surgery; there rarely is an infection prior to surgery. Although infections can become evident within 1 day in a grossly contaminated wound, they generally first emerge 5–10 days postoperatively. Operative wounds are classified as clean (no gross contamination), clean-contaminated (e.g., in gastric or biliary tract surgery), contaminated (e.g., in unprepared colon surgery), or dirty and infected (infection encountered during the surgery). The risk for wound infection increases if the wound is located in the abdomen, the surgery lasts longer than 2 hours, or contamination of the wound is encountered during surgery. One of the key factors that predisposes to infection is decreased oxygen tension in the tissues. Attention to careful surgical techniques (reduced trauma to tissue, less suture material, removal of foreign bodies) and prophylactic use of antibiotics in certain types of surgeries reduce the chance of infection. Cefazolin is the drug of choice for prophylaxis during surgery when both aerobes and anaerobes are a concern. Antibiotic prophylaxis is only given in selected clean or clean-contaminated procedures because antibiotic use in contaminated and dirty wounds is considered therapeutic. A single preoperative dose should be administered intravenously at the time of induction of anesthesia. Additional doses may be given after surgery but are usually discontinued within 24 hours. Treatment of wound infection involves opening the wound and allowing drainage. Antibiotics are reserved for invasive infections.

Atelectasis (choice **C**) is the most common cause of fever within 24 hours of surgery. Endotoxic shock (choice **B**) would be accompanied by warm shock, due to vasodilation of peripheral vessels, and would be an unlikely cause of this woman's fever. Resorption of blood (choice **A**) is not associated with fever. Renal failure (choice **E**) is associated with oliguria, not fever.

### 6 The answer is C *Pediatrics*

With an incidence of 1 case per 400 births, sickle cell disease is the most common hemoglobinopathy in the African American population. The blood smear illustrated as part of the case history confirms a diagnosis of sickle cell disease in this girl, since it shows numerous boat-shaped sickle cells. Dactylitis is the most frequent initial manifestation of sickle cell disease, with a typical onset of symptoms at an age of 4–12 months; this time range approximately coincides with the replacement of hemoglobin (Hb) F with Hb A (choice **C**). Dactylitis is characterized by soft-tissue swelling of the hands, feet, or both, with associated heat and tenderness over the metacarpals, tarsals, and proximal phalanges. Radiographs made at the onset of disease only show soft-tissue swelling. After 1–2 weeks, infarction and necrosis of the underlying bones are noted secondary to sickling of red blood cells (RBCs) in the sinusoids. This is followed by subperiosteal new bone formation. Absorption of the infarcted bone results in radiolucent areas. These areas of infarction are restored to normal within a few months, but recurrent disease is common.

A hemolytic crisis induced by an aberrant G6PD (choice **A**) may be caused by infection (most common) or by oxidizing drugs. The mutation resulting in this aberrant enzyme occurs on the X chromosome and is inherited as a recessive trait; consequently, it is very unlikely to occur in a female infant. The G6PD gene is very susceptible to mutation; over 400 hundred different genetic variants of G6PD have been described. Nonetheless, most black Africans express the "normal" A variant, whereas most Caucasians carry the "normal" B variant. However, about 11% of African Americans express the A$^-$ variant, which affords protection against falciparum malaria. Individuals carrying the A$^-$ form are essentially normal except when their red cells are exposed to oxidative stress. This is because the primary function of the hexose monophosphate shunt in red cells is to produce NADPH via the G6PD reaction to keep glutathione (GSH) in the reduced state; this GSH protects the red cell membrane and the Hb from oxidative denaturation. The residual activity of the A$^-$ variant suffices to maintain healthy red cell function for almost their full normal lifespan. However, as red cells age, the activity of their enzymes declines, and G6PD activity falls below a critical limit at which NADPH production can no longer maintain GSH levels in stressed cells. Consequently, some of the Hb is denatured, forming Heinz bodies that react with the cell membrane, causing a distortion that is recognized by and destroyed in the spleen; this causes a hemolytic crisis. This crisis is self-limiting, even in the continued presence of the agent causing the stress, because only a variable population of older cells is affected.

The B$^-$ variant, also known as the Mediterranean form, is commonly expressed by people originating from the malaria zones abutting the northern, southwestern, and western Mediterranean Sea. It too protects against malaria, but the residual activity is lower, and a hemolytic crisis can be life-threatening; the mutation sometimes also makes itself evident in the newborn via excessive jaundice. Individuals carrying the B$^-$ variant also suffer severe crises when exposed to fava beans, the common Mediterranean flat bean.

As noted above, there are more than 400 known variants of this enzyme. Expressions of many of these produce symptoms, some incompatible with life; others, a chronic hemolytic anemia or chronic granulomatous disease. However, since most of these impart severe symptoms and have no benefit, they are very rare conditions.

*Salmonella paratyphi* is the most common cause of osteomyelitis (choice **B**) in sickle cell disease, and infection tends to occur when functional hyposplenism is present from autoinfarction of the spleen. However, hyposplenism is unlikely to occur in a 6-month-old infant. The highest risk of infection is after age 1 year to 10 years of age. Coxsackievirus (choice **D**), an enterovirus, is associated with hand, foot, and mouth disease, a highly contagious condition that primarily affects children in pre-elementary school groups. It is called hand, foot, and mouth disease because of the typical ulcers on the tongue and oral mucosa and vesicles that do not ulcerate on the palms and soles. It is also accompanied by a temperature of 101–104°F (38.3–40°C), and although most often self-limiting, in rare cases, usually in neonates, it causes life-threatening myocarditis or encephalitis. Turner syndrome, a sex chromosome abnormality with an XO pattern (choice **E**), is associated with nuchal lymphedema and painless lymphedema of the hands and feet in newborns; there is no fever, and no sickle cells are seen in a peripheral smear.

### 7 The answer is B *Psychiatry*

The phenotype described for the boy is typical of fragile X syndrome, the most prevalent inherited cause of mental retardation in males. It is caused by the expansion of a CGG repeat near a gene located on the X chromosome. Once the number of repeats goes beyond 52, chance of further expansion during oogeneses or spermatogenesis is great. Because it is X-linked, males are generally more severely affected than females, but females sometimes do show psychologic symptoms, such as autism and mild mental retardation (choice **B**).

In this family, the grandfather was a so-called premutation carrier, with minimal expansion, the only obvious symptom being tremor. The number of repeats probably increased in the mother and then again in her children. The mother was completely protected by her second X chromosome, and the daughter was partly protected.

Cri du chat syndrome (partial deletion of the short arm of chromosome 5) (choice **A**) is associated with severe mental retardation. Klinefelter syndrome (XXY) (choice **C**) is associated with cognitive and emotional difficulties. Down syndrome (trisomy 21) (choice **D**) is associated with mental retardation and early Alzheimer disease. Turner syndrome (XO) (choice **E**) is associated with various cognitive, social, and behavioral problems.

### 8 The answer is C *Medicine*

The patient has acromegaly secondary to a benign pituitary adenoma with excess secretion of growth hormone (not decreased [choice **E**]) by the anterior pituitary and of insulin-like growth factor-1 (not decreased [choice **D**]) from the liver. If the condition occurs before fusion of the epiphysis, gigantism occurs.

Clinical findings associated with acromegaly include:

- Generalized enlargement of bone, cartilage, and soft tissue, resulting in large hands and feet, frontal bossing, a prominent jaw, an increase in hat size, spaces between the teeth, and hypertrophy of the left ventricle observed by chest radiography (not a normal-sized heart [choice **A**]). This hypertrophy may lead to cardiomegaly and cardiomyopathy with congestive heart failure (the most common cause of death).
- Diastolic hypertension (observed blood pressure is 135/95 mm Hg)
- Muscle weakness (his perception confirmed by the physician)
- Peripheral neuropathies (he can't be sure where his feet are, loss of proprioception)
- Diabetes mellitus from the gluconeogenic properties of growth hormone
- Headaches and visual field defects from encroachment on the optic chiasm

The laboratory findings include:

- Hyperglycemia (40%) (his serum glucose level is 195 mg/dL)
- Inability to suppress glucose with an oral glucose tolerance test (choice **C**)
- A paradoxical increase of serum growth hormone concentration with injection of thyrotropin-releasing hormone (TRH)
- No stimulation of growth hormone release with L-dopa (normal persons have an increase in GH)
- Before fusion of the epiphysis occurs, increased serum phosphate associated with growth spurts
- Enlargement of the sella turcica in more than 90% of patients (not a normal-sized sella turcica [choice **B**])

Treatment consists of transsphenoidal surgery or the use of a somatostatin analogue called octreotide, which produces clinical improvement in 70% of cases.

### 9 The answer is D *Medicine*

The differential diagnosis of this patient includes gastroesophageal reflux disorder (GERD), peptic ulcer with associated reflux disease, an esophageal motility disorder, panic disorder, and some type of myocardial disease. GERD is suggested by pain that is not induced by exercise and is relieved by antacids. However, a myocardial disorder (e.g., atypical angina) is still a possibility and could be life-threatening. Therefore, an electrocardiogram (ECG) should be performed immediately (choice **D**).

Referral to a psychologist (choice **A**) would be a proper course of action for panic disorder, which is often associated with chest discomfort. However, the absence of other symptoms makes this an unlikely diagnosis. Cisapride (choice **B**) decreases reflux activity by acting as a prokinetic motility agent that increases the strength of esophageal peristalsis, raises the lower esophageal sphincter pressure, and increases the rate of gastric emptying; however, not only should potential cardiac problems be ruled out first, but cisapride was voluntarily withdrawn from the market in 2000 because of potential side effects. The histamine blockers mentioned in choice **C** or the proton pump inhibitors listed in choice **F** lower acid secretion. However, after heart problems are ruled out, the first line of treatment recommended by the American College of Gastroenterology is a series of lifestyle changes. Controlling gastric *Helicobacter pylori* infection (choice **E**) is part of the standard treatment used to cure peptic ulcers, not GERD.

### 10 The answer is B *Surgery*

Bruising about the orbit (raccoon sign) and blood in the external auditory meatus indicate that the patient has a basilar skull fracture. Cerebrospinal fluid (CSF) is an ultrafiltrate of plasma primarily derived from the choroid plexus in the lateral ventricles and is resorbed by the arachnoid granulations. The patient has otorrhea with suspected loss of CSF. When compared with serum concentrations, CSF has a higher chloride (118–132 vs. 94–106 mEq/L) (choice **B**), a lower protein (<4 vs. 6.0–7.8 g/dL) (choice **A** is wrong), a lower glucose concentration (about 60% of the plasma; 40–70 vs. 70–110 mg/dL) (choice **C** is wrong), and fewer white blood cells (0–5 vs. 4,500–11,000 leukocytes/μL) (choice **D** is wrong). Prealbumin is present in CSF electrophoresis (choice **E**) but cannot be distinguished on routine serum protein electrophoresis.

### 11 The answer is E *Pediatrics*

Live vaccines, such as measles-mumps-rubella (MMR), should not be administered to pregnant woman, immunocompromised patients, persons with moderate to severe fever, and those with allergy to neomycin causing anaphylaxis (choice **E**).

Persons with fever and upper respiratory infection (choice **A**) and persons with no fever and upper respiratory infections (choice **C**) are not contraindications to the MMR vaccine. Likewise, persons with allergy to neomycin causing contact dermatitis (choices **A**, **B**, **C**, **D**) should receive the MMR vaccine. However, the MMR vaccine should not be administered to persons with allergy to neomycin causing anaphylaxis (choice **E**). Live-virus vaccines may be administered to persons with leukemia in remission (choice **B**) who have not received chemotherapy in 3 months. The not severely immunocompromised human immunodeficiency virus (HIV) (choice **D**) positive patient should receive the MMR vaccine because of the increased risk associated with measles infection in this population, as well as the absence of serious adverse events after measles vaccination among this group.

### 12 The answer is E *Surgery*

Pneumothorax (choice **E**) can inadvertently occur while introducing a subclavian venous catheter. The patient will complain of sudden dyspnea. A chest x-ray film should always be taken after subclavian catheter placement, to determine the position of the tip of the catheter and to exclude the possibility of pneumothorax.

Air embolism (choice **A**) is not usually seen during introduction of a subclavian venous catheter, because the patient is placed in a Trendelenburg position (head end down, foot end up) so that venous pressure is increased, and air cannot be sucked into the right atrium. However, should this be attempted with the patient lying flat, or if the line is disconnected when the patient is upright, a fatal air embolism could result. The patient will have tachypnea, hypotension, and a continuous murmur. Pulmonary embolism (choice **B**) is unlikely, as no particulate matter has been introduced through the catheter at this point in time. Fat embolism (choice **C**) most often results from fractures of the long bone. If acute anxiety were to cause the dyspnea (choice **D**), an attack would be expected to precede the introduction of the catheter.

### 13 The answer is E *Psychiatry*

This woman's symptoms are most suggestive of shared psychotic disorder, characterized by the acceptance of delusional beliefs from a psychotic individual with whom one has a close relationship, often called the inducer. Shared psychotic disorder most often occurs in individuals who are in close company of a dominant person with delusional beliefs and who are isolated from others. She is less likely to suffer from delusional disorder in so much as there is little evidence of delusions not connected with those of the husband. Shared psychotic disorder is most successfully treated by separation from the inducer (choice **E**). When this is accomplished, symptoms usually fade quickly. Separation may be difficult or impossible because of the wishes of the patient.

There is little evidence to suggest that behavioral psychotherapy (choice **A**), cognitive psychotherapy (choice **B**), conjoint psychotherapy (choice **C**), or ziprasidone (choice **D**) or other antipsychotic medications are useful treatments for this disorder.

### 14 The answer is A *Pediatrics*

As the patient is dehydrated, fluid replacement is warranted. However, since total body water loss is minimal, aggressive therapy is not called for, and a bolus of 20 mL/kg of isotonic crystalloid (choice **A**) is the most appropriate choice.

Accordingly, more aggressive fluid management (answer **B**) is not warranted. Likewise, administering maintenance fluids (answer **C**) would be inappropriate for this patient and for the emergency medicine setting. Most likely, an initial bolus will be adequate therapy; therefore, giving an antiemetic (choice **D**) would not be the next best step. Additionally, antiemetics are not widely used in the pediatric population. Antibiotic therapy (answer **E**) is also incorrect because the first step in management is to administer fluids and because antibiotics should not be administered until it is determined that there is a bacterial infection.

### 15 The answer is C *Psychiatry*

Dissociative fugue (choice **C**) is characterized by sudden travel away from home, inability to recall one's past, and a disturbance of identity. It often occurs during the course of severe stress.

Memory impairment may or may not be present with psychosis due to a general medical condition (choice **A**), but no psychotic symptoms are present in the case description. Conversion disorder (choice **B**) is characterized by loss of sensory or motor function—not simply memory loss. Subjective memory problems sometimes occur during major depressive disorder (choice **D**), but identity disturbance would be very unusual in this condition. Delirium (choice **E**) may present with memory impairment but also involves a disturbed level of awareness.

### 16 The answer is A *Surgery*

The clinical presentation of a young adult female with fever, left-sided abdominal pain, multiple daily bowel movements, bloody diarrhea with mucus, and rectal bleeding is strongly suggestive of ulcerative colitis (choice **A**). This diagnosis will be confirmed by sigmoidoscopy (colonoscopy is not recommended for fear of perforation). Sigmoidoscopy will reveal a granular, hyperemic, and friable mucosa that bleeds easily on minimal contact. The disease is confined to the rectum in up to 50% of cases. However, in about 30% of patients, inflammation extends up the left colon in a continuous fashion (no skip lesions) to the splenic flexure, and 20% will have even more extensive colitis. The disease is slightly more common in females than males, and surprisingly, smoking seems to impart some protection against this disease. Its etiology is unknown, and the clinical profile is highly variable. Mild cases are defined as having fewer than four bloody bowel movements per day, moderate case have four to six, and severe cases more than six. The severity of the anemia, the elevation of the sedimentation rate, and the decrease in serum albumin level also reflect the severity of the disease. Typically, ulcerative colitis is a recurring disease with attacks precipitated by stress.

There are several goals in the treatment of ulcerative colitis. First is to stop an attack in progress. In the typical case limited to the distal part of the tract, this is done using mesalamine and hydrocortisone suppositories or enemas. In more extensive cases, mesalamine tablets are used along with sulfasalazine and balsalazide. Very severe cases are treated with IV methylprednisolone. The second aim of treatment is to return the patient to a more healthy state by evaluating and treating the anemia, hypovolemia, and malnourishment that is likely to have developed. A final goal is to try to prevent further sudden attacks. This is done by a high-fiber diet, which also limits the intake of caffeine and gas-producing vegetables. Prophylactic use of antidiarrheal agents is sometimes recommended, and a maintenance daily dose of sulfasalazine with mesalamine has been shown to reduce the relapse rate to about 33%, compared with a rate of 75% for patients not on maintenance therapy. Although medical management permits most patients to live an almost normal life, some 25% will need surgery to remove the affected segment of rectum and colon or to remove observed dysplasia or carcinoma. (The disease makes patients more prone to develop colon cancer.)

Crohn disease (choice **B**) is an ulcer-causing inflammatory bowel disease. About half the cases involve the small bowel, usually the terminal ileum and the adjacent colon (ileocolitis). Crohn disease usually presents with right lower quadrant pain, fever, and diarrhea. However, in other cases, more distal areas are affected, and in about 30% of cases, there is perianal involvement. In contrast to ulcerative colitis, the diarrhea is nonbloody and cigarette smoking is a definite risk factor. Anal fissures (choice **C**) produce severe rectal pain on defecation, bleeding, and anal tenderness. Ischemic bowel disease (choice **D**) presents with diffuse abdominal pain and bloody diarrhea. The solitary ulcer syndrome (choice **E**) is characterized by mucosal prolapse with ischemic ulceration.

### 17 The answer is D *Medicine*

These data indicate that this man has prediabetic metabolic syndrome; contemporary standards recommend aggressive treatment. However, recent summaries of several studies conclude that lifestyle modification (choice **D**) should be the first choice to prevent or delay diabetes. Moreover, such lifestyle changes will also help alleviate risk factors such as hypertension and excess weight. The data in the table that support the conclusion of prediabetic metabolic syndrome include the following:

- He has a fasting blood glucose value of 119 mg/dL, which is less than the 125 mg/dL value needed to diagnose diabetes upon a repeat determination, but is also well above the high normal value of 99 mg/dL. This strongly suggests he is prediabetic.
- His HbA1c value of 6.0% and his Hispanic heritage are findings also consistent with this idea; the latter suggests that he is genetically susceptible for type 2 diabetes.
- Similarly, his blood pressure value of 135/80 mg Hg falls into the pre-hypertensive range (normal systolic being defined as <120 mm Hg, frank hypertension as ≥140, normal diastolic as <80 mm Hg, and hypertensive as ≥89).
- He also has dyslipidemia (total cholesterol 220 mg/dL [desirable <200 mg/dL, high risk >240 mg/dL], triglycerides 150 mg/dL [desirable <150 mg/dL, high risk >200 mg/dL], HDL 45 mg/dL [desirable >60 mg/dL, high risk <40 mg/dL], LDL 145 mg/dL [optional <100 mg/dL, desirable <130 mg/dL, high risk >160 mg/dL]).

These facts, plus the observation that he is slightly overweight (BMI 25.4, normal 18.5–24.9, overweight 25–29.9, obese over 30), add to the diagnostic picture.

Clearly, he does not have frank diabetes (choice **A**), hypertension (choice **B**), or nephropathy (choice **C**), let alone diabetes and hypertension (choice **D**); thus, these choices are not correct. However, the physician clearly should discuss a dietary regime, which, if adhered to, could lower both his circulating glucose levels and his blood pressure, thus preventing or at least delaying the development of diabetes. It would appear that this patient also has osteoarthritis of the knees. His physician might prescribe an analgesic for this but not a disease-modifying antirheumatic drug (DMARD), which would be reserved for treatment of rheumatoid arthritis; he has osteoarthritis (choice **E** is incorrect).

### 18 The answer is D *Surgery*

This patient has a mechanical obstruction of the bowel caused by a large gallstone (>2.5 cm) lodged within the lumen of the ileus: i.e., gallstone ileus (choice **D**). These stones are usually radiopaque. Gallstone ileus is most commonly seen in elderly women who have a chronically inflamed gallbladder that adheres to the bowel. This results in a cholecystenteric fistula, which connects the gallbladder with either the duodenum or hepatic flexure of the colon, both of which are in the vicinity of the gallbladder. In 40% of cases, air is seen in the biliary tree because bowel air is transported to that location via the fistula. Emergency laparotomy and enterotomy to remove the stone should be undertaken. A second stone may be present proximally and should be removed to avoid recurrence. The fistula should be left alone, because it is not the cause of this patient's symptoms, and it closes off by itself. Cholecystectomy might be undertaken at a later date, if the patient has symptoms.

Tumors of the small bowel (e.g., lymphoma of the small bowel [choice **A**]) are rare. The most common location is the terminal ileum, and they are not radiopaque. Lymphoma is the most common primary malignant tumor of the small intestine. It may present with rectal bleeding or intussusception. Acute pancreatitis (choice **B**) presents as an acute abdomen, but it is not associated with a radiopaque mass in the small bowel. It is more common in males and in a younger age group. A plain abdominal x-ray film shows a sentinel loop, which represents a dilated proximal loop of jejunum adjoining the pancreas. Intussusception (choice **E**) is a telescoping of a segment of the bowel into the adjacent segment. This usually involves the terminal ileum telescoping into the proximal large bowel. It is the most common cause of intestinal obstruction in children. It is associated with a sausage-shaped mass in the midabdomen and red, currant-jelly stool. If it cannot be reduced by barium enema, surgery is required. Acute appendicitis with radiopaque fecalith (choice **C**) has a different clinical presentation. The patient would complain of nausea, vomiting, constipation, and periumbilical pain that radiates and settles in the right lower quadrant. Physical examination would elicit tenderness and guarding in the right lower quadrant. Finally, fecaliths are not radiopaque.

### 19 The answer is B *Medicine*

The patient has a glioblastoma multiforme (choice **B**). This is the most common primary cancer of the brain in adults (peaks in the 40- to 70-year-old age bracket) and either arises de novo or from a preexisting low-grade astrocytoma. The tumors are located predominantly in the cerebral hemispheres and are classified as grade IV astrocytomas. There is no causal relationship with cigarette smoking. The distribution of this lesion and the history of headache, projectile vomiting, and bilateral papilledema are classic signs and symptoms of glioblastoma multiforme. The magnetic resonance imaging (MRI) scan shows a mass lesion extending across the splenium of the corpus callosum and into the adjacent cerebral hemisphere bilaterally. These tumors rarely metastasize out of the neuraxis. Radiation and chemotherapy are used for treatment. There is a 25%–40% 5-year survival rate.

Cerebral infarctions (choice **A**) are most commonly caused by a thrombus overlying an atheromatous plaque, which causes a pale infarction that extends to the periphery of the cerebral cortex. The lesion in this patient does not adhere to this distribution. Intracerebral hemorrhages (choice **C**) usually are due to hypertension (not recorded in this patient), which produces small-vessel aneurysms that result in rupture of the vessel and hemorrhage into the brain. The basal ganglia area is the most common site for the hemorrhage. Medulloblastomas (choice **D**) usually are located in the midline of the cerebellum in children. Metastases to the brain (choice **E**) usually are multifocal and occur primarily at the junction of the gray and white matter near the periphery of the brain.

### 20 The answer is B *Preventive Medicine and Public Health*

The question relates to assessing differences among three groups of a continuous variable, which in this question is systolic blood pressure. To assess the significance of differences in data derived from three or more groups it is necessary to use analysis of variance (choice **B**).

If the comparison were between only two groups, a Student's *t*-test (choice **A**) would be correct. A correlation coefficient (choice **C**) assesses the strength of association, not the differences between groups. The chi-squared test (choice **D**) assesses differences among groups of categorical variables. Logistic regression (choice **E**) is used to assess a categorical outcome for a continuous predictor.

### 21 The answer is A *Psychiatry*

Social withdrawal and a family history of psychopathology (choice **A**) are both more commonly associated with schizophrenia than with delirium.

Memory impairment and waxing and waning of confusion within a period of hours (choice **B**) are both more suggestive of delirium. Hallucinations (choice **C**) are common in both delirium and schizophrenia. Visual hallucinations are more commonly associated with delirium, while auditory hallucinations are more often described in schizophrenia, but there is much overlap. A family history of schizophrenia is more common in schizophrenia than in the general population, but rapid waxing and waning of confusion is a characteristic of delirium and is much less common in schizophrenia; hence choice **D** is incorrect. Similarly, choice **E** is wrong because social withdrawal suggests schizophrenia, whereas rapid fluctuation of confusion much more strongly suggests delirium.

### 22 The answer is C *Medicine*

Clearly, this young man has a polydipsia/polyuria (excessive drinking/urinating) problem. Desmopressin (choice **C**) is a vasopressin (also known as, the antidiuretic hormone) analog (1-deamino-8-*D*-arginine vasopressin) and is the only choice presented that would directly inhibit water loss into the urine. The word *diabetes* means to have an abnormal need to urinate. There are two basic types of diabetes, the more common "sweet" type, *diabetes mellitus*, and the insipid, or "tasteless" type *diabetes insipidus*. Physicians presented with such a patient would order an electrolyte panel to help diagnose his condition, but even without additional data, common sense indicates this patient does not have diabetes mellitus (and therefore does not need metformin choice **A**) since he has had this condition for many years and is healthy except for his abnormal thirst; it follows he must have diabetes insipidus. However, there are five recognized types of diabetes insipidus:

1. Central (also known as, neurogenic or pituitary), in which the hypothalamus has lost the capacity to synthesize vasopressin; this condition may be idiopathic or due to some sort of injury, physical or pathological (tumors or infection).
2. Nephrogenic, in which the kidney tubules have lost functional binding sites for vasopressin; this may be caused by kidney disease, drugs that inhibit binding, or in very rare cases, it is inherited.
3. Dipsogenic, in which the thirst-regulating part of the brain is damaged.
4. Gestational, caused by the placenta's destruction of vasopressin. As a rule, recovery is spontaneous within 24 days after birth, although an affected woman is at high risk to develop another case of diabetes insipidus during subsequent pregnancies.
5. Psychogenic, in which a patient has an obsessive compulsion to drink large quantities of water.

Usually, a physician will measure blood glucose, bicarbonate, and electrolyte levels, as well as urinary osmolarity, as the first step in confirming diabetes insipidus. Typically, urine osmolarity and electrolyte levels are lower than normal and the degree to which hypernatremia occurs reflects the degree of dehydration. A fluid deprivation test helps determine if the diabetes is due to lack of vasopressin (central), to the kidney's insensitivity to vasopressin (nephrogenic), or to excessive fluid ingestion (dipso- or psychogenic). Normally, as fluid deprivation proceeds, dehydration starts to occur and the kidney compensates by excreting a lesser volume of more concentrated urine; consequently, the body retains a greater volume of water. Patients with diabetes insipidus fail to concentrate their urine; however, patients having central diabetes insipidus will start to concentrate their urine after the administration of desmopressin. This will not occur if the patient has nephrogenic, dipsogenic, or psychogenic diabetic insipidus.

Foscarnet (choice **B**), an antibiotic used to treat cytomegalovirus infection, has recently been shown to cause nephrogenic diabetes insipidus in certain patients and consequently will not likely be used to treat any form of diabetes insipidus. Increasing his daily water intake (choice **D**) also would be counterproductive and might lead to water intoxication caused by hyponatremia. Demeclocycline (choice **E**) is a broad-spectrum tetracycline antibiotic and the only tetracycline with the property of competing with vasopressin for its binding sites on the renal tubules, thus it too may cause a transient diabetes insipidus and will not likely be used to treat diabetes insipidus.

### 23 The answer is C *Surgery*

This patient has developed a compression fracture of the vertebra (choice **C**). She probably has osteoporosis, which makes it possible for a compression fracture to occur. Sudden onset of pain that radiates to the front of the abdomen like a belt is a characteristic presentation. This, together with tenderness in the vertebra to palpation, should suggest the diagnosis. Additional features include neurologic deficits secondary to spinal cord compression. The sensory deficits in the legs of this patient and the absent ankle jerks are due to diabetic neuropathy.

A spinal cord tumor (choice **A**) is usually associated with chronic pain, and there may be tenderness on palpation of the vertebra. Clonus has to be sustained to be pathologic and signifies involvement of the corticospinal pathway. Thus, there are no neurologic findings in this patient to support a spinal cord tumor. An epidural abscess (choice **B**) can present with pain over a few days and tenderness in the spine, together with pyrexia, which is absent in this patient. Furthermore, the patient may have neurologic deficits as well. A posterolateral lumbar disk herniation (choice **D**) is associated with radicular pain (i.e., pain going down one lower extremity) together with sensory loss over the distribution of the appropriate dermatome in the leg. There may be motor weakness, either weak dorsiflexion or weak plantar flexion of the appropriate foot, depending on which nerve root is involved. No spinal tenderness will be elicited. A central lumbar disk herniation (choice **E**) is associated with saddle anesthesia and an absent or weakened anal wink reflex, or weakness of the lower extremity with partial saddle anesthesia. The former is due to involvement of the conus medullaris, whereas the latter is due to involvement of the cauda equina. In neither case will there be tenderness of the vertebral spine.

### 24 The answer is D *Pediatrics*

Mastitis is not a contraindication to breastfeeding (choice D). The infant will not become ill if nursed on the affected breast (choice A). The most important fact to remember about mastitis is that early antibiotic treatment and continued breastfeeding or pumping are essential to its cure. However, the mother should be treated with antibiotic therapy and analgesics that do not put the infant at risk (choice B). Frequent nursing on the affected breast will keep the breast from becoming engorged (choice C). In many cases, this will keep mastitis from progressing to a breast abscess. Changing to a commercially prepared formula (choice E) is not necessary because mastitis is not a contraindication to breastfeeding and breast milk is superior to commercial milk. Other supportive therapy for mastitis may include rest, plenty of fluids, and cold packs on the painful breast.

### 25 The answer is C *Preventive Medicine and Public Health*

Despite the fact that this woman is young and has no signs or symptoms of coronary artery disease (CAD), her obesity, lipid profile, and family history put her at risk for early disease; therefore, she is a prime subject for preventive measures. Regardless of the serum cholesterol level, high-density lipoprotein (HDL) level, or any other relevant laboratory value, the first step in management for primary prevention is 6 months of diet and aerobic exercise (choice C).

The patient should always begin with the American Heart Association step 1 diet, not the step 2 diet (choice **D**). If after 3 months there is no change in lipid profile, the patient should be changed to the step 2 diet. Pharmacologic intervention (choices **A**, **B**, and **E**) should be considered only after 6 months of aerobic exercise and diet.

### 26 The answer is A *Psychiatry*

Family dynamics are strongly implicated in the development of anorexia nervosa (choice **A**). Patients' mothers are often seen as overly controlling and fathers are seen as inhibited and compulsive. Food restriction and weight loss are postulated to be attempts to regain some control and perhaps avoid sexual issues by retaining a more juvenile appearance. Psychotherapeutic intervention often involves family therapy.

Dissociative identity disorder (choice **B**) is associated with childhood sexual abuse. Narcissistic personality disorder (choice **C**) and schizophrenia (choice **D**) are not associated with a particular set of family dynamics. The onset of separation anxiety disorder (choice **E**) in childhood is sometimes associated with the death or other loss of a primary family member.

### 27 The answer is D *Preventative Medicine and Public Health*

Osteoporosis is the most common metabolic abnormality of bone in the United States; it is estimated that some 10 million individuals in the United States presently have osteoporosis, of these about 2 million are males. Consequently, the prevalence of osteoporosis in males is about 20% that of females (choice **D**). Moreover, 20%–30% of hip fractures occur in men, who also have twice the first-year post-fracture mortality rate as do women. Thus, choice **B** is incorrect. Additionally, approximately 30% of men lose their independence and move into a nursing facility or into a relative's home. Unlike women, the onset of osteoporosis in men does not have a defined beginning point, such as menopause, but the rate of bone loss gradually increases with age and because physicians in general do not look for it the condition it is likely under diagnosed. In women, the relationship between the onset of menopause and the accompanying decrease in estrogen production clearly points to the decrease in estrogen levels as the primary underlying mechanism responsible for the rapid development of osteoporosis. Although this does not occur in males, estrogen levels also decline with age in males, and some investigators postulate that this decline is responsible for the age-related loss of bone in males. Thus, choice C is incorrect. Circulating testosterone in both sexes supports the production of estradiol by aromatization of testosterone in bone as well as in other estrogen-dependent tissues. In premenopausal women, this local production of estrogen is minuscule relative to the amounts produced by the ovaries, but after menopause, this becomes the major mechanism of estrogen production and because testosterone levels are low, estrogen production in various tissues may be suboptimal; in bone, this upsets the normal equilibrium between bone synthesis and bone destruction, causing the rate of bone loss to exceed the rate of synthesis. Consequently, bone thins and first osteopenia and eventually osteoporosis may ensue. However, in males, this local mode is the major normal route of estrogen production throughout most of life. During the first six or seven decades of adult life, most men produce sufficient testosterone to permit sufficient production of estrogen to meet the needs of local tissues, but as testosterone production declines with age estrogen production also declines, accounting for the decline in circulating estrogen in aging males.

It is important that older males be screened for osteopenia and osteoporosis because several treatments are available that may reduce the risk of fractures. If men are hypogonadal, testosterone supplementation has been found to be beneficial for the reasons discussed above. Another treatment with a long history, albeit mainly in females, is use of bisphosphonates. A more recent development is use of teriparatide, a recombinant copy of the 34 amino acids on the N-terminus of human parathyroid hormone. Unlike the bisphosphonates, and testosterone as well, teriparatide acts to stimulate osteoblastic activity rather than inhibit osteoclastic activity. There are also a few small studies reporting that thiazide diuretics improve bone density in about 20% of males having osteoporosis and hypercalciuria; however, pharmaceutical companies are not anxious to engage in large, expensive clinical trials because these drugs are so inexpensive. Calcitonin is still another drug that theoretically should combat osteoporosis but few, if any, reliable studies have been published regarding male use of calcitonin.

In osteoporosis, the organic bone matrix is deficient but the matrix that is there is fully calcified; thus choice **A** is incorrect. Although older individuals may absorb vitamin D less efficiently and are less prone to obtain as much sun exposure as younger persons, choice **E** is incorrect. In children, vitamin D deficiency is called *rickets* and in adults *osteomalacia*; in both cases, an excess of noncalcified bone matrix results in soft, malleable bones, not the fully calcified but brittle ones that characterize osteoporosis.

**28 The answer is B** *Medicine*

The patient has herpes simplex keratoconjunctivitis. A fluorescein stain exhibits the classic dendritic type of shallow ulcer with an irregular edge. Herpes labialis may or may not be present. Corneal involvement is frequently precipitated by topical corticosteroids or systemic corticosteroid therapy. Steroid therapy frequently results in deeper penetration of the ulcer. Topical trifluridine (choice **B**) is used for treatment. Ophthalmologists frequently denude the infected corneal epithelium to enhance recovery.

Topical phenylephrine (choice **C**) is a decongestant. Topical ketoconazole (choice **A**) is used in fungal corneal ulcers, which are rare. Topical erythromycin (choice **D**) and sulfacetamide (choice **E**) are both useful for bacterial conjunctivitis.

**29 The answer is A** *Medicine*

Bacteria that infected this man's wound multiplied, entered his circulatory system, and localized in one of his heart valves. Initially, this caused a case of subacute endocarditis marked by a low-grade fever. The infection then fulminated, causing symptoms commonly associated with acute infectious endocarditis, including a higher temperature, excessive sweating, chills, fatigue, muscle and joint pains, night sweats, and painful lesions, called Osler's nodes, on the pads of the fingers. Infections initiated by breaks in the skin are often caused by *Staphylococcus aureus* (choice **A**). In this case, because the shot of penicillin received at the ER did not prevent the development of endocarditis, it is likely that this was a methicillin-resistant strain. Unless faced with a massive infusion of organisms, skin breaks as a rule do not cause endocarditis because healthy valves are smooth and don't provide a surface for organisms to adhere to. However, in older individuals, one or more valves are sometimes affected by arthrosclerosis and become roughened by calcification; this provides a place for organisms to anchor and proliferate, as presumably happened in this gentleman. This is the reason why the incidence of endocarditis is higher in the elderly.

*Streptococcus viridans* is an organism found in the mouth and is associated with endocarditis after dental work (choice **B**). Prior to October 2007, dentists were advised to administer penicillin to patients at risk for heart infection as prophylaxis to prevent endocarditis. However, at that time, the American Heart Association published an article in *Circulation* recommending that most of these patients no longer get short-term antibiotics as a preventive measure before their dental treatment. The consensus was that the risks of taking preventive antibiotics outweigh the benefits for most patients. These risks include adverse reactions to antibiotics that range from mild to potentially severe and, in very rare cases, death. Inappropriate use of antibiotics can also lead to the development of drug-resistant bacteria. Infection by the yeast *Candida albicans* most commonly occurs in IV drug users; these infections commonly enter the right heart and often infect the tricuspid valve (choice **C**). *Streptococcus bovis* (choice **D**) and *Clostridium septicum* (choice **E**) are part of the natural flora of the colon and cause endocarditis if the bowel is pierced or in colon cancers, rarely from skin punctures.

**30 The answer is E** *Preventive Medicine and Public Health*

Medicaid eligibility is a means-tested program, and eligibility is generally determined by the presence of financial hardship. Rules vary from state to state, but in most states this means that to be eligible, a person's net worth must be less than $2,000 (choice **E**). This often requires an individual to expend personal resources for health care before Medicaid can be used. A potential loophole is that a sum of money, usually $10,000 or less, can be transferred to a family member not sooner than 3 years before residence is established. The 3-year requirement can sometimes be at least partially averted if it can be shown that a person, usually a family member, has been providing nursing care and can document valid expenses.

In contrast to Medicaid, Medicare is a Social Security–linked program, and all persons or spouses of persons who paid into Social Security are eligible for benefits at age 65. There is no financial requirement, but Medicare will only pay for doctor care, hospital stays, and usually 10–20 days of posthospitalization rehabilitation care. Since 2006, it contributes to payment of prescription drugs. It will not contribute toward the cost of residential care (choice **F**). In contrast, Medicaid almost always covers the cost of medications (choice **A**) and the cost of long-term residential care (choice **B**). It also differs from Medicare in that eligibility does not depend on prior payment into the system (choice **C**) or on reaching a particular age (choice **D**). Specific regulations for Medicaid vary by state, but the federal aspects of both programs are run by the Centers for Medicare and Medicaid Services (CMS), a division of the U.S. Department of Health and Human Services.

**31 The answer is F** *Psychiatry*

About 20% of adult sons of alcoholics are also alcoholic. That this is due to a component of heritability is supported by twin studies and studies of adopted children in which the biologic parent does not raise the child (choice **F**).

Although there is speculation about heritability of other substance dependencies, including cocaine (choice **B**), heroin (choice **C**), and benzodiazepines (choice **E**), the data are much less compelling. Social factors, rather than genetics, appear to be of great significance in causing opiate (choice **A**), psychostimulant (choice **G**), and tobacco (choice **D**) dependency.

**32 The answer is C** *Psychiatry*

Patients with dissociative identity disorder (choice **C**) (formerly called multiple personality disorder) report an incidence of childhood sexual abuse that is much higher than that reported by the general population. A history of childhood sexual abuse is also commonly associated with the subsequent development of borderline personality disorder and antisocial traits.

Dependent personality disorder (choice **A**), hypochondriasis (choice **D**), and major depressive disorder (choice **E**) are not so clearly associated with a history of childhood sexual abuse. Children with existing emotional disturbances are more likely to be abused than other children; however, autistic disorder (choice **B**) is not known to be a sequela of abuse.

**33 The answer is B** *Surgery*

Infection is the most common complication of burns. *Pseudomonas aeruginosa* (choice **B**) is the organism most frequently involved and the most common cause of death in burn patients. This organism will cause black patches; however, charred fat can also result in black patches. Burn patients who develop fever do not always have an infection. Thermal injury releases interleukin-1 (IL-1), which can produce fever by stimulating the hypothalamus to synthesize prostaglandins, which in turn stimulate the thermoregulatory center in the brain. This underscores the need for biopsy of suspicious burn wounds for culture to ascertain whether infection is the cause of fever. Antibiotics are not recommended for prophylaxis in burn patients.

*Staphylococcus aureus* (choice **A**), *Candida albicans* (choice **C**) (usually involved in catheter-related sepsis), and group A streptococcus (choice **D**) are less common offenders. *Staphylococcus pneumoniae* (choice **E**) is rarely involved.

**34 The answer is B** *Psychiatry*

The signs and symptoms are most suggestive of "type A" behavior, described as a constellation of personality traits that include anger, ambition, competitiveness, hostility, and impatience. Such behavior has been associated with an increased risk for coronary artery disease (CAD), at least in middle-aged U.S. citizens (choice **B**).

Cancer (choice **A**), emphysema (choice **C**), migraine (choice **D**), and peptic ulcer disease (choice **E**) have not been as convincingly associated with these traits. However, these illnesses, along with other disabling medical conditions, can be exacerbated by stress and may cause anxiety, depression, and difficulties with interpersonal relationships.

**35 The answer is (D)** *Medicine*

There are three inborn errors of copper metabolism: Wilson disease, Menkes disease, and occipital horn syndrome (choice **D**). Both occipital horn syndrome (once known as Ehlers-Danlos syndrome IX and sometimes called X-linked cutis laxa) and Menkes syndrome (also known as, kinky hair syndrome) are caused by mutations in *ATP7A* located on Xq12-13. The normal gene has 23 exons and encodes a P-type copper transport protein with ATPase activity. Mutations in the splicing sites may result in insertions or deletions and nonsense rearrangements. Such errors result in greater distortion of the protein product in patients having Menkes disease than they do in patients with occipital horn syndrome; thus, boys afflicted with Menkes disease are by definition sicker than those with occipital horn syndrome.

Male Menkes babies tend to be born a little prematurely; they seem normal at first, but then spiral into a tragic decline. Usually by about the third month, the child has an epileptic event and his appearance takes on the typical manifestation of the disease, which includes light, often steely colored, kinky hair that is sparse on the sides, plus an unusual appearance. From that time on, the child fails to thrive and degenerates neurologically and physically, eventually dying, generally by the third year.

The normal Menkes gene product exists in both a long and short form, with different tissue distribution. The shorter form is expressed in occipital horn syndrome, and this probably accounts for the milder phenotype, which is similar to the one described in the case history. Formerly, most afflicted boys died in their early teens but now commonly live well into their 20s.

The normal Menkes and Wilson disease genes have about 55% identity, and both code for copper-transporting proteins, but their distribution and the function of their gene products are different. The underlying function of the normal Menkes gene product is to bring copper ion into the body and distribute it among cells; in contrast, the function of the normal Wilson gene product is to remove excess copper ion from the body. Consequently, the normal Wilson disease gene is expressed predominantly in the liver, whereas the normal Menkes disease gene is not expressed to a significant extent in liver but is in most other tissues; moreover, serum copper ion levels are lower than normal in both Menkes disease and occipital horn syndrome, but raised in Wilson disease.

A rare autosomal recessive condition called *acrodermatitis enteropathica* (also known as, Brandt syndrome, Danbolt-Cross syndrome or congenital zinc deficiency) causes a congenital form of zinc deficiency (choice **A**). Zinc and copper are the only trace elements associated with known inborn errors of metabolism. Zinc is a cofactor for as many as 300 enzymatic reactions; hence, a deficiency can have profound effects. Patients having acrodermatitis enteropathica who are not treated by lifelong dietary zinc supplementation die within a few years. Acquired deficiencies are more common; the deficiency may be due to dietary insufficiency (either because of poor nutrition or to conditions such as anorexia nervosa or alcohol abuse), a decreased ability to absorb the ion (either because of intestinal disorders or sometimes associated with aging), and in patients on complete parenteral nutrition, insufficient zinc allowance. Deficiency states in developed counties are generally modest and the effects subtle. An obvious effect is in limiting the growth of children. Earlier studies in several U.S. communities showed that dietary supplementation with zinc induced growth spurts, thus indicating that these children had a nutritional deficiency. Dermatologic changes (e.g., rashes) are another readily recognized consequence of zinc deficiency. Loss of acuity of taste (dysgeusia) or smell (anosmia) caused by a reduced ability to absorb zinc has been observed among aged individuals. Chronic zinc deficiency also increases susceptibility to infection by reducing immunologic efficiency and also by reducing the efficiency of wound healing because it is a cofactor for collagenase, which is required to resorb type III collagen so that it may be replaced by type I collagen. As a rule, these acquired deficiencies can be reversed by zinc supplementation, but with a note of caution: taking large quantities of zinc can reduce the bioavailability of copper because zinc induces the synthesis of a metallothionein that binds copper within intestinal cells and prevents its absorption. Thus, individuals taking zinc supplements are advised to also take a copper supplement.

Selenium (choice **B**) is a cofactor for glutathione peroxidase (which neutralizes hydrogen peroxide and peroxide free radicals in cells), thioredoxin reductase (which indirectly reduces certain oxidized molecules), and three deiodinase enzymes (which interconvert forms of thyroid hormone). Its glutathione peroxidase activity helps reduce free radicals and is thought to act to reduce the risk of cancer. A frank selenium deficiency also predisposes patients to Keshan disease, an endemic viral cardiomyopathy primarily affecting children and young women. At high doses, selenium is toxic, causing hair loss, abnormal nails, dermatitis, peripheral neuropathy, nausea, diarrhea, fatigue, irritability, and a garlicky breath odor. Chromium (choice **C**) is another essential trace element required by humans. It is almost ubiquitous in nature, making deficiency states essentially unknown. Promotional literature from supplement distributors may claim chromium supplements can reduce serum cholesterol levels, prevent or help alleviate symptoms associated with diabetes, reduce body fat, and help build muscle, but there is little evidence to substantiate such claims. Nonetheless, chromium is a component of glucose tolerance factor, and consequently does help insulin make glucose available to cells by facilitating the binding of insulin to its receptors located in adipose and muscle. Thus, if a deficiency of chromium truly did exist, it might be associated with impaired glucose tolerance. The human requirement for cobalt (choice **E**) is not for the ionic form of the metal, but for a preformed metallovitamin that cannot be synthesized from dietary metal. Therefore, it is the vitamin $B_{12}$ content of foods in the diet that is of importance in human nutrition. Manganese (choice **F**) is a cofactor for arginase, pyruvate carboxylase, glutamine synthetase, and manganese superoxide dismutase (SOD), and is the preferred metal cofactor for glycosyltransferases. No deficiency states for manganese have been established.

### 36 **The answer is E** *Medicine*

This patient has herpes simplex encephalitis (HSE). The data presented do not definitely point to this diagnosis but they do raise the suspicion. Historically, the definitive test for HSE was a brain biopsy, but for the past two decades the preferred diagnostic modality is identification by a polymerase chain reaction (PCR) (choice **E**). After DNA amplification, a Southern blot technique can identify herpes simplex early in the disease, with a turnaround time of 24 hours or less. This test is now considered the definitive standard for the diagnosis of HSE, having a specificity and sensitivity of 98%–99%. HSE is the most common cause of sporadic lethal encephalitis, occurring in about 1 person per 250,000–500,000 population per year. The frequency distribution is bimodal, peaking among individuals younger than 20 years of age and again among persons older than 50 years. In younger individuals, cases are generally caused by primary infections, whereas in older individuals the encephalitis is generally caused by reactivation of latent infections in cranial nerve ganglia (often in the trigeminal ganglion) or sometimes in the brain itself. In adults, essentially all cases are caused by herpes simplex 1, whereas in neonates herpes simplex 2 is the more common culprit, the infection being transmitted from the mother's genitalia. Early treatment is crucial to a good outcome, and empiric acyclovir therapy can be initiated before a definitive diagnosis is established. The mortality rate is as high as 70% in untreated patients and is reduced to about 19% in treated patients; however, approximately 50% of survivors are left with significant neurological deficits.

Serologic analysis (choice **A**) of blood or CSF has no role in the acute diagnosis and treatment of HSE patients. However, it may have value in retrospective diagnosis. Similarly, strategies based on increases in antibody levels and on the ratio of antibody levels in serum and CSF (choice **B**) also have not proven to be clinically useful. Magnetic resonance imaging (MRI) (choice **C**) is more useful than computed tomography (CT) scans in permitting visualization of changes in the brain's anatomy, but these images do not provide specific information concerning the etiology of these changes. Electroencephalography (choice **D**) will, in an analogous way, provide information concerning changes in the brain's function, but once again, does not point definitively to a causative agent.

### 37 **The answer is A** *Preventive Medicine and Public Health*

Several clinical studies report that regular consumption of fatty fish or fish oil supplements reduces the risk of heart attacks, sudden death, and deaths due to any cause in people with histories of heart attacks, whereas other clinical studies have shown that a daily dose of low-dose aspirin helps lower the risk of a heart attack for people otherwise at risk. Most patients in these studies were also using standard heart drugs, suggesting that the benefits of aspirin and fish oils may add to the effects of other therapies. The effects of both aspirin and fish oil are in large part mediated by their effects on prostaglandin (PG) metabolism. Aspirin inhibits synthesis of series 2 PGs by covalently binding to the cyclo-oxygenase (COX) isoenzymes; this reduces platelet clumping, thereby helping to prevent or reduce formation of blood clots. Fish oil contains long-chain omega-3 fatty acids that are converted to series 3 PGs, which as a whole counter the action of series 2 PGs and inhibit inflammation (choice **A**).

Although it is true that aspirin covalently binds to the COX isoenzymes that convert arachidonic acid to PG $H_2$, which then serves as an intermediate to several products including the series 2 PGs, PG $E_2$, and PG $D_2$, as well as to several others of the eicosanoid family, it is not true that fish oil contains omega-3 fatty acids that are converted to arachidonic acid (choice **B**). The relatively unique fatty acids of importance in fish oils are eicosatetraenoic acid, a 20-carbon quintuple unsaturated omega-3 fatty acid and docosahexaenoic acid, a 22-carbon omega-3 fatty acid with six double bonds. These are potential precursors to series 3 PGs, which tend to counterbalance the inflammatory effects of the series 2 PGs synthesized via the arachidonic acid pathway and also appear to play important roles in the stabilization of cell membranes and central nervous tissue white matter. These long-chain polyunsaturated fatty acids are obtained preformed in fish oil but can in theory be synthesized by mammals, starting with α-linolenic acid, an 18-carbon triple unsaturated omega-3 essential fatty acid primarily found in flax seed and walnuts; the α-linolenic acid is then desaturated and elongated in a series of reactions that does not include arachidonic acid. However, it generally is conceded that this latter series of reactions is not able to provide optimal amounts of the longer polyunsaturated fatty acids. Although aspirin and the other nonsteroidal anti-inflammatory drugs block the COX enzymes, acetaminophen has a different mode of action (choice **C**). The prevailing hypothesis is that there is a third COX isozyme located in the brain that is acetaminophen sensitive. Aspirin covalently, not noncovalently, blocks the COX enzymes, and fish oil does not contain omega 3-fatty acids that are converted to series 2 PGs (choice **D**).

Series 1 PGs have been called the "good" PGs, but fish oil does not contains significant quantities of omega-3 fatty acids that are converted to series 1 PGs (choice **E**). The series 1 PGs are diverted off of the arachidonic pathway before the latter is produced. The immediate fatty acid precursor is di-homo-γ-linolenic acid, a triple-unsaturated C-20 omega-6 fatty acid, which in turn is formed from γ-linolic acid, a triple-unsaturated C-18 omega-6 fatty acid, found in high concentration in evening primrose, borage, and black currant oils, and recommended by some advocates of alterative medicine to ease menstrual cramps and relieve itchy skin. Series 1 PGs may also lower blood pressure.

### 38 **The answer is C** *Medicine*

This lady most likely suffers from an anal fissure, for which the classical treatment is application of a local steroid cream twice daily, plus use of stool softeners and hot sitz baths (choice **C**). Such a fissure results from the passage of a large, hard bolus of stool and is a common cause of rectal bleeding. Severe pain is an important symptom, and the condition is confirmed by observation of a semiepileptical defect in the anal skin running in a radial direction. The treatment described usually results in complete recovery.

A mass protruding from the patient's anus is usually due to a prolapsed internal hemorrhoid and generally is caused by straining to defecate. The mass generally retracts spontaneously and is rarely accompanied by pain unless it is thrombosed (choice **A**). There is no call for a sigmoidoscopy, and polyps cannot be removed during a sigmoidoscopy (choice **B**). Prescription of antihypertensive drugs and antibiotics is a therapy used to treat relatively mild cases of ischemic colitis (choice **D**). Control of hypertension will facilitate blood flow into the colon, while the antibiotics will help prevent infection. Idiopathic bleeding from the bowel due to dilated blood vessels in the mucosa is called *angiodysplasia* and may be initially treated by cautery employing argon plasma coagulation applied via an endoscope (choice **E**).

### 39 **The answer is B** *Medicine*

Phyllodes tumors, formally called cystosarcoma phyllodes (choice **B**), account for about 1% of all breast cancers and are recognized by the fact they usually develop in the fourth or fifth decade, on the left breast away from nipple, can be moved freely, and have sharply discernible borders and a firm smooth texture; they also grow very rapidly and can become large (up to 30 cm have been reported) and bulky. Some 70%–90% of the tumors are benign, although even benign ones tend to recur locally at about a 20% rate. When cross-sectioned, the tumor's internal structure looks like a leaf. Histologically, phyllodes tumors can be recognized by their stromal component. They are not staged in the usual way, but are classified as benign, intermediate, or malignant on the basis of the number of cells undergoing mitosis and the fraction of irregularly shaped cells in the biopsy sample. Some 10% of the malignant ones prove to be fatal. However, some intermediate tumors are difficult to classify. The tumors are resistant to radiation or chemotherapy; consequently, treatment must be surgical, and to ensure complete removal, at least 2 cm of nontumorous tissue is generally excised along with the tumor itself.

Fibroadenoma (choice **A**) shares a few superficial characteristics with phyllodes tumor. Both are mobile upon palpitation, spherical or ovoid, elastic, nodular, have well-demarcated capsules, and are more commonly are found in the left breast. However, a fibroadenoma does not grow rapidly, is often located close to the areola, but rarely behind the nipple, and most often is found in younger females, those in their late teens or early 20s. A final diagnosis, however, generally depends upon ultrasound, mammography, and usually a biopsy. Because a fibroadenoma is a benign tumor, surgery may not be required. However, the tumor is generally excised if the diagnosis is in doubt, particularly in older women, or if the fibroadenoma is larger than usual. Follow-up chemotherapy is not required. Invasive (also known as, infiltrating) ductal carcinoma (choice **C**) accounts for about 78% of all breast neoplasms. Upon mammography, they may be well circumscribed or stellate. The latter have a poorer prognosis. Invasive (also known as, infiltrating) lobular carcinoma (choice **D**) represent about 15% of all breast neoplasms and generally are found in the upper outer quadrant as a subtle thickening rather than a lump. Inflammatory breast cancer (choice **E**) is a rare but very aggressive type of breast cancer, in which the lymph vessels in the skin of the breast are blocked by cancer cells. It is called "inflammatory" because the breast often looks swollen and red or "inflamed." It accounts for 1%–5% of all breast cancer cases in the United States.

**40** **The answer is B** *Medicine*

The clinical findings in this patient are due to hypoglycemia. The most common overall cause of hypoglycemia is excessive insulin in a person with insulin-dependent diabetes. Hypoglycemia is precipitated by administration of an excessive dose of insulin, increased physical activity, delay in eating a meal, fluctuations in absorption in various administration sites, and autonomic neuropathy impairing counterregulatory mechanisms. The adrenergic symptoms of hypoglycemia include perspiration, tachycardia, increased salivation, and restlessness. These symptoms can be blunted if the patient is taking a β-blocker (e.g., propranolol), thus making the diagnosis more difficult. Lack of Kussmaul's respiration (deep respiration) and no smell of ketones on the breath are clues that ketoacidosis is not present in this patient. Immediate measurement of blood glucose (choice **B**) with glucose oxidase–impregnated paper strips or a glucometer is easily accomplished in the emergency department, so that therapy can be initiated. Patients who are conscious should be given oral feedings of fruit juice or, if available, glucose pills. Comatose patients are usually given an IV infusion of 50% dextrose in water. If IV glucose is not available, 1 mg of glucagon is given intramuscularly. Hypoglycemia presenting with similar symptoms and requiring similar treatment can also be induced in persons with non–insulin-dependent diabetes who are taking an antidiabetic pill that promotes insulin secretion (e.g., the sulfonylureas).

A complete blood count (CBC) (choice **A**), serum electrolytes (choice **C**), a drug screen (choice **D**), and arterial blood gas (ABG) determination (choice **E**) are not appropriate initial steps in the management of patients with the classic adrenergic symptoms of hypoglycemia.

**41** **The answer is H** *Obstetrics and Gynecology*

The most common cause of vaginal bleeding in a prepubertal girl is a vaginal foreign body. However, a cystic grapelike mass at the introitus suggests a more worrisome cause. Sarcoma botryoides (choice **H**) (also known as, rhabdomyosarcoma of the vagina) is a malignancy in infants and young children that arises from embryonal rhabdomyoblasts (ancestral muscle cells). The tumor resembles a bunch of grapes. It has a generally good prognosis with conservative surgery followed by chemotherapy. It is a rare malignant tumor of the female reproductive tract, most commonly seen in girls younger than 8 years of age. The most common symptom is abnormal vaginal bleeding.

**42** **The answer is D** *Obstetrics and Gynecology*

Intermittent vaginal bleeding between normal menses is suggestive of an anatomic lesion. The absence of postcoital bleeding makes it unlikely that the bleeding is caused by invasive cervical carcinoma. The normal pelvic examination rules out a lower genital tract lesion such as vulvar neoplasms, vaginal varicosities, or cervical polyps. Upper tract causes of vaginal bleeding include endometrial polyps or submucosal leiomyomas. The presence of an asymmetrically enlarged, firm, nontender uterus is suggestive of subserosal or intramural uterine myomas. The presence of bleeding suggests the likelihood of a submucosal leiomyoma (choice **D**) as the cause.

**43** **The answer is I** *Obstetrics and Gynecology*

The key to identifying the most likely cause of the increasing vaginal bleeding in this case is its linkage to increasing pain with menses. Pain with menses is known as dysmenorrhea, and this scenario describes secondary dysmenorrhea. Secondary dysmenorrhea is caused by anatomic abnormalities such as endometriosis, chronic pelvic inflammatory disease, leiomyomas, or adenomyosis. The finding of a diffusely enlarged, globular, soft, tender uterus is classic for adenomyosis (choice **I**). Ordering a β-human chorionic gonadotropin (β-hCG) test is critical to rule out pregnancy, the most common cause of an enlarged uterus in the reproductive years. The history of treatment for cervical dysplasia is only an incidental historical finding.

**44** **The answer is G** *Obstetrics and Gynecology*

The history of irregular, unpredictable menstrual bleeding is strongly suggestive of an anovulatory cause. The absence of cramping and pain is consistent with anovulation. (Ovulatory cycles typically are associated with cramping, from the release of prostaglandins triggered by the necrosis that is endometrial spiral arteriolar spasm caused by the decrease in progesterone production from the corpus luteum.) With anovulation, the unopposed estrogen results in simple endometrial hyperplasia without atypia (choice **G**). Management is by administering cyclic progestins or combination oral contraceptives to reverse the hyperplasia.

**45** **The answer is F** *Obstetrics and Gynecology*

A history of intermittent vaginal bleeding between normal menses is suggestive of an anatomic lesion. The additional finding of painless postcoital bleeding makes one highly suspicious for a cervical lesion, such as cervical polyps or invasive cervical carcinoma (choice **F**). She has many risk factors for cervical neoplasia including multiple sexual partners and a long history of cigarette smoking. The long gap to the present from her last Pap smear is troublesome. She will need colposcopy and a cervical biopsy for diagnosis.

**46** **The answer is B** *Obstetrics and Gynecology*

The most common cause of vaginal bleeding in a prepubertal girl is a vaginal foreign body (choice **B**). To confirm that this is the case requires visual inspection of the vagina by a speculum or a fiberoptic scope, usually under sedation. In this case, the lack of pubertal changes on examination (e.g., breast budding, pubic hair) makes precocious puberty unlikely and the absence of a cystic tissue (as in case 41) tends to rule out other possible causes of bleeding such as a tumor. Although an unlikely possibility in a 6-year-old, the ingestion of steroid contraceptives could stimulate the endometrium, resulting in bleeding; this possibility could be checked by obtaining a medical history.

**47** **The answer is C** *Obstetrics and Gynecology*

Vaginal bleeding in a postmenopausal woman must be assumed to be endometrial carcinoma (choice **C**) until proven otherwise. A complete workup will require endometrial biopsy and hysteroscopy. The presence of a normal-sized uterus on pelvic examination cannot rule out endometrial cancer that is confined to the endometrium. The most likely cause of endometrial carcinoma is long periods of unopposed estrogen. This patient has many risk factors that include never being pregnant (with 9 months of high progesterone levels), absence of oral contraceptive use (which provides regular progestin effects that stabilize the endometrium), and obesity (with peripheral adipose cell conversion of adrenal androgens to estrogens).

**48** **The answer is A** *Obstetrics and Gynecology*

This scenario displays the classic triad of ectopic pregnancy (choice **A**): vaginal bleeding, unilateral lower abdominal pelvic pain, and amenorrhea. If this triad is accompanied by hypotension and tachycardia, the diagnosis would be ruptured ectopic pregnancy with hemoperitoneum, and the management would be emergency laparotomy to stop the bleeding. With stable vital signs, this case is suggestive of unruptured ectopic pregnancy. The diagnosis is confirmed by failure to see an intrauterine gestational sac with transvaginal sonography, plus the presence of a quantitative serum β-human chorionic gonadotropin (β-hCG) titer above 1,500 mIU. (A gestational sac from a normal intrauterine pregnancy would be visible when the serum β-hCG titer is above 1,500 mIU.) The most likely site of the ectopic pregnancy is in the distal oviduct. Management is by parenteral methotrexate if the pregnancy is early (serum β-hCG titer below 6,000 mIU) and by laparoscopy surgery if the pregnancy is advanced (serum β-hCG titer above 6,500 mIU). Follow-up with serial serum β-hCG titers is essential to ensure complete destruction or removal of the ectopic pregnancy tissue.

**49** **The answer is E** *Obstetrics and Gynecology*

This woman shows the classic symptoms of gestational trophoblastic disease and is probably carrying a complete hydatiform mole (choice **E**). In the United States, the frequency of trophoblastic disease is 1 per 1,500 pregnancies. However, in Taiwan and the Philippines, the rate is 1 per 125 pregnancies. The risk is increased with lower economic status and age below 18 or above 40 years. Management involves obtaining a baseline serum β-human chorionic gonadotropin (β-hCG) titer, chest x-ray to rule out lung metastasis, and then evacuating the uterine contents with a suction dilation and curettage. Benign pathologic findings are followed with serial serum β-hCG titers for 1 year to ensure no recurrence of the disease.

**50** **The answer is J** *Obstetrics and Gynecology*

This woman has an advanced case of an ovarian carcinoma (choice **J**). The overall lifetime risk of a woman developing ovarian cancer is 1.6%; if one first-degree relative has had it, the risk is 5%; with two affected first-degree relatives, the risk is 7%; if a woman carries a BRCA2 gene, her lifetime risk is 25%, but a BRCA1 gene raises the risk to 45%. Unfortunately, most early ovarian neoplasms, whether benign or malignant, are essentially asymptomatic. Some are discovered during routine physicals, and many benign ones resolve without treatment. Transvaginal sonography and cancer antigen 125 (CA 125) testing are used to screen very high risk women but are too insensitive to use on the general population. As a consequence of all these factors, some 75% of women are first diagnosed with ovarian cancer at an advanced stage. The overall 5-year survival is 17% with advanced disease with distal spread, 36% with local metastases, and 89% if discovered early.

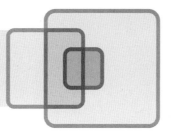

# test 6

# Questions

***Single Best Choice Directions:*** *This section consists of numbered statements or questions followed by a list of potential answers; you are to select the ONE best answer.*

**1** An 87-year-old woman was brought into the emergency department by the paramedics in response to her daughter's 911 call stating that her mother has acute abdominal pain and also is acting in a confused way and feels faint and very weak. The paramedic personnel found her pulse rate to be 120/min and her blood pressure to be 89/45 mm Hg; moreover, she was barely conscious, seemed confused, and complained of feeling nauseous and of having a profound thirst. Her skin appeared pale and felt cold and clammy; in addition, she was hyperventilating. Her daughter volunteered that her mother had been doing fairly well considering her age, but she had chronic lower back pain, as well as osteoarthritis in her knees and other joints. However, she rarely complained and instead treated herself with aspirin. These first responders suspected this lady was undergoing hypovolemic shock. Assuming this is the proper diagnosis, which of the following is the most likely cause?

(A) Esophageal varices
(B) Crohn's disease
(C) A Mallory-Weiss tear
(D) Bleeding hemorrhoids
(E) Peptic ulcer

**2** A 79-year-old man with a long history of systolic hypertension was enrolled in a physical therapy session because of chronic back pain. For a reason that was unknown at the time, it was becoming increasing difficult for him to perform exercises involving raising his legs. As a result, the therapist decided to massage his legs and noted they were distended with edema. Consequently, he made an appointment with his primary care physician, who performed an electrocardiogram (ECG); this was essentially normal. The physician also prescribed a diuretic and several tests, and referred him to a cardiologist. Which one of the following tests will best provide quantitative evidence defining the severity of the problem suspected by the primary care physician?

(A) Atrial natriuretic peptide (ANP)
(B) Brain type (B-type) natriuretic peptide (BNP)
(C) C-type natriuretic peptide
(D) A chest x-ray
(E) A complete blood count (CBC)

**3** Five days ago, a 10-year-old child had an upper respiratory infection and was given symptomatic treatment and an antipyretic (i.e., aspirin for fever). She had seemingly recovered but now presents with fever, protracted vomiting, and lethargy. Physical examination reveals mild hepatomegaly. Serum analysis found total bilirubin, serum transaminases, and serum ammonia to be increased. Cerebrospinal fluid (CSF) was then obtained; it is normal, except for elevated pressure. Which of the following is the most likely diagnosis?

(A) Hepatitis A virus (HAV)
(B) Drug-induced hepatitis
(C) Reye syndrome
(D) Infectious mononucleosis
(E) Gilbert syndrome

**4** During a routine visit to his primary care physician, a 71-year-old man complains about a persistent pain in his back and abdomen that started some weeks ago and has been getting progressively worse. He adds that he "sometimes feels a heart beat around his belly button." In reviewing his history, the physician notes that this patient has smoked since his teens, has hypertension, and although he finally brought his total cholesterol level down below 200 mg/dL by taking a statin, he did have hypercholesterolemia for many years. After determining that his vital signs were stable, the physician has his patient lie on his back on the examination table with his knees slightly flexed and palpates his abdomen; a pulsating mass near the midline between the xiphoid process umbilicus is felt. Which of the following tests is best to conduct next?

(A) A computed tomographic (CT) scan
(B) Abdominal radiography
(C) A magnetic resonance imaging (MRI) study
(D) Abdominal ultrasonography
(E) An upper gastrointestinal series

**5** A 26-day-old infant is brought to the emergency department with a temperature of 39.0°C (102.2°F). The mother is a 25-year-old gravida 2, para 2 who had good prenatal care. Samples of the cerebrospinal fluid (CSF), blood, and urine are sent for culture and analysis. In addition, prophylactic antibiotics are started. It is of paramount importance that the antibiotic treatment provides protection against which of the following pathogens?

(A) *Escherichia coli, Streptococcus pneumoniae,* and *Listeria monocytogenes*
(B) *Streptococcus pneumoniae, Neisseria meningitides,* and *Listeria monocytogenes*
(C) *Streptococcus agalactiae, Escherichia coli,* and *Listeria monocytogenes*
(D) *Streptococcus agalactiae, Escherichia coli,* and *Neisseria meningitides*
(E) *Neisseria meningitides, Streptococcus pneumoniae,* and *Streptococcus agalactiae*

**6** A 5 ft 2 in (1.57 m), 31-year-old woman who weighs 186 pounds (84.4 kg) (body mass index [BMI] = 34 kg/m²) complains to her physician that she has been trying to get pregnant for the past 5 years, and while she has stopped having periods and has gained a lot of weight, it is all fat, no baby. Examination shows no other major physical disorder except hirsutism. Ultrasonography of the ovaries reveals bilaterally enlarged ovaries with subcortical cysts. Which of the following laboratory findings will most likely also be found?

(A) Decreased serum estrone
(B) Increased dehydroepiandrosterone (DHEA) sulfate
(C) Increased follicle-stimulating hormone (FSH)
(D) Increased luteinizing hormone (LH)
(E) Increased serum prolactin

**7** Ten years ago, a 79-year-old female with a 25-year history of type 2 diabetes was diagnosed with diabetic nephropathy. At this time, she is overweight but not obese and she smokes about three packs of cigarettes per week. Despite being diagnosed with diabetic nephropathy, she had not stopped smoking and in general had not tightly controlled her blood glucose levels; consequently, her renal function has steadily deteriorated and her physician now believes she has end-stage renal disease (ESRD). He arranges for her to undergo hemodialysis. Before undergoing hemodialysis, it was also recommended that she have an operation. Which one of the following choices describes the surgical procedure most likely recommended?

(A) A renal biopsy
(B) Insertion of a special, soft catheter through a small slit made adjacent to the naval under local anesthesia
(C) Performing open surgery and inserting a catheter under general anesthetic
(D) Formation of an arteriovenous (AV) fistula
(E) Removal of a renal stone

**8** A 48-year-old patient presents to the emergency room with a history of tiredness, vomiting, and abdominal pain. He has a long history of hypertension, diabetes mellitus, and hyperlipidemia, and during this past year, he developed end-stage renal disease. He admits to being depressed of late and has not kept his appointment with the nephrologist for renal dialysis, which he used to go to three times a week. The patient is on medications for hypertension, diabetes, and hyperlipidemia, in addition to medications for renal failure. Which of the following is the initial medication that should be administered to reverse the clinical condition reflected by the accompanying electrocardiogram pattern?

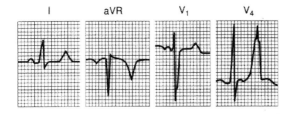

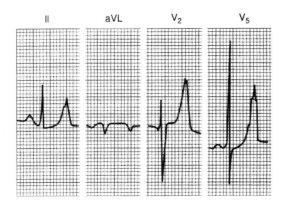

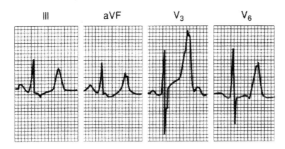

(A) Sodium bicarbonate
(B) Furosemide
(C) Calcium gluconate
(D) Glucose plus insulin
(E) Cation-exchange resin

**9** A 40-year-old man presents to a physician complaining of erectile dysfunction. In taking a history, it is determined that he started drinking alcohol at the age of 14 years and has continued since. Presently, he starts his day by having a beer or two with his breakfast, and he carries a flask of whiskey with him to help him get thorough the day. In the evening, he often polishes off a pint of whiskey before going to bed. However, he also states that he has a "hollow leg," and the alcohol doesn't affect his functioning in any way. Physical examination reveals a distended abdomen and dependent pitting edema. He also has numerous radially oriented vessels around a central

core on his face, neck, and upper trunk. Which additional physical finding in this patient has the same pathogenesis as the skin lesion?

(A) Ascites
(B) Asterixis
(C) Caput medusae
(D) Esophageal varices
(E) Gynecomastia

**10** During her visit to a primary care physician, a 39-year-old woman relates that she has recently had bouts of hoarseness often associated with difficulty in swallowing and breathing. Upon taking a history, the physician also determines that she immigrated with her parents from the Ukraine in 1988 at the age of 17 years, married a 40-year-old American citizen a year ago, and gave birth to her first child 8 months ago. Upon examination, the physician discovers a firm nodule near her Adam's apple. The next step in obtaining a diagnosis is which of the following?

(A) Analyzing the results of an ultrasound scan
(B) Doing a fine needle aspiration biopsy
(C) A thyroid nuclear scan using $^{123}$I
(D) Determining the serum thyroid level
(E) A formal surgical biopsy

**11** A married couple who are second cousins and who recently immigrated from Turkey now live in Santa Monica, California, had a child who is now almost 3 months old. When the child was tested and then retested for possible phenylketonuria (PKU), the values obtained for serum phenylalanine were 11 mg/dL (0.665 mM) and 14 mg/dL (0.847 mM) (for interpretation, see the table below). Upon taking a history, it was revealed that the father had a paternal uncle who died in infancy. Although he lacked precise information about this uncle, he did recall relatives talking about the fact he had reddish colored hair, which caused gossip among his maiden aunts on his mother's side of the family regarding the child's true paternity. In addition to recommending a special diet for the infant, the pediatrician also prescribed a drug. Which of the following choices most likely represents the drug prescribed?

(A) Rosiglitazone
(B) Infliximab
(C) Sapropterin
(D) 5-Hydroxyindoleacetic acid
(E) Amlodipine

**Relationship Between Serum Phenylalanine Concentration and Diagnostic Categorization**

| Categorization | Normal | Benign HSPA[a] | Variant HSPA[a] | Classic PKU[a] |
|---|---|---|---|---|
| Phenylalanine concentration | <1 mg/dL (0.061 mM) | ~4–10 mg/dL (0.242–0.605 mM) | ~10–20 mg/dL (0.605–1.21 mM) | ≥20 mg/dL (1.21 mM) |

[a]PKU, phenylketonuria; HSPA, hyper serum phenylalanine values.

**12** A 56-year-old alcoholic man with chronic pancreatitis has recurrent attacks of abdominal pain that radiates into his back. The pain is controlled with medical therapy. He has lost 30 lb (13.6 kg) in the past 3 months because of chronic diarrhea. Examination of the abdomen reveals no masses. Computerized tomography (CT) of the pancreas reveals multiple calcifications but no mass lesions. The serum glucose value is normal. A qualitative stool test for fat is positive. Antigliadin antibodies are not present. Which of the following would be the most appropriate treatment?

(A) Total pancreatectomy
(B) Broad-spectrum antibiotic therapy
(C) Gluten-free diet
(D) Oral pancreatic enzymes before, during, and after meals
(E) Administration of lactulose

**13** A 23-year-old male prelaw student presents to the ER with the complaint of an itch and rash in his genital region. In providing a history, he states that the itching is worse at night, making avoidance of scratching almost impossible. He adds that the morning after his first night of discomfort, he noted a few small red blisters and bumps on his penis and while trying to treat the condition he bathed and applied hand lotion. The next night, the itching was even more intense, and in the morning, he noted the head of his penis was fully involved and the rash had spread to the surrounding genital area. This induced him to seek medical help. The attending physician asks if the student had had sex within the past 4–8 weeks? The student tells him that he did have sex with a young woman he met at a bar about a month ago; however, he felt he was protected since he wore a condom. The attending physician replies, "I am 99% sure I know what ails you, and I am going to write a prescription. If I am correct and you follow the directions, your condition should clear up within a few days. If it doesn't, let me know; otherwise, there should be no problem. I would also like to talk to the young lady if that is possible." Which of the following choices most likely describes the prescription given?

(A) Topical permethrin 5%
(B) Oral azithromycin
(C) Oral ivermectin
(D) Topical lindane (γ-benzene hexachloride) 1%
(E) Parental penicillin G

**14** A 36-year-old woman complains of severe episodes of headache, tremulousness, palpitations, and anxiety. The patient has noted a change in her voice, and she has difficulty swallowing solids. On physical examination, there is a palpable, nontender swelling in front of her neck that moves with deglutition. No cervical lymphadenopathy is noted. Laboratory studies show serum hypercalcemia. An x-ray film of the cervical region reveals irregular calcification in the mass, while magnetic resonance imaging (MRI) of the abdomen confirms the presence of bilateral adrenal lesions. Which of the following would be the best screening test for the thyroid mass in this patient?

(A) An iodine-123 ($^{123}$I) scan
(B) Measurement of the serum thyroid-stimulating hormone (TSH) level
(C) Measurement of the serum thyroxine ($T_4$) level
(D) Measurement of the serum calcitonin level
(E) Measurement of the serum parathormone level

**15** A 35-year old woman was taking a shower while vacationing in Hawaii. While applying soap onto her body, she felt a lump in her left breast. She was alarmed, as she had never felt the lump before, and it seemed to have crept up on her without causing any pain or discomfort. The patient was nulliparous, had a healthy lifestyle, and exercised regularly. She had no medical illness, did not smoke, and imbibed alcohol sparingly. Physical examination revealed a healthy slim woman who was rather anxious. Apart from a moderate tachycardia brought on by anxiety, her vital signs were normal. The left breast revealed an indrawn nipple. However, no nipple discharge was noted. A nontender hard lump that was immobile and measured approximately 2 × 3 cm was felt in the left breast. Examination of the axilla revealed no palpable lymph nodes. Examination of the right breast and axilla yielded normal findings. Examination of the cardiovascular and respiratory systems also yielded normal findings. Abdominal examination was unremarkable. The most likely location where the lump was discovered would be:

(A) Lower inner quadrant of the breast
(B) Upper inner quadrant of the breast
(C) Lower outer quadrant of the breast
(D) Upper outer quadrant of the breast
(E) Subjacent to the areola

**16** For approximately the past two decades, a 62-year-old man had been a successful office manager at a new car dealership; for most of this time, he had his first alcoholic drink of the day upon arising and one or two more before arriving at work, then easily finishing off another pint of bourbon after leaving work and before going to bed. He felt alcoholic drinks had little effect on his ability to function and bragged about having a "hollow leg." Until recently, he had never had anything to drink while at work, and despite his extreme drinking habits, his work had not suffered. Lately, however, he has had an irresistible urge to indulge in a drink or two or more, even during the workday, and he began to exhibit symptoms of impaired performance. Moreover, he had been caught telling untruths to cover up shortcomings in his performance. Consequently, the owner of the dealership threatened to fire him unless he admitted himself into an alcohol and drug rehabilitation center. As part of his admission to such a center, he underwent a thorough physical examination during which an abnormality present in most heavy drinkers—one that may be reversed by abstinence—was uncovered. This abnormality most likely was which one of the following?

(A) Alcoholic hepatitis
(B) Liver cirrhosis
(C) Portal hypertension
(D) An increase in the serum alanine aminotransferase (ALT) activity greater than an increase in the serum aspartate aminotransferase (AST) activity
(E) Wernicke disease (Wernicke's encephalopathy)
(F) Korsakoff psychosis (Korsakoff syndrome)
(G) Fatty liver

**17** A 30-year-old man with a history of chronic diarrhea describes his stools as greasy and foul smelling. He recently developed pruritic vesicular lesions involving the elbows. A quantitative stool test for fat shows an increased amount of fat. An oral D-xylose absorption test reveals decreased reabsorption of xylose into the blood. Which of the following tests would be most useful in identifying the cause of the diarrhea?

(A) Antigliadin antibodies
(B) Antinuclear antibodies
(C) Fecal smear for leukocytes
(D) Stool for ova and parasites
(E) Stool osmotic gap

**18** A 65-year old man presents to a primary care physician for his pre-Medicare physical examination. He is 5 feet, 10 inches tall and weighs 225 pounds, making his body mass index (BMI) 32.3; consequently, he is classified as being overweight but not obese. His physical appearance shows that he has a belly. In addition, the following laboratory data were obtained: fasting blood glucose value 115 mg/dL; blood pressure 180/95 mm Hg; total cholesterol 275 mg/dL, low-density lipoprotein 155 mg/dL, and high-density lipoprotein 25 mg/dL. The examining physician concluded that this man has metabolic syndrome and is likely to be prediabetic. Consequently, he subjected his patient to an oral glucose tolerance test by measuring the patient's fasting serum level, giving him a standard glucose drink, and then determining his blood glucose 2 hours later; the 2-hour value was 175 mg/dL, resulting in a diagnosis of prediabetes. He informed his patient that clinical studies have shown that the best way to reverse such a prediabetic state is by choosing to undergo a lifestyle change that includes eating a carefully controlled diet and exercising regularly; however, since many patients quickly fall away from such a regime, he also prescribed a drug that had been shown help prevent progression to full-blown diabetes when given to prediabetic patients. Moreover, this drug will not cause hypoglycemia, promote weight gain, or increase the risk of heart failure. Which one of the following drugs did the physician choose?

(A) Sitagliptin phosphate
(B) Glyburide
(C) Metformin
(D) Rosiglitazone
(E) Nateglinide

**19** A 19-year-old Caucasian woman appears at a walk-in clinic complaining of weakness and general malaise. In presenting her history, she informs the physician that, over the past month, these symptoms have grown progressively worse and that she lost 20 lb (9 kg) during this period and had no appetite. In addition, she states that she has pains in her wrist and finger joints, a stomach ache, and a funny rash on her cheeks that causes her a great deal of embarrassment (illustrated below). Upon examination, the physician notes her vital signs are as follows: temperature, 40°C (100°F); blood pressure, 135/70 mm Hg; pulse, 76/min. Which of the following pairs of antibody tests would be the most specific for diagnosing this patient's disease?

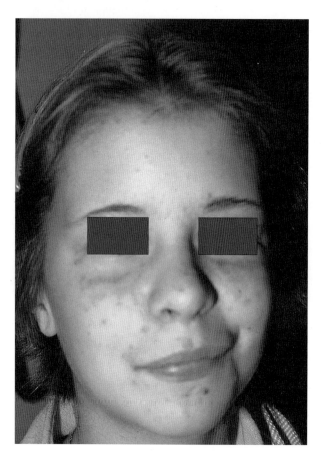

(A) Anti-SSA (Ro) and semi-Sm (Smith)
(B) Antinuclear and anti-ds (double-stranded) DNA
(C) Anti-SSB (La) and anti-ds DNA
(D) Anticentromere and antiribonucleoprotein
(E) Lupus anticoagulant test
(F) Antihistone antibody test

**20** The son of a 79-year-old woman whose husband died more than 6 months ago after 60 years of marriage consults a physician about his mother's current behavior. She had her husband's body cremated and keeps the urn in their bedroom, spending what the son perceives as an inordinate time there talking to his ashes. She also has ceased socializing with her friends and in fact doesn't get dressed or sometimes even get up out of bed. Which of the following behaviors would the physician most likely consider normal after 6 months of bereavement?

(A) Brief periods of longing for her husband
(B) Feelings of worthlessness
(C) A suicide attempt
(D) Inability to work
(E) Despair

**21** A 21-year-old soldier returns from a 15-month overseas tour of duty during which time he participated in close-quarter and bloody combat. Since returning home 3 months ago, his parents note that he stays in his room all day and does not return calls from friends. They find him awake in the kitchen at night, looking anxious and sweaty. He says he can't sleep because he keeps thinking about his war experiences. Which of the following might be the medication with which to treat him?

(A) Olanzapine
(B) Sertraline
(C) Eszopiclone
(D) Topiramate
(E) Atomoxetine

**22** A bereaved family just returned from a funeral for their 20-year-old son. In her grief, the mother began to reminisce to her mother. "He was such a healthy baby until he reached his third birthday. Then he stopped running and started walking like a duck. Next, he couldn't stand without climbing up on somebody or something, and by his 11th birthday, we had to get him a motorized wheelchair. Even then he was doing well, finished high school, enrolled in City College, was a member of the chess team, and took an interest in politics. Then he caught what seemed just to be a cold and died." The grandmother replied, "Yes, it is so tragic. I can't understand what happened. Nobody else in the family ever had anything like his disease. Not his sisters, your sisters, or my sisters." Which of the following diseases did this young man have?

(A) Becker muscular dystrophy
(B) Myotonic muscular dystrophy
(C) Facioscapulohumeral muscular dystrophy
(D) Limb girdle muscular dystrophy
(E) Welander distal myopathy
(F) Duchenne muscular dystrophy

**23** A pediatrician performs a physical examination on a newborn he is asked to evaluate. The pertinent findings he notes include severe hypotonia, generalized weakness, and absent tendon stretch reflexes. The baby lies flaccid with little movement, but there appears to be preservation of the extraocular muscles. The patient is also observed to have fasciculations of the tongue, and the nurse informs the pediatrician that the infant has had trouble feeding. Which of the following is the most likely diagnosis?

(A) Myotonic dystrophy
(B) Werdnig-Hoffmann disease
(C) Infant botulism
(D) Infantile myasthenia gravis
(E) Duchenne's muscular dystrophy

**24** The pediatric intern is called to the nursery to examine a small-for-gestational-age newborn. The mother had one prenatal visit during her entire pregnancy. Physical examination is pertinent for hepatosplenomegaly, jaundice, cataracts, and widespread maculopapular lesions of a reddish-blue color. Diagnostic studies are indicative of hepatitis and thrombocytopenia. The mother most likely developed which one of the following diseases during her pregnancy?

(A) Toxoplasmosis
(B) Rubeola
(C) Rubella
(D) Varicella
(E) Syphilis

**25** A 74-year-old widow who lived alone fell at home and hurt her left wrist. She could immediately see that it was broken because of the way it dangled. Consequently, she called 911. The paramedics set her arm in splints and took her to the nearest emergency clinic. While the attending physician treated the fracture, he also took a history. Among the questions he asked was: "Why do you think you fell?" She responded that she became dizzy; she felt the room was spinning while she was standing in one place; consequently, she lost her balance. The physician probed further and subsequently discovered that she had been having similar spells of dizziness intermittently at various times both during the day or night for the past several months. The dizziness could occur while she was lying down, sitting, or standing without her changing her position. He further determined that her left ear often felt full and that she sometimes had a faint but annoying ringing in her ears. She denied ever vomiting during these dizzy spells but did say she often felt nauseated. Her

dizziness was most likely caused by which of the following?

(A) Shy-Drager syndrome
(B) Ménière disease
(C) Essential hypertension
(D) Orthostatic hypotension
(E) Benign positional vertigo

**26** A 55-year-old man presents to the emergency department with massive hematemesis. Physical examination reveals abdominal distention, shifting dullness on percussion of the abdomen, and spider angiomata over the face and upper chest. An emergency endoscopic examination reveals blood rapidly filling the distal esophagus. The hematemesis is most likely due to which of the following?

(A) Pyloric obstruction
(B) Ruptured esophageal varices
(C) Gastric ulcer
(D) Esophageal carcinoma
(E) Duodenal ulcer

**27** An 18-year-old male student who was suffering from bipolar disorder was admitted to a local hospital for treatment. At that time he was manic. Unfortunately, he got into an altercation with another mental patient and, in the scuffle, was bitten on the arm. There was a breach in the skin and treatment for a human bite was initiated. The hospital protocol involved ruling out transmission of human immunodeficiency virus (HIV) and hepatitis C in the perpetrator and the victim. The perpetrator turned out to be HIV negative and hepatitis C antibody (HCVAb) positive. However, careful history from the family suggested that he had never suffered from hepatitis C, and they were surprised that he had tested positive for the disease. The best way to establish if he was really positive for hepatitis C would be to:

(A) Repeat HCVAb test in a week
(B) Repeat HCVAb test after a month
(C) Order a genotype
(D) Order a recombinant immunoblot assay (RIBA) test
(E) Order serial liver enzyme analyses and evaluate for increasing activity levels

**28** A 40-year-old man came to see his primary care doctor as he had been feeling very fatigued of late. He stated that he was tired all the time, had difficulty walking the distance that he could only a month or so ago, and he also noticed some swelling of his feet, usually at the end of the day. Physical examination revealed a medium-built well-nourished man with conjunctival pallor. The sclera appeared mildly icteric. His temperature was 98.6°F (37.0°C), pulse 88/min regular, respirations 18/min, and his blood pressure was 120/86 mm Hg. Oxygen saturation using room air was 90%. His lungs were clear to auscultation, bilaterally; he had a soft murmur in the precordial area without a thrill, and no gallops or rubs were noted. The abdomen was soft to palpation, and he had mild tenderness without guarding or rigidity in the right upper quadrant. No organomegaly was noted, and bowel sounds were present in all four quadrants. A complete blood count revealed a low hematocrit and a corrected reticulocyte count of greater than 3%. Which one of the following changes in serum levels also would most likely occur?

(A) Conjugated bilirubin, haptoglobin, and lactic acid dehydrogenase levels would all be elevated

(B) Conjugated bilirubin would be elevated; haptoglobin and lactic acid dehydrogenase levels would be decreased

(C) Unconjugated bilirubin and haptoglobin levels would decrease; the lactic acid dehydrogenase level would increase

(D) Unconjugated bilirubin, haptoglobin, and lactic acid dehydrogenase levels would all increase

(E) Only the haptoglobin level would increase

**29** A 28-year-old woman presents to her doctor's office with a painless lump in the neck. She has a 10-year history of smoking cigarettes, and consumes three to four cigarettes per day. Physical examination reveals a nontender, firm, mobile lymph node in the right mid-cervical region. An excision biopsy of the node was carried out, and the specimen revealed well-differentiated, branching structures with blue-staining concretions. Which of the following is the most likely source of this lesion?

(A) Vocal cord
(B) Parotid gland
(C) Thyroid gland
(D) Lung
(E) Breast

**30** A 77-year-old man who prides himself as having been in prime physical health all his life despite seldom seeing a doctor, and who claims the only medication he ever takes is aspirin, suddenly is plagued by severe headaches, vertigo, and a loss of balance that makes standing and walking difficult. Consequently, he has a fall and bumps his head. His worried daughter takes

him to the nearest emergency department, where he is examined. He is found to be a thin man who is relatively muscular for his age. Although still unable to stand or walk without losing his balance, there is no evidence of muscle weakness. He remains fully conscious, is fully cognizant of his surroundings, and can answer questions quickly and lucidly. His heart and lungs are normal, as is an electrocardiogram (ECG). A nonfasting finger stick blood glucose determination reads 152 mg/dL of glucose. His blood pressure remains between 165 and 185 mm Hg systolic over 75–85 mm Hg diastolic. Which of the following is the most likely underlying cause of his problem?

(A) An epidural hemorrhage
(B) Ménière syndrome
(C) Isolated systolic hypertension
(D) A cerebral infarct
(E) A pulmonary thromboembolism

**31** A low-birth-weight infant presents to his pediatrician at 2 months of age. The mother states that the infant has not been eating well. Upon physical examination, the infant is noted to be pale and tachycardic. The lungs are clear to auscultation, and there is no hepatosplenomegaly. A complete blood count shows the hemoglobin level to be 6 g/dL. Which one of the following is the most likely cause of anemia in this infant?

(A) Megaloblastic anemia
(B) Sickle cell anemia
(C) Anemia of prematurity
(D) α-Thalassemia
(E) Homozygous β-thalassemia

**32** A 51-year-old woman presents with an episode of dysphoria, sleep difficulty, psychomotor agitation, and rumination about mistakes she has made in her life. She has delusions of guilt about indirectly causing the deaths of many people. She has a history of two previous episodes with similar symptoms, but no history of unusually elevated mood or increased activity. Between episodes, she is asymptomatic. Which of the following is the most likely diagnosis?

(A) Bipolar II disorder, depressed phase
(B) Dysthymic disorder
(C) Major depressive disorder, recurrent
(D) Schizoaffective disorder, depressive type
(E) Schizophrenia

**33** A child was in her usual state of good health when she first developed a focal seizure while playing with her sister. The mother, a registered nurse, states that the seizure lasted approximately 5 minutes. The 911 Emergency Services were called, and the child arrived postictal to the emergency department approximately 1 hour after the seizure first occurred. On physical examination, her vital signs are stable, but the patient is noted to have weakness and hemiparesis. Remarkably, within 24 hours, the weakness and neurologic deficits disappear. Which of the following is the most likely diagnosis?

(A) Hemiplegia complicating a migraine headache
(B) Spastic hemiplegia
(C) Postviral encephalitis
(D) Todd's paralysis
(E) Infratentorial tumor

**34** A 38-year-old woman, gravida 1, para 0, delivers an appropriate-for-gestational-age infant by spontaneous vaginal delivery in the vertex position. The mother had excellent prenatal care and denies any history of tobacco, alcohol, or drug use. The infant weighs 8 lb 6 oz (3.8 kg). The Apgar score is 8 at 1 minute and 9 at 5 minutes. On physical examination, the infant is noted to have edematous swelling of the soft tissue of the scalp that crosses the midline. Which of the following is the most likely diagnosis?

(A) Cephalohematoma
(B) Subcutaneous fat necrosis
(C) Fracture of the skull
(D) Caput succedaneum
(E) Overriding of the parietal bones

**35** A blue-eyed, Caucasian, 75-year-old man has had gradual loss of vision for the past 5 years. He initially had trouble reading fine print and road signs, and similar distant objects appeared blurred. The vision loss has progressed to the point at which, if he looks directly at a book or an object, he cannot make out what it is. However, he found that he can compensate to a large extent by looking at things using side vision. As a consequence, he can still walk around and even cross a street safely unaided. Which of the following is the most likely cause of his visual loss?

(A) Macular degeneration
(B) Trauma
(C) Cataract surgery
(D) Optic neuritis
(E) Diabetic retinopathy

**36** A 25-year-old man presents to the emergency room with a history of swelling around the left eye, which has become very painful. He states that initially he had noted double vision and that it hurts to move his eye. He was in considerable distress due to pain. The vital signs were as follows: temperature 101°F (38.3°C), pulse 86/min regular, respirations 18/min, blood pressure 128/78 mm Hg and, oxygen saturation 98% on room air. There was considerable swelling around the left eye, which was boggy and tender to touch. Ocular movements were present in all directions but were painful. The pupils were equal and reacting appropriately to light and accommodation, and funduscopy was unremarkable. The most likely cause for this problem is:

(A) Cavernous sinus thrombosis
(B) Corneal ulcer
(C) Sinusitis
(D) Orbital abscess
(E) Ocular trauma

**37** An 82-year-old retired university professor of Scott-Irish ancestry has had gastroesophageal reflux disease (GERD) and hypertension for a number of decades. Lately, he has been having increasing difficulty walking; his gait has become more and more shuffling and hesitant. More recently, he has also complained of excessive fatigue; for example, he might doze off in his chair while eating breakfast. His wife thought this might be because he did not get a good night's sleep—in fact, she complained that she couldn't sleep well either because of his loud snoring. His primary care physician is treating his GERD with omeprazole and is using six different antihypertension drugs (enalapril, labetalol, clonidine, doxazosin mesylate, amlodipine besylate, and hydrochlorothiazide) to control his systolic hypertension, but his systolic pressure remains, at best, in the 140–160 mm Hg range. Frustrated, the physician arranges for his patient to be tested for possible obstructive sleep apnea, which theoretically could cause fatigue and muscle weakness, and contribute to the hypertension. Testing shows that he had an inadequate amount of rapid eye movement (REM) sleep, and his oxygen saturation dropped below 90% on a regular basis. He was provided with a continuous positive airway pressure (CPAP) device, so that he could treat himself at home. However, his systolic blood pressure stubbornly remained above 140 mm Hg, and he continued to walk poorly and doze off during the day.

Looking for some other source for his patient's hypertension and fatigue, the physician ordered a battery of blood tests including a complete blood count (CBC). Which of the following patterns could best explain this patient's symptoms?

(A) Normal hemoglobin levels and a mixture of normal-looking red cells mixed in with some abnormally large erythrocytes, some poikilocytes, a few hypersegmented neutrophils, and a reduced the reticulocyte count
(B) Normal red cells mixed in with a substantial fraction of schistocytes and normal leucocytes and a decrease reticulocyte count
(C) Primarily spherocytic red cells, normal white cells, and a decreased reticulocyte count
(D) Normal red cells mixed in with some sickled cells and a decreased reticulocyte count
(E) A reduced number of normal red cells with normal white cells and a decreased reticulocyte count

**[38]** A 49-year-old man comes to the emergency department complaining that a worm is eating the bone marrow in his "leg bone." He indicates a small scab over his right tibia and insists this is where the worm entered while he was asleep several days ago. There is no previous history of psychiatric hospitalization or substance abuse. Mental status examination reveals an alert, oriented individual whose thought processes are coherent. Which of the following is the most likely diagnosis?

(A) Body dysmorphic disorder
(B) Delusional disorder, somatic type
(C) Hypochondriasis
(D) Schizophrenia
(E) Somatization disorder

**[39]** A 14-year-old previously well patient is diagnosed with clinical sinusitis by his physician. A prescription for antibiotics was made out for the patient and given to his parents to treat this condition. The patient's parents had the prescription filled at the pharmacy. Unfortunately, the teenager, who does not like to take medication, was not always compliant and missed many doses of the antibiotic. Presently, he is being evaluated in the emergency department for fever, confusion, extraocular palsies, and proptosis of the eye. Which of the following is the most likely diagnosis?

(A) Hand-Schüller-Christian disease
(B) Graves disease
(C) Cavernous sinus thrombosis
(D) Acute bacterial conjunctivitis
(E) Temporal lobe abscess

*Directions for Matching Questions (40 through 50): Each set of matching questions is preceded by a list of 4 to 26 lettered options followed by a brief explanation of the required task and then by a series of numbered statements. For each lettered statement, you are to select ONE lettered option that best fulfills the task as it relates to that statement. Remember that each of the listed options might be correctly selected once, more than once, or not at all.*

## Question 40–46

*The following questions relate to the frequency of dosing and duration of action of steroid contraceptives.*

(A) Levonorgestrel intrauterine system
(B) Estrogen-progestin combination pill
(C) Subdermal progestin subdermal implant
(D) Estrogen-progestin vaginal ring
(E) Progestin-only pill
(F) Progestin-only intramuscular injection
(G) Estrogen-progestin transdermal patch
(H) Progestin-only "morning-after" pill

**[40]** Must be taken at the same time every day

**[41]** Has to be taken in two doses 12 hours apart

**[42]** If a dose is missed, it is OK to double up the next day

**[43]** Has to be replaced weekly for 3 weeks a month

**[44]** Effective for only 3 weeks

**[45]** Effective for only 3 months

**[46]** Has to be replaced every 3 years

## Questions 47–50

*Match each drug with the related graph from those below, which illustrate sleep patterns. Graph A represents normal sleep architecture.*

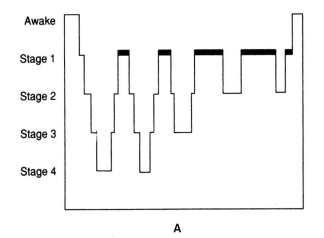

A

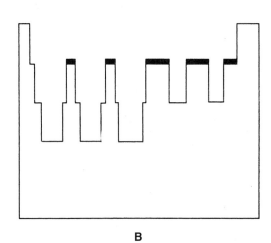

B

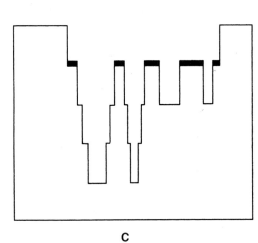

C

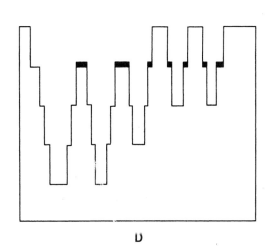

D

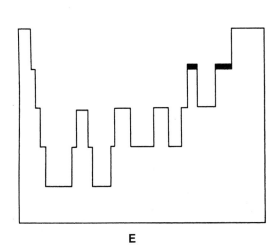

E

**47** Often associated with major depressive disorders

**48** Diazepam

**49** Benzodiazepine rebound

**50** Barbiturates

# *Answer Key*

| | | | | | | | | | |
|---|---|---|---|---|---|---|---|---|---|
| **1** | E | **11** | C | **21** | B | **31** | C | **41** | H |
| **2** | B | **12** | D | **22** | F | **32** | C | **42** | B |
| **3** | C | **13** | A | **23** | B | **33** | D | **43** | G |
| **4** | D | **14** | D | **24** | C | **34** | D | **44** | D |
| **5** | C | **15** | D | **25** | B | **35** | A | **45** | F |
| **6** | D | **16** | G | **26** | B | **36** | C | **46** | C |
| **7** | D | **17** | A | **27** | D | **37** | A | **47** | D |
| **8** | C | **18** | C | **28** | D | **38** | B | **48** | B |
| **9** | E | **19** | B | **29** | C | **39** | C | **49** | C |
| **10** | B | **20** | A | **30** | C | **40** | E | **50** | E |

# Answers and Explanations

### 1 The answer is E   *Surgery*

The stomach and upper duodenum are subject to potential injury from chronic exposure to gastric acid, as well as to other potential toxic agents (most commonly nicotine from smoking, hot liquids, and alcohol) that might be ingested. Normally, the gastric intestinal mucosa provides protection against such toxic agents, but aspirin and other nonsteroidal anti-inflammatory drugs (NSAIDs) damage the mucosa, permitting erosive disease and peptic ulcer to occur (choice **E**). The mode of action by which these drugs do their damage is to inhibit the cyclo-oxygenase (COX) enzymes and consequently impede synthesis of the prostaglandins that normally promote development of a healthy mucosa. The erosion of the mucosa may induce bleeding, which can be severe enough to produce anemia and eventually lead to hemorrhagic shock, as in the case described. This is a fairly common cause of death among persons older than 80 years of age. Studies have also demonstrated that *Helicobacter pylori* infection increases the susceptibility to NSAID-induced damage. Although several studies have shown that aspirin lowers the levels of series 2 prostaglandins, misoprostol, a synthetic $E_1$ prostaglandin analog, is approved by the U.S. Food and Drug Administration for use in protecting the mucosa of patients at high risk of ulceration because of chronic NSAID therapy.

The superficial veins lining the esophagus can become distended, causing esophageal varices in individuals with portal hypertension, which is most commonly associated with cirrhosis of the liver. Esophageal varices are prone to bleeding, but this patient has no symptoms of portal hypertension or cirrhosis (choice **A**). Crohn disease (choice **B**) is an autoimmune inflammatory disease of the gastrointestinal tract that primarily causes abdominal pain, bloody diarrhea, vomiting, and weight loss rather than the symptoms described. Mallory-Weiss tears (choice **C**) occur in the mucosa at the junction of the esophagus and stomach, usually in persons subject to violent chronic vomiting or coughing, but sometimes also in person having an epileptic seizure. Such a tear will cause bleeding, but in the case described, there was no mention of coughing, sneezing, or epilepsy. Bleeding hemorrhoids (choice **D**), as the name indicates, also cause bleeding, which can in atypical instances cause anemia but rarely is severe enough to induce hypovolemic shock.

### 2 The answer is B   *Medicine*

The onset of edema is a possible symptom of congestive heart failure, which in turn may be caused by long-term hypertension and/or arthrosclerosis. This probable diagnosis needs to be confirmed, as must the degree of the problem. Among the tests outlined, this can best be done by determining the level of brain type (B-type) natriuretic peptide (BNP) in the serum (choice **B**). The natriuretic peptides are a family of polypeptides that cause the excretion of sodium into the urine; that is, they promote natriuresis. The different forms of the natriuretic peptides are named by the tissues from which they were first isolated. Even though BNP was first isolated from brain, its medical significance lies in the fact that this peptide is released from the heart's ventricles in response to excess stretching of the ventricular myocytes as often occurs in the stressed heart in congestive heart failure. In addition to stimulating natriuresis, this peptide also decreases systemic vascular resistance, thus causing a decrease in central vascular pressure, inducing and permitting a decrease in cardiac output.

At first, it was thought that measuring the serum level of BNP would provide a quantitative estimate of the degree to which the heart is damaged, but at best it is semiquantitative and conditions other than congestive heart failure may also increase the activity. The most definitive test of heart function and thus the best test to estimate the extent to which the heart is damaged is a stress echocardiogram. However, the measurement of the serum level of the BNP can be done in the doctor's office or at the bedside while an echocardiogram, in particular a stress echocardiogram, takes special equipment that is not always readily available, particularly in a primary care physician's office or in remote areas and Third World countries. In addition to using BNP as a diagnostic aid, a recombinant human BNP, nesiritide, has been approved for use in the acute treatment of decompensated congestive heart failure caused by systolic dysfunction. Unfortunately, it must be administered IV and has a very short half-life.

Atrial natriuretic peptide (ANP) (choice **A**) acts similarly to BNP but is released from the atrium. However, its half-life in the serum is much shorter than that of BNP, which limits its usefulness as a diagnostic tool. C-type natriuretic peptide (choice **C**) is also found in brain and may play a role similar to BNP but its medical value has not yet been established. A chest x-ray (choice **D**) can show an enlarged heart but that in itself is not diagnostic of congestive heart failure nor does it provide even semiquantitative information concerning severity. A complete blood count (CBC) (choice **E**) is irrelevant.

### 3 The answer is C *Pediatrics*

Reye syndrome (choice **C**) is a secondary mitochondrial hepatopathy that, in genetically susceptible individuals, has a very high association with the ingestion of aspirin-containing medicines during influenza-like illnesses or varicella. The number of cases peaked in the 1970s, with a mortality rate of greater than 40%. Because the relationship between aspirin and Reye syndrome was discovered, aspirin is no longer recommended for treatment of children; consequently, the prevalence has since significantly decreased, but unless diagnosed and treated promptly the mortality rate has not changed. Reye syndrome has a biphasic course. It usually presents in a previously healthy child who had an upper respiratory infection or varicella. After the child seems to have recovered, the symptoms of vomiting, lethargy, and confusion appears and progress quickly. The patient may also be combative. Liver enzymes and the serum ammonia level are elevated. Treatment requires early recognition and control of increased intracranial pressure. Prognosis depends on duration of disordered cerebral function. Early diagnosis and treatment increases the likelihood for recovery to 90%.

Hepatitis A virus (HAV) (choice **A**) is an RNA-containing virus. It is a member of the Picornaviridae family and is spread predominantly by the fecal–oral route. In the United States, there is increased risk of infection with HAV in day care centers, in contacts of children who attend day care centers, and in the homosexual population. The diagnosis of HAV infection should be considered when a history of jaundice exists in the patient's contacts, or if the patient or his or her family has traveled to an endemic area. The acute infection is diagnosed by the presence of immunoglobulin M (IgM) anti-HAV. Although elevation may be found in the bilirubin and serum transaminase levels, they do not help to differentiate the cause. Drug-induced hepatitis (choice **B**) is not the correct answer, because the patient in this scenario has a history of aspirin usage, and aspirin is excreted by the kidney. Infectious mononucleosis (choice **D**) is a clinical syndrome caused by the Epstein-Barr virus (EBV). Clinical symptoms in children are often mild, but patients may have fatigue, fever, sore throat, and generalized lymphadenopathy. Splenomegaly may be prominent, causing left upper quadrant abdominal tenderness. Hepatomegaly may be present in a small number of patients. Symptomatic hepatitis or jaundice is uncommon. A mononuclear lymphocytosis with atypical-appearing lymphocytes is associated with infectious mononucleosis. Gilbert syndrome (choice **E**) is an inherited, benign, unconjugated hyperbilirubinemia that is transmitted as an autosomal dominant disease. The hyperbilirubinemia is mild, and the bilirubin level may fluctuate. Jaundice is intermittent and may be noted on routine physical examination. Results of liver biopsy and other liver function tests are normal.

### 4 The answer is D *Medicine*

The described symptoms suggest an expanding abdominal aortic aneurysm, and the patient has the primary risk factors, namely: age, a long history of smoking, hypertension, and probable arthrosclerosis (high cholesterol for years). In addition, the finding of a palpable pulsatile mass in the abdomen is almost diagnostic. The most appropriate next test is abdominal ultrasonography (choice **D**), which indeed has been recommended by the U.S. Preventative Task Force (USPSTF) as a screening test for all men over 65 years old who have smoked for years, particularly if the risk has been compounded by hypertension or arthrosclerosis or if a first-degree relative has had an aneurysm. Ultrasonography is available at most hospitals, is relatively inexpensive, does not require exposure to radiation, reveals details of the aortic wall, and permits accurate measurement of shape and size of the aneurysm. An aneurism larger than 5.5 cm (2.14 in) is in danger of rupture and is usually surgically repaired as soon as possible, either by open surgery or more recently by less invasive endo-surgery procedures. One less than 3 cm (1.12 in) is generally committed to watchful waiting. Whether surgery should be done on aneurysms of intermediate size depends upon the assessment of risk of rupture, including size, evidence of recent expansion, family history, and the patient's general health. The goal is to avoid rupture because once ruptured, there is a 90% fatality rate. Approximately 9,000–15,000 Americans are estimated to die from an abdominal aortic aneurysm annually.

A computed tomographic (CT) scan (choice **A**), abdominal radiography (choice **B**), or a magnetic resonance imaging (MRI) study (choice **C**) all can be used to diagnose an aneurism but are either more expensive, are less convenient, or provide less information and are therefore no longer recommended as first-choice diagnostic modalities. An upper gastrointestinal series (choice **E**) would be inappropriate.

### 5 The answer is C *Pediatrics*

The infectious disease that the physician would be most concerned about is meningitis. The treatment must be designed to prevent or, if already fulminating, cure this disease. *Streptococcus agalactiae* (group B streptococcus) is a common inhabitant of the maternal genitourinary tract. It is acquired by newborns via vertical transmission, and it is the most common cause of neonatal meningitis, followed by *Escherichia coli* and *Listeria monocytogenes*. Early-onset disease is associated with sepsis; late onset is associated with meningitis. Consequently, *S. agalactiae*, *E. coli*, and *L. monocytogenes* (choice **C**) is the correct answer.

*Streptococcus pneumoniae* (part of choice **A**, **B**, and **E**) and *Neisseria meningitidis* (part of choice **B**, **D**, and **E**) are more commonly seen in older age groups.

### 6 The answer is D *Medicine*

The patient has polycystic ovary syndrome (PCOS), which affects 4%–6% of reproductive-age women. In this disorder, patients have a steady production of estrogen rather than the normal fluctuating rate that occurs during the menstrual cycle. Commonly, this excess estrogen is due to conversion of ovarian and adrenal androgens to estrogen in the body fat, although there also may be an underlying endocrine disorder. The excess synthesis of estrogen causes a steady rate of luteinizing hormone (LH) production, leading to a relative increase (choice **D**); this causes excessive stimulation of the ovaries with increased synthesis of 17-ketosteroids (dehydroepiandrosterone [DHEA] and androstenedione) and testosterone. An increase in these androgen compounds causes hirsutism (excess hair in normal hair-bearing areas). Thus, in obese patients, a vicious circle is established; this androgen excess is converted to still more estrogen by the aromatase in the excess number of adipose cells (e.g., androstenedione is converted to estrone and testosterone is converted to estradiol). An increase in estrogen has a negative feedback on the release of follicle-stimulating hormone (FSH) and a positive feedback on the release of LH; therefore, LH is still further increased and FSH is decreased (not increased [choice **C**]). Decreased FSH causes degeneration of the ovarian follicles, which results in the formation of subcortical cysts. In PCOS, the LH-to-FSH ratio usually exceeds 2:1, and 80% of cases present with amenorrhea or abnormal menstruation, 50% with hirsutism, 40% with obesity, and 20% with virilization. In addition, these patients are generally infertile (although they may ovulate on occasion); show insulin resistance, which puts them at risk for type 2 diabetes; and are at risk for endometrial and breast cancer because of the unopposed action of estrogen. In obese patients, weight loss will often break the vicious circle and restore normal ovulatory function.

Serum estrone is increased in PCOS (not decreased [choice **A**]) because of increased conversion of androstenedione to estrone by aromatase in the adipose cells. Dehydroepiandrosterone (DHEA) sulfate (choice **B**) is a 17-ketosteroid that is primarily synthesized in the adrenal cortex (95%) and is not increased in PCOS. However, there is an increase in DHEA in PCOS, because the nonsulfated form is synthesized in the ovaries. This explains why an increase in DHEA sulfate is used as a marker for hirsutism caused by adrenal cortical hyperfunction (e.g., Cushing syndrome). Prolactin levels (choice **E**) are not altered in PCOS.

### 7 The answer is D *Surgery*

To preform hemodialysis, it is necessary to surgically form an arteriovenous (AV) fistula (choice **D**). This is accomplished by creating an opening in which the artery is sewn onto a vein; this is usually is done in an arm. In hemodialysis, blood is withdrawn from an artery and returned via a vein. However, veins are typically too small to accommodate the amount of fluid returned and therefore must be enlarged. In an AV fistula, the arterial blood pressure eventually enlarges the vein, thus permitting insertion of a large needle or cannula. Nonsurgical AV fistulas also do occur. These may be congenital or acquired, caused by trauma or by erosion of an arterial aneurism into an adjacent vein. Congenital AV fistulas are uncommon but acquired AV fistulas can be caused by any injury that damages an artery and a vein that lie next to each other. Most often the injury is a piercing wound caused by a knife or a bullet. Symptoms of the fistula may show up immediately or after several hours. If the fistula is superficial, escaping blood often causes swelling. However, in a large, spontaneously acquired AV fistula, the flow of blood under pressure into the venous system stretches the veins and more blood flows through the venous system than through the arterial system. This causes the blood pressure to fall, making the heart pump more vigorously and potentially resulting in high output failure.

A renal biopsy (choice **A**) is performed by inserting a long needle into a kidney from the back, usually in a lightly sedated individual. Most commonly, three samples are obtained and evaluated for possible pathologies. Such biopsies are sometimes recommended to help evaluate hematuria, proteinuria, and/or elevated creatinine or blood urea nitrogen (BUN) levels. Insertion of a catheter, whether by making a small incision in the abdomen (choice **B**) or by performing more invasive surgery (choice **C**), are operations used to perform peritoneal dialysis in which a hypertonic dialysis fluid is added into the patient's peritoneal cavity via an implanted catheter. The hypertonicity of the dialysis solution draws low-molecular-weight molecules (e.g., water, salts, and waste products) from the blood system into the peritoneum, which soon becomes saturated; consequently, the old solution must be drained and replaced by fresh dialysis solution.

Removal of a renal stone (choice **E**) is not likely to play a role in treatment of chronic renal failure, although it may play a role in treatment of postrenal acute kidney failure.

### 8 The answer is C *Medicine*

The electrocardiogram (ECG) pattern shown indicates that this patient has hyperkalemia. It reveals tall, slender, tented T waves in leads I, II, aVF, and $V_2$ through $V_6$. Other findings suggesting hyperkalemia include a widened QRS complex and even biphasic QRS-T complexes. Although hyperkalemia produces these characteristic patterns, the ECG is not a sensitive indicator of hyperkalemia, as almost 50% of patients with serum potassium levels above 6.5 mEq/L do not show any changes in the ECG pattern. This is because atrial cells are more sensitive than ventricular cells to elevated levels of potassium, permitting normal conduction even if atrial depolarization is inhibited; as a result, a junctional rhythm can result. To avoid dangerous arrhythmias and asystole, hyperkalemia above 6.5 mEq/L warrants immediate correction. In this case, hyperkalemia also is suspected clinically because the patient has end-stage renal disease, has not been undergoing dialysis, and has a history of tiredness, vomiting, and abdominal pain. Hyperkalemia could, in addition, have caused motor paralysis. Calcium gluconate 10% (choice **C**) or 5% calcium chloride is the initial drug of choice. Approximately 5–30 mL of either administered intravenously provides calcium ion, which acts within minutes to antagonize cardiac conduction abnormalities; the effect lasts approximately an hour. In patients who are on digoxin, one must ensure that they do not have digoxin toxicity; if that were the case, calcium would only increase its toxic effects on the myocardium.

Although administering calcium has a rapid effect, it does not promote the shift of potassium into the cells; consequently, its effect is transitory. To secure a more permanent effect, one usually follows up with insulin and glucose (choice **D**). This drives potassium into the cells, thereby lowering serum potassium levels. Regular insulin (5–10 units) combined with 25 g of 50% glucose is administered intravenously. Insulin takes about 15 minutes to an hour to act, and the action lasts anywhere from 4 to 6 hours. Use of sodium bicarbonate (choice **A**) is an alternative to insulin plus glucose. It creates a metabolic alkalosis, causing potassium ion to enter the cells in exchange for hydrogen ions. One or two ampules of sodium bicarbonate (approximately 44 mEq each) can be administered intravenously. Its effects begin in approximately 15–30 minutes and last anywhere from 1 to 2 hours. Thus, it is not as long lasting as insulin. The use of furosemide (choice **B**) is inappropriate in an emergency situation because it takes anywhere from 30 minutes to 2 hours to lower potassium levels, and one may very well not have the luxury of time. It is a loop diuretic that exchanges sodium for potassium, expelling the latter in the urine. Like loop diuretics, sodium polystyrene sulfonate in 20% sorbitol, a cation-exchange resin (choice **E**), may be used in nonemergency situations; 15–30 mL is administered orally or rectally. Potassium ions bind to the resin, lowering serum potassium levels. Due to the mode of administration, it takes much longer to act; its action lasts approximately 3 hours.

### 9 The answer is E *Medicine*

The patient has cirrhosis of the liver (history of alcohol abuse, ascites, and dependent pitting edema). The skin lesions are spider angiomas, which have a central spiral arteriole with a group of small vessels radiating from the arteriole. Spider angiomas are associated with hyperestrinism, which is a complication of cirrhosis. In cirrhosis, the dysfunctional liver is unable to metabolize estrogen, which produces hyperestrinism. Hyperestrinism in men causes gynecomastia (development of breast tissue in males; choice **E**) and female secondary sex characteristics (palmar erythema, soft skin, and female hair distribution).

Although the distended abdomen is due to ascites, the question asks for additional symptoms having the same pathogenesis as the skin lesion. The factors that contribute to the development of ascites (choice **A**) include portal hypertension (increase in hydrostatic pressure), hypoalbuminemia (decrease in oncotic pressure), secondary aldosteronism (salt retention), and increased lymphatic drainage into the peritoneal cavity. Asterixis (choice **B**), or flapping tremor, refers to the inability to sustain posture. It is a sign of hepatic encephalopathy, which is caused by an increase in ammonia and false neurotransmitters (e.g., γ-aminobenzoic acid).

Caput medusae (choice **C**) are dilated periumbilical veins that are associated with increased venous pressure caused by portal hypertension. Esophageal varices (choice **D**) are dilated left gastric coronary veins, which normally drain the distal esophagus and proximal stomach and empty into the portal vein. An increase in portal vein pressure leads to dilation of the gastric veins (varices), which commonly rupture.

## 10 The answer is B *Surgery*

Although several procedures provide clues concerning whether a thyroid nodule is benign or cancerous, a definitive answer requires a biopsy and histological analysis by a pathologist; thyroid fine needle aspiration (FNA) biopsy (choice **B**) is a nonsurgical method that usually can definitely differentiate between benign and malignant nodules. Consequently, it commonly is the first and only test used to evaluate the potential malignancy of a nodule. Performing a successful fine needle aspiration biopsy early in the workup of a nodule typically provides a rapid and unambiguous diagnosis, thus reducing cost and saving the patient anxiety. That she immigrated from the Ukraine is relevant because of the accident at Chernobyl.

Analyzing the results of an ultrasound scan (choice **A**) and/or a thyroid nuclear scan using $^{123}$I (choice **C**) are generally reserved for the approximately 5% of fine needle aspiration biopsies that are reported to be nondiagnostic or the approximately 10% of results categorized as suspicious. A report of nondiagnostic biopsy generally results from an inability to obtain a sufficient number of thyroid cells using FNA, whereas about 75% of the nodules identified as suspicious are benign follicular adenomas that cannot be distinguished from follicular or Hürthle cell cancers. A solid or complex ultrasound scan result implies that the nodule is malignant, and a cold area after a thyroid scan (i.e., where $^{123}$I is not taken up) indicates possible malignancy since about 95% of hot nodules are benign. Consequently, a cold nodule found suspicious by FNA is generally removed surgically. In addition to being an aid in diagnosis, an ultrasound scan is also carried out to help in the placement of the needle while performing FNA.

Determining the serum thyroid level (choice **D**) is generally an early test done to obtain an overview of the patient's thyroid function, but it is not able to diagnose the potential malignancy of a nodule. A formal surgical biopsy (choice **E**) is reserved for the diagnosis of nodules labeled nondiagnosable or suspicious after FNA.

## 11 The answer is C *Medicine*

Phenylketonuria (PKU) is an autosomal recessive disease causing toxic amounts of phenylalanine (Phe) and some of its metabolic products to accumulate in the blood; it affects about 1 newborn in every 15,000 births. Presently, all U.S. states and territories require measurement of Phe within a few days after birth; consequently, essentially all cases of classic PKU are diagnosed and treated by putting the affected infants on a low Phe diet. This diet alleviates symptoms, but does not cure the condition; hence, affected individuals must remain on this very limited diet throughout their lifetimes. In addition to these classic cases of PKU that respond well to a low Phe diet, there is a group of infants who suffer from "malignant" PKU, so called because the usual low-Phe diets do not adequately relieve symptoms. As illustrated in the Variant HSPA group in the table accompanying this question, most of these infants have higher than normal levels of Phe but lower levels than required for a clear diagnosis of PKU. While classic PKU is caused by low Phe-hydroxylase activity due to mutations in the enzyme itself, most variant cases of hyperphenylalaninemia are due to low levels of tetrahydrobiopterin (BH4), a cofactor required by this enzyme. In December 2007, the U.S. FDA approved sapropterin (choice **C**), a synthetic BH4 analog for treatment of such cases. In the United States, these variant cases only represent 1.5%–2% of all cases of hyperphenylalaninemia, but the rate is considerably higher among certain ethic groups, including the Taiwanese (2%–30% reported to fall into the variant range), Saudi Arabians (66% reported to be variant cases), and Turks, who have a well-documented rate of 15% of all hyperphenylalaninemia cases falling into the variant range.

Since one of the symptoms associated with PKU is hypopigmentation, which among other things causes a reddish tint to hair, it seems likely that the father's uncle died because of PKU, and since Turkey has such a high prevalence of the variant variety, there is a good chance he had the variant variety. Moreover, since the reference couple was closely related, it is possible that the child in question inherited a copy of this aberrant gene from each parent. Moreover, the analytical data clearly show that this child falls into the "variant" category. It follows that he would be a likely candidate for treatment with sapropterin (choice **C**). Cases of hyperphenylalaninemia due to BH4 deficiency do not respond to a low-Phe diet as well as do infants with classic PKU because BH4 is a required cofactor for several other enzymes, including tyrosine-3-hydroxylase, needed to convert tyrosine to L-dopa; tryptophan-5-hydroxylase, which converts tryptophan to 5-hydroxythryptophan and which is further metabolized to serotonin; and also for nitric oxide synthase, required to form nitric oxide.

Rosiglitazone (choice **A**) is a drug used to treat type 2 diabetes. It functions by increasing the sensitivity of muscle cells to insulin. However, it has been reported to also increase the risk of heart failure and of hip and spine fractures. Infliximab (choice **B**) is an antitumor necrosis factor (TNF)α drug. TNFα is a cytokine that induces and maintains inflammation. Consequently, this drug is used to treat rheumatoid and psoric arthritis, psoriasis, Crohn disease, ankylosing spondylitis, sarcosis, and ulcerative colitis. 5-Hydroxyindoleacetic acid (choice **D**) is not a drug, but rather an end-product of serotonin metabolism, which is increased in patients having carcinoid syndrome. Amlodipine (choice **E**) is a calcium channel inhibitor used to treat hypertension and/or angina.

### 12 The answer is D *Surgery*

Chronic pancreatitis produces steatorrhea (increased fat in the stool) because the intestine is lipase deficient. Consequently, undigested lipid and fat-soluble vitamins are lost in the stool. Oral pancreatic enzyme preparations (choice **D**) have high lipase activity; thus, administration before, during, and after a meal, will help hydrolyze ingested fats, thereby facilitating their absorption. Concurrent administration of a histamine ($H_2$) antagonist will assist this process by blocking inactivation of the enzyme by acid. In addition, the patient should be on a low-fat diet.

Total pancreatectomy (choice **A**) is a treatment option in chronic pancreatitis if intractable pain is present and is not amenable to medical therapy. However, normally the patient's pain is controlled with medical therapy. A broad-spectrum antibiotic (choice **B**) does not enhance lipid absorption because bacterial overgrowth is not part of the pathophysiology of chronic pancreatitis. Bacterial overgrowth produces bile salt deficiency, which leads to steatorrhea. A gluten-free diet (choice **C**) is the therapy of choice for celiac disease, which is an autoimmune disease that has antibodies directed against the gliadin fraction in gluten. These antibodies are not present in the patient. Lactulose (choice **E**) is a synthetic sugar used to treat constipation and to lower blood ammonia levels resulting from hepatic encephalopathy; it has no role in the treatment of steatorrhea.

### 13 The answer is A *Medicine*

The patient suffers from a case of scabies caused by a small, almost microscopic (0.3–0.9 mm) mite called *Sarcoptes scabei*, variety *hominis*. The recommended treatment for adults is 5% permethrin lotion (choice **A**), applied on a clean body from the neck to the toes and left for at least 8 hours, after which it can be washed off. A second treatment is recommended a week later. To ensure that all eggs and mites are killed, all clothing, bedding, towels, etc. used by the infected person should be washed in hot water and dried in a hot dryer before treatment begins. No special cleaning is needed for rugs, floors, coats, and furniture because the mites cannot survive away from a human body. When patients are infested, pregnant female mites burrow into the stratum corneum and deposit eggs. In 3–10 days, the eggs hatch into larvae, which then molt and mature into a new generation of adults via a nymphal stage. The eggs produce an allergic reaction that is intensified by the action of the maturing mites; this induces the rash and the itch. A first-time infection may take as long as 8 weeks for the full-blown allergic reaction to develop. On the other hand, a person sensitized by a previous infection will develop symptoms much more rapidly. The mites, and consequently scabies, are transmitted readily by skin-to-skin contact with an infected person. Thus, clusters of cases often occur within a household or a health care facility. Obviously, sexual intercourse involves skin-to-skin contact, thus causing scabies to be classified as a sexually transmitted disease. It is quite possible that this patient's partner picked up a few mites while working as a nurse and has already shown signs of scabies on her hands, a common site for early scabies to appear. Perhaps she only recognizes it as unusually red and rough hands and is spreading the disease among other patients; hence, the value of informing her that she is a vector. An epidemic of scabies in a health care facility can create havoc. Absolute diagnosis depends upon isolation and microscopic identification of active mites. However, it is more practical to make a tentative diagnosis based upon appearance and confirmed by response to treatment. Treatment as described above results in a 100% cure rate

Topical lindane (γ-benzene hexachloride) 1% (choice **D**) is an organochlorine insecticide once used as the primary treatment for scabies. It functions as a neurotoxin by interacting with γ-aminobutyric acid (GABA)$_A$ receptor. In humans, it has a dermal $LD_{50}$ of 1,000 mg/kg and has also been reported to be a carcinogen in rodents. Because of potential toxicity, it is now banned in 50 countries and approved by the U.S. Food and Drug Administration only as a second-line treatment for scabies or for pubic (crabs) and head lice. Oral azithromycin (choice **B**) is an antibiotic commonly used to treated chlamydial infections. Scratching a scabies infection can sometimes lead to thick scaling, particularly in immunocompromised persons. Such a condition is called *Norwegian scabies,* and the extensive scaling makes topical medication ineffective.

Consequently, Norwegian scabies is treated with ivermectin (choice **C**), a broad-spectrum antiparasitic medication. Parental penicillin G (choice **E**) is an antibiotic often used to treat primary syphilis infections but has no role in treating primary scabies infections.

**14** **The answer is D** *Surgery*

This woman has bilateral pheochromocytoma (bilateral adrenal lesions), a parathyroid adenoma (hypercalcemia and ectopic calcium deposits), and an oversized thyroid (a palpable, nontender swelling in front of her neck). This by definition is an example of multiple endocrine neoplasias (MEN). There are three such multigland syndromes, called MEN 1 (aka, Wermer syndrome), MEN 2a (aka, Sipple syndrome), and MEN 2b. All are inherited as autosomal dominant traits. MEN 1 is caused by a mutation in a tumor suppressor gene on chromosome 11; in this germline mutation, tumors form in cells in which the normal allele is suppressed. Both MEN 2a and 2b are due to mutations in a gene that codes for a protooncogene called *RET*, which is only expressed in cells with a neurocrest origin, such as medullary thyroid C-cells and chromaffin cells. (C-cells are sometimes also found in parathyroid tissue.) The RET gene is located on chromosome 10, and a given kindred will have a mutation in a specific codon that will correlate with a variation in clinical expression, such as age first expressed. This probably also accounts for the unique characteristics of MEN 2b, which include gastrointestinal and mucosal neuromas, a Marfan-like phenotype with skeletal abnormalities, as well as medullary carcinoma and pheochromocytoma. Genetic testing can identify 95% of persons with a mutated gene and is of value for genetic counseling and for identification of affected family members before symptoms arise; the latter permits a prophylactic thyroidectomy. Among adults worldwide, the prevalence of all three types of MEN is estimated to be between 0.2 and 2 cases per $10^5$ individuals; about 90% of cases are MEN 1, and MEN 2a makes up almost all of the remainder (MEN 2b is extremely rare). There is a 2:1 male-to-female ratio. The approximate degree to which the various organs are affected is as follows: MEN 1, parathyroid more than 80%, pancreas 75%, pituitary, 60%; MEN 2a, medullary thyroid carcinoma more than 90%, parathyroid 20%–50%, pheochromocytoma 20%–35%; MEN 2b, mucosal and gastrointestinal gangliomas more than 90%; medullary thyroid carcinoma 80%, pheochromocytoma, 60%, and parathyroid, rarely. Accordingly, the woman described in the vignette has MEN 2a. Medullary carcinomas of the thyroid derive from C cells, which synthesize calcitonin. For MEN 2a, serum calcitonin is the best screen (choice **D**). A provocative stimulation test using omeprazole, pentagastrin, or calcium can be used on family members to identify those who are at risk for developing medullary carcinoma. Although medullary carcinomas of the thyroid arising from MEN 2a are usually not highly aggressive, eventually death will ensue unless the thyroid is removed; thus, early identification by genetic screening of children in affected families is important.

Serum thyroid-stimulating hormone (TSH) (choice **B**) and serum thyroxine ($T_4$) (choice **C**) levels are normal in patients with medullary carcinoma. An iodine-123 ($^{123}$I) scan (choice **A**) and measurement of the serum parathyroid hormone level (choice **E**) are of no additional value in determining a diagnosis in this patient and would only identify half the cases.

**15** **The answer is D** *Surgery*

The upper outer quadrant of the breast is the most common location for a breast carcinoma (choice **D**); 60% of lesions are located here. In contrast, 6% of breast carcinomas reside in the lower inner quadrant of the breast (choice **A**), 12% of breast carcinomas in the upper inner quadrant (choice **B**), 10% in the lower outer quadrant of the breast (choice **C**), and 12% are located subjacent to the areola (choice **E**). Therefore, it is imperative to examine every quadrant of the breast, including the axillary tail, when ruling out a breast mass, keeping in mind the most common location. The examiner should use the flat of his or her hand to examine the breast. The pectoral muscles must be relaxed, as they are immediately deep to the breast. Failure to do so may result in missing a small lesion. Likewise, it is important to relax the axilla, so as not to miss lymphadenopathy here. Most breast carcinomas manifest themselves as a hard lump, and an indrawn nipple may be an added feature. Carcinoma affects the left breast more often than it does the right. Patients often discover them while they are showering.

**16** **The answer is G** *Medicine*

Alcohol abuse and alcoholism are major problems in the United States, estimated to affect over 8% of the adult population. Alcoholism, also known as alcohol dependence, is a disease that includes an almost irresistible craving for a drink; an inability to stop drinking once started; physical dependance marked by withdrawal symptoms such as nausea, sweating, shaking, and profound anxiety once drinking is stopped; and, a requirement to drink greater amounts to get a high as time progress, a phenomena called tolerance. Alcohol abuse is defined as drinking alcohol to such a degree that it causes personal harm, socially, physically, or with the law as in accumulating drinking under the influence of alcohol (DUIs); however, in contrast to true alcoholism, physical dependance is not a characteristic. Whether a person is afflicted with alcoholism or abuse, drinking large quantities of alcohol causes many different pathological changes in the drinker's body. These abnormalities probably affect all heavy drinkers, although there is great variability regarding individual responses; thus, the pattern of symptoms shown varies among different individuals. Fatty liver (choice **G**) is an abnormality found to be present in almost all heavy drinkers; fortunately, it frequently can be reversed by abstinence. Although fatty liver itself may not cause permanent damage, it is a symptom of abuse and a strong warning indicating a person should stop drinking before permanent damage is done. Generally, it is indicated by a slightly enlarged liver accompanied by higher than normal activity levels of liver enzymes in the serum. A computed tomography scan will show a liver that is less dense than normal, whereas an ultrasound test will produce a bright image in a ripple pattern. However, an absolute diagnosis requires a biopsy.

Up to 35% of chronic drinkers develop an inflammation of the liver know as alcoholic hepatis (choice **A**). This is caused by the oxidative metabolism of alcohol by the liver that produces free radicals as a side product and also by reaction to acetaldehyde, a toxic intermediate. Alcohol also permits the passage of bacterial endotoxins from the intestine to the small intestine via the portal vein. These toxins further damage liver cells causing the release of inflammation-promoting cytokines, which set up a vicious cycle by stimulating the release of additional cytokines. These inflammatory processes deplete oxygen levels, inducing cell death, and cause fibrous scarring, a condition known as cirrhosis (choice **B**). Early hepatis may be reversed by abstinence, but cirrhosis is not reversible and in 10%–20% of drinkers, these inflammatory processes lead to cirrhosis severe enough to eventually cause death if the patient is not given a liver transplant.

The fibrous scar tissue of cirrhosis also blocks the flow of blood through the branches of the portal vein that traverses the liver. This causes portal hypertension (choice **C**); when the portal pressure becomes high enough, blood is forced into other veins en route to the heart. These include veins in the esophagus, causing esophageal varices, and veins in the skin over the abdomen, leading to the appearance of spider veins. Esophageal varices are prone to bleeding, which may result in an anemia and may contribute to eventual death. Liver disease is almost always associated with leakage of enzymes from affected liver cells, causing an increase of these enzymes in the serum. Two of the liver enzymes are serum alanine aminotransferase (ALT) and serum aspartate aminotransferase (AST); however, in cases involving alcohol abuse, the increase in AST activity is always greater than that of ALT; thus choice **D** is incorrect.

Chronic excess alcohol consumption of course damages additional organs, the brain being one of the more critical. Wernicke disease (choice **E**) affects nerves in both the central and peripheral nervous systems. The underlying cause is believed to be malnutrition, primarily a lack of thiamine. Heavy drinking is often associated with a poor diet, but individuals who maintain a balanced diet may still suffer from a lack of thiamine because alcohol inhibits thiamine absorption from the gut. Symptoms associated with Wernicke disease include confusion, nystagmus, ophthalmoplegia, anisocoria, ataxia, poor pupillary reflexes, and in extreme cases, coma and death. Korsakoff psychosis (choice **F**) often follows Wernicke disease, and although it too may involve thiamine deficiency, Korsakoff psychosis is associated with a direct toxic effect of alcohol on the brain that causes general cerebral deterioration, particularly affecting the medial thalamus and the mammary bodies of the hippocampus. The six major symptoms of Korsakoff's psychosis are blackouts after a bout of drinking, known as anterograde amnesia; loss of memory of people and/or effects occurring prior to a bout of drinking, known as retrograde amnesia (this symptom often follows delirium tremens); invention of memories to fill in gaps associated with blackouts or other losses of memory, known as confabulation (confabulation may not be purposeful, and the false accounts are often believed by the teller); evasion of meaningful conversation; loss of insight; and increased apathy. These changes involve loss of neural function and bleeding within the mammary bodies. Although some improvement may occur during abstinence and treatment with thiamine supplementation, the condition cannot be reversed. It has been hypothesized that individuals genetically susceptible to symptoms associated with thiamine deficiency are more susceptible to acquiring the Wernicke and Korsakoff conditions.

### ☐17 The answer is A *Medicine*

The patient has celiac disease, an autoimmune disease with antibodies directed against the gliadin fraction in gluten (choice **A**), which is present in wheat products. The antibodies cause an inflammatory reaction in the villi, resulting in villous atrophy (flat mucosa) leading to malabsorption of fat (greasy stools), carbohydrates, and protein. In addition, this patient has an increased quantitative stool test result for fat and abnormal results in the D-xylose reabsorption test, which is an excellent screening test for documenting small bowel disease as a cause of malabsorption. The vesicular lesion on the patient's elbow is dermatitis herpetiformis, which is an autoimmune skin disease that has an almost 100% correlation with underlying celiac disease. Other antibodies present in celiac disease include antiendomysial and antireticulin antibodies. The treatment of choice is to eliminate gluten from the diet.

Antinuclear antibodies (choice **B**) directed against nuclear proteins are not present in celiac disease. A fecal smear for leukocytes (choice **C**) is used for evaluating diarrhea that may be caused by invasive microbial pathogens (e.g., *Campylobacter jejuni, Shigella sonnei*). The presence of leukocytes presumes an invasive enterocolitis and would not be expected in celiac disease. Testing the stool for ova and parasites (choice **D**) is always recommended in the workup of a patient with chronic diarrhea. Giardiasis is the most common cause of chronic diarrhea associated with malabsorption; however, the presence of dermatitis herpetiformis excludes a parasitic cause of the chronic diarrhea. A stool sample to calculate the osmotic gap (choice **E**) is used for high-volume diarrheal states when a secretory or osmotic type of diarrhea is suspected rather than malabsorption. The stool osmotic gap is obtained by measuring potassium and sodium in the diarrheal fluid, adding them together, and multiplying the number by 2 (i.e., $2 \times \{[\text{potassium}] + [\text{sodium}]\}$). This value is then subtracted from 300 mOsm/kg, which represents the osmolality of plasma. Secretory diarrheas are characterized by isotonic diarrheal fluid, therefore, the osmotic gap in stool will be less than 50 mOsm/kg. Causes of a secretory type of diarrhea include certain types of laxatives and enterotoxigenic bacteria such as enterotoxigenic *Escherichia coli* and *Vibrio cholerae*. Osmotic diarrhea is characterized by a hypotonic stool due to the presence of osmotically active solutes drawing more water than electrolytes out of the enterocytes. The classic example of an osmotic diarrhea is lactase deficiency, leading to an increase in lactose, which is osmotically active. The osmotic gap in osmotic diarrheas exceeds 100 mOsm/kg.

### 18 The correct answer is C

As indicated in the case study, this man shows the classic symptoms of metabolic syndrome (once called syndrome X). This includes a fasting glucose value higher than normal but below that required to diagnose diabetes (i.e., between 100 and 126 mg/dL), overweight, hypertension, and an abnormal serum lipid panel. Individuals having this syndrome feel well but are at high risk of developing full-blown diabetes. Even before becoming diabetic, they may be undergoing pathological changes that will lead to the typical complication of diabetes including retinopathy, nephropathy, and cardiovascular disease. Indeed, prediabetes likely should be considered a less severe form of diabetes rather than a unique condition in itself. The biguanide metformin (choice **C**) is one of several oral diabetic drugs demonstrated to have the potential of reversing this prediabetic state; moreover, metformin operates primarily by inhibiting liver gluconeogenesis, as well as having a secondary ability to promote the uptake of glucose into muscle cells. In addition, it does not cause hypoglycemia or weight gain or increase the risk of heart failure, although it very rarely causes lactic acidosis. The potential ability of metformin to reverse the prediabetic state was evaluated in the Diabetic Prevention Program (DPP), a major clinical research program involving 27 research centers; in this study, overweight prediabetics persons were divided into three groups: the first group, called the lifestyle intervention group, received counseling, plus intensive training and supervised dietary and physical conditioning training as well as motivational therapy. The second and third group also received lifestyle counseling but not intensive training, supervision, or motivational therapy. The second group also received 850 mg metformin twice a day and the third group a placebo. In comparison to the placebo group, diabetes development was reduced 58% in the lifestyle intervention group and 31% in the metformin group.

Sitagliptin phosphate (choice **A**) is the first drug in a relatively new drug class called dipeptidyl peptidase IV (DPP-4) inhibitors. DPP-4 normally breaks down the proteins that stimulate insulin production after a meal. Thus, a DPP-4 inhibitor permits insulin production to continue for a longer time, limiting the postmeal increase in glucose. Sitagliptin phosphate does not cause hypoglycemia or weight gain; however, it has not yet been evaluated for its ability to reverse prediabetes, and sitagliptin may inflame the pancreas, conceivably worsening diabetes. Glyburide (choice **B**) is one of the many sulfonylureas that act by stimulating the pancreatic β cells to excrete more insulin. This class of drugs is liable to cause weight gain as well as bouts of hypoglycemia. Rosiglitazone (choice **D**) and the other thiazolidinedione, pioglitazone, work by promoting the uptake of insulin by muscle cells, thereby decreasing insulin resistance in type 2 diabetics. It was reported at the 2008 meeting of the American Diabetic Association that pioglitazone lowered the progression from pre- to full diabetes by 81%; however, these thiazolidinediones promote water retention with concomitant weight gain and are suspected of inducing heart failure and therefore represent a false choice.

Nateglinide (choice **E**) and repaglinide are the two medications presently approved for treatment of type 2 diabetes. These drugs, like the sulfonylureas, stimulate the β cells to produce insulin; in contrast to the sulfonylureas, however, they only do so when blood glucose concentrations are elevated. Thus, they are taken usually three times a day, before a meal; as a result, they reduce the postprandial glucose high. Like sitagliptin phosphate, neither nateglinide nor repaglinide have yet been evaluated with respect to their potential for reversing prediabetes.

### 19 The answer is B *Medicine*

The illustrated malar rash, arthralgia, fever, and anorexia are all common symptoms of systemic lupus erythematosus (SLE). The serum antinuclear antibody (ANA) test is the gold standard screening test used to rule out SLE and other collagen vascular diseases. The major groups of ANAs are antibodies against DNA (both double- and single-stranded), histones and nonhistone proteins, and nucleolar antigens. Approximately 95%–100% of all cases of SLE test positive. However, although sensitive, this test is far from specific; it also will give a positive test in patients with Sjögren syndrome (95%), diffuse and limited (CREST syndrome), scleroderma (80%–95%), polymyositis and dermatomyositis (80%–95%), rheumatoid arthritis (30%–60%), and Wegner's granulomatosis (0%–15%). As a consequence, a positive ANA test result needs to be confirmed using a more specific test. The most specific autoantibody test available for SLE is the anti-native DNA test, also known as the anti–double-stranded (ds) DNA test, which has a positive result in some 60% of the patients with SLE and a positive result in fewer than 5% of rheumatoid arthritis cases and in no other of the major autoimmune diseases. Thus, positive results obtained with the antinuclear and anti-ds (double-stranded) DNA tests (choice **B**) will almost definitely confirm a case of SLE. Further confirmation can be obtained using an anti-Sm (Smith) test, which is 100% specific for SLE, but its sensitivity is only about 10%–25%. Obviously, some true cases of SLE will not be confirmed using these tests (false negatives), and as a consequence, the diagnosis will depend upon clinical criteria.

Anti-SSA (Ro) (choice **A**) and anti-SSB (La) (choice **C**) results are both positive in fewer than 20% of SLE patients but are also positive in 60%–70% of Sjögren syndrome patients and in a small minority of patients with rheumatoid arthritis; thus, these tests add little to the diagnosis of SLE. Anticentromere antibodies are present in 50% of patients with CREST syndrome, and antiribonucleoprotein antibodies are seen in most cases of patients with so-called mixed connective tissue disease (choice **D**), which is also called *overlap connective tissue disease*, since a case will often resolve into one or the other connective tissue autoantibody conditions; however, this test is neither as sensitive as the ANA nor very specific for SLE. Despite its name, the lupus anticoagulant test (choice **E**) result is only positive in about 7% of SLE patients. The term is a misnomer in a sense because the anticoagulant is directed against a phospholipid and not against any specific factor. Hence, the test result is positive in a number of disorders, including rheumatoid arthritis, infections including *Pneumocystis carinii*, lymphoproliferative disorders, drugs, and toxemia of pregnancy. Antihistone antibodies (choice **F**) are present in more than 95% of cases of drug-induced lupus but are not found in lupus caused in other ways.

### 20 The answer is A *Psychiatry*

Brief periods of longing for the lost person are seen in normal bereavement (choice **A**), even many years after the event, especially on holidays or on the anniversary of the death. Feelings of worthlessness (choice **B**), suicide attempts (choice **C**), inability to work, or as in this case, to socialize and get out of bed (choice **D**), or feelings of despair (choice **E**) indicate depression rather than a normal grief reaction.

### 21 The answer is B *Psychiatry*

The patient's symptoms are most suggestive of posttraumatic stress disorder (PTSD), characterized by traumatic recollections, emotional numbing, and increased arousal that follow a traumatic event and persist for at least 1 month. Although treatment involves psychotherapy and emotional support, sertraline (choice **B**) and other selective serotonin reuptake inhibitors have been shown to be effective pharmacologic interventions. Other antidepressants may also be useful.

Olanzapine (choice **A**) is an antipsychotic medication that has not been demonstrated to be useful for PTSD. Eszopiclone (choice **C**) is a nonbenzodiazepine hypnotic that can be used for chronic insomnia but has not been studied as a treatment for PTSD. Topiramate (choice **D**) is an anticonvulsant that may be useful for treating bipolar disorders but not PTSD. Atomoxetine (choice **E**) is a treatment for attention-deficit/hyperactivity disorder (ADHD) and may exacerbate insomnia.

## 22 The answer is F *Medicine*

At least nine major variant types of muscular dystrophy exist, with several subtypes. The common feature is a progressive form of muscular weakness. The most common of these is Duchenne (choice **F**), the disease that killed the boy described in the vignette. It has an estimated incidence of 1 case per every 3,500 male live births in the United States and is due to a major deletion on the short arm of the X-chromosome (Xp21). It is inherited as a sex-linked recessive trait and results in the nonproduction of dystrophin, a very large protein (427 kDa) that is part of the contractile apparatus of muscle cells. In addition to making the muscles weak, the absence of a dystrophin molecule makes the muscle cell leaky, which leads to a marked increase in serum creatine kinase activity and contributes to the ultimate death of muscle cells. Affected boys seem normal until the age of 2–5 years, when they develop a peculiar duck-like waddling gait caused by weakness of the pelvic girdle muscles. The weakness then progresses throughout the legs, forcing them into a wheelchair by their teens, and then to the upper body. During the early period, their lower legs often increase in diameter, not from muscle, but from fat and connective tissue causing psuedo-hypertrophy. By their late teens, the respiratory muscles and/or heart also weaken, and these patients succumb to a respiratory disease or cardiac failure not long afterward. There is no treatment. The literature often reports mild retardation (an average IQ of 85), but there are many exceptions to this, as in the chess-playing boy described here.

Becker muscular dystrophy (choice **A**) also results from a mutation in the dystrophin gene, but the mutation permits production of a defective dystrophin protein that has limited function. The result is a muscular dystrophy similar to Duchenne but not as severe. First symptoms usually occur during the late teens or early 20s, and affected persons are able to walk into their 30s. However, they too will eventually die from either respiratory or cardiac failure. Duchenne muscular dystrophy is also inherited as an X-linked recessive disorder. The incidence in the United States is about 1 case per 30,000 live male births. Type 1 myotonic muscular dystrophy (choice **B**) is the most common adult dystrophy and takes its name from the tendency for affected persons have progressive muscle wasting and weakness, coupled with myotonia, the inability to relax muscles after use; thus, for example, a person may not be able to put down a fork after using it. At least two distinct forms of myotonic muscular dystrophy exist, type 1 (DM1) and type 2 (DM2); DM1 accounts for as many as 98% of the cases and affects about 1 in 8,000 individuals. Both forms are inherited as autosomal dominant diseases and DM1 in particular shows anticipation—the disease appears earlier and become more severe with each successive generation. DM1 is caused by a trinucleotide repeat on chromosome 19 that results in a defective myotonin protein kinase, whereas DM2 is caused by a tetra-nucleotide repeat on chromosome 3. Additional poorly characterized variants of myotonic muscular dystrophy might also exist. Diagnosis of the myotonic muscular dystrophies is difficult to make because not only do symptoms vary from family to family, the range and severity of symptoms can vary greatly among patients even in the same family. At one extreme, a patient may only develop mild muscle weakness and/or cataracts late in life, whereas at the other extreme, a child might be born with the congenital form of the disease and have early-onset life-threatening disease. All patients with the condition are at risk of severe reactions to anesthesia and should be monitored carefully if subjected to anesthesia. Facioscapulohumeral muscular dystrophy (choice **C**) is an autosomal dominant condition that usually starts in the teens or early 20s. It first affects the face and shoulder girdle and then the pelvic girdle, legs, and abdomen. Clinically, its effects vary from very mild to severe; about 50% of patients can walk until they die at a normal age. Limb girdle muscular dystrophy (choice **D**) can be inherited in an autosomal dominant or more commonly in an autosomal recessive fashion. First symptoms usually start in the teens or early adulthood as weakness in the hips. It then slowly progresses, first to the shoulders, then to the arms and legs. Some 20 years after the first onset of symptoms, walking becomes very difficult. Welander distal myopathy (choice **E**) is a rare autosomal dominant condition most commonly is found among persons of Swedish or Finnish ancestry, having a prevalence of about 1 in 4,000 in mid-Sweden. It is one of a group of heterogeneous myopathies classified as distal myopathies, characterized clinically by muscular weakness and atrophy beginning in the hands and feet. The disease generally then progresses in severity and to muscles elsewhere in the body. As many as two dozen suspected distinct types of distal myopathies have been described (at least five of which have been identified as mutations in a specific gene), making diagnosis difficult. Most have adult onset, a major exception being Laing myopathy, which can be identified in infancy. In addition, individuals in the same family can be affected to markedly different degrees. One member may live a long, essentially normal life with little more than what appears to be arthritis of the hands, whereas another may be bedridden by mid-adulthood.

### 23 The answer is B *Pediatrics*

Werdnig-Hoffmann disease (choice **B**) is a spinal muscular atrophy caused by a pathologic continuation of a process of programmed cell death that normally occurs in embryonic life, but should cease at birth. It is inherited in an autosomal recessive fashion. Infants can be symptomatic at birth. Sparing of the extraocular muscles and sphincters is characteristic. Fasciculations are a sign of denervation of muscle and are best seen in the tongue. Infants assume a flaccid "frog-leg" posture. Most die by 2 years of age.

A neonatal form of myotonic dystrophy (choice **A**) appears in infants born to mothers with myotonic dystrophy. Clubfoot and contractures are common. Fasciculations are not seen. Infant botulism (choice **C**) has a peak onset at 2–6 months of age. Sources for spores include honey, corn syrup, soil, and dust. Infantile myasthenia gravis (choice **D**) can be transient—as in those infants born of mothers with myasthenia gravis—or, very rarely, a congenital manifestation of the disease itself. Fasciculations are not seen, and the extraocular muscles are not spared. Duchenne's muscular dystrophy (choice **E**) is rarely symptomatic at birth.

### 24 The answer is C *Pediatrics*

Congenital rubella syndrome (choice **C**) occurs after German measles infection during pregnancy and causes a variety of congenital malformations. These manifestations may include hepatosplenomegaly, thrombocytopenia, hepatitis, jaundice, cataracts, widespread maculopapular lesions of reddish blue color (i.e., "blueberry muffin" rash), and neurologic depression.

Clinical manifestations of congenital toxoplasmosis (choice **A**) are chorioretinitis, hepatosplenomegaly, jaundice, convulsions, and cerebral calcifications. Rubeola (choice **B**; aka, measles) during pregnancy is not associated with congenital abnormalities. Congenital varicella (choice **D**) acquired during the first half of pregnancy may cause limb hypoplasia, microcephaly, seizures, and cataracts in the newborn. If transmitted in the last 3 weeks of pregnancy, varicella can be mild or can involve fever and pneumonia. Hepatosplenomegaly and generalized lymphadenopathy may be seen in a newborn with congenital syphilis (choice **E**). In addition, the mucocutaneous lesion of syphilis produce snuffles (a purulent and blood-tinged nasal discharge).

### 25 The answer is B *Medicine*

Ménière disease (choice **B**) is one of a host of conditions that can cause dizziness. Characteristics in the case history described that point to Ménière disease are the description of the room spinning while the patient stood still, tinnitus, and a sensation of fullness in one or both ears. It is also often also accompanied by nausea and vomiting. Since there is no specific test, it is diagnosed by clinical symptoms and response to treatment. Specifically, acute attacks usually respond to the antivertigo drug meclizine and/or benzodiazepines but not to treatment used to prevent other causes of dizziness.

Shy-Drager syndrome (choice **A**; aka, neurologic orthostatic hypotension or multiple system atrophy) is a rare disease that, among a host of other symptoms, causes a feeling of dizziness. The disease starts gradually, often manifesting with frequent falls caused by dizziness due to a drop in blood pressure upon standing up. It progresses into a parkinsonian-like condition that includes slowness of movement, muscle rigidity, bladder dysfunction, and poor balance; ultimately, it causes death. Commonly, it affects males more than females, and symptoms start at about the age of 50 60 years. The patient described is female, and by the age of 74 years, had she had Shy-Drager syndrome she would likely had symptoms more severe than dizziness. Essential hypertension (choice **C**) should not of itself cause dizziness, nor does the case history mention hypertension. Orthostatic hypotension (choice **D**) is a common cause of dizziness provoked by rapidly standing, particularly from a supine position; typically, the patient feels faint. Moreover, the dizziness described by the lady in this question occurred while she was lying down, sitting, or standing, and was not provoked by a change in position. Benign positional vertigo (choice **E**) is the most common cause of peripheral vertigo. Normally, tiny mineral particles help maintain balance by rotating within the semicircular canals. In benign positional vertigo, some of these get stuck in one place. Most patients get relief by body repositioning maneuvers that can be performed in the physician's office or even at home. Benign positional vertigo is not associated with tinnitus (although a patient may have had tinnitus before being troubled by vertigo), or with a feeling of fullness in an ear; nor is it likely a patient will describe the room as spinning. A patient with benign positional vertigo is more likely to describe the dizziness as an unsteady feeling and/or faintness rather than a spinning room.

### 26 The answer is B *Surgery*

The patient has cirrhosis of the liver complicated by ascites (shifting dullness in the abdomen) and portal hypertension, the latter causing esophageal varices that have ruptured (choice **B**), producing hematemesis.

The most common cause of portal hypertension is alcoholic cirrhosis. Approximately 50% of the deaths in cirrhosis are due to ruptured varices. The left gastric coronary vein, a branch of the portal vein, normally drains blood from the distal esophagus and proximal stomach to the portal vein for drainage into the liver. However, in portal hypertension, caused by blocked blood flow due to tissue scarring, as in alcoholic cirrhosis, blood backs up into the vein causing distention (varices) and the potential for rupture. Bleeding varices cannot be diagnosed on the clinical presentation alone and require an emergency endoscopy to localize the source of bleeding. Endoscopy also is useful in therapy with variceal ligation, banding, or sclerotherapy. Ancillary management may include the use of intravenous octreotide, which decreases splanchnic blood flow and portal vein pressure. Intravenous vasopressin plus nitroglycerin may also be used; the nitroglycerine reduces the cardiac afterload and coronary artery resistance induced by the vasopressin. In recalcitrant cases, a transjugular intrahepatic portosystemic shunt (TIPS) may be required to stop the bleeding. A metal stent is inserted that connects the hepatic vein with the portal vein. This reduces portal pressure; however, it increases the risk for developing hepatic encephalopathy by increasing blood ammonia levels. Other options include caval shunting, in which the portal vein is anastomosed to the inferior vena cava (side-to-side or end-to-side), or a distal splenorenal shunt.

Pyloric obstruction (choice **A**) is associated with vomiting due to retention of food in the stomach. Hematemesis is not a feature of the disease. Although hematemesis is most frequently associated with peptic ulcer disease (most commonly duodenal ulcers [choice **E**] followed by gastric ulcers [choice **C**]), the endoscopic findings described are most compatible with bleeding varices. Esophageal carcinoma (choice **D**) does not usually present with massive hematemesis. Dysphagia for solids, weakness, and weight loss are the usual presenting signs and symptoms.

### [27] The answer is D *Medicine*

In the case presented, the family's history casts doubt on the diagnosis of hepatitis C. Moreover, because the enzyme-linked immunosorbent assay (ELISA) test that is currently used has a significant fraction of false-positive results, it may well be true that the patient is hepatitis C free. A recombinant immunoblot assay (choice **D**) will confirm the presence or absence of disease. This assay has a claimed specificity of 99%; consequently, a negative result essentially excludes infection by the hepatitis C virus. At the time of this writing, a third-generation ELSIA test allegedly more specific than the one presently employed is awaiting U.S. Food and Drug Administration approval.

Repeating the test in a week (choice **A**) or after a month (choice **B**) probably would not confirm the diagnosis since whatever led to a false-positive test is likely still present. Ordering a genotype (choice **C**) is usually reserved for confirmed cases of hepatitis C, in order to establish duration of treatment and likelihood of success. Serial liver enzyme analyses to evaluate for increasing activity levels (choice **E**), along with other tests, are usually carried out to assess response to treatment.

### [28] The answer is D *Medicine*

This patient has a hemolytic anemia. Hemolytic anemia occurs when more red blood cells are destroyed than are being produced. It could result from immune or nonimmune disorders; the defect could be intrinsic or extrinsic. Causes include intrinsic red cell anomalies; premature destruction of otherwise normal cells, as occurs in mismatched transfusion; drug interaction; infection due to some strains of streptococci; and hypersplenism. Intrinsic abnormalities of red blood cells that may cause a hemolytic anemia include hereditary spherocytosis, in which there usually is an abnormality in spectrin, a protein that provides most of the scaffolding for the red cell membrane and enables it to deform; deficiencies in one of several of the enzymes involved in glucose metabolism; and abnormal hemoglobins, such as hemoglobin S, which causes sickle cell disease, an autosomal recessive disorder leading to sickling of red cells under conditions of local hypo-oxygenation. A peripheral blood smear will help distinguish between spherocytes and sickle cells. If sickle cells are found, hemoglobin electrophoresis is required to establish whether the sickling is due to sickle cell disease. In hemolytic anemia, the levels of unconjugated bilirubin, haptoglobin, and lactic dehydrogenase are increased (choice **D**). Bilirubin is a breakdown product of hemoglobin and is usually transported to the liver via the circulation. For this to happen, bilirubin has to be noncovalently associated with albumin. This complexed form is called *unconjugated* or *indirect bilirubin*. Once it reaches the liver, it is metabolized and albumin is no longer required. Most of this bilirubin freed from albumin is covalently bound to glucuronic acid is now called *conjugated* or *direct bilirubin*. However, in cases of hemolysis, a large quantity of unconjugated bilirubin remains circulating in the blood because the liver is unable to conjugate such a large quantity; hence, the level of circulating unconjugated bilirubin increases. Haptoglobin is a circulating protein and is an acute-phase reactant, meaning its concentration is increased in the serum in conditions in which stress, infection, or inflammation occurs. In cases of hemolysis, haptoglobins bind the hemoglobin that is released, thus minimizing its accumulation in the plasma. The hemoglobin–haptoglobin complex is then eliminated by the reticuloendothelial system. Lactic dehydrogenase is present in the cytoplasm of red cells and is released into the circulation when cells undergo hemolysis, resulting in its elevation. Obviously if choice **D** is correct, then choices **A**, **B**, **C**, and **E** are incorrect.

### 29 The answer is C *Surgery*

The patient has a papillary adenocarcinoma of the thyroid (choice **C**) that has metastasized to the cervical lymph nodes. These are the most common thyroid cancers and are usually found in women between 20 and 60 years of age. They are papillary tumors that are often mixed with follicles. Psammoma bodies (blue-staining calcium concretions) are an excellent marker for the cancer. Most patients initially present with palpable lymphadenopathy in the neck, which represents nodal metastasis via permeation of the lymphatics. They can produce a miliary pattern of metastasis to lung resembling miliary tuberculosis.

Carcinomas of the larynx may involve the vocal cord (choice **A**); approximately 70% of these are found in the glottic area, 20% are found in the supraglottic region, and the remaining 10% are located in the subglottic or hypopharynx regions. Laryngeal carcinomas are usually squamous-celled. Those involving the glottic fold (i.e., true vocal cords) usually arise in the anterior half of one of the true vocal cords. They are usually papillary and rarely ulcerative. Due to the paucity of lymphatics in this area, the tumor tends to be locally malignant for a long time, and hence has a relatively good outcome. Often it is symptom free until the fifth or sixth decade of life; although cigarette smoking is a definite contributory factor, the greatest risk factor is consumption of alcohol. The most frequent and initial symptom is a change in voice—a huskiness that becomes progressive. Thereafter, the patient can barely whisper, until finally, aphonia develops as the vocal cord becomes fixed. Although supraglottic tumors (which involve the false cords, laryngeal ventricles, or the base of the epiglottis) metastasize early to the cervical lymph nodes, those that involve the glottis remain localized for a long time. Subglottic carcinomas occur beneath the vocal folds, and the patient presents with difficulty in breathing. Metastasis occurs to the paratracheal and lower deep cervical nodes, and even the thyroid gland. Laryngeal carcinoma located in the hypopharynx is associated with dysphagia and pain on swallowing. The most common malignant parotid gland tumor (choice **B**) is mucoepidermoid carcinoma. The most common primary lung cancer (choice **D**) is an adenocarcinoma with the formation of glandular structures. The most common breast cancer (choice **E**) is an infiltrating ductal carcinoma. Papillary cancers are very uncommon.

### 30 The answer is C *Medicine*

Isolated systolic hypertension (choice **C**) is a condition that often affects the elderly; in fact, it is so common that it was once believed that normal systolic pressure is equal to 100 plus a person's age. However, trial studies have conclusively demonstrated that elevated systolic blood pressure is a more significant underlying cause of cardiac disease and stroke than is elevated diastolic pressure; 30% of women and 20% of men older than 65 years have this condition. The underlying reason is a loss of arterial elasticity that occurs with aging, and the condition becomes more common with advancing age. The man described most likely is suffering from a cerebellar stroke, which typically is associated with headache and ataxia.

An epidural hemorrhage (choice **A**) is a consequence of trauma and could conceivably have resulted from his fall. However, his fall occurred after the symptoms first appeared; typically, an epidural hematoma is characterized by coma after a lucid interval, and there is no mention of loss of consciousness. Ménière syndrome (choice **B**) is a cause of vertigo induced by distention of the endolymphatic compartment of the inner ear. Although usually idiopathic, it can be caused by head trauma or syphilis. It is not age associated, and there is no evidence presented in the vignette that this patient might have Ménière syndrome. A cerebral infarct (choice **D**) would not have only primary symptoms relating to ataxia but would rather have loss of muscular strength or cognitive function. A pulmonary thromboembolism (choice **E**) is usually accompanied with signs of dyspnea, chest pain, hemoptysis, and/or syncope. Except for syncope, the man had none of these symptoms. Moreover, there is no indication of a predisposition for venous thrombosis, and the one drug this man uses is aspirin.

### 31 The answer is C *Pediatrics*

Anemia of prematurity (choice **C**) occurs in low-birthweight infants approximately 1–3 months after birth. It is caused by the physiologic effects of the transition from fetal to neonatal life, as well as by factors such as shortened red blood cell survival, rapid growth, and frequent phlebotomy for blood tests. Hemoglobin (Hb) levels in anemia of prematurity are below 7–10 g/dL. Clinical manifestations may include feeding problems, tachypnea, tachycardia, and pallor.

Megaloblastic anemia of infancy (choice **A**) usually is caused by a deficiency of folic acid and has its peak incidence between 4–7 months of age. Infants with folate deficiency are irritable, have poor weight gain, and have chronic diarrhea. Newborns with sickle cell anemia (choice **B**) rarely exhibit clinical manifestations until 5–6 months of age, when the γ-globin of fetal Hb is replaced by the β-globin of adult Hb. Acute sickle dactylitis (i.e., painful swelling of the hands and feet) is usually the first evidence that sickle cell disease is present in an infant. The thalassemias are a group of heritable, hypochromic anemias. α-Thalassemia (choice **D**) is caused by abnormalities in the synthesis of the α-chains of Hb and is manifested as microcytosis of the newborn (mean corpuscular volume [MCV] <95 pg). Homozygous β-thalassemia (choice **E**) usually manifests as a severe, progressive hemolytic anemia in the second 6 months of life (after Hb A replaces Hb F) and requires regular blood transfusion.

### 32 The answer is C *Psychiatry*

The history and findings are most suggestive of major depressive disorder, recurrent (choice **C**), with mood-congruent psychosis. The absence of a history of abnormally elevated moods makes bipolar disorder (choice **A**) unlikely. Dysthymic disorder (choice **B**) is less likely because it is usually characterized by long periods of depressed mood, but without the full features of a depressive episode or psychosis present in this case. Schizoaffective disorder (choice **D**) is diagnosed only when psychosis persists for at least 2 weeks in the absence of mood episodes. In schizophrenia (choice **E**), psychotic symptoms and emotional blunting persist in the absence of mood symptoms, and these symptoms are usually more prominent than any associated mood pathology.

### 33 The answer is D *Pediatrics*

Todd's paralysis (choice **D**) commonly occurs after a seizure. The hemiparesis lasts minutes to hours but resolves within 24 hours. It can easily be confused with a stroke except for its duration.

Hemiplegia complicating migraine headaches (choice **A**) also shows recovery within a few hours without seizures, but residual neurologic effects are associated with transient hemiparesis/plegia. The disorder usually involves a strong maternal history of classic migraine. Neurologic deficits would not disappear after 24 hours in patients with infratentorial tumor (choice **E**). In postviral encephalitis (choice **C**), focal neurologic signs may be stationary, fluctuating, or progressive. Spastic hemiplegia (choice **B**) occurs in patients with cerebral palsy who have decreased spontaneous movements on one side of their body. These patients may also demonstrate hand preference at a very early age. This problem is not transient.

### 34 The answer is D *Pediatrics*

Caput succedaneum (choice **D**) is a diffuse swelling of the soft tissues of the scalp. It extends across suture lines, and the edema starts to resolve over the first few days.

Underlying skull fractures (choice **C**), not seen in caput succedaneum, are occasionally associated with cephalohematomas (choice **A**). The hemorrhages caused by cephalohematomas are subperiosteal; therefore, they are limited to one bone and do not cross suture lines. Cephalohematomas tend to increase in size over the first few days and resorb in approximately 3 months. Subcutaneous fat necrosis (choice **B**) of facial or scalp tissue may be associated with a forceps delivery. Overriding of the parietal bones (choice **E**) occurs when the bones of the scalp overlap at the suture line. The examiner would feel the overlap of bone, not a soft-tissue swelling.

### 35 The answer is A *Surgery*

Macular degeneration (choice **A**) is the most common cause of permanent loss of visual acuity in the elderly. It is a strongly age-related phenomenon (prevalence of 25%–30% by 75 years of age). Predisposing conditions include: sex (slightly more common in females than in males), Caucasian ethnicity, a genetic propensity as demonstrated by family history, occupational exposure to chemicals, blue eyes, cardiovascular disease, smoking, diastolic hypertension, and left ventricular hypertrophy. There are two basic types: atrophic (or dry) and exudative (or wet). The dry form progresses slowly and is usually bilateral. The wet form progresses more rapidly, and affects the eyes sequentially. The wet form is usually more severe and is accompanied by accumulation of serous fluid or blood that separates the retina. The wet form is responsible for 90% of the blindness associated with macular degeneration, but if caught earlier can be treated by laser therapy.

Diabetic retinopathy (choice **E**) is the most common cause of blindness in the United States, but its development is associated with uncontrolled diabetes, either type 1 or 2, and it does not have a primary predilection for the elderly population. Neovascularization of the retinal vessels portends a poor prognosis. Optic neuritis (choice **D**) is a cause of sudden, unilateral loss of vision. The vignette provides no reason to suspect trauma (choice **B**) or cataract surgery (choice **C**), and neither of these are associated with a high rate of permanent loss of visual acuity.

## 36  The Answer is C  *Medicine*

This patient has orbital cellulitis, which is most commonly due to sinusitis (choice **C**). Patients will often give a history of prior upper respiratory infection. Orbital cellulitis can lead to life-threatening complications, including cavernous sinus thrombosis and orbital abscess. This is an emergency and should be treated with intravenous broad-spectrum antibiotics. Sinusitis, if present, should be treated,

Although cavernous sinus thrombosis (choice **A**) is a potential complication of orbital cellulitis, this patient as not yet developed this condition. In addition to fever and diplopia, it usually presents with a history of nausea, vomiting, and headache. Alteration in mental status also may be present, and the pupil is dilated. Corneal ulcer (choice **B**) is associated with blepharospasm (the eyelid is squeezed shut, as if squinting), epiphora (increased tear secretion), and ocular pain. Diplopia and fever are not features. Orbital abscess (choice **D**) results from ulitis (inflammation of the gums) and is a potential complication of orbital cellulitis. The patient does not give a history of trauma (choice **E**), and if trauma were responsible for the symptoms, ocular hemorrhage would probably have been associated with it and noted on examination.

## 37  The Answer is A  *Medicine*

The pattern described in answer **A** describes a macrocytic/normochromic anemia (i.e., an anemia that produces abnormally large red cells that have a normal hemoglobin content); this is also known as a *megaloblastic anemia*. This condition occurs whenever DNA synthesis is inhibited in an otherwise viable developing cell. The inhibition of DNA synthesis delays nuclear maturation and induces an imbalanced rate of development in which cell division is inhibited, thus permitting the erythroblasts in the bone marrow to grow to an abnormal size and often an aberrant shape. (The generic term for such irregularly shaped cells is poikilocytes.) Although cell division is inhibited cytoplasmic functions continue permitting the maturing red cell to take up hemoglobin. As development continues, the unusually small nucleus of the blast cell is lost, and the malformed red cell is transport into the circulation, where it is readily recognized. Folate is required for DNA synthesis, and consequently, this type of abnormal development always occurs under conditions of absolute or functional folate deficiency. Functional deficiency of folate can occur when sufficient vitamin $B_{12}$ is not available because vitamin $B_{12}$ is a cofactor in the homocysteine methyltransferase reaction, which methylates $N^5$-methyltetrahydrofolate to form tetrahydrofolate, an active form of folate used in DNA synthesis. ($N^5$-methyltetrahydrofolate is the end-product of all metabolically active forms of folate and has no other catalytic function; thus if vitamin $B_{12}$ levels are insufficient to permit this methylation reaction, a functional deficiency of folate will occur, provided dietary intake of folate is not adequate enough to overcome its loss via conversion of the active forms to the $N^5$-methyltetrahydrofolate derivative.)

As ingested, dietary vitamin $B_{12}$ passes through the stomach, where it attaches to a glycoprotein called the *intrinsic factor*, which is synthesized by the gastric parietal cells; this binding requires a low pH. The vitamin $B_{12}$ intrinsic factor complex then binds to specific receptors in the mucosal cells of the ilium and subsequently is transported into the general circulation. Pernicious anemia results when this complex mechanism of vitamin $B_{12}$ absorption goes awry. Such malfunction may result from an autoimmune reaction disabling the production or function of the intrinsic factor, an autoimmune reaction or surgery causing the loss of parietal cells, or a lower than normal gastric pH. Pernicious anemia has been reported to be most commonly found among persons of Celtic or Scandinavian ancestry but in the past few decades, people from other ethnic groups have been reported to have a similar prevalence. This may be because in modern developed societies the hematologic symptoms of pernicious anemia have become more difficult to observe because they are commonly made imperceptible by excess folate in the diet, which makes the conversion to $N^5$-methyltetrahydrofolate largely inconsequential. One might think this would make the reduced ability to absorb vitamin $B_{12}$ unimportant; however, this vitamin has one additional function in normal metabolism and that is as a cofactor in the methylmalonyl CoA mutase reaction that converts methylmalonyl CoA to succinyl CoA. This reaction permits the conversion of propionyl CoA to succinate; this propionyl CoA is produced by the final β-oxidation step during the oxidation of odd-carbon fatty acids, as well as from valine, leucine, and methionine. Thus, a deficiency of vitamin $B_{12}$ inhibits the methylmalonyl CoA mutase reaction and leads to an accumulation of propionyl CoA, which can get incorporated into fatty acids during fatty acid synthesis; this will produce odd-carbon fatty acids that then get incorporated into neural myelin causing neuropathy, a relatively early symptom of which is loss of proprioceptor function. However, over the long-term it may cause more severe symptoms, including psychiatric symptoms resulting in senile dementia. In addition to showing some hematologic symptoms, namely signs of a macrocytic-normochromic anemia, the patient described shows signs of neuropathy, namely loss of proprioceptor function marked by a shuffling hesitant gait. In addition, he might be genetically prone to develop pernicious anemia because of his Celtic ancestry and because his gastroesophageal reflux disease (GERD) is being treated with a protein pump inhibitor.

Choices **B**, **C**, **D**, and **E** are incorrect because the root part of the answer is irrelevant and because each condition described should result in increased not decreased reticulocyte formation.

### 38 The answer is B *Psychiatry*

This patient's symptoms are most suggestive of delusional disorder, somatic type (choice **B**), which is characterized by clearly false beliefs involving bodily symptoms, sensations, or functions.

Unlike individuals with schizophrenia (choice **D**), individuals with delusional disorder are often coherent and show no other signs of thought disturbance. Body dysmorphic disorder (choice **A**) is characterized by an exaggerated perception of a slight physical anomaly. Hypochondriasis (choice **C**) is characterized by a misinterpretation of physical symptoms. Somatization disorder (choice **E**) is characterized by multiple physical complaints.

### 39 The answer is C *Pediatrics*

Cavernous sinus thrombosis (choice **C**) is a complication of sinusitis. Symptoms of cavernous sinus thrombosis include ophthalmoplegia and loss of accommodation. Sinusitis also can be complicated by meningitis, epidural or subdural abscesses, optic neuritis, periorbital and orbital cellulitis and abscess, and osteomyelitis of surrounding bones. Complications develop secondary to local extension of the infection.

Hand-Schüller-Christian disease (choice **A**) has a variable presentation. It may involve skeletal abnormalities, skin lesions, exophthalmos, hepatosplenomegaly, or pituitary dysfunction. Proptosis is not a feature. Graves disease (choice **B**) is a hyperthyroid state characterized by irritability, excitability, crying easily, restlessness, and tremors of the fingers. Acute bacterial conjunctivitis (choice **D**) presents with generalized conjunctival hyperemia, edema, mucopurulent exudate, and various degrees of ocular discomfort. Temporal lobe abscess (choice **E**) does not present with proptosis.

### 40 The answer is E *Obstetrics and Gynecology*

The progestin-only pill is different from the standard contraceptive pill in that it contains only one hormone. Many brands are available. It must be taken every day because its effectiveness depends on altering cervical mucus to make it hostile to sperm entry. It must be taken at the same time each day in order to maintain its impact on cervical mucus. It does not suppress gonadotropins, so has only a limited duration of effect. This also explains why it cannot be used to suppress functional ovarian cysts, like the combination estrogen-progestin pill can.

### 41 The answer is H *Obstetrics and Gynecology*

The progestin-only "morning-after" pill contains levonorgestrel and is 90% effective in preventing pregnancy if taken within 72 hours of unprotected intercourse. It is often referred to as the "emergency" or "postcoital" contraceptive. It must be taken in two doses 12 hours apart. It does not alter an implanted pregnancy. The mechanism of action is multiple and may include delaying ovulation, preventing fertilization, and preventing implantation.

### 42 The answer is B *Obstetrics and Gynecology*

The estrogen–progestin combination pill is the earliest form of steroid contraception was developed. Many brands are available. Its main mechanism of action is by suppressing gonadotropins, thus preventing the luteinizing hormone (LH) surge and ovulation. This is largely due to the effect of the estrogen component. The impact on the hypothalamic-pituitary axis does not wear off rapidly. Therefore, missing a daily dose will not alter the contraceptive effect; rather, a double dose the next day will maintain its contraceptive effectiveness. The estrogen dose used today is much lower than was used in years past.

### 43 The answer is G *Obstetrics and Gynecology*

The estrogen–progestin dermal patch is a relatively new form of steroidal contraception. The trade name is Ortho Evra. The patch is applied onto the upper outer arm, buttocks, abdomen, or thigh. Its effectiveness is similar to the estrogen–progestin combination pill. Because release of the hormones rapidly declines on the seventh day of skin application, the patch must be replaced consecutively for 3 weeks. No patch is used for the fourth week, thus allowing for the withdrawal bleed of the menstrual period.

**44 The answer is D** *Obstetrics and Gynecology*

The estrogen–progestin vaginal ring, a relatively new form of steroidal contraception, is a thin, transparent, flexible ring that is inserted into the vagina. The trade name is Nuva Ring. It does not need to fitted like a vaginal diaphragm or cervical cap does. It slowly releases estrogen and progestin into the vagina, which is then absorbed systemically to provide continuous contraception. It is left in place for 3 weeks and then removed to allow for the withdrawal bleed of the menstrual period. The mechanism of action is to suppress ovulation and thicken the cervical mucus, thus creating a barrier to prevent sperm from fertilizing an egg. It has an effectiveness similar to the estrogen–progestin combination pill. Each vaginal ring provides 1 month of birth control.

**45 The answer is F** *Obstetrics and Gynecology*

This progestin-only intramuscular injection is placed into the buttocks or the upper arm and contains depot medroxyprogesterone acetate (DMPA). The trade name is Depo Provera. It is one of the most effective contraceptive methods available. Because the release of the hormone takes place slowly, it must be readministered only every 12–13 weeks. Like other progestins, it makes cervical mucus unfavorable for sperm entry. Unlike other progestins, it does suppress gonadotropins. The suppression of follicle-stimulating hormone (FSH) lowers estrogen levels and this can, over time, result in decreased bone density. Other side effects include weight gain and breakthrough bleeding.

**46 The answer is C** *Obstetrics and Gynecology*

This progestin-only subdermal implant is a flexible plastic rod measuring 40 × 2 mm, about the size of a matchstick. The trade name is Implanon. It contains a progestin hormone called etonogestrel and is effective for up to 3 years. The mechanism of action is similar to depot medroxyprogesterone acetate (DMPA), with suppression of ovulation and alteration of cervical mucus. Placement is under the skin of the underside of the upper arm; implantation requires a local anesthetic and takes 1 minute. Removal takes a little longer, about 2 minutes, and also requires a local anesthetic.

**REMAINING INCORRECT CHOICE**

Choice **A**, the levonorgestrel (LNG) intrauterine system, is a progestin-only intrauterine contraceptive. It is T-shaped, with a reservoir in the stem of the device that contains LNG. The trade name is Mirena. The LNG is released gradually over 5 years, after which time the device needs to be replaced. The mechanism of action is primarily local in the uterus rather than systemic, although serum levels are measurable. Contraceptive effectiveness is high and is mediated through alteration of cervical mucus, interference with sperm transport, and endometrial atrophy. Menstrual flow is decreased and some women may become amenorrheic.

**47 The answer is D** *Psychiatry*

Graph **D** represents early morning awakenings, which are often associated with major depressive disorder.

**48 The answer is B** *Psychiatry*

Diazepam decreases stage 4 sleep (graph **B**), which makes this medication useful in treating sleep disorders characterized by pathology during this stage. Sleep terror and sleepwalking are examples of such pathologies.

**49 The answer is C** *Psychiatry*

Benzodiazepine rebound causes increased sleep latency (time to fall asleep) (Graph **C**), which is one mechanism that leads to addiction.

**50 The answer is E** *Psychiatry*

Graph **E** represents suppression of rapid eye movement (REM) sleep, which is caused by barbiturates and some antidepressants.

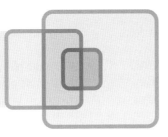

# test **7**

# Questions

*Single Best Choice Directions: This section consists of numbered statements or questions followed by a list of potential answers; you are to select the ONE best answer.*

**1** A 23-year-old man presents to the emergency department with bizarre delusions, a blunted affect, and tangential thought processes. He has no history of mood episodes and no history of substance abuse. Results of his laboratory studies are unremarkable. Which of the following possible findings from a subsequent, more extensive evaluation would most strongly indicate a favorable prognosis?

(A) An extensive premorbid history of social withdrawal
(B) A family history of schizophrenia
(C) A sudden and dramatic onset of illness
(D) Magnetic resonance imaging (MRI) studies that show gross changes in brain morphology
(E) Catatonic symptomatology

**2** A 43-year-old Caucasian man of northern European descent had been feeling a rapidly escalating degree of fatigue for the past several weeks and consequently consulted his primary care physician. Upon taking a history, his physician confirmed that, in addition to feeling tired, the patient has noted a shortness of breath and heart palpitations. Laboratory analyses showed low serum hemoglobin and haptoglobin levels and raised serum reticulocyte, lactic acid dehydrogenase, and bilirubin concentrations. Deducing that her patient may have a hemolytic anemia, the physician referred him to a hematologist, who determined that there was no family history of anemia. The hematologist asked the patient to void a midday urine sample into a prelabeled Erlenmeyer flask, and to also provide her with a second urine sample obtained immediately after rising in the morning; she also and told him to bring both samples into her office the following day. The patient did as requested; the midday urine sample had a deep orange-yellow color typical of concentrated normal urine, but the early morning sample was a bright reddish color. The patient most likely suffered from which one of the following conditions?

(A) A drug-induced nonautoimmune hemolytic anemia
(B) Paroxysmal nocturnal hemolytic anemia
(C) Paroxysmal cold hemoglobinuria
(D) Warm autoimmune hemolytic anemia
(E) Acute intermittent porphyria

**3** A 31-year-old man presents to the emergency department with the sudden onset of weakness in his right hand. Two weeks ago, his wife filed a complaint of spousal abuse with the local police, and yesterday, he gave several guns to a friend of his because he "didn't trust himself with them." Mental status examination reveals a peculiar calmness and lack of concern about his weakness. Which of the following is the most likely diagnosis?

(A) Conversion disorder
(B) Specific phobia
(C) Obsessive-compulsive disorder
(D) Hypochondriasis
(E) Melancholic depression

**4** Morrisville (population 150,000) had 3,000 deaths in 2009 from all causes, including meningitis. At the beginning 2009, 25 patients with meningitis diagnosed the previous year were under treatment. During 2009, 200 new cases of meningitis were diagnosed. There were 11 deaths from this cohort of newly diagnosed patients; seven patients died in 2009, and four patients died in 2010. Which of the following represents the meningitis case-fatality rate during 2009 for Morrisville?

(A) $(7 \div 11) \times 100$
(B) $(7 \div 200) \times 100$
(C) $(200 \div 3{,}000) \times 100$
(D) $[(200 - 11) \div 3{,}000] \times 100$
(E) $[(7 + 11) \div 11] \times 100$

**5** After recovering from his third episode of psychosis, a 22-year-old man returns home to live with his parents and his younger siblings. The family asks what they can do to improve his adjustment. Which of the following would be the best advice?

(A) Insist that the patient abstain from social interaction.

(B) Encourage the patient to participate in an assertive community treatment program.

(C) Encourage animated discussions at dinner, with an emphasis on exploring areas of friction among family members.

(D) Strongly encourage the patient to return to school or get a job.

(E) Keep the patient at home as much as possible.

**6** A 39-year-old man presented to his physician with a history of back pain that started 2 weeks previously. The patient stated that he had been cleaning the garage for a yard sale when he felt a little pain in his "lower back." He decided to use some hot packs and analgesics that were available over the counter. Unfortunately, over the past few days, he noticed that the pain had gotten worse. He had stiffness of his back and could not sit for long periods. Walking seemed to help. Whenever he coughed or sneezed, the pain would shoot down his right leg. Physical examination revealed that the patient was in moderate distress. He had spasm and tenderness of the paraspinal muscles on the right lumbar region. His straight-leg raising test was 50 degrees on the right, but full on the left. Additional examination of the right foot revealed weak dorsiflexion and hypesthesia over the first web space. The rest of the neurologic examination was normal. The most likely reason for his symptoms is which one of the following?

(A) Epidural hematoma

(B) Spinal cord astrocytoma

(C) Epidural abscess

(D) Prolapsed intervertebral disk at L4–5 level

(E) Prolapsed intervertebral disk at L5–S1 level

**7** At a routine well-child visit, a mother reports that her infant is able to babble, coo, and form a social smile. When supine, the infant is able to follow an object 90 degrees from the midline through an arc of 180 degree. When prone, the infant is able to lift its head 45 degrees. The infant is also able to roll from the prone to the supine position. Which of the following is the most likely age of this infant?

(A) Newborn

(B) 1 month

(C) 2 months

(D) 3 months

(E) 4 months

**8** A 55-year-old man presented to his family physician with a history of tiredness, aching, tingling, and cramps in his left leg. These symptoms got progressively worse toward the end of the day, but elevating the leg relieved them. The problem has become worse over the last several weeks, and he is now unable to walk a city block without extreme pain, which lingers even after he sits down and rests for a few minutes. He has tried over-the-counter analgesics, which have given him temporary relief. The patient has noticed that his foot is swollen by the end of the day, when he has to loosen the shoelace to feel comfortable. He is a factory worker and must stand for long hours at his job. Physical examination revealed soft-tissue swelling of the left ankle. A reddish brown discoloration of the skin was noted behind the medial malleolus of the left ankle, together with a small area of ulceration in the center. No calf tenderness was elicited, but he did have some scattered areas of venous dilatation under the skin of the leg. No abnormality was noted in the right leg. The femoral, popliteal, and dorsalis pedis pulses were normal and equal in both lower extremities. The most likely condition this patient is suffering from is which one of the following?

(A) Superficial thrombophlebitis

(B) Embolic disease

(C) Arterial insufficiency

(D) Immune vasculitis

(E) Deep venous insufficiency

**9** A 31-year-old woman, gravida 4, para 2, abortus 1, was seen at the outpatient clinic with a chief complaint of missing her menstrual period. She had been using barrier methods of contraception. Her most recent pregnancy ended in a spontaneous first trimester loss requiring dilation and curettage. Her two previous successful pregnancies were unremarkable, resulting in spontaneous-onset labor at term, followed by uncomplicated spontaneous vaginal deliveries of healthy neonates who are alive and well. Her last menstrual period was June 10. A qualitative serum β-human chorionic gonadotropin (β-hCG) test had positive results. Assuming her usual cycle length is 32 days, which of the following is her most likely due date?

(A) March 12

(B) March 17

(C) March 21

(D) November 13

(E) November 17

**10** A 65-year-old man was seen by his family physician with a 6-month history of constipation and a recent history of pain in the left lower quadrant of his abdomen. The patient complained of weakness and fever as well. He smoked approximately two packs of cigarettes per month and consumed a six-pack of beer during weekends. Physical examination revealed a moderately obese man. His blood pressure was 138/90, pulse 76/min regular, respirations 16/min, and temperature 100°F (37.8°C). His cardiovascular and respiratory systems were normal. Examination of the abdomen revealed tenderness in the left lower quadrant with a positive rebound. In addition, a tender mass was felt on rectal examination. A complete blood count revealed neutrophilic leukocytosis, and the stool guaiac test result was negative. The most likely diagnosis in this patient is:

(A) Ulcerative colitis
(B) Irritable bowel syndrome
(C) Acute diverticulitis
(D) Carcinoma colon
(E) Ischemic colitis

**11** A 35-year-old Caucasian man with neurofibromatosis presents to his physician with a complaint of nausea and vomiting, vertigo, nystagmus, tinnitus, and nerve deafness in the right ear. These symptoms had gradually worsened over the past month or so. Upon examination, the physician noted hemianesthesia on the right side of the face. Which of the following is the most likely diagnosis?

(A) Mastoiditis
(B) Cerebellar tumor
(C) Vertebrobasilar arterial insufficiency
(D) Glioblastoma multiforme
(E) Acoustic Schwannoma

**12** An afebrile 12-week-old infant is brought to the pediatrician by his mother because of a persistent cough. Upon physical examination, the patient is found to have a temperature of 100°F (37.8°C) per rectum and is noted to have bilateral conjunctivitis. Other pertinent findings include tachypnea, inspiratory rales, and scattered expiratory wheezing. The rest of the physical examination is unremarkable. A complete blood count reveals eosinophilia. The chest x-ray film shows hyperinflation and patchy interstitial infiltrates bilaterally. Which of the following is the most likely diagnosis?

(A) Respiratory syncytial viral pneumonia
(B) Bronchiolitis
(C) Chlamydial pneumonia
(D) Cystic fibrosis
(E) The larval phase of ascariasis

**13** A 45-year-old woman sees her primary care doctor for fatigue. She states that she used to be able to walk a mile "with ease," but of late has been having problems doing so. She feels tired and winded, and has noticed some problems eating as her tongue "feels raw." This patient most likely has which one of the following conditions?

(A) Microcytic anemia
(B) Macrocytic anemia
(C) Thalassemia
(D) Sideroblastic anemia
(E) Anemia of chronic disease

**14** A 2-year-old boy is brought to the emergency department because of increasing and profound lethargy during the past 4 hours. The past medical history is unremarkable. However a 7-year-old brother who is a bed wetter has an upper respiratory infection. There have been no other contacts with individuals who are sick. On physical examination, the child's temperature is 37.4°C (99.3°F), and he is noted to be hypotensive. There is no history or evidence of trauma. The cardiac monitor demonstrates a ventricular dysrhythmia, and the child begins to have a seizure. Which of the following is the most likely cause for this child's problem?

(A) Shaken baby syndrome
(B) Meningitis
(C) Imipramine
(D) Congenital heart disease
(E) Febrile seizure

**15** A 68-year-old man with intermittent, cramping abdominal pain also has difficulty defecating. He manages a bowel movement every third or fourth day only with a great deal of straining and then only passes small hard feces with a lot of mucous and sometimes fresh blood. His physician suspects obstipation and orders a barium enema that reveals a massively dilated sigmoid colon with a column of barium resembling a "bird's beak." Which of the following is the most likely diagnosis?

(A) Intussusception
(B) Volvulus of the sigmoid colon
(C) Toxic megacolon
(D) Ogilvie syndrome
(E) Impacted stool

**16** A 45-year-old man made an appointment to see his family physician because he noted bleeding per rectum. In providing a history, he disclosed that his father had died of cancer of the bowel at age 54 years. He also stated that the bleeding had started about 6 weeks ago and was in small amounts. Although he did not complain of abdominal pain, he did feel somewhat tired and said he had "lost energy." He did not smoke, consumed alcohol in moderation, and avoided red meat. He included a large amount of vegetables and fruits in his diet "for fiber." Anoscopy revealed internal hemorrhoids. Laboratory test results were positive for microcytic hypochromic anemia, and stool samples tested positive for blood. Colonoscopy revealed a moderately large lesion at the splenic flexure of the colon, which was biopsied. The pathology report indicated penetration of the muscle wall and infiltration into serosal fat by sheets of malignant cells without gland or mucin formation. The liver and spleen are of normal size, and a computed tomography scan shows no evidence of distant metastasis, but 3 of 10 lymph nodes contain metastatic tumor. Based on the forgoing data, which of the following choices best describe the most probable prognosis?

(A) He has an 80% or better chance of surviving for 5 years.

(B) He has a 60% chance of surviving for 5 more years.

(C) He has a 55% chance of surviving for 5 more years.

(D) He has a 30% chance of surviving for 5 more years.

(E) He has a 20% chance of surviving for 5 more years.

(F) His has less than a 5% chance of surviving for 5 more years.

**17** A recently retired 67-year-old man makes an appointment to see his physician because his hands are beginning to tremble in an uncontrollable manner. During the examination, the physician notes that he does have an obvious resting tremor of both hands. However, he had no difficulty in picking up a quarter, and during that process the tremor ceased. When asked to hold his hand out, palm up, his fingers underwent an involuntary movement as if he was rolling a pill across his palm. He states that although the tremor is annoying and sometimes embarrassing, it makes little difference in his lifestyle; it has not even interfered with playing golf. At this time, which of the following is the best first step in treatment?

(A) Amantadine

(B) An anticholinergic drug

(C) Levodopa

(D) Carbidopa

(E) A dopamine agonist

(F) Selegiline

(G) Watchful waiting

**18** A 65-year-old woman has an 8-year history of involuntary loss of urine: she leaks small amounts of urine when she coughs, sneezes, or laughs. In providing a history to her physician, she complains about feeling pelvic pressure, but denies feeling a burning sensation upon urinating or having an abnormally strong urinary urgency or frequency. She has no loss of urine at night; however, the symptoms occur frequently enough that she needs to wear a perineal pad. She underwent menopause 12 years ago. For treatment of hot flashes, she initially used oral estrogen hormone replacement along with 7 days of medroxyprogesterone acetate 1 week of every month. For the last 8 years, she has not used any hormone therapy. Speculum examination reveals an atrophic vagina and cervix without lesions. Bimanual examination reveals a small, symmetrical, midline, mobile, nontender uterus. There are no adnexal masses. With the Valsalva maneuver, there is protrusion of her anterior vaginal wall. Which one of the following is the most likely diagnosis for the physical finding?

(A) Cystocele

(B) Urethral diverticulum

(C) Gartner's duct cyst

(D) Rectocele

(E) Enterocele

**19** A pediatrician is requested to attend the delivery of a 25-year-old primigravida, with a history of good prenatal care. The patient tells the pediatrician that she is expecting a full-term single delivery. She denies any history of sexually transmitted diseases, alcohol, or illicit drug use. Her physical examination is pertinent for a malar rash, alopecia, and polyarticular arthritis. In addition, she has a history of renal disease. This patient's newborn will have an increased risk for which of the following disorders?

(A) Complete heart block

(B) Coarctation of the aorta

(C) Open neural tube defects

(D) Microcephaly

(E) Polycystic kidney disease

**20** One night, a 75-year-old man was driving his wife home from a concert when he realized he was having great difficulty in discerning the lines designating the lanes. In fact, he almost hit another car when he accidently made a lane change where the road suddenly curved. His wife was greatly upset and insisted that he should not drive at night until he has been cleared by a doctor. Consequently, he made an appointment to see his primary care physician, who had been treating him for type 2 diabetes and hypertension for over a decade; in providing a history, he informed the physician that he had become aware of gradually deteriorating vision; he stated that he had been noticing some difficulty in reading and that he also saw halos around light fixtures and headlights from oncoming cars during the night. Given this history, the most likely diagnosis would be which one of the following?

(A) Retinal detachment
(B) Age-related macular degeneration
(C) Diabetic retinopathy
(D) Hypertensive retinopathy
(E) Cataract

**21** A 55-year-old man who suffered a stroke 6 months ago is administered a Folstein Mini Mental Status Examination. Although he devotes much effort to the task, he is unable to successfully copy intersecting pentagons. Based on this finding, which of the following areas of the brain is most likely to have been affected by the stroke?

(A) Nondominant frontal lobe
(B) Nondominant temporal lobe
(C) Nondominant parietal lobe
(D) Dominant temporal lobe
(E) Dominant frontal lobe

**22** A 4-day-old infant born by spontaneous vaginal delivery without complications is brought to the pediatric emergency department. The parents report that the child is vomiting and feeding poorly. Physical examination reveals muscular rigidity with alternating bouts of flaccidity and severe opisthotonos. A bedside glucose determination shows that the infant is hypoglycemic; however, correcting the blood glucose concentration does not improve the patient's clinical condition. The urinalysis does not show evidence of infection, but the urine has a distinct odor. Other routine laboratory studies are unremarkable, except for evidence of severe acidosis. Which of the following is the most likely diagnosis?

(A) Sepsis
(B) Neonatal seizure
(C) Maple syrup urine disease
(D) Trauma
(E) Phenylketonuria

**23** During 2006, the five leading causes of death in the United States across age groups in descending order were which one of the following?

(A) Cancer, heart disease, stroke, accidents, and acquired immune deficiency syndrome (AIDS)
(B) Cancer, chronic lower respiratory disease, accidents, stroke, heart disease
(C) Stroke, heart disease, cancer, AIDS, stroke
(D) Heart disease, cancer, stroke, chronic lower respiratory disease, accidents
(E) Malignancy, stroke, heart disease, diabetes, accidents
(F) Heart disease, stroke, chronic lower respiratory disease, accidents

**24** A 25-year-old man being evaluated for social withdrawal says that he has no friends, is not really interested in other people, and does not feel particularly lonely. A mental status examination reveals no peculiar thought processes. Which of the following is the most likely personality diagnosis?

(A) Schizotypal personality disorder
(B) Paranoid personality disorder
(C) Narcissistic personality disorder
(D) Avoidant personality disorder
(E) Schizoid personality disorder

**25** A 6-year-old girl who appears healthy is brought to the primary care physician by her mother because of a rash. The mother states that the patient had been in her usual state of good health until 2 days earlier, when she developed a tactile fever and mild upper respiratory symptoms. Yesterday, the patient had erythematous facial flushing that spread as a macular red lesion to her proximal extremities and trunk, which now has a lacy appearance. Which of the following is the most likely diagnosis?

(A) Erythema infectiosum
(B) Roseola
(C) German measles
(D) Measles
(E) Scarlet fever

**26** A 54-year-old white woman presented to her family physician with a recent history of pain in the upper right quadrant of the abdomen associated with nausea, vomiting, and fever. She did have a prior history of discomfort in the stomach, especially after eating a fatty meal, but this lessened after she started eating salads and avoiding butter and fried foods. She had no other relevant medical history. She did not smoke and consumed alcohol only on social or religious occasions. On physical examination, she appeared to be in moderate distress, blood pressure 130/90 mm, pulse 78/min regular, respirations 18/min regular, and temperature 101°F (38.3°C). She was moderately obese and had minimal guarding and tenderness in the right upper quadrant. Examination of the rest of the abdomen was normal. Examination of the cardiovascular and respiratory systems was noncontributory. A complete blood count showed leukocytosis; a chemistry panel showed mildly elevated liver enzymes, but was otherwise unremarkable. X-ray films of the chest and abdomen were normal. Ultrasonography of the abdomen revealed a thickened gallbladder wall with a solitary calculus within. The bile ducts were not dilated. The pancreas and the terminal ducts were normal. Conservative treatment with nasogastric suction, analgesics, and antibiotics provided no relief, and she underwent laparoscopic cholecystectomy. Within 24 hours following surgery, the patient developed a temperature of 102°F (38.9°C); blood pressure 90/60 mm Hg; pulse 100/min regular; respirations 22/min, rapid and shallow; and urine output less than 30 mL/h. Her skin was clammy and cold. She complained about some chest discomfort and pain. The most likely cause for this development is which one of the following?

(A) Hemoperitoneum
(B) Gram-negative sepsis
(C) Acute myocardial infarction
(D) Pulmonary embolus
(E) Pneumothorax

**27** A 45-year-old man who is a conforming Seventh-Day Adventist who works as a technician in the laboratory of a Veterans Administration Hospital complains of increasing fatigue over the past few months. He has had to buy new trousers as his waist has been increasing in size, and he has difficulty in putting on his shoes. Recently, he also has noticed swelling of his breasts. These physical changes are most likely due to which one of the following causes?

(A) Medication
(B) Alcohol
(C) Hepatitis A
(D) Hepatitis B
(E) Hepatitis C

**28** Parents bring their internationally adopted 2-year-old child to the pediatrician's office because he has a temperature of 40°C (104°F) and a morbilliform rash. The parents state that the patient has been in the United States for only 5 days and was scheduled for a well-child visit at the end of the week. They report that they thought the child had an upper respiratory infection until the rash began this morning. According to the father, the confluent maculopapular rash started cephalad and spread caudad to include the palms and soles. The mother also notes that, prior to developing the rash, the child had a dry cough, clear discharge from his nose, and conjunctivitis. The immunization status is unknown. Which of the following complications is most likely to develop in this child?

(A) Acute appendicitis
(B) Subacute sclerosing panencephalitis
(C) Interstitial pneumonia
(D) Myocarditis
(E) Otitis media

**29** A 21-year-old woman, primigravida, presents at 39 weeks' gestation in active labor. She is 155 cm tall and weighs 75 kg. Her pregnancy weight gain has been 20 kg. On digital vaginal examination, the fetus is in cephalic presentation at −1 station. Her cervix is 5 cm dilated, 90% effaced, soft, midposition. Onset of regular uterine contractions was 8 hours ago, and she is now experiencing regular contractions every 3 minutes, lasting 45 seconds, which are firm to palpation. Clinical pelvimetry shows her pelvic dimensions as follows: pelvic sidewalls are straight, ischial spines are not prominent, pubic arch is wide, sacrum is hollow, and sacrosciatic notch is well rounded. Based on general bony architecture, the characteristics of this woman's pelvis identify it as which one of the following common female bony shapes?

(A) Gynecoid
(B) Android
(C) Anthropoid
(D) Platypelloid
(E) Obstetroid

**30** On a hot August day in North Carolina, a 35-year-old Hispanic woman is seen by her primary care physician for progressive fatigue and a feeling of general malaise. She informs him that, over the past few days, she has been noticing difficulty in walking up a brush-covered slope leading to her home where she lives in the country, and she suspects she may be coming down with the flu. She has no history of chest pain, but did complain of some difficulty in breathing. She stated that she bruises easily. Apart from taking ibuprofen fairly regularly, which she purchases over the counter for arthritis, she has not been on any other any long-term medications. She had taken one ibuprofen a few hours prior to seeing her physician. She has no allergies. Physical examination reveals a moderately built and well-nourished female who has a low-grade fever and a yellowish tinge in the sclera. Her vital signs are within normal limits. She has normal heart sounds and no murmurs, gallops, or rubs. A few basal rales are present, but the lungs are clear otherwise. Examination of the abdomen is unremarkable except for mild tenderness in the right upper quadrant. She does have mild pitting edema in the pretibial area. The most likely cause for her problem is which one of the following?

(A) Lyme disease
(B) West Nile virus
(C) Rocky mountain spotted fever
(D) Sarcoidosis
(E) Q fever

**31** A 20-year-old man comes to his family physician with a complaint concerning fainting attacks. He states that he has started going to the gym where he uses the treadmill and lifts some weights. He feels faint and sometimes actually passes out after being on the treadmill for some time; even more distressing, he almost always passes out soon after he begins to lift heavy weights. His father also had episodes of fainting; furthermore, he died following a heart attack at the age of 54 years. The present patient has had a "double pulse" for a long time, and it has never bothered him. In fact, he likes to show off his special pulse to his friends. He denies chest pain, but does complain of some breathing difficulty. Upon examination, the physician observed a distinct cardiac murmur. This murmur would be expected to do which of the following?

(A) Increase when he sits upright or when he squats
(B) Decrease when he sits upright and remain unchanged when he squats
(C) Increase when he holds his breath or when he squats
(D) Decrease when he holds his breath or when he squats
(E) Increase when he sits upright and decrease when he squats

**32** A 65-year-old man who recently moved to a new town consulted a family physician concerning a 2-week history of tiredness and weakness. Moreover, he recently noticed blood in his urine, pain on the right side of his back, fever, and shortness of breath, especially when walking further than 100 yards. In addition, he has a history of chronic headache, which had been attributed to high blood pressure by his previous physician, who had prescribed medication. However, he admitted his compliance was poor and he seldom remembered to take the prescribed medications regularly. He also provided a history of smoking one pack of cigarettes per week for more than 20 years and has had a longstanding "smoker's cough" with intermittent purulent expectoration. He did have some blood in his sputum a few months previously, and he has also noticed a loss of weight. He consumes alcohol in moderation, and although not diabetic himself, he has a family history of diabetes mellitus. Vital signs are blood pressure 170/100 mm Hg (repeatedly elevated), pulse 78/min regular, respirations 18/min, and temperature 101°F (38.3°C). He weighs 170 lb and is 6 feet tall. His oxygen saturation was observed to be 98% on room air. He has no pallor or cyanosis. Examination of his respiratory system reveals a midline trachea, absence of clubbing or cyanosis, and a few scattered crepitations in both lung fields, but no rales and rhonchi. His cardiovascular system appears to be normal, except for sinus tachycardia and hypertension. He has no peripheral pitting edema. Examination of the abdomen reveals a tender palpable mass in the right lower quadrant, which can be easily felt on ballottement. A complete blood count was normal; a chemistry panel revealed borderline high blood urea nitrogen (BUN) and creatinine levels but was otherwise unremarkable. Urinalysis revealed a few red and white blood cells per high-power field. The posteroanterior and lateral chest x-ray views revealed multiple well-differentiated masses of homogenous density in both lung fields, changes due to emphysema, and evidence suggesting chronic bronchitis. Which one of the following is the most likely diagnosis?

(A) Renal tuberculosis
(B) Transitional cell carcinoma of the bladder with metastasis to the lung
(C) Primary lung cancer with metastasis to the kidney
(D) Renal adenocarcinoma
(E) Acute pyelonephritis with metastatic abscesses in the lung

**33** A 17-year-old boy made an appointment to see his parent's primary care physician because he has had repeated episodes of waking during the night due to lower back pain. In addition, he finds his spine to be very stiff in the morning, as if he were an old man. He described the pain as being centered over the sacrum. Examination showed tenderness during percussion over the sacroiliac joints and a pain response upon springing the pelvis. In addition, he was unable to bend forward to touch his toes. The patient denied a history of trauma, pain going down his legs, muscle weakness, or problems with his urinary bladder or bowel. Serology showed that he expressed human leukocyte antigen B27. In addition to his complaint about his back, he complained of pain in his eye. Examination of the pupils would most likely reveal which one of the following?

(A) The pupil was unequal.
(B) The pupils would react to light but not accommodate.
(C) The pupils would react to accommodation but not react to light.
(D) Consensual light reflex was painful.
(E) No abnormality was noted in the pupils.

**34** A 4-day-old girl is brought to the pediatrician because she has a blood-tinged discharge from her vagina. The patient was born at 38 weeks' gestational age to a 22-year-old primigravida. The infant weighed 7 lb 6 oz at birth and had no complications at birth. The infant was discharged home with her mother 24 hours after delivery. The mother reports that, since that time, the child has been afebrile and is feeding and sleeping well. At this point, the physician should do which of the following?

(A) Draw blood for a hematocrit determination.
(B) Notify the Child Protective Services.
(C) Reassure the mother that this is normal.
(D) Call the endocrinologist.
(E) Obtain a urinalysis.

**35** A 56-year-old man presents himself to a walk-in clinic complaining about tiredness, muscle weakness, polyuria, and nocturia. The triage nurse finds his blood pressure is 220/125 mm Hg. Recognizing a potential medical emergency, she immediately introduces him to the physician on duty. That physician treats him with nitroglycerine, which brings the readings down to 175/90 mm Hg. He also gives him a few extra nitroglycerine pills, plus prescriptions for hydrochlorothiazide and verapamil and tells him to make an appointment with a physician who can treat him on a regular basis because he suspects that he may be suffering from a serious condition. Taking his advice, the patient makes an appointment at a local free clinic. At this time, his sense of muscle weakness has increased, as has his general feeling of fatigue. In addition to the symptoms above, he now also suffers from muscle cramps and constipation. His new physician finds his blood pressure to be 190/95 mm Hg, and he also notes a mild cardiac arrhythmia; blood serum analysis was normal except for his serum $K^+$ level, which is 3.1 mm/L. The patient claims he has been taking the pills prescribed by the doctor at the walk-in clinic on a regular basis. Which of the following conditions does this patient most likely suffer from?

(A) Essential hypertension
(B) Conn syndrome
(C) Addison disease
(D) Cushing syndrome
(E) Pheochromocytoma

**36** A 55-year-old man recently consulted a physician for the first time in several decades because he felt "poorly." The physician determined he had a body mass index (BMI) of 38, a fasting plasma glucose level of 215 mg/dL, and a systolic blood pressure of 185 mm Hg. He immediately recommended a diet and a regimen of drugs that included metformin, hydrochlorothiazide, and acetaminophen; the latter because of mild joint pains associated with incipient osteoarthritis. A series of follow-up appointments were made, during which it was determined that the patient was becoming increasingly withdrawn and apathetic. Over a period of a month, he has become insomniac; has lost interest in his family, sex, work, eating, and hobbies; and he spends much time brooding about his perceived loss of health. He informs his physician that sometimes he feels as if life is no longer worthwhile. Administration of which of the following is most likely to be prescribed as the initial line of treatment used for his psychiatric symptoms?

(A) A monoamine oxidase inhibitor
(B) A selective serotonin reuptake inhibitor
(C) A tertiary amine tricyclic antidepressant
(D) A secondary amine tricyclic antidepressant
(E) A heterocyclic antidepressant
(F) A mixed reuptake inhibitor
(G) Electroconvulsive therapy

**37** A 67-year-old man consults his physician because of difficulties while urinating. His major concern is that he has trouble completely emptying his bladder and that after concluding the act, urine sometimes dribbles across the head of his penis, irritating the skin. When asked, he admits that the flow is weaker and slower than it had been and that sometimes it is interrupted. Moreover, he is often awakened during the night by an overpowering urge to urinate. Otherwise, he is healthy. A physical examination was unremarkable, except for findings on a digital rectal examination. This revealed a nontender, smooth but enlarged prostate gland that felt firm but not hard. Routine laboratory workup showed no abnormalities. The prostate-specific antigen (PSA) level was 3.5 ng/dL. Among the following alternatives, which is the best initial treatment to prescribe for this patient?

(A) Transurethral resection of the prostate
(B) Trimethoprim-sulfamethiazole
(C) Finasteride
(D) Radical prostatectomy
(E) Interstitial radiotherapy

38 A 28-year-old female, para 0 gravida 1, underwent routine sonography at gestational age 18 weeks. The ultrasound revealed a twin pregnancy, one of which was male, the other female. The fetuses were appropriate for gestational age, and no congenital deformities were detected. The woman did not have a history of bleeding diathesis, but her husband was known to suffer from hemophilia A. The woman's mother is of Scottish descent, and her father, a Ukrainian Jew. Both of her parents are alive and in their 70s. Her mother suffers from hypertension, and the father from diabetes mellitus and hyperlipidemia. Neither

suffers from bleeding diathesis. Two of her paternal uncles died at a young age from complications associated with hemophilia. Assuming both parents carry the normal number of chromosomes, which one of the following statements about the fetuses she is carrying is factual?

(A) The female fetus has a 50% probability of being a carrier but no possibility of expressing the disease; the male, on the other hand, has no possibility of being a carrier but a 50% probability of expressing the disease.
(B) Both the female and the male fetuses have no prospect of either being carriers or expressing the disease.
(C) The female fetus has a 75% probability of being a carrier and a 25% probability of expressing the disease; the male fetus cannot be a carrier, but has a 50% possibility of expressing the disease.
(D) The female fetus has a 50% likelihood of being a carrier, and a 50% likelihood of expressing the disease; the male fetus, on the other hand, has no chance of being a carrier, but a 50% chance of expressing the disease.
(E) The female fetus has a 100% chance of being a carrier, but no possibility of expressing the disease; the male fetus has no chance of either being a carrier or of expressing the disease.

*Directions for Matching Questions (39 through 50): Each set of matching questions is preceded by a list of 4 to 26 lettered options followed by a brief explanation of the required task and then by a series of numbered statements. For each numbered statement, you are to select ONE lettered option that best fulfills the task as it relates to that statement. Remember, each of the listed options might be correctly selected once, more than once, or not at all.*

## Questions 39–47

(A) Paraovarian cyst of Morgagni
(B) Hydrosalpinx
(C) Tubo-ovarian abscess
(D) Chronic pelvic inflammatory disease (PID)
(E) Pregnancy
(F) Follicular cyst
(G) Corpus luteum cyst
(H) Theca-lutein cyst
(I) Luteoma of pregnancy
(J) Endometrioma
(K) Polycystic ovaries
(L) Mucinous cystadenoma
(M) Benign cystic teratoma
(N) Granulosa cell tumor
(O) Sertoli-Leydig cell tumor
(P) Gonadoblastoma

*For each of the following descriptions, select the ONE most appropriate diagnosis in reference to female pelvic masses.*

39 A 23-year-old woman, gravida 2, para 1, underwent first-trimester sonography at 10 weeks to rule out twins. A 6-cm, unilateral, fluid-filled, smooth-walled, unilocular pelvic mass was found. The mass is separate from the uterus and is essentially unchanged on serial sonograms. However, it is variable in location, being noted anterior, posterior, and lateral to the uterus.

40 A 34-year-old woman, gravida 1, para 0, at 18 weeks' gestation with severe hyperemesis has a blood pressure of 150/95 mm Hg and 2+ proteinuria. Pelvic examination reveals bilateral adnexal masses that are 8–10 cm in diameter and appear multiloculated on a sonogram.

**41** An 18-year-old woman, gravida 1, now para 1, just delivered a 3,500 g (7 lb 12 oz) healthy male neonate without complications. At the beginning of this pregnancy, at 8 weeks' gestation, she was noted to have a 5-cm right adnexal cystic mass that appeared as a simple, thin-walled, round, fluid-filled cyst structure. The mass spontaneously involuted and was no longer seen on sonogram at 16 weeks' gestation.

**42** A 29-year-old woman experienced her last menses 9 weeks ago. On her first prenatal visit, she is noted to have a 9–10 cm soft, smooth, symmetrical, mid-line pelvic mass. The mass is mobile and not tender to palpation. She has experienced morning nausea but no vomiting.

**43** A mother brings her 5-year-old daughter to the family physician. The girl is of appropriate height and weight for age. The girl shows changes of early breast development and has had vaginal bleeding. These changes have occurred suddenly. Pelvic examination under sedation reveals a normal vagina, but a sonogram shows a 4 cm unilateral, solid pelvic mass. There is no family history of such events.

**44** A 55-year-old postmenopausal woman shows evidence of temporal balding, clitoromegaly, and increased facial hair that began 6 months ago and had a rapid onset. She is noted to have a 5 cm unilateral, solid pelvic mass. Family history is negative for these findings.

**45** A 28-year-old nulligravid woman is found on routine annual examination to have an asymptomatic, mobile, nontender, 6 cm unilateral pelvic mass. On sonogram, the mass is partially solid and partially cystic, with foci of calcifications. She is sexually active with her husband of 5 years. She has used combination oral contraceptives for the past 3 years.

**46** A 32-year-old infertile, obese nulligravida complains of secondary dysmenorrhea as well as pain with intercourse and bowel movements. She is sexually active but has never used any contraceptive methods. Bimanual pelvic examination reveals a 7 cm right adnexal mass. On rectovaginal examination, she is found to have uterosacral ligament nodularity and a fixed retroverted uterus.

## Questions 47–50

(A) Altruism
(B) Blocking
(C) Denial
(D) Displacement
(E) Dissociation
(F) Distortion
(G) Humor
(H) Projection
(I) Rationalization
(J) Reaction formation
(K) Regression
(L) Repression
(M) Suppression
(N) Undoing

*Match each patient with the ONE associated defense mechanism.*

**47** A political figure is engaged in a televised debate and comes under increasing pressure from his opponent. As his anxiety mounts, he begins to lose poise, interrupt his opponent, and attack his character. He finally resists an urge to throw down his papers and angrily stalk offstage by telling a self-disparaging joke.

**48** A man with a dubious record of compliance with Internal Revenue Service (IRS) regulations faces a tax audit. However, he twice missed appointments with the agent after becoming involved with projects at work.

**49** A 19-year-old star football player celebrated his graduation from high school by partying with his friends. While celebrating, he drank a six-pack of beer, and while driving home, he lost control of his car, crashing into a tree. As a result, he shattered his left ankle. An orthopedic surgeon repaired the ankle by ankylosing it; however, the young man could no longer play football well enough to hope of becoming a professional. He consulted a lawyer about suing the surgeon, blaming him for ruining his chances to become a professional football player.

**50** A 66-year-old woman sees a physician for a growth on her breast that she neglected until it broke through the skin, creating a weeping, smelly mess. When the physician asked why she waited so long before coming to see him, she replied "I just forgot about it."

# Answer Key

| | | | | | | | | | |
|---|---|---|---|---|---|---|---|---|---|
| 1 | C | 11 | E | 21 | C | 31 | E | 41 | G |
| 2 | B | 12 | C | 22 | C | 32 | D | 42 | E |
| 3 | A | 13 | B | 23 | D | 33 | D | 43 | N |
| 4 | B | 14 | C | 24 | E | 34 | C | 44 | O |
| 5 | B | 15 | B | 25 | A | 35 | B | 45 | M |
| 6 | D | 16 | E | 26 | A | 36 | B | 46 | J |
| 7 | E | 17 | G | 27 | E | 37 | C | 47 | G |
| 8 | E | 18 | A | 28 | E | 38 | E | 48 | M |
| 9 | C | 19 | A | 29 | A | 39 | A | 49 | D |
| 10 | C | 20 | E | 30 | C | 40 | H | 50 | L |

# Answers and Explanations

**1** **The answer is C** *Psychiatry*

The symptoms are suggestive of schizophrenia or schizophreniform disorder. In these disorders, the sudden onset of illness (choice **C**), especially with symptoms of agitation and psychosis, has a more favorable prognosis than an insidious onset.

A premorbid history of social withdrawal (choice **A**) is predictive of more severe and long-lasting psychopathology. A family history of schizophrenia (choice **B**) is commonly found in second-degree relatives and has little prognostic significance. Magnetic resonance imaging (MRI) changes (choice **D**) are associated with more severe symptoms and clinical course in schizophrenia. The presence of catatonic symptomatology (choice **E**) is not associated with any particular clinical course.

**2** **The answer is B** *Medicine*

Paroxysmal nocturnal hemolytic anemia (PNHA) (choice **B**) is a rare acquired form of hemolytic anemia. It is characterized by hemolysis that typically occurs during the night, resulting in excretion of early morning urine colored dark red by hemoglobin released from lysed red cells. The first symptoms may present at any age from infancy into the 80s, but it most frequently affects adults between 17 and 75 years old, with a mean age of presentation of 42 years. It is caused by the loss of membrane surface proteins due to an apparent mutation that inhibits the ability to synthesize glycosyl-phosphatidylinositol, which normally serves to anchor these surface proteins to the cell. The responsible gene is called phosphatidylinositol glycan class A (PIGA) and the mutations may be of several types, including frame shifts, point mutations, and deletions. This defect is believed to be a stem cell mutation because all cells in the hemopoietic line are affected; it is hypothesized that the mutations are caused by autoimmune reactions. The critical membrane proteins involved in PNHA symptomlogy normally react with members of the complement family, including those that normally act to impede the amplification of complement action; consequently, such a mutation acts to inhibit the normal dampening control in the complement cascade, permitting the action of complement to run amok and resulting in cell lysis. Because all hematopoietic cell lines are affected, symptoms extend beyond lysis of erythrocytes, causing a generalized pancytopenia that reduces the number of white cells and platelets, as well as causing an anemia. Thus, in addition to the anemia, thrombi often occur, particularly in large veins; these may cause severe disease, resulting in death. In theory, the ideal treatment is stem cell replacement; unfortunately, this process is not yet practical. Presently, treatment includes anticoagulants plus an anticomplement antibody called eculizumab. Use of this drug dramatically improves all almost all symptoms of PNHA.

Whenever anemia is found in a patient, it is important to ascertain whether the anemia is due to a disorder in the bone marrow, to hemolysis, or to loss of blood. A corrected reticulocyte count will help make the differentiation. The formula for a corrected reticulocyte count is the patient's reticulocyte count, multiplied by the patient's hematocrit, divided by the expected hematocrit. If the corrected reticulocyte count is below 2%, the most likely cause of anemia is decreased red blood cell production due to a hypoproliferative bone marrow. On the other hand, if the corrected reticulocyte count is greater than 3%, the most likely cause is hemolysis. In this patient, who has hemolytic anemia, it is important to establish if the etiology is due to an immune or a nonimmune disorder. This can be achieved by the Coombs test. The classic example of a drug-induced nonautoimmune hemolytic anemia (choice **A**) is a glucose-6 phosphate dehydrogenase deficiency. It can be ruled out in the case described because the onset of glucose-6 phosphate dehydrogenase deficiency is sudden and dependent upon ingestion of a drug, rather than a gradually worsening fatigue; moreover, the patient most likely would be African American or of Mediterranean descent. Paroxysmal cold hemoglobinuria (choice **C**) is a rare condition characterized by an abrupt onset of a severe hemolytic anemia and hemoglobinuria when a patient is exposed to cold temperatures. (The hemolysis usually occurs in a limb or digit exposed to a cold temperature.) Induction of this phenomenon involves the attachment of a foreign antibody to the red cell, which is promoted by the reduced temperature; hemolysis is then induced by activation of the complement system when cells are warmed. The phenomenon commonly manifests itself as a sudden transitory development induced by infections, usually a postviral episode. Before the advent of antibiotics, it was more commonly observed, often among patients suffering the tertiary stage of syphilis. Warm autoimmune hemolytic anemia (choice **D**) is the most common type of hemolytic anemia and is usually found in mature adults. In this condition, the patient's body makes auto-antibodies against their own red blood cells, and hemolysis occurs under warm conditions (i.e., normal body temperature). Diagnosis is generally made by the direct Coombs test. Acute intermittent porphyria (choice **E**) is a rare dominant disease caused by a deficiency of porphobilinogen deaminase. Insufficient activity of this enzyme leads to the accumulation of porphobilinogen in the cytoplasms of cells in various organs in the body. This accumulation may be influenced by various hormones and external stimuli, causing intermittent attacks. These attacks may include various digestive, muscular, or even mental aberrations and the voiding of a port wine–colored urine, which turns to purple when exposed to ultraviolet light for a period of time.

**3** **The answer is A** *Psychiatry*

Conversion disorder (choice **A**) is suggested by loss of motor control or sensory function that is not fully explained by physiologic mechanisms and is associated with psychologic conflict. Affected individuals often demonstrate an emotional blandness that is sometimes referred to as *la belle indifférence.*

Specific phobias (choice **B**), obsessive-compulsive disorder (choice **C**), and hypochondriasis (choice **D**) are often associated with anxiety. Melancholic depression (choice **E**) may be associated with decreased psychomotor activity.

**4** **The answer is B** *Preventive Medicine and Public Health*

The case-fatality rate expresses the probability of death from a disease over a specified period of time:

$$\text{Case-fatality rate} = \frac{\text{Number of deaths due to a disease per during a specified time period}}{\text{The number of new cases diagnosed during the same time period}} \times 100$$

In the situation described, the number of cases of meningitis diagnosed in 2010 was 200. Even though 11 deaths occurred from this group, the calculation is based only on the seven deaths that occurred during the year under consideration. Therefore, the answer is 7/200 × 100 (choice **B**).

Choice **A** (7 ÷ 11) × 100; choice **C** (200 ÷ 3,000) × 100; choice **D** [(200 − 11) ÷ 3,000] × 100; and choice **E** [(7 + 11) ÷ 11] × 100, do not represent the case-fatality rate.

**5** **The answer is B** *Psychiatry*

This description suggests schizophrenia. Many studies indicate that assertive community treatment (ACT) programs (choice **B**), which provide a wide variety of counseling, peer support, medication, and supported employment significantly improves social rehabilitation and recovery from disabling symptoms of illness. This standard of care supersedes older treatment methods that shielded the patient from social interaction (choice **A**) and focused primarily on symptom reduction, low stress, and minimally challenging environments. Such methods do not promote social rehabilitation. Animated and stressful discussions at dinner (choice **C**) or strong pressures to return to school or find a job (choice **D**) would likely increase stress and conflict and would tend to aggravate him. Keeping him home (choice **D**) is liable to subvert his social rehabilitation.

**6** **The answer is D** *Surgery*

This patient has a prolapsed intervertebral disk involving the L4–5 level (choice **D**). A herniated disk at this level will typically compress the fifth lumbar nerve root. The distribution of sensory deficit in such cases would be along the medial side of the leg and in the web space between the first and second toes. Since the fifth lumbar nerve root is required for effective dorsiflexion of the foot, weak dorsiflexion is to be expected, and is indeed noted on the vignette. These patients have difficulty standing on their heels. The initial management is conservative, bed rest, nonsteroidal analgesics, muscle relaxants, and physiotherapy usually fracture of the temporal bone. It may also occur in patients on anticoagulants or who have bleeding diathesis, but these patients usually have suprachoroid hemorrhage.

Choice **A** is incorrect; epidural hematoma is an acute event. This can result from trauma or in patients who have been on anticoagulants or have bleeding diathesis. The patients usually have sudden localized pain, which could result in cord compression. A computed tomographic (CT) scan will reveal the hemorrhage. Treatment is surgical decompression. Choice **B** is incorrect; a spinal cord astrocytoma is intradural and intramedullary in location. It usually affects people between the ages of 25 and 40. This is a slow-growing tumor that is associated with a long history of slowly progressive backache. The pain is usually localized, and in some cases may be radicular, namely spreading down along the path of a sensory nerve root. The tumor arises from the gray or white matter of the spinal cord. Pain is followed by motor weakness of the lower extremities, and sensory symptoms are usually the last to occur. Treatment is surgical resection. Choice **C** is incorrect; an epidural abscess is an acute event and is rare. The patient would have severe localized pain, and tenderness would be noted over the vertebral spine where the abscess is located. In addition, fever may be present. Radiculopathy is unusual. Treatment is surgical. Choice **E** is incorrect; an L5–S1 prolapsed intervertebral disk compresses the S1 nerve root. Such patients have pain along the lateral side of the leg and hypesthesia over this region and along the little toe. They also have difficulty with plantar flexion and standing on their toes. The ankle jerk is depressed or absent, as the S1 nerve root innervates it. The initial management is the same as that for a prolapsed L4–5 intervertebral disk.

**7** **The answer is E** *Pediatrics*

Rolling over from the prone to supine position usually does not occur until 4–6 months of age (choice **E**).

From the age of newborn (choice **A**) to 1 month, an infant (choice **B**) may be able to regard a face, respond to a bell, and have equal movements. In addition, a 1-month-old may follow to midline. Babbling and cooing occur by 2 months of age (choice **C**). The social smile also is present by this time. Lifting the head and chest occurs by 3 months of age (choice **D**). A 2-month-old infant can use the eyes well enough to follow an object through 180 degrees.

**8** **The answer is E** *Surgery*

The patient has deep venous insufficiency (choice **E**), as indicated by the history of venous symptoms stated in the vignette, including stasis dermatitis and superficial varicosities. Stasis dermatitis is a rusty discoloration of the skin, with or without ulceration, which usually is located behind the medial malleolus. Venous blood from the skin and superficial tissues that lie external to the deep fascia of the leg drains via perforators (communicating veins), into the deep veins in the calf and is then returned to the right atrium. When the calf muscles contract, valves prevent retrograde flow into the superficial system. Incompetence of the venous valves leads to retrograde flow, increased venous pressure in the dorsal vein of the foot, and ensuing changes to the skin around the ankle. Persistently elevated venous pressure leads to capillary leakage. As a result, blood and fibrin is deposited in surrounding tissues. Breakdown of blood into hemosiderin leads to pigmentation of the skin, while fibrin deposition around capillaries leads to the formation of a barrier. Ischemia predisposes to ulceration of the skin. Finally, the retrograde blood flow from the deep to the superficial venous system causes varicosities as well.

Choice **A** is incorrect; superficial thrombophlebitis presents with pain and erythema along the course of the superficial saphenous vein. Fever may be present. It is not associated with stasis dermatitis. Superficial thrombophlebitis may occur spontaneously in polycythemia or polyarthritis, or may herald the presence of a visceral tumor, such as carcinoma of the pancreas. The condition is known as thrombophlebitis migrans. Choice **B** is incorrect; in embolic disease, the history would suggest an embolus to the lungs and physical findings suggestive of deep venous thrombosis. Deep vein thrombosis may be asymptomatic, presenting as pulmonary embolus, or it may be symptomatic. In the latter case, the patient will have low-grade fever, pain, swelling, redness, and dilated superficial veins. Stasis dermatitis is not a feature. Choice **C** is incorrect; arterial insufficiency is not associated with stasis dermatitis. However, varicose veins may coexist in patients with arterial insufficiency. The presence of normal arterial pulses and the lack of claudication pain that is characteristic of arterial insufficiency rules out this diagnosis. Choice **D** is incorrect; rheumatoid arthritis is three times more common in women than in men. Rheumatoid arthritis may be associated with vasculitis. However, varicosities, or stasis dermatitis, are absent. Furthermore, the patient would have evidence of joint involvement, which is absent in the case described.

**9** **The answer is C** *Obstetrics and Gynecology*

A good menstrual history is essential for calculating the estimated due date. Nägele's rule is a convenient method that uses the last menstrual period to calculate an estimated due date. Assuming a 28-day menstrual cycle, 3 months are subtracted from, and 7 days are added to, the date of the last normal menstrual period. This would result in an estimated due date of March 17 (choice **B**). However, adjustments must be made for cycles that are longer or shorter than 28 days. In the given scenario, the cycle length was 4 days over 28 days; therefore, ovulation took place 4 days later than the usual day 14, thus moving the due date 4 days forward. Instead of subtracting 3 months and adding 7 days, in this case one would need to subtract 3 months and add 11 days, thus yielding an estimated due date of March 21 (choice **C**). March 12 (choice **A**), November 13 (choice **D**), and November 17 (choice **E**) are therefore incorrect.

**10** **The answer is C** *Surgery*

The patient has acute diverticulitis (choice **C**). Herniation of the colonic mucosa through the circular muscles of the colon leads to the formation of diverticula. In the United States, about 95% of these are located in the sigmoid colon, but among Koreans, Japanese, Chinese, and Malaysians, they are twice as likely to form in the ascending colon. In some severely affected individuals, the entire colon may be involved; however, diverticula are not found in the rectum because it has a complete circular layer of muscle. Diverticula usually form due to a lack of roughage in the diet. The high fiber content of typical African and Indian diets makes diverticular disease a rarity in these cultures. When one or more diverticula get inflamed, the term *diverticulitis* applies. The clinical presentation in diverticulitis is similar to that of acute appendicitis, except that it is on the left side. Pyrexia, malaise, and leukocytosis are features. Sometimes a tender mass may be palpable on rectal examination. Presence of urinary symptoms, such as dysuria, may be a forerunner to the formation of a vesicocolic fistula. In such cases, the patient would develop pneumaturia and pass flatus or even fecal material in the urine. The diagnosis is made on clinical grounds. Computed tomography (CT) confirms the diagnosis and also delineates associated pericolic abscesses. Although very mild cases may be treated at home with oral antibiotics and a liquid diet, more commonly, acute diverticulitis is treated in a hospital setting with intravenous antibiotics, a combination of cefuroxime and metronidazole. Once the acute attack has resolved, a barium enema and flexible sigmoidoscopy or colonoscopy should be performed. Doing so in the acute phase could result in perforation and peritonitis. Surgery is indicated in approximately 10% of patients. Such surgery is performed during a quiescent period after careful bowel preparation; it consists of a one-stage resection and end-to-end anastomosis. If there is bowel obstruction, a Hartmann's procedure is performed. If the patient has fecal peritonitis, the options include primary resection and Hartmann's procedure or, in rare cases, primary resection and anastomosis.

Choice **A** is incorrect; ulcerative colitis is a nonspecific inflammatory disease that usually affects adults between the ages of 20 and 40. Both sexes are equally affected. In approximately 95% of cases, it commences in the rectum and spreads proximally. In chronic cases, pseudopolyps occur (chronic inflammatory polyps). The sine qua non of this disease is bloody diarrhea and rectal discharge that may be blood-stained or foul smelling. Pain is not an early symptom of the disease. The disease is characterized by exacerbations and remissions. In severe cases, mild-grade fever, tachycardia, and hypoalbuminemia could occur. Other complications include toxic megacolon, perforation, and rarely, severe hemorrhage. Carcinoma can occur in those who develop the disease early in life or if the malady involves the whole colon. Colonoscopy and biopsy have an important role to play in the diagnosis of ulcerative colitis. Choice **B** is incorrect. Irritable bowel syndrome (IBS) is the most common gastrointestinal disease seen in clinical practice. It usually begins before the age of 30. Women are twice as likely to suffer from it as are men. Patients with IBS may have psychiatric disorders such as hysteria, obsessive-compulsive disorder, and depression. There are three types of presentation: (a) chronic abdominal pain and constipation (spastic colon), (b) alternating constipation and diarrhea, and (c) chronic painless diarrhea. The patients may also complain of abdominal distention, a feeling of incomplete evacuation, and relief of abdominal pain with evacuation. The diagnosis is based on the Rome criteria and is one of exclusion. Barium enema and colonoscopy are required to exclude inflammatory or neoplastic disease. Treatment includes a high-fiber diet, psyllium extract, and anticholinergics. Psychiatric consultation is indicated in appropriate cases. Choice **D** is incorrect; carcinoma of the colon is most commonly seen on the left side. It is usually of the stenosing type. Thus, the predominant symptoms are that of progressive intestinal obstruction. In approximately 15% of cases, diverticular disease and colon carcinoma coexist. Loss of weight, positive occult blood test result, and a falling hematocrit should raise concerns about this possibility. Additional features include change in bowel habit, such as alternating constipation and diarrhea, colicky pain, and tenesmus (need for evacuation), especially if the tumor is located low in the descending colon. In the latter case, patients may pass blood and mucus, mucus being more common in the morning. If a mass is felt on rectal examination, it will not be tender. Double-contrast barium enema is carried out in patients who have such altered bowel habits, and colonoscopy is indicated in those who have bleeding per rectum. Ultrasonography is used to exclude the presence of hepatic metastases, while CT is indicated in patients who have large palpable masses in the abdomen. Choice **E** also is incorrect; ischemic colitis results from paucity of blood flow to the colon. The most common location is at the splenic flexure. The patient is usually in the sixth decade of life and has degenerative vascular disease. Rectal bleeding and infrequent colicky abdominal pain and vomiting may precede a dramatic onset. Pain may occur several hours after a meal. The onset is usually abrupt, with severe lower abdominal pain, vomiting, fever, and bleeding per rectum. Tenderness and guarding of the abdomen will be noted, and bowel sounds may be decreased. An arteriogram confirms the diagnosis. Most cases resolve spontaneously. Treatment is supportive. Some of these patients could develop strictures that would require surgery.

## 11 The answer is E *Medicine*

An acoustic schwannoma (choice **E**) is associated with tinnitus, nausea and vomiting, vertigo, nystagmus, and eighth-nerve deafness. It arises in the cerebellopontine angle and may involve the trigeminal nerve, producing ipsilateral sensory changes in the face. It is most commonly a schwannoma a benign —which is a benign, encapsulated tumor arising from Schwann cells. Patients with neurofibromatosis have an increased incidence of acoustic schwannomas.

Untreated mastoiditis (choice **A**) that erodes through bone to produce acoustic nerve damage is rare. Cerebellar tumors (choice **B**) and vertebrobasilar artery insufficiency (choice **C**) produce ataxia. Furthermore, they are not usually associated with eighth-nerve damage. A glioblastoma multiforme (choice **D**) is the most common primary malignancy of the brain in adults and usually involves the frontal lobes. It would not be expected to produce eighth-nerve damage.

## 12 The answer is C *Pediatrics*

Chlamydial pneumonia (choice **C**) in infants characteristically presents at 3–16 weeks of age. Typically, the infants appear quite well, are afebrile, but have been ill with tachypnea and a repetitive staccato cough. Rales, and sometimes wheezing, can be heard. Conjunctivitis is present in approximately 50% of patients. Hyperinflation and patchy infiltrates are seen on chest x-ray films, and eosinophilia ($>400$ cells/mm$^3$) is apparent upon a complete blood count (CBC).

Respiratory syncytial virus (RSV) pneumonia (choice **A**) may present with temperature instability, respiratory distress, wheezing, apnea, clear nasal discharge, and poor feeding. Bronchiolitis (choice **B**) causes inflammation of the bronchioles with narrowing of the bronchial diameter. It is a viral disease caused by RSV in 50% of cases, but also by *Mycoplasma*, parainfluenza viruses, adenoviruses, and other viruses. It manifests with low-grade fever, tachypnea, nasal flaring, rales, and expiratory wheezing. Chest radiography shows hyperinflation or atelectasis without infiltration. Cystic fibrosis (choice **D**) commonly presents as respiratory insufficiency with cough, dyspnea, bronchiectasis, and pulmonary fibrosis. The affected child also shows signs of malabsorption and failure to thrive. The larval stage of ascariasis (choice **E**) is asymptomatic. However, if a large parasite load penetrates the lungs, it may manifest with cough, hematemesis, eosinophilia, and pulmonary infiltrates.

## 13 The Answer is B *Medicine*

This patient has pernicious anemia due to vitamin B$_{12}$ deficiency. In younger patients such as this, the most common cause of pernicious anemia is an autoimmune reaction in which antibodies destroy the stomach's parietal cells, which normally manufacture intrinsic factor. Intrinsic factor is required for B$_{12}$ absorption in the terminal ileum. As in this case, patients may have glossitis, as well as neurological symptoms such as tingling in the fingers, loss of vibration and position sense, and in extreme cases, dementia. Other causes of B$_{12}$ deficiency anemia in include inadequate dietary intake of vitamin B$_{12}$, alcoholism, partial gastrectomy, malabsorption syndromes, Crohn's disease, and infestation with the fish tape worm (*Diphyllobothrium latum*), which is present in fresh water fish in the northern hemisphere. Antiparietal cell antibodies will be present in autoimmune cases of pernicious anemia. In the presence of macrocytic anemia, it is important to check both B$_{12}$ and folate levels, as folic acid deficiency could lead to macrocytic anemia as well. Red blood cell folate level is more accurate than serum folate level. Whether a macrocytic anemia is due to lack of B$_{12}$ or folic acid can be resolved by ascertaining the levels of serum methylmalonic acid and homocysteine. Both levels are increased in B$_{12}$ deficiency, but in the case of folic acid deficiency, only homocysteine levels are elevated. Methylmalonic acid is an intermediate in fatty acid metabolism that is derived from malonate, while homocysteine, an amino acid not found in diet, is derived from methionine. It is involved in the metabolism of cysteine. A Schilling test will distinguish between nutritional or absorptive cause of macrocytic anemia. Conversely, it is also possible that high intake of folate will prevent signs of a macrocytic anemia even if a patient has a vitamin B$_{12}$ deficiency. Thus, one should pay careful attention to neurological symptoms that may be the only sign of a vitamin B$_{12}$ deficiency and could easily be overlooked; unfortunately, these may in the long run cause severe permanent neurological damage, including psychological aberrations.

Microcytic anemia (choice **A**) is seen in iron deficiency that can result from inadequate intake or absorption of iron, or excessive blood loss, with the most common cause being inadequate intake. Clinical features include cheilosis, in which the lips are cracked at the angles of the mouth, dysphagia, brittle nails, and in extreme cases, koilonychia, also known as spooning of the nails. Thalassemia (choice **C**) is the most common genetic disorder worldwide. It is due to abnormal hemoglobin. Mature hemoglobin is a tetramer of two α and two β chains. If there is an aberration in this combination, interaction with oxygen will result in precipitation of hemoglobin and destruction of the abnormal red blood cell by the spleen, with resultant hemolytic anemia. Patients will have microcytic hypochromic red blood cells in the peripheral smear. Thalassemia can affect either the α or β chains, hence hemoglobin electrophoresis is required to uncover the malady. Sideroblastic anemia (choice **D**) is usually an acquired form of anemia in which there is an inability to incorporate heme into protoporphyrin to create hemoglobin. Causes include myelodysplasia, which may progress to acute leukemia; chronic alcoholism; and lead poisoning. Patients have mild to moderate anemia, and usually present with fatigue. Mean corpuscular volume (MCV) is usually normal. In some instances, it may be decreased, causing confusion with iron deficiency anemia. The distinction can be made by the peripheral blood smear, which shows two kinds of red blood cell populations, some normal and others hypochromic. In addition, iron stores are increased due to the primary anomaly, which is that heme cannot be adequately utilized. The diagnosis is best made by examining the bone marrow, which will reveal ineffective erythropoiesis as noted by the presence of marked erythroid hyperplasia, increased iron stores, and the presence of ringed sideroblasts. The serum iron and transferrin saturation will be markedly elevated, and iron may be deposited in mitochondria as well. Sideroblastic anemia due to lead poisoning will reveal basophil stippling in the red blood cells and elevated lead levels in the serum. Anemia of chronic disease (choice **E**), as the name suggests, occurs in chronic systemic disorders such as infection, inflammation, hepatic disease, and malignancy. Chronic renal failure is also a notable cause. In cases other than chronic renal failure, anemia results from reduced red cell survival rate, and the inability of the bone marrow to step up production as iron is stashed away in the reticuloendothelial system where it has been delivered by haptoglobin. In chronic renal failure, on the other hand, anemia is due to inadequate production of erythropoietin, which is essential to prime the bone marrow to produce red blood cells. The diagnosis of anemia of chronic disease is confirmed by the presence of low serum iron, low total iron binding capacity, and normal or elevated levels of ferritin, and in the case of anemia of chronic disease, low erythropoietin levels.

### 14 The answer is C  *Pediatrics*

The patient is a toddler and at risk for accidental ingestion. Imipramine (choice **C**) is an antidepressant sometimes used to treat nocturnal enuresis. Children who have ingested tricyclic antidepressants primarily present with status epilepticus, coma, and dysrhythmias.

Seizures may also be associated with shaken baby syndrome (choice **A**), but retinal hemorrhages are usually noted on physical examination. Congenital heart disease (choice **D**) usually manifests itself earlier than 2 years of age. Febrile seizures (choice **E**) are associated with a rapid rise in temperature and usually develop when the core temperature reaches 39.0°C (102.2°F) or above. This patient is afebrile. Although meningitis (choice **B**) should be included in the differential diagnosis of a lethargic child, it is less likely given the fact that the child presents with symptoms associated with tricyclic antidepressant ingestion, and the child's brother is a bed wetter.

### 15 The answer is B  *Surgery*

The patient has volvulus of the sigmoid colon (choice **B**). Volvulus is a twisting of the bowel around the mesenteric root. It is most common in the sigmoid colon (65%) and is most often seen in the elderly population. Obstruction and strangulation with infarction are potential sequelae. Clinical signs include colicky abdominal pain, abdominal distention, and vomiting. In sigmoid volvulus, there is a single dilated loop of bowel resembling a "coffee bean" rising up out of the pelvis. The concavity of the coffee bean points toward the left lower quadrant. Barium studies reveal a "bird's beak" or "ace of spades" appearance, with the lumen of the bowel tapering toward the volvulus. A volvulus can frequently be decompressed with a flexible colonoscope, but it often recurs. If it cannot be decompressed, then surgery should be performed with resection of the redundant bowel.

Intussusception (choice **A**) is uncommon in adults. It refers to the telescoping of one segment of proximal bowel into the distal bowel. In adults, it commonly results from an underlying mucosal lesion that serves as the nidus for the intussusception, producing obstruction and strangulation of the bowel. Bloody diarrhea and a palpable mass are usually present. Toxic megacolon (choice **C**) is associated primarily with ulcerative colitis. The diameter of the descending colon exceeds 6 cm. Perforation is a common complication. The patient does not have a history compatible with ulcerative colitis (e.g., intermittent bouts of bloody diarrhea). Ogilvie syndrome (choice **D**) is a pseudo-obstruction of the ascending colon in elderly persons. There is a sudden, massive distention of the colon without pain or tenderness. The right colon is distended with a cutoff at the splenic flexure. Barium studies are negative for obstruction. An impacted stool (choice **E**) would not likely result in complete obstruction.

### 16 The answer is E *Surgery*

Two parameters are taken into account when dealing with cancers of the colon. The first, judged histologically, is the grade: Are they well differentiated or not (the less anaplastic the cells, the lower the grade)? The second parameter is stage, the depth of penetration and degree of invasion by the tumor: the smaller the depth of penetration and the less the evidence of metastatic activity, the lower the stage. Although both parameters are used to establish treatment and prognosis, staging is the more important factor for patient prognosis, because it describes the size of the tumor and whether it has metastasized to lymph nodes or further on. In the case described, the microscopic appearance described in the pathology report indicates a high-grade colon cancer: the cells are bereft of mucin and glands and appear to be undifferentiated (i.e., it is anaplastic). Colorectal cancers are commonly staged by use of the modified Dukes' staging system as summarized in the table below.

**Dukes' Staging System for Colorectal Cancer**

| Stage | Description Survival Rate | |
|-------|--------------------------|------|
| A | Tumor limited to mucosa and submucosa | 80% |
| B1 | Tumor into, but not through, muscle wall; no lymph node or distant involvement | 60% |
| B2 | Tumor penetrates entire wall; no lymph nodes involved | 55% |
| C1 | Tumor into, but not through, muscle wall; lymph node involvement | 30% |
| C2 | Tumor penetrates entire wall; lymph node involvement | 20% |
| D | Distant metastasis; any level of invasion; may or may not be lymph node involvement | <5% |

Note that the key difference between stages B and C is lymph node involvement and that the key criterion for stage D is distant metastasis.

According to this system, the cancer described belongs to modified Dukes' stage C2, because it has penetrated the muscle wall, infiltrated the serosa, and involved the lymph nodes, but has not undergone distal metastasis. Accordingly, the most probable prognosis is that the patient has a 20% chance of surviving an additional 5 years (choice **E**). That this tumor is also anaplastic (high grade) does not improve his chances. The overall average 5-year survival rate for colorectal cancer is 35%; obviously, the earlier the diagnosis, the better the prognosis.

The tumor was not limited to mucosa and submucosa; as a consequence choice **A** is incorrect. The tumor did penetrate the muscle wall and did involve lymph nodes, thus choice **B** is wrong. Choice **C** is incorrect because lymph nodes are involved. Choice **D** is wrong because the cancer did penetrate the wall, and choice **F** is erroneous because there is no evidence of distant metastasis.

### 17 The answer is G *Medicine*

This man is suffering from early parkinsonism. Most commonly, this is due to Parkinson disease, a condition of unknown etiology that generally starts between the ages of 45 and 65. Parkinson disease is a heterogenous and progressive condition that has tremor, rigidity, bradykinesia, and postural instability as its cardinal features. Cases tend to fall into one of two major subtypes. In one group, tremor is the major symptom; in the other, postural instability and gait difficulty predominate. Even though symptoms do overlap, most patients clearly fall to the greatest extent into one or the other subcategory. Patients with predominantly tremor-type symptoms tend to have a slower progression of symptoms, have less trouble with bradykinesis, and less often develop severe mental symptoms. Other symptoms in more advanced cases include infrequent blinking, a blank stare, a shuffling gait with rapid acceleration and difficulty stopping once started, increased salivation, and severe depression or even dementia. No one patient needs to develop all symptoms to meet the diagnostic criteria, and patients who have early symptoms of gait disturbances progress more rapidly and are more apt to develop the more severe symptoms. The underlying pathology is dopamine depletion due to degeneration of the nigrostriatal system. This leads to an imbalance between acetylcholine and dopamine neurotransmission. The cornerstone of treatment is dopamine replacement coupled to blockage of the acetylcholine system. Unfortunately, resistance to ceratin key drugs develops with use. Therefore, an attempt is made to refrain from using them as long as possible. Thus, watchful waiting (choice **G**) is typically used until symptoms interfere with the patient's normal lifestyle. This patient clearly states that his tremor does not impinge upon his normal lifestyle.

Once it is decided that some medical intervention will be of value, amantadine (choice **A**) is typically the first drug to be used while symptoms are still minimal. This antiviral drug helps to improve muscle control and reduce stiffness; its mode of action is not understood, but it is hypothesized to help release dopamine from nerve endings. Its effect is always less than profound, and the benefit further decreases with use. Anticholinergics (choice **B**) also are used to treat early parkinsonism, sometimes in conjunction with amantadine. Again, drug resistance develops, and these drugs are generally administered in increasing doses until the adverse effects outweigh the benefits. Thus, eventually, it becomes necessary to use the most effective treatment—namely, dopamine replacement. However, dopamine cannot cross the blood–brain barrier. Consequently, it is usually administered as Sinemet, a preparation that contains levodopa (choice **C**) and carbidopa (choice **D**) in fixed proportions. The levodopa is converted to dopamine in the body, and the carbidopa inhibits the enzyme that converts levodopa to dopamine. But carbidopa cannot cross the blood–brain barrier; thus, by administering the two together there is both more levodopa available, and some of the adverse peripheral effects of dopamine—such as nausea, vomiting, hypotension, and cardiac irregularities—are avoided. Long-term administration of levodopa induces untoward central nervous system effects including dyskinesias, restlessness, confusion, and behavioral changes. Still later during therapy, the so-called on–off phenomena may occur, in which severity of parkinsonism may quickly increase at any time of the day. Dopamine agonists (choice **E**) that act directly on dopamine receptors were once only used to reduce the symptoms associated with this on–off action associated with long-term levodopa use. However, with the advent of newer dopamine agonists that are not derived from ergot, such agonists are now used to help treat early Parkinson disease and to keep the levodopa dose (via Sinemet) at a minimal level as long as possible. Selegiline (choice **F**) is an irreversible monoamine oxidase B (MAO-B) inhibitor. MAO-B selectively deaminates dopamine and phenethylamine (chocolate's amphetamine). Selegiline is sometimes used as an adjunct treatment, with the idea of reducing symptom fluctuations associated with long-term levodopa therapy. During the past decade, an ever-increasing number of otherwise refractory patients have been treated with *deep brain stimulation*, which has proven to be a relatively safe and effective treatment for the involuntary movements associated with Parkinson disease.

### 18 The answer is A *Obstetrics and Gynecology*

Urinary stress incontinence is an anatomic problem that develops when the proximal urethra and bladder neck drop below the pelvic floor because of lack of support due to pelvic relaxation. The increase in intraabdominal pressure is transmitted more to the bladder than to the urethra, resulting in involuntary urine loss with laughing, coughing, or sneezing. This condition may be associated with a cystocele (choice **A**), the bulging of the bladder into the upper anterior vaginal wall. However, the incontinence is not caused by the cystocele itself.

A urethral diverticulum (choice **B**) is a localized outpouching of the urethra into the anterior vaginal wall; it is diagnosed via urethroscopy. Although it causes increased urinary frequency it does not lead to stress leakage. Rectocele (choice **D**) is associated with bulging of the posterior vaginal wall. Enterocele (choice **E**) is herniation of the pouch of Douglas into the upper posterior vaginal wall. Gartner's duct cysts (choice **C**) are found in the lateral vaginal wall and are remnants of the embryologic mesonephric duct.

### 19 The answer is A *Pediatrics*

The mother has systemic lupus erythematosus (SLE). Neonatal lupus syndrome consists of rash, thrombocytopenia, and congenital heart block. Liver disease, hemolytic anemia, and leukopenia occur less frequently. Maternal SLE is the most common cause of congenital complete heart block (choice **A**) in the newborn. Injury is caused by maternal immunoglobulin G (IgG). The exact mechanism of damage is unknown. Most infants with congenital heart block have mothers with antibodies to Ro/SSA or La/SSB. The heart damage may be permanent.

Coarctation of the aorta (choice **B**), open neural tube defects (choice **C**), microcephaly (choice **D**), and polycystic kidney disease (choice **E**) have not been associated with SLE.

### 20 The Answer is E *Medicine*

This patient has cataracts (choice **E**). Although cataracts can be congenital or acquired (due to diseases like diabetes mellitus or from medications such as long-term steroids), they most commonly occur with advancing age as "senile cataracts" (by the age of 80 years most person have had cataracts or at least precataract changes in their lens). Cataracts may be central or peripherally located (i.e., nuclear or cortical). Patients complain of a gradual loss of vision, blurred vision, and difficulty in driving a car at night, as in this case.

Some of them will state that they have a problem with perceiving colors, while others may state that their vision has improved such that they require reading glasses with less power. This is often called "second sight," and results from a nuclear cataract. On the other hand, patients who develop posterior subcapsular cataract will complain of deterioration in near vision. Although cataracts are often perceived as an advent normally associated with aging, they are due to denaturation of proteins in the lens; depending upon the major protein affected, they may be hard or soft, partial or more complete, unchanging or progressive. Additionally, any action or substance that promotes protein denaturation will accelerate cataract formation. Treatment is surgery, in which the old lens is removed and is replaced by a plastic one.

Retinal detachment (choice **A**) presents as a sudden loss of vision, which is not the presentation in this case. Age-related macular degeneration (choice **B**) is associated with progressive loss of central vision, which can appear gradually or suddenly. Although diabetes can promote diabetic retinopathy (choice **C**) that may lead to deteriorating vision culminating in blindness, glare halos from headlights or light fixtures are not a feature. Hypertensive retinopathy (choice **D**) is associated with deteriorating vision, but once again, halos caused by glare from bright lights are not a feature.

### 21 **The answer is C** *Psychiatry*

The construction apraxia seen in this patient is associated with damage to the nondominant parietal lobe (choice **C**).

Damage to the nondominant frontal and temporal lobes (choices **A** and **B**) is associated with problems of mood, orientation, concentration, and memory. Damage to the dominant temporal lobe (choice **D**) is associated with receptive (Wernicke's) aphasia. Damage to the dominant frontal lobe (choice **E**) is associated with expressive (Broca's) aphasia.

### 22 **The answer is C** *Pediatrics*

The abnormality in classical maple syrup urine disease (MSUD) (choice **C**) is a deficiency of branched chain α-keto dehydrogenase, the enzyme responsible for decarboxylation the three branched-chain amino acids (B-CAAs): leucine, isoleucine, and valine. It is characterized by the presence of high concentrations of the B-CAAs in urine. Screening is accomplished by the addition of 2,4-dinitrophenylhydrazine (DNPH) to a sample of urine, which will cause the ketoacids of the B-CAAs to precipitate. Additionally, the urine, skin, or hair has a characteristic smell of maple syrup or caramel. Infants present with symptoms 3–5 days after birth; these include feeding difficulties, hypoglycemia, seizures, opisthotonos, and muscular rigidity with or without intermittent flaccidity. Cortical atrophy is seen on computed tomography (CT) or magnetic resonance imaging (MRI) scans. Dietary management of intake of branched-chain amino acids is the cornerstone of therapy. However, most patients with the classical form of the disease have already suffered permanent brain damage by the time diagnosis is made and treatment is initiated. Some patients have less severe variants.

Neonatal seizures (choice **B**) are a disorder of the central nervous system (CNS) that suggests hypoxic ischemic encephalopathy resulting from asphyxia, intracranial hemorrhage, hypoglycemia, infarction, or meningitis. Bruising and retinal hemorrhages might be seen if the patient had been a victim of trauma (choice **D**). Phenylketonuria (PKU; choice **E**) results from a defect in the metabolism of the amino acid phenylalanine. The infant is normal at birth, but gradually develops mental retardation. Vomiting may be an early symptom of PKU. Children with PKU are fair skinned and have eczematous rash. Some will develop a seizure disorder. A newborn with sepsis (choice **A**) may have vomiting, poor feeding, and hypoglycemia, but the fact that this patient has a distinct odor to the urine, acidosis, no response to glucose, and bouts of flaccidity and opisthotonos makes MSUD the best answer.

### 23 **The answer is D** *Preventive Medicine and Public Health*

According to the National Vital Statistics Report, April 17, 2009, during 2006, there were 2,426,264 deaths in the United States. This amounts to a death rate of 810.4 per 100,000 people with a life expectancy of 77.7 years. (Infant mortality was 6.69 deaths per 1,000 live births). The number of deaths for the ten leading causes of death in the United States across all age groups in descending order is:

- Heart disease: 631,636
- Cancer: 559,888
- Stroke (cerebrovascular diseases): 137,119
- Chronic lower respiratory diseases: 124,583

- Accidents (unintentional injuries): 121,599
- Diabetes: 72,449
- Alzheimer disease: 72,432
- Influenza and pneumonia: 56,326
- Nephritis, nephrotic syndrome, and nephrosis: 45,344
- Septicemia: 34,234

These data indicate that heart disease (choice **D**) once again has become the leading cause of death, surpassing cancer, which was the leader in 2005.

Choices **A** and **C** include acquired immune deficiency syndrome (AIDS), which no longer is included in the ten leading causes of death across age groups in the United States. Choices **B**, **E**, and **F** list the leading causes of death, but in the wrong order.

### 24 The answer is E *Psychiatry*

This case is most consistent with schizoid personality disorder (choice **E**), characterized by emotional aloofness, indifference to praise or criticism, and the absence of any bizarre or idiosyncratic thinking.

Individuals with schizotypal personality disorder (choice **A**) are often withdrawn and aloof, but they also demonstrate peculiar thinking. Paranoid personality disorder (choice **B**) is characterized by unwarranted suspiciousness. Narcissistic personality disorder (choice **C**) involves disdain for most people, but extreme idealization or denigration of a few. Avoidant personality disorder (choice **D**) implies that the individual has a need for human contact and feels lonely.

### 25 The answer is A *Pediatrics*

Erythema infectiosum (choice **A**; also known as Fifth disease) is a mild exanthematous disease caused by parvovirus B19. Usually, there is no prodrome, and fever is low-grade or absent. The rash usually starts on the cheeks, which appear to have been slapped. Following the bright-red and confluent rash, an erythematous maculopapular rash appears on the trunk, although it can precede the facial rash. The rash then fades, giving a lacy or reticular appearance. The rash is often pruritic, but does not desquamate, as seen with measles. Other symptoms include headache, rhinitis, and arthralgia, but these symptoms are more common in adults.

In most cases, roseola (choice **B**) is caused by herpesvirus 6. Children with roseola present with the differential diagnosis of a fever of unknown origin until the temperature drops precipitously and the rash appears. The rash is maculopapular and nonpruritic, and it blanches on pressure. It first appears on the trunk and spreads to the arms and neck (mild on legs and face). Rubella (also known as German measles; choice **C**), or three-day measles, is another viral exanthematous disease of children and adults, with worldwide distribution. The signs and symptoms include adenopathy (posterior auricular), low-grade fever, arthralgias, coryza, and conjunctivitis. The exanthem is descending, beginning on the face or neck and spreading in hours to the trunk and extremities. The lesions are maculopapular and may desquamate. The rash fades in 24–48 hours. Measles (choice **D**) is a highly contagious viral infection transmitted by respiratory droplets. Prodromal symptoms include brassy cough, coryza, conjunctivitis, and fever. Koplik's spots (grayish white spots with a red halo) appear on the buccal mucous membrane 24–48 hours before the rash. The rash begins on the face and ears and spreads to the trunk and extremities in 24–36 hours. The lesion is maculopapular and may become confluent on the face and body (a distinct characteristic of measles). Scarlet fever (choice **E**) is an upper respiratory infection associated with a characteristic diffuse maculopapular "sandpaper"-type rash and group A streptococcal pharyngitis. The face is usually spared, but the cheeks may be erythematous and the area around the mouth spared. Pastia's lines (prominence of the rash in the creases of the elbow, axillae, and groin) and strawberry tongue (in which the tongue is coated and the papillae may be swollen and reddened) are also associated with scarlet fever.

### 26 The answer is A *Surgery*

This patient has the classic symptoms of hypovolemic shock, namely, hypotension, tachycardia, tachypnea, oliguria, and peripheral vasoconstriction resulting in cold clammy skin. Hemoperitoneum (choice **A**; i.e., intraabdominal hemorrhage) is the most common cause of shock in the first 24 hours following abdominal surgery. The most likely cause is a slipped ligature from an artery, for example, the cystic artery. The hematocrit will not fall until several hours after the primary event. Management involves restoration of blood volume and immediate surgical intervention to secure the vessel and arrest the hemorrhage.

Gram-negative sepsis (choice **B**) results in endotoxic shock. Toxins released by gram-negative bacteria lead to vasodilatation of blood vessels. As a result, the patient would have a bounding pulse and warm skin. Other features include high fever and hypotension. Acute myocardial infarction (choice **C**) is associated with chest pain. Cardiogenic shock could result from a massive myocardial infarction. In that case, the patient would have hypotension, tachycardia, and a weak pulse. The skin would not be warm, and fever, if present, would be low grade. Pulmonary embolus (choice **D**) usually presents several days after surgery. It is seen in patients who have been lying immobile for a few days in bed and then develop deep vein thrombosis. There may be calf swelling and tenderness, but pulmonary embolus without clinical symptoms of deep venous thrombosis has been known to occur. The patient would have sudden chest pain, hemoptysis, hypotension, and tachycardia. A pneumothorax (choice **E**) is associated with stabbing chest pain, tachypnea, tachycardia, and, in the case of tension pneumothorax, hypotension. Physical findings will include absent breath sounds, hyperresonance to percussion, and a tracheal shift to the contralateral side. This could follow insertion of a line into the subclavian vein.

### 27 The Answer is E   *Medicine*

This patient has cirrhosis of the liver with portal hypertension. The expanding waist line is due to ascites, while swollen feet cause him to have difficulty in putting on his shoes. He has breast enlargement (gynecomastia) because the small amount of estrogen normally present in a male could not be metabolized by the failing liver. Other features would include palmar erythema and spider nevi. In the United States, the most common cause of liver cirrhosis is chronic hepatitis C (choice **E**). Approximately 20% of patients with chronic hepatitis C will end up with cirrhosis around 20 years after infection. Hepatitis C is most commonly transmitted via IV drug use. Other modes of transmission include sex, snorting cocaine, body piercing, tattoos, hemodialysis, blood transfusion, and upon occasion, an accidental finger stick by a laboratory worker. Unfortunately, there is no vaccine against hepatitis C, and the number of cases that would result in mortality and development of hepatocellular carcinoma is expected to increase threefold within the next one or two decades.

Choice **A** medication is incorrect. Drugs such as isoniazid can induce hepatitis, but this is not very common, and nor is it common for medication-induced hepatitis to lead to cirrhosis. Alcoholic hepatitis (choice **B**) is a major problem, but a conforming Seventh-Day Adventist is not likely to be an alcoholic. Moreover, not all alcoholics with hepatitis develop cirrhosis of the liver. The incidence of chronic alcoholics who end up with cirrhosis of the liver is in the range of 10%–15%. Hepatitis A (choice **C**) is transmitted from the fecal–oral route and usually resolves spontaneously. Chronic hepatitis and cirrhosis does not occur, and immunization is available. Hepatitis B (choice **D**) can lead to cirrhosis of the liver, but the incidence is not as great as it is for hepatis C, and immunization against it is available.

### 28 The answer is E   *Pediatrics*

The symptoms in this patient clearly describe a case of measles. Otitis media (choice **E**) is the most common complication of measles.

Because of mesenteric node involvement, diffuse lymphadenopathy can cause abdominal pain mimicking appendicitis (choice **A**). Subacute sclerosing panencephalitis (choice **B**) is a rare neurologic complication, with fewer than five new cases per year registered with the U.S. National Sub-Acute Sclerosing Panencephalitis (SSPE) Registry each year since 1982. Interstitial pneumonia (choice **C**) is caused by the measles virus itself and is more common in immunocompromised patients. Bronchopneumonia is more common than interstitial pneumonia and is usually caused by pneumococcus, group A *Streptococcus*, *Staphylococcus aureus*, or *Haemophilus influenzae* type b. Myocarditis (choice **D**) is a rare but serious complication of measles.

### 29 The answer is A   *Obstetrics and Gynecology*

The classification of female bony pelvis types is based on the work of Caldwell and Moloy, who examined large numbers of x-ray pelvimetry films. These procedures hark back to the days when radiographs of the pelvis were obtained in cases of protracted labors. The pelvis described in this question is characteristic of the gynecoid shape (choice **A**). It is the most common shape, occurring in approximately 50% of women. The dimensions of the gynecoid shape allow optimal use of the pelvic diameters in obtaining a vaginal delivery.

Android pelvises (choice **B**) predispose to arrest of descent, anthropoid pelvises (choice **C**) predispose to occiput posterior position at delivery, and platypelloid pelvises (choice **D**) predispose to occiput transverse position at delivery. These pelvic shapes occur with frequencies of 30%, 20%, and 3%, respectively. Some women have combinations of features from more than one pelvic shape. Obstetroid (choice **E**) is not a formally described pelvic shape.

## 30  The Answer is C  *Medicine*

Several factors provided in the case history are consistent with a diagnosis of Rocky Mountain Spotted Fever (RMSF; choice **C**), a disease caused by the transmission of *Rickettsia rickettsii* via a bite by a tick. These factors include the following:

- The possibility of a tick bite is suggested by the statement that the patient had to walk up a brush-covered slope in order to get home and that it was August, a time when ticks are most prevalent.
- The patient lives in North Carolina (despite the name, only about 3% of all cases occur in a Rocky Mountain state, and most cases occur in the South Atlantic states—with North Carolina having the greatest incidence).
- Difficulty in breathing is likely an early sign of pneumonitis, as part of the acute respiratory distress syndrome (ARDS) often found in association with RMSF.
- Pitting edema is present, which is a common sign of interstitial nephritis, a disease often induced by *R. rickettsii*.
- There is tenderness in the right upper quadrant, possibly an early sign of hepatomegaly, also a trait commonly associated with RMSF.
- Yellowing of the sclera is likely an early sign of jaundice caused by excess hyperbilirubinemia due to hemolysis induced by RMSF.

As in the case described, initially, patients will have symptoms akin to influenza, such as fever, headache and myalgia. However, careful observation will discern early signs of some of the typical complications described above. After about the first week of the illness, a defining macular rash that progresses centripetally is usually seen. The initial rashes are at the wrists and ankles, and these may become petechial as they progress and as thrombocytopenia supervenes. In addition to the complications mentioned, a necrotizing vasculitis and uremia can also result. The diagnosis is confirmed by serology. Other laboratory finding suggestive of RMSF include elevated liver enzymes, thrombocytopenia, and hyponatremia. Treatment most typically is a tetracycline.

Although Lyme disease (choice **A**) is also transmitted by a tick, the incidence of new cases is highest in the New England states and is relatively low in North Carolina; even more significant to the contention that this is an incorrect choice is that early signs do not include hepatomegaly, respiratory problems, interstitial nephritis, or jaundice. Similarly, although interstitial nephritis and consequently pitting edema can be caused by several entities in addition to RMSF—including prolonged use of nonsteroidal anti-inflammatory drugs (NSAIDs); some antibiotics, such as penicillin and cephalosporins; and infections other than RMSF, such as those caused by cytomegalovirus and streptococcus—none of these factors is included among the choices nor do they cause the other symptoms described as associated with RMSF.

West Nile virus (choice **B**) is a flavivirus transmitted to humans by a mosquito bite and may cause encephalitis. The key features are neurological in nature, such as headache, fever, nuchal rigidity, stupor, and coma. Spastic paralysis and upper motor neuron signs and presence of lymphocytosis and elevated proteins on cerebrospinal fluid examination are present as well. Sarcoidosis (choice **D**) is a disease of unknown etiology that primarily causes granulomatous inflammation in the lungs. It is more common in women than in men and among African American and Northern European populations. Being a systemic disease, it can target various organs, including the skin (causing erythema nodosum), heart, liver, spleen, kidneys, salivary glands, and peripheral nerves. Diagnosis is by histology, in which noncaseating granulomas are found on biopsy. Q fever (choice **E**) is a rickettsial disease caused by *Coxiella burnetii*; it is transmitted by inhalation and not by vectors, as are many rickettsial diseases. It is usually seen in patients who are exposed to farm animals such as goats, sheep, and cattle. The patient presents with fever, headache, cough, and abdominal pain. Pneumonitis, hepatitis, and in some cases, endocarditis and encephalitis can ensue. The diagnosis is confirmed by serology.

### 31 **The Answer is E** *Medicine*

This patient has hypertrophic cardiomyopathy. Hypertrophic cardiomyopathy is a condition in which the left ventricular space is decreased due to the disproportionate hypertrophy of the interventricular septum. The restricted space reduces the amount of outflow. Performing a Valsalva maneuver or sitting upright increases the loudness of the murmur, whereas squatting reduces it (choice **E**). This is because a Valsalva maneuver or sitting upright decreases left ventricular filling and obstructs outflow. Likewise, sympathetic stimulation (as occurs during exercise) does the same, leading to symptoms such as syncope and even dangerous arrhythmias. Patients with hypertrophic cardiomyopathy have pulsus bisferiens, in which two peaks are felt, one following the other—the "double pulse" described by the patient. Chest pain and dyspnea may be symptoms as well. Hypertrophic cardiomyopathy can be inherited as an autosomal dominant trait. It can result in dangerous arrhythmias and sudden death. His father must have died from sudden arrhythmias. The fact that the patient has the same disorder points to a genetic cause. A defibrillator should be implanted in patients who have a history of syncope, recurrent ventricular arrhythmias, or a family history of sudden death.

Since choice **E** is correct choices **A**, **B**, **C**, and **D** are incorrect.

### 32 **The answer is D** *Surgery*

The patient has renal adenocarcinoma (choice **D**) and hypertension secondary to ectopic production of renin by the tumor. Renal adenocarcinoma is the most common neoplasm of the kidney. It affects men twice as often as women, usually in the sixth to seventh decade of life. The neoplasm arises from renal tubular cells. Smoking is a predisposing factor. The tumor affects the poles of the kidney, more commonly the upper. Hematuria is the most consistent sign (90%), sometimes associated with colic due to clot formation, followed by a dragging discomfort in the loin (45%), a palpable mass (30%), and fever (20%). "Cannonball" metastases to the lung occur in 60% of cases. Fever is not related to infection but results from chemicals released by the tumor. The tumors can ectopically secrete erythropoietin (leading to secondary polycythemia), parathormone-like peptide (leading to hypercalcemia), renin (leading to hypertension as noted in this case), gonadotropins (leading to feminization or masculinization), and/or cortisol (leading to Cushing syndrome). Serum levels of these hormones should be determined to confirm potentially elevated levels. A plain x-ray of the abdomen may show abnormal calcification in the tumor and distortion of the renal outline. An intravenous pyelogram (IVP) will reveal the mass, and the calyces may be stretched and distorted. Ultrasonography will show if the lesion is solid or cystic, and computed tomography (CT) with enhancement will demonstrate the extent of the lesion, including presence of hilar lymphadenopathy or involvement of the renal vein. Needle aspiration of the mass using CT for needle guidance is usually performed to obtain a histologic diagnosis. Angiograms are rarely done, as CT scans with contrast are adequate. Occasionally, an inferior venacavagram is indicated to establish extent of inferior vena caval involvement by the tumor. Radical nephrectomy is the treatment of choice if the tumor is confined to the kidney. The presence or absence of the renal vein or capsular invasion affects overall survival; 45% of patients without renal vein or capsular invasion achieve a 5-year survival, as opposed to 15%–30% of those with invasion. Adenocarcinoma of the kidney does not respond well to radiotherapy or conventional chemotherapy.

Although the kidney is the most common extrapulmonary site for tuberculosis (TB), choice **A** is incorrect; the homogeneous nodular masses in the lung go against this diagnosis. Furthermore, renal tuberculosis usually occurs between the ages of 20 and 40. Other properties of renal TB include that it is 50% more likely to occur in men than in women, urinary frequency is the most common and earliest symptom, and the urine remains negative for bacteria in the early stages. Dysuria sets in when the patient develops cystitis. Hematuria occurs in less than 5% of cases, and it is very uncommon to be able to palpate a renal mass in TB of the kidney. Transitional cell carcinomas of the bladder (choice **B**) usually involve the renal pelvis and produce obstruction. They are not as common as renal cell adenocarcinoma. Primary lung cancer (choice **C**) is not multifocal, and metastasis to the kidney is rare. Choice **E** is incorrect; acute pyelonephritis is more common in females. The patient may have headache, nausea, and fatigue. Pain is usually sudden in onset and is associated with fever and chills. Soon after onset, the patient develops cystitis, which causes enhanced urinary frequency and urgency, as well as dysuria. The patient has tenderness in the loin and in the hypochondrium, but no mass is felt. A midstream specimen of urine will reveal a few pus cells and bacteria. In some cases, the blood urea nitrogen (BUN) and creatinine levels may be elevated. Although acute pyelonephritis is usually unilateral, it could be bilateral. Acute pyelonephritis does not produce metastatic abscesses; however, if untreated, it could cause pyonephrosis that could be life-threatening.

## 33 The answer is D  *Medicine*

It is very likely that this patient has ankylosing spondylitis, an autoimmune disease. Approximately 90%–95% of patients with ankylosing spondylitis have the tissue antigen human leukocyte antigen B27 (HLA-B27); by comparison, HLA-B27 is present in 7% of the general population. However, because only 1% of individuals who have HLA-B27 develop ankylosing spondylitis, the disease is likely triggered by an unknown environmental factor in persons who are genetically predisposed. However, this genetic predisposition also makes the patient vulnerable to other autoimmune diseases, such as anterior uveitis, which is found in some 20% of the patients with ankylosing spondylitis. Anterior uveitis, an ophthalmic emergency, is also found in conjunction with other autoimmune diseases, including ulcerative colitis, Crohn's disease, and juvenile rheumatoid arthritis. It is also seen as a co-occurrence with cases of psoriatic arthritis, infections such as Lyme disease, sarcoidosis, and in some malignancies such as leukemia. Anterior uveitis used to be known as iridocyclitis. Inflammation involves the iris and ciliary bodies. Hence, pupillary contraction is painful. The patient usually has photophobia and a painful, red eye with decreasing vision. Redness around the cornea (circumcorneal injection) is also seen. The pupil will be small, and the globe will be tender to palpation. Light shone in the uninvolved eye will evoke pain in the affected eye when it attempts to react to the consensual light reflex (choice **D**). Treatment with a topical corticosteroids and a cycloplegic agent should be started immediately.

Unequal pupils (anisocoria) (choice **A**) may be seen in trauma. Failure of accommodation in pupils that react (choice **B**) is due to involvement of Perlia's nucleus in the midbrain. Failure of light reflex but presence of accommodation (choice **C**) is due to involvement of the Edinger-Westphal nucleus in the midbrain. Choice **E** obviously is incorrect.

## 34 The answer is C  *Pediatrics*

Vaginal bleeding, or pseudo-menses, may occur in a newborn female. In utero, the vaginal epithelium is stimulated by circulating maternal estrogens, which diffuse across the placenta. After birth, these hormone levels rapidly fall, which results in endometrial sloughing. There may be a thick mucoid discharge from the newborn's vagina, which is sometimes bloody. The discharge will usually resolve within 10 days after birth. No testing or treatment is necessary (choices **A** and **E**), only reassurance (choice **C**). Because the vaginal bleeding is not related to abuse, the Child Protective Services need not be informed (choice **B**). It is not necessary to call an endocrinologist (choice **D**) because this is not an endocrinopathy.

## 35 The answer is B  *Medicine*

Conn syndrome (choice **B**) is an important example of a secondary hypertension, in this case caused by aldosteronism. Although some studies suggest it is a rare condition, careful studies find it to be the cause of up to 15% of the cases of hypertension and should be suspected in all cases resistant to treatment or accompanied by low serum $K^+$ levels. It is caused by either an adenoma (a nonmalignant aldosterone-producing tumor in one of the adrenals), or by bilateral adrenal hyperplasia. The former is readily treated by surgery, while the latter generally may be treated with spironolactone, an aldosterone antagonist. The condition is diagnosed by measuring serum aldosterone and renin levels. In Conn syndrome, aldosterone concentration is elevated while the renin level is not—in fact, it usually is very low.

As people age, their blood pressure tends to increase. In fact, in the 1940s, normal systolic blood pressure was regarded to be 100 mm Hg plus a person's age. Now, normal pressure is defined in terms of the risk for organ damage. Thus, normal pressure for otherwise healthy adults is defined as shown in the following table:

|  | Systolic |  | Diastolic |
| --- | --- | --- | --- |
| Normal | <120 | *And* | <80 |
| Prehypertension | 120–139 | *Or* | 80–89 |
| High blood pressure |  |  |  |
| Stage 1 | 140–159 | *Or* | 90–99 |
| Stage 2 | ≥160 | *Or* | ≥100 |

For persons with diabetes or chronic renal disease, high blood pressure is defined as greater than 130/80 mm Hg because of the greater potential for end-organ damage. Roughly about 30% of adults over the age of 18 years have hypertension as defined in this table. In most cases, there is no specific cause for these higher-than-normal values, and this is called essential hypertension (choice **A**). In general, essential hypertension can be distinguished from Conn syndrome by the observations that (a) the degree to which the pressure is raised is not as great as in Conn syndrome, (b) the pressure responds more readily to medication, and (c) the serum $K^+$ level stays within normal limits. Thus, patients with essential hypertension are less likely to have symptoms due to serum $K^+$ deficiency.

Addison disease (choice **C**) is caused by the underproduction of adrenal gland hormones, usually due to an autoimmune reaction. Symptoms usually develop gradually and include low blood pressure, muscle weakness, bronzing of the skin, weight loss, and fatigue. Cushing syndrome (choice **D**) is caused by chronic exposure of the body to excess cortisol. It sometimes occurs as a consequence of long-term treatment of various conditions with cortisol; when it occurs spontaneously, it is due to a pituitary adenoma in 70% of the cases. These benign tumors secrete excess adrenocorticotropic hormone (ACTH). Usually, a single tumor is present, and the disorder is called Cushing disease. The syndrome may also be caused by ACTH-producing tumors found outside the pituitary. These ectopic tumors are found in association with small-cell lung cancers more than half the time, but may also be caused by thymomas, medullary carcinomas of the thyroid, and pancreatic islet cell cancers. Excess cortisol may also arise from carcinoid cells, essentially developmentally misplaced adrenal tissue. Cushing syndrome also may arise from an adrenal adenoma; these nonmalignant tumors are approximately five times more common in females than males and usually first appear at about the age of 40 years. Malignant adrenal cortical tumors are the least common cause of Cushing syndrome. In addition to secreting very high levels of cortisol, such tumors also usually secret adrenal androgens. Unlike the other choices, a pheochromocytoma (choice **E**) is a tumor located in the adrenal medulla rather than the cortex; consequently, these tumors secrete excess amounts of the catecholamines (epinephrine, norepinephrine, and dopamine) and their metabolic products. Symptoms of a pheochromocytoma are those expected to be caused by excess levels of circulating catecholamines, including high blood pressure, but generally also including other symptoms, such as severe headaches, tachycardia and palpitations, severe anxiety including feelings of impending death, tremors, chest and/or abdominal pain, nausea, weight loss, and heat intolerance. The classical diagnosis is analysis of a 24-hour urine sample for excreted catecholamines plus their metabolic products. More recently, a blood test has been developed. Although not as sensitive and not as widely available, this test is simpler for the patient to take.

## 36 The answer is B *Psychiatry*

The symptoms are most strongly suggestive of a depressive episode. Although it may have been precipitated by the realization that he had medical problems, they are not likely to provide a physiologic basis for his depression, nor are any of the drugs listed likely to cause depression. His symptoms, in particular his somewhat oblique references to possible suicide, indicate that antidepressive therapy should be started at once. This would most likely consist of cognitive counseling plus the administration of an antidepressant. The most probable initial choice would be a selective serotonin reuptake inhibitor (an SSRI; choice **B**) such as fluoxetine, sertraline, paroxetine, fluvoxamine, or escitalopram. These drugs have significantly fewer adverse effects than the other antidepressants, and treatment is effective 70%–75% of the time. However, it usually takes about 4 weeks for the treatment to become fully effective, and doses may have to be adjusted. Combining cognitive therapy with drug treatment will potentially enhance the therapeutic effect and make it longer-lasting.

Monoamine oxidase inhibitors (MAOIs; choice **A**) were developed in the 1950s; they have antidepressive activity and still are used to treat resistant cases of depression. However, they have lost popularity as a first line of treatment because of adverse effects. A particularly worrisome adverse effect, especially in this already hypertensive patient, is a tendency to provoke a hypertensive crisis. This is most likely to occur when the drug is used in combination with certain foods, such as red wine or aged cheese, or as a result of interaction with a multitude of different drugs. Other common adverse effects include dizziness, orthostatic hypotension, insomnia (with daytime sleepiness), and sexual malfunction. Tertiary amine tricyclic antidepressants (TCAs; choice **C**) were among the earliest antidepressants to be developed. Adverse effects include sedation, orthostatic hypotension, and anticholinergic effects. Overdosing readily induces death and consequently, they should not be used if there is danger of the patient committing suicide. They are converted to secondary amines in the body, and not surprisingly, secondary amine tricyclic antidepressants (choice **D**) act similarly to the tertiary amine TCAs but are less prone to cause sedation or orthostatic hypotension or to have anticholinergic effects; however, they are more likely to exacerbate psychosis. Heterocyclic antidepressants (choice **E**) act on dopamine receptors and may have a tendency to provoke convulsions. Mixed reuptake inhibitors (choice **F**) block the action of norepinephrine, 5-hydroxyytrptamine (5HT), and dopamine. They are sometimes used as a first-line treatment but less often than SSRIs. Bupropion (Wellbutrin) especially may be prescribed if decreased libido is an important primary concern. Electroconvulsive therapy (ECT; choice **G**) may be used if the patient is resistant to other forms of treatment, cannot tolerate antidepressant drugs, or is in immediate danger of committing suicide. An advantage of ECT is that positive effects are immediately evident. In the hands of an experienced psychiatrist, the current procedure is far less traumatic than it was years ago.

## 37 The answer is C  *Surgery*

The symptoms described in the case history clearly suggest a diagnosis of benign prostatic hypertrophy (BPH) since his PSA level is 3.5 ng/dl, below the 4.0 ng/dl level considered to be non malignant. Normally, the prostate is a walnut-sized gland situated just below the bladder and is wrapped around the urethra. With age, it tends to enlarge and constrict the urethra, making urination more difficult. BPH affects about 50% of men in their 50s and as many as 80% after the age of 70 years. Initially only a nuisance, if left untreated too long, BPH can become a serious medical problem: nonvoided urine can lead to infection, and relentless back pressure can irreversibly damage bladder muscles and even the kidney. Normally, the first line of treatment is medical. Finasteride (choice **C**) has proved to effectively reduce prostate size by as much as 20% and to effectively relieve mild to moderate symptoms over the long term, with few adverse effects. It is an inhibitor of 5α-reductase, the enzyme that converts testosterone to its more active derivative dihydrotestosterone, the hormone that promotes the abnormal growth of the prostate, causing BPH. The major shortcoming of finasteride is that it takes up to a year to become fully effective. As a consequence, a selective $\alpha_1$-blocker such as doxazosin, terazosin, or prazosin often is also prescribed. The $\alpha_1$-blocker acts more rapidly to relax prostatic smooth muscle tone, resulting in reduction of urethral resistance and permitting urine to flow more freely. Thus, the two classes of drugs act synergistically short term; however, it is not clear if that is also true long term.

Transurethral resection of the prostate (TURP; choice **A**) remains the gold standard for treatment for BPH, against which other treatments are compared. It is relatively safe and effective about 80% of the time; however, as with any surgical procedure, complications, sometimes severe, may arise, and some patients are left with urinary incontinence and/or impotence, and a smaller fraction with infection and other more serious problems. Therefore, it is not usually the first line of treatment and is generally reserved for cases more severe than the one described, such as chronic cases, and cases in which medical treatment is ruled out or has proved ineffective. Trimethoprim-sulfamethiazole (TMP-SMX; choice **B**) is one of the several antibiotics that might be used to treat prostatitis. It has no role in treating BPH unless a secondary infection has set in. Radical prostatectomy (choice **D**), interstitial radiotherapy (choice **E**), or external beam radiotherapy are three of the more common therapies used to treat prostatic cancer. Prostate carcinoma is the most common malignancy in males. The prevalence is estimated to be 30% for men in their 60s, close to 70% for those in their 80s, and approaching 100% for men in their 90s. However, because it often is slow growing, older men often die from causes other than problems arising from prostatic carcinoma. Early symptoms of BPH and prostatic cancer are similar. However, the digital rectal examination can often help distinguish between the two, since the cancerous prostate tends to be hard and nodular, not smooth and firm as in BPH. Although both conditions tend to elevate the PSA, the value in cancer is often above 10 ng/dL. Unfortunately, PSA values for both BPH and cancer can sometimes fall into a gray area, between 4 and 10 ng/dL, adding possible ambiguity to the diagnosis. The ultimate confirmatory test is biopsy.

## 38 The answer is E  *Preventive Medicine and Public Health*

Hemophilia A is a sex-linked recessive disease carried on the X chromosome. Normally, males inherit an X chromosome from their mother and a Y chromosome from their father, while females inherit one X chromosome from their mother and the other from their father. Therefore, a male cannot pass an X-linked disease to a son, but has a 100% chance of passing the defective gene to a daughter.

In the genealogy described, there is no reason to suspect that the mother has a defective gene. Despite the fact that her paternal uncles had hemophilia, her father is a healthy male; therefore, the solitary X chromosome that he possesses is normal. In addition, the fact that the woman's mother is of Scottish ancestry and her father is a Ukrainian Jew eliminates consanguinity in that generation. This heritage reduces the chances of the twin's mother carrying a recessive gene even further. On the other hand, the father suffered from hemophilia A; as a consequence, his X chromosome carried the mutant gene. Therefore, the female fetus has a 100% chance of being a carrier, but she will not express the disease, and the male fetus will neither be a carrier nor will he express the disease (choice **E**).

If the mother was a carrier and the father did not have the disease, the male fetus would have a 50% chance of expressing the disease, but none of being a carrier. The female fetus on the other hand, would have a 50% chance of being a carrier, but have no chance of expressing the disease (choice **A**). If both parents carried normal X genes, neither the female nor the male fetus would have a possibility of being a carrier or expressing the disease (choice **B**). Choice **C** is highly improbable because if one X chromosome is affected, she has a 50% chance of passing it on; if both are affected, she has the disease herself. To have a 75% chance of being a carrier, she would require three X chromosomes, two of which would have to be abnormal. If the father had the disease and the mother was a carrier, the female fetus would have a 50% probability of being a carrier (one normal X gene from the mother and one defective X gene from the father) and a 50% probability of expressing the disease (one defective X gene from each parent). The male fetus would have a 50% likelihood of expressing the disease, but none of being a carrier (choice **D**).

### 39 The answer is A  *Obstetrics and Gynecology*

The case scenario describes a hydatid cyst of Morgagni (choice **A**), also known as a paraovarian cyst. They are thin-walled, pedunculated, benign cysts attached to the tubal fimbria. They are of paramesonephric origin and are usually small and asymptomatic, but they can grow to 10 cm in size; they can be very mobile because of their long stalk and can even undergo torsion of the pedicle.

### 40 The answer is H  *Obstetrics and Gynecology*

The case scenario describes theca-lutein cysts (choice **H**), which occur as a response of normal ovaries to excessively high β-human chorionic gonadotropin (β-hCG) titers produced by the trophoblastic tissue of a molar pregnancy. Preeclampsia before 20 weeks' gestation, as is seen in this scenario, is common with a hydatidiform mole. The cysts are bilateral and fluid-filled, growing to massive size. They disappear when the source of the increased β-hCG levels is removed by a suction dilation and curettage. Follow-up with serial β-hCG titers is essential for at least a year. With a complete molar pregnancy, no fetus is seen within the uterus, which is filled with avascular cystic dilated villi. Karyotype of the placental tissue will be 46,XX with both X chromosomes paternally derived. With an incomplete mole, a nonviable aneuploidy fetus with 69,XXY karyotype will be seen.

### 41 The answer is G  *Obstetrics and Gynecology*

The case scenario describes a classic corpus luteum cyst of pregnancy (choice **G**) that resolved spontaneously when the placenta took over the function of progesterone production. This typically occurs around 10 weeks' gestation. These are unilateral, simple cysts that are an exaggerated response to a normal physiologic event. Management is conservative observation.

### 42 The answer is E  *Obstetrics and Gynecology*

The case scenario describes a normal intrauterine pregnancy (choice **E**). This is the most common cause of an enlarged pelvic mass in the reproductive years. Confirmation by sonogram is appropriate. A pelvic mass in the reproductive years is always an indication for a β-hCG test.

### 43 The answer is N  *Obstetrics and Gynecology*

The case scenario describes a child undergoing isosexual (in the expected direction for a female), complete (evidence of all pubertal changes), precocious (prior to the age of 8) puberty with the finding of a unilateral pelvic mass. This must be assumed to be a hormonally functional ovarian tumor producing estrogen, such as a granulosa cell tumor (choice **N**), until proved otherwise. Management is exploratory laparotomy for possible ovarian cancer staging and surgical removal.

### 44 The answer is O  *Obstetrics and Gynecology*

The case scenario describes a postmenopausal woman with virilization and a unilateral pelvic mass. Until proved otherwise, this must be assumed to be a hormonally functional ovarian tumor producing androgens, such as a Sertoli-Leydig cell tumor (choice **O**). Clitoromegaly is suggestive of high levels of peripheral androgens most often produced by an ovarian or adrenal tumor.

**45** **The answer is M** *Obstetrics and Gynecology*

The case scenario describes a benign cystic teratoma (choice **M**). Because these tumors derive from primordial germ cells, they may contain any combination of well-differentiated ectodermal, mesodermal, and endodermal elements. Foci of calcification, even the presence of teeth, are common. Management is surgical removal by laparoscopy.

**46** **The answer is J** *Obstetrics and Gynecology*

The case scenario is characteristic for endometriosis (choice **J**). Endometriomas are cysts on the ovary that result from accumulation of menstrual-like detritus from endometriosis. These "chocolate cysts" can enlarge to several centimeters in size. Endometriosis is responsible for 75% of chronic pelvic pain in women and is implicated in 40% of infertility cases.

**REMAINING INCORRECT CHOICES**

Hydrosalpinx (choice **B**) is a condition in which the fallopian tube is occluded at both ends, leading to collection of fluid within it. Sexually transmitted bacterial or viral infections lead to inflammation and scarring of the fallopian tubes and their subsequent closure. The patient may have infertility as a result of it. Diagnosis is made by pelvic ultrasonography.

Tubo-ovarian abscess (choice **C**) is an advanced form of pelvic inflammatory disease (PID), which is usually caused by anaerobic bacteria that spread in a retrograde manner from the lower genital tract. Sexually transmitted disease, douching, and multiple sexual partners are risk factors. Patients usually present with pelvic pain. Complications include infertility, a greater risk for ectopic pregnancy, and chronic pelvic pain secondary to adhesions. Diagnosis is made by pelvic ultrasonography, which shows complex, fluctuant, enlarged adnexal masses. The mass often involves the tubes, ovaries, bowel, and omentum.

Chronic pelvic inflammatory disease (PID; choice **D**) is caused by adhesions, usually the result of sexually transmitted disease. The most common bacterial etiology is *Chlamydia trachomatis*. The patient typically has dull, aching, constant, chronic pelvic pain. Menorrhagia or intermenstrual irregular bleeding can occur, and infertility is the invariable result. Treatment includes removal of adhesions by surgery, or in severe cases with extensive fallopian tube involvement, the tubes may have to be sacrificed. If unrelenting chronic pelvic pain is the main complaint, it may be necessary to perform a total abdominal hysterectomy and bilateral salpingo-oophorectomy. In these cases, estrogen replacement therapy is essential.

Follicular cyst (choice **F**) is usually seen in early pregnancy and resolves by the second trimester. It usually results from failed ovulation. Most cases are asymptomatic. However, if hemorrhage occurs within the cyst, the patient presents with acute pelvic pain, which, if on the right side, could be mistaken for acute appendicitis. Diagnosis is made by ultrasonography.

Luteoma of pregnancy (choice **I**) is a rare non-neoplastic condition usually affecting both ovaries, which show enlargement during pregnancy. It is more common in black multiparous women than in others. The patients are usually asymptomatic, and the condition is usually noted at cesarean section. The characteristic finding is replacement of normal ovarian parenchyma by a solid mass made up of luteinized stromal cells. These cells are under the influence of human chorionic gonadotrophin. However, unlike patients with gestational trophoblastic disease, these patients do not have elevated levels of human chorionic gonadotrophin levels. Virilization of the mother and fetus could occur because stromal cells secrete androgens. No treatment is necessary, as the disorder is self-limiting.

Polycystic ovaries (choice **K**) and polycystic ovarian syndrome are the most common hormonal reproductive disorders in women of childbearing age. Patients usually have pelvic pain, absent or irregular periods (which are usually anovulatory), increased androgen production leading to hirsutism, dandruff, acne, and increased body weight, and, in many cases, cysts in their ovaries. Other features include hypertension, hypercholesterolemia, and type 2 diabetes mellitus. Progesterone is essential for the shedding of the endometrium at the end of a menstrual cycle. The absence of menstruation, therefore, leads to thickening of the endometrium over time. As a result, endometrial hyperplasia or carcinoma could occur. Diagnosis is made by ultrasonography. Other tests include measuring serum hormone and blood glucose levels. Treatment includes combination oral contraceptive pills to suppress gonadotropins, decrease androgen production, increase sex-hormone binding globulin, and normalize menstrual periods. Clomiphene citrate is used to induce ovulation in women who desire fertility. If fertility medications do not work, surgery is an option. Diabetes mellitus should be treated; metformin is a good drug to choose. Not only will it lower blood sugar levels, it will decrease testosterone production too. The latter effect will slow down androgenic effects such as hirsutism.

Mucinous cystadenoma (choice **L**) is a benign ovarian neoplasm that is slow growing and usually affects women between the ages of 30 and 50. The tumor may be bilateral. The patient presents with heaviness and distention of the abdomen, which can grow to a very large size. Ultrasonography usually reveals a multiloculated cyst. Rupture of the cyst leads to pseudomyxoma peritonei. Treatment is surgical.

Gonadoblastoma (choice **P**) is a rare benign tumor that can turn malignant, especially in patients with intersex disorders. Phenotypically, 80% are females, while 20% are males. Gonadoblastoma are usually found within the second decade of life. The usual presentation is primary amenorrhea following puberty. Gonadoblastoma could develop in patients with male pseudohermaphroditism (46, XY), mixed gonadal dysgenesis (45, X/46, XY), and Turner syndrome (45, XO).

## 47 The answer is G *Psychiatry*

His initial impulses are most suggestive of regression (choice **K**), characterized by a return to less mature levels of functioning. However, he instead lowered his high anxiety levels by using humor (choice **G**), a more mature defense mechanism.

## 48 The answer is M *Psychiatry*

These behaviors are most suggestive of suppression (choice **M**), a defense mechanism that involves forcing anxiety-provoking feelings into the unconscious by substituting other feelings or thoughts. Denial (choice **C**) differs in that it is simply the failure to acknowledge the disturbing effects of an external reality.

## 49 The answer is D *Psychiatry*

Displacement (choice **D**) occurs when the emotions associated with a psychologically unacceptable object, idea, or activity is transferred to another object or situation. The new object or situation is often symbolically related to the original.

## 50 The answer is L *Psychiatry*

Repression (choice **L**) is the complete separation of aspects of reality (e.g., memories, cognitions, impulses, and/or conditions) from conscious awareness.

### REMAINING INCORRECT CHOICES

Altruism (choice **A**) involves decreasing one's own internal fears or anxiety by caring for others.

Blocking (choice **B**) is defined as the sudden repression of anxiety-provoking thoughts in midsentence. Conversation, if it resumes, is usually about another topic.

Dissociation (choice **E**) involves sealing off disturbing thoughts or emotions from consciousness.

Distortion (choice **F**) is altering the perception of disturbing aspects of external reality to make it more palatable.

Rationalization (choice **I**) is a distortion of reality that makes an undesirable act or event seem more desirable.

Reaction formation (choice **J**) occurs when an unacceptable thought or feeling is transformed into its opposite.

Sublimation (choice **M**) occurs when unacceptable impulses are channeled into more acceptable activities.

Undoing (choice **N**) involves performing an activity that symbolically reverses a previous behavior or thought.

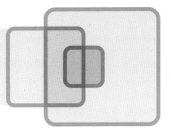

# test 8

# *Questions*

**Single Best Choice Directions:** *This section consists of numbered statements or questions followed by a list of potential answers; you are to select the ONE best answer.*

**1** A 33-year-old woman, gravida 4, para 3, presents to the obstetric unit at 29 weeks' gestation by dates with painless vaginal bleeding. The bleeding began 2 hours ago and has been accompanied by passage of a significant amount of blood and clots. An intravenous infusion of normal saline is in place. No record of her prenatal obstetric ultrasound examination is available. Her vital signs are as follows: temperature, 37.4°C (99.3°F); pulse, 105/min; respiration, 16/min; blood pressure, 100/70 mm Hg. The baseline fetal heart rate on electronic fetal monitoring is 150/min with frequent accelerations and no decelerations. Uterine contractions are absent, and the patient appears very anxious. Her last pregnancy was delivered by emergency cesarean section at 37 weeks' gestation due to double-footling breech presentation in labor. The type of uterine incision is unknown. Which of the following is the best working diagnosis?

(A) Placenta previa
(B) Abruptio placenta
(C) Vasa previa
(D) Bloody show
(E) Uterine rupture

**2** Parents present to the emergency department carrying their 4-year-old child, who is lethargic and has excessive oral secretions, miosis, tearing, and "soiled" trousers from urination and defecation. Remnants of emesis are seen on his clothing. Tremors, fasciculations, and hypertension are also present. The parents tell the physician that the child had been in his usual state of good health until that afternoon. The patient's symptoms developed while playing in a field recently sprayed with insecticides. The physician suspects organophosphate poisoning. To treat the nicotinic effects, the physician should use which of the following?

(A) Atropine
(B) British antilewisite
(C) Pralidoxime
(D) Calcium disodium ethylenediaminetetraacetate
(E) Naloxone

**3** In response to a community-wide influenza A epidemic, residents of a nursing home were vaccinated with inactivated (killed virus) influenza vaccine containing antigens identical or similar to the influenza A and B viruses circulating the previous year. Six days later, an ambulatory and sociable 74-year-old resident developed a temperature of 38.8°C (102°F), severe headache, myalgia, nausea, and weakness over a 24-hour period. Which of the following would be the most appropriate response on the part of the nursing home administration?

(A) Take no further prophylactic measures, because the residents have already been vaccinated.
(B) Prophylactically treat all residents with ampicillin.
(C) Prophylactically treat all residents with amantadine or rimantadine.
(D) Attempt to isolate all residents with whom the patient had been in contact during the past week.
(E) Give all residents a booster influenza vaccination to ensure that their antibody titer is high.

**4** A 68-year-old man presents to the emergency room of a small-town hospital with a history of crushing substernal chest pain that occurred while he was watching television. The patient gave a history of chest pains that came and went, which he had chosen to ignore, but this was his first severe episode. He did not smoke, drank alcohol in moderation, and had been retired for 4 years. He had no past history of medical illness or long-term medications. In the emergency room, his temperature was 37°C (98.4°F), pulse was 100/min regular, and blood pressure was 140/60 mm Hg. His respirations were 20/min. The patient was diaphoretic and had pallor and a hint of peripheral cyanosis. He was given 100% oxygen by nasal canula at 4 L/min, morphine for pain, sublingual nitroglycerin, and aspirin. An electrocardiogram (ECG) showed an inferior myocardial infarct (MI) based on ST changes in leads II, III, and AVF. As percutaneous coronary intervention was unavailable, and the event was less than 6 hours in duration, thrombolytic therapy was carried out. Thereafter, he was transferred to the coronary intensive care unit. On the fourth day post-MI, he complained of severe substernal pain similar in intensity and character to the one that heralded the first event. Positive physical findings included a third heart sound and bibasilar rales. Pertinent negative findings included the absence of a murmur and friction rub. Laboratory studies revealed the presence of creatine phosphokinase isoenzyme CKMB and a lactate dehydrogenase (LDH) isoenzyme study with an $LDH_1/LDH_2$ flip. Which of the following findings is the most specific indication of reinfarction?

(A) Recurrent pain
(B) A third heart sound
(C) Bibasilar rales
(D) The presence of creatine phosphokinase isoenzyme CKMB
(E) A lactate dehydrogenase (LDH) isoenzyme $LDH_1/LDH_2$ flip

**5** A 9-month-old child presents for a well-care examination. The mother states that the child has not been feeding well and seems to be less active than usual. The patient's vital signs are within normal limits, and the patient is afebrile. On physical examination, the head circumference is found to be two standard deviations above the norm. The child has frontal bossing, the skin is translucent, and the eyes manifest a "setting sun" sign. The child also has a meningomyelocele. A computed tomography (CT) scan of the head would show which of the following?

(A) Epidural hematoma
(B) Chronic subdural hematoma
(C) Shaken baby syndrome
(D) Noncommunicating hydrocephalus
(E) Leptomeningeal cyst

**6** A 19-year-old woman becomes very concerned that a small lump in her left breast is malignant cancer. Workup and biopsy show it to be entirely benign, but she remains excessively worried, in spite of reassurance by her physician. Which of the following is the best treatment in this case?

(A) A careful explanation of the benign nature of the physical complaint
(B) Use of benzodiazepine
(C) Skillful physician reassurance and frequent follow-up
(D) Use of placebo medication
(E) Psychotherapy to explore her current life circumstances

**7** An 18-year-old woman presents to the emergency department with a history of severe retrosternal chest pain that is aggravated by swallowing and deep breathing. The patient appears anxious. She is afebrile, has sinus tachycardia, slightly elevated blood pressure, and tachypnea. Mild pallor is noted, but she seems well hydrated and has no icterus. Examination of the cardiovascular system had normal findings, except for sinus tachycardia. The abdomen is scaphoid, and no tenderness, masses, or organomegaly is noted. Her weight is less than the norm for her age and height. The patient, however, feels that she is obese and has taken to binge eating followed by self-induced vomiting. Which of the following is the most probable cause of her pain?

(A) Gastroesophageal reflux
(B) Boerhaave syndrome
(C) Tension pneumothorax
(D) Gastric ulcer disease
(E) Esophageal cancer

**8** For the past few months, a 62-year-old woman has been feeling poorly. She complains about recurring cramps and apparent arthritic pains, and she adds that she feels weaker than usual: she can no longer lift the 24-pound bags of cat litter that she used to buy, and her bridge partner is upset with her because she seems unable to concentrate. In addition, although her chronic bipolar disorder had been kept under good control for years with lithium, recently her bouts of depression have increased. However, the incident that brought her to the emergency department of a local hospital was the fact that, the previous night, she was awakened by a pain in her left flank that was so severe that she called 911. In the ER, they gave her analgesics; during the night, she passed a small stone, providing her with immediate relief from pain. Prior to this treatment, the emergency physician ran a metabolic panel. The resultant analyses are summarized in the following table.

| Measurement | Value | Units | Normal or Desirable Range |
|---|---|---|---|
| Na$^+$ | 142 | mmol/L | 135–147 |
| K$^+$ | 5.0 | mmol/L | 3.5–5.5 |
| Cl$^-$ | 102 | mmol/L | 96–108 |
| CO$_2$ | 26 | mmol/L | 22–29 |
| Nonfasting glucose | 160 | mg/dL | 65–99 |
| Calcium | 10.4 | mg/dL | 8.5–10.4 |
| Blood urea nitrogen (BUN) | 20 | mmol/L | 9–23 |
| Serum creatinine | 1.10 | mg/dL | 0.70–1.25 |
| Urea/Creatinine | 18.2 | Ratio | 10–22 |
| Osmolarity calculated | 288 | milliosmolar /kg | 268–292 |
| SGOT/AST$^a$ | 33 | Units/Liter (U/L) | 0–44 |
| GPT/ALT$^a$ | 30 | U/L | 0–44 |
| Alkaline phosphatase | 127 | U/L | 40–129 |
| Total protein | 7.0 | gm/dL | 6.3–8.3 |
| Albumin (A) | 3.0 | gm/dL | 3.6–5.0 |
| Total bilirubin | 0.7 | mg/dL | 0.2–1.2 |
| Conjugated bilirubin | 0.3 | mg/dL | 0.0–0.3 |
| Globulin (G) | 2.6 | gm/dL | 2.4–4.4 |
| A/G ratio | 1.2 | Ratio | 0.7–2.5 |
| Total cholesterol | 104 | mg/dL | >199 |
| Triglycerides | 88 | mg/dL | >149 |
| High-density lipoprotein (HDL) | 48 | mg/dL | <40 |
| Total cholesterol/HDL | 2.2 | Ratio | >6 |

$^a$SGOT, serum glutamic oxaloacetic transaminase; AST, aspartate aminotransferase; GPT, glutamate pyruvate transaminase; ALT, alanine aminotransferase

This patient most likely is suffering from which one of the following conditions?

(A) Sarcoidosis
(B) Production of parathyroid hormone by ectopic tumors
(C) Hyperparathyroidism
(D Familial hypocalciuric hypercalcemia (aka, familial benign hypercalcemia)
(E) Milk-alkali syndrome

**9** A 45-year-old man went skiing in Aspen, Colorado, and met with an unfortunate accident, following which he was airlifted to a hospital. He had a swollen left thigh, after having bled into it. An x-ray revealed multiple fractures of the left femur. He was transfused with blood and underwent emergency reduction and internal fixation of the fractures. Following surgery, he was transferred to the intensive care unit, and a few days later, to a step-down unit. Unfortunately, the patient developed a pulmonary embolus, which was successfully treated. The most common early presentation of a pulmonary embolus is which one of the following?

(A) Swelling of the calf
(B) Calf tenderness
(C) Chest pain on deep inspiration
(D) Fever
(E) Increased pulse rate

**10** A first-year pediatric resident is called to the newborn nursery to evaluate a 2-day-old who has passed a bloody stool. The patient was born by normal spontaneous vaginal delivery to a 34-year-old primigravida. The birth weight was 8 lb 3 oz (3.7 kg), and Apgar scores were 8 at 1 minute and 9 at 5 minutes. The mother had good prenatal care throughout the entire pregnancy. She denied using tobacco, alcohol, or drugs during her pregnancy. The patient has been sleeping, feeding, defecating, and urinating well since birth. Vital signs are stable, and the rest of the physical examination findings are within normal limits. Which of the following tests would best determine the cause of the bloody stool?

(A) Apt test on the blood in the stool
(B) Hemoglobin electrophoresis of the blood from the stool
(C) Barium enema
(D) Clinitest examination of the stool
(E) Methylene blue stain of the stool

**11** An 18-year-old nulligravid woman complains of painful menses for the past 3 years. These symptoms are associated with cramping located in her lower abdomen and radiating to her lower back and inner thighs. She also has nausea and vomiting. She experienced menarche at age 13. Initially, her menses were irregular and not associated with any cramping or pain. She is not sexually active and is not requesting contraception. The only medication she is taking is thyroid hormone replacement for a diagnosis of hypothyroidism that was made 2 years ago. General and pelvic examinations are unremarkable. Her uterus is midline, symmetrical, not enlarged, nontender, and freely mobile. She has no cervical motion tenderness. Which of the following is the most likely mechanism causing this patient's symptoms?

(A) Excessive prostaglandin-induced myometrial contractions
(B) Myometrial irritation from ectopic endometrial glands
(C) Pelvic congestion from dilated spiral arterioles
(D) Excessive endometrial proliferation from unopposed estrogen
(E) Bleeding into rapidly growing uterine leiomyomas

**12** A 56-year-old grandmother whose hobby is gardening presents with a red swelling in her right ring finger. She does not remember any specific trauma to the area, but frequently sustains small cuts on her hands while tending to her garden. Physical examination reveals a small, red, nontender papule on the right ring finger, which shows erythema and swelling, with a small draining pustule on the lateral side. There are ascending erythematous streaks up the right arm, with several draining pustules along their course. Bacterial cultures are negative. Which one of the following is the most effective medication, and most likely to be well-tolerated by this patient?

(A) Itraconazole
(B) Saturated solution of potassium iodide
(C) Amphotericin B
(D) Erythromycin
(E) Dicloxacillin
(F) Cephalexin

**13** A 2-week-old infant is brought to the emergency department because of diarrhea, poor feeding, abdominal distention, and vomiting for the past 3 days. Physical examination is pertinent for temperature (39°C [102.2°F]), cataracts, hepatomegaly, and jaundice. The patient has poor skin turgor and a capillary refill of 3 seconds. The physician suspects that the infant is septic and has galactosemia. Which of the following would be the most probable pathogen involved in the sepsis?

(A) Group B streptococcus
(B) *Listeria monocytogenes*
(C) *Escherichia coli*
(D) *Staphylococcus aureus*
(E) Pneumococcus (*Streptococcus pneumoniae*)

**14** A 35-year-old businessman comes to see his primary care physician for a complete physical. The patient has no medical history suggestive of hypertension, diabetes, seizures, or other chronic disease. He does consume ibuprofen tablets for "tension headaches" due to pressures caused by his job. He does not have chest pain, nor does he have a history of shortness of breath. There is no family history of chronic medical illness. Physical examination reveals a well-nourished male, who is afebrile and has normal vital signs. He has no pallor, cyanosis, or icterus. Examinations of his cardiovascular and respiratory systems show normal findings. Findings of his abdominal examination are normal as well. During his interaction with his primary care physician, he stated, rather warily, that he visited a prostitute on one of his travels and did not use protection. Examination of his genitalia did not reveal any abnormal physical findings. He was tested for sexually transmitted disease. His human immunodeficiency virus (HIV) enzyme-linked immunosorbent assay (ELISA) test result was negative, as were results of the tests for chlamydia and herpes genitalis. His serum rapid plasmin reagin test result (RPR) showed a reaction at 1:10, and the microhemagglutination-*Treponema pallidum* (MHA-TP) showed a reaction as well. Which one of the following statements about this patient is true?

(A) He should be treated with procaine penicillin.
(B) He must have syphilis because the RPR test is specific.
(C) The RPR assay should become nonreactive between 12 and 24 months after treatment.
(D) His disease is not communicable, and his sexual partners do not need testing.
(E) The MHA-TP should become nonreactive within 6 months after treatment.

**15** A 2-year-old male child from a Vietnamese immigrant family is brought to the emergency department by a Child Protective Services (CPS) worker for suspected physical abuse. The worker states that, earlier that morning, she received a call from a day care facility that the child attends. According to the CPS worker, the day care employee stated that she thought that the child had been physically abused. The physician performs a thorough history and physical examination to determine evidence of maltreatment. Which one of the following would be specific evidence of child abuse in this case?

(A) Bruises on the back in a fir-tree pattern from "coining"

(B) A blue, nontender macular lesion in the presacral area

(C) Weight less than the fifth percentile

(D) Bruised knees

(E) A circular burn restricted to the buttocks

**16** A 24-year-old man presents to the emergency room with fever, severe myalgias, and headache. He just returned from a trip to Alaska, where he ate a variety of foods, including walrus meat. The patient has a temperature of 39°C (102.2°F), his blood pressure is 120/90 mm Hg, pulse is 95/min regular, and his respiratory rate is 20/min regular. The patient is in moderate distress. He has some pallor but no cyanosis. He has periorbital edema and subconjunctival hemorrhages affecting both eyes. There is evidence of blood under the bed of his fingernails. His heart sounds are normal, and he has sinus tachycardia. Findings of an examination of the respiratory system are normal. His abdominal examination also is unremarkable. Laboratory examination reveals a white blood cell (WBC) count of 9.5 cells/μL with 25% eosinophils. Which of the following is the best diagnostic test to first perform on this patient?

(A) Blood culture

(B) Stool examination for ova and parasites

(C) Muscle biopsy for histologic examination

(D) Echocardiogram

(E) Serologic test for febrile agglutinins

**17** 55-year-old man is being treated for diabetes, hypertension, and degenerative joint disease. His physician prescribed metformin for the diabetes; methyldopa, propranolol, and hydrochlorothiazide for his hypertension; and acetaminophen to treat the pain associated with degenerative joint disease. Over several months, he becomes increasingly withdrawn and apathetic. He loses interest in his family, work, and hobbies, and he spends much time brooding about his loss of health. Which of the following medications has been most consistently associated with his psychiatric symptoms?

(A) Hydrochlorothiazide

(B) Metformin

(C) Acetaminophen

(D) Methyldopa

(E) Propranolol

**18** A 25-year-old woman comes to the emergency room of a local hospital with severe right-sided headache that has not responded to treatment with ibuprofen or acetaminophen. She states that she has been having these headaches for quite some time and that the

stress at her job makes them worse. During the attacks, she also becomes nauseated and vomits, and she sees bright flashes of light during the attacks. She prefers quiet. The most distressing symptom in this patient is most likely which one of the following?

(A) Headache

(B) Nausea

(C) Vomiting

(D) Flashing lights

(E) Increased sensitivity to sound

**19** A 13-year-old basketball player presents to the pediatrician with a limp and right knee pain, which he states to have had for the last week. He tells the pediatrician that the basketball season has just begun and the training is physically demanding. The patient thinks that he may have pushed himself too hard during workouts. He reports that running, jumping, or climbing stairs exacerbates his knee pain. On physical examination, the tibial tuberosity is enlarged. However, there is no synovial effusion or thickening of the knee joint. Which one of the following is the most likely diagnosis?

(A) Legg-Calvé-Perthes disease

(B) Slipped capital femoral epiphysis

(C) Osgood-Schlatter disease

(D) Septic arthritis of the knee

(E) Idiopathic adolescent anterior knee pain syndrome

**20** A 24-year-old female college student presents to the physician's office with complaints of watery diarrhea, abdominal cramping and bloating, and nausea. She returned from a backpacking trip in the mountains 4 days previously. The patient was in moderate distress, had mild pyrexia, moderate tachycardia, and normal blood pressure and respiratory rate. There was no pallor or cyanosis. She was mildly dehydrated, and showed no signs of icterus. The cardiovascular system was normal except for sinus tachycardia. The respiratory system was normal. The abdomen was soft, and there was diffuse tenderness without guarding. No masses were felt, and there was no organomegaly. Bowel sounds were increased. A complete blood count revealed leukocytosis, and the hematocrit was elevated. Her serum electrolytes revealed moderate hypernatremia but were otherwise unremarkable. Microscopic examination of stool revealed pear-shaped, dorsally convex, flattened parasites with two nuclei and four pairs of flagella. Which of the following represents the best treatment for this patient?

(A) Reassurance

(B) Penicillin

(C) Tetracycline

(D) Azidothymidine (AZT)

(E) Metronidazole

**21** A 29-year-old woman, gravida 2, para 2, had a liquid-based thin-layer cervical Pap smear performed in the office a week ago. A high-grade squamous intraepithelial lesion was reported. Human papilloma virus (HPV) typing was positive for serotypes 16 and 18. She returned to the office and underwent colposcopically directed cervical biopsy. The entire transformation zone was seen with no lesion entering the endocervical canal. A specimen from a biopsy of a lesion at 6 o'clock on the cervix exhibited abnormal vessels and mosaicism. The histologic report showed full-thickness dysplastic epithelial changes with malignant cells that had penetrated the basement membrane and had invaded lymphatics. Which of the following procedures would be considered appropriate in identifying the stage of her disease?

(A) Intravenous pyelogram
(B) Laparoscopy
(C) Exploratory laparotomy
(D) Lymphangiogram
(E) Lymphadenectomy

**22** A 25-year-old man presents with complaints of dysuria for the past 6 days. He has had multiple female sexual partners in the past 2 months. Physical examination shows a yellowish penile discharge with inguinal adenopathy but no genital ulcers. Gram's stain of the discharge shows intracellular gram-negative diplococci in leukocytes. Which one of the following should be used in the treatment of this patient?

(A) Ceftriaxone
(B) Ciprofloxacin
(C) Procaine penicillin
(D) Ceftriaxone plus doxycycline
(E) Doxycycline

**23** A 15-year-old boy is brought to the pediatrician for a school physical examination. The mother states that they have just moved to this area from Georgia. According to the mother, the child, who is mentally retarded, has been in his usual state of good health. His past medical history is pertinent for a few ear infections and upper respiratory tract infections. Although the mother did not bring the child's previous medical record with her, she believes that the patient's immunizations are current. Pertinent findings on the physical examination include a prominent jaw, protruding ears, macroorchidism, and developmental delay. Which of the following is the most likely diagnosis?

(A) Klinefelter syndrome
(B) Trisomy 18
(C) Prader-Willi syndrome
(D) Trisomy 21
(E) Fragile X syndrome

**24** A 44-year-old woman presents complaining of lower left leg pain. Three weeks ago, she started intensive training in preparation for an upcoming 10-kilometer race. Her pain becomes more severe while she is running and intermittently occurs while she is walking. On physical examination, there is localized tenderness at the junction of the middle and distal portions of the tibia. Which of the following is the most likely diagnosis?

(A) Stress fracture of the tibia
(B) Chronic exertional compartment syndrome
(C) Overuse myositis
(D) Acute compartment syndrome
(E) Anterior tibialis tendinitis

**25** Prostate cancer is a very common malignancy in males; according to an August 2008 report from the U.S. Preventive Services Task Force (USPSTF), it is the second leading cause of cancer-related morbidity (following skin cancer) and the second most common cause of mortality (following lung cancer). Approximately 17% of adult men will receive a diagnosis of prostate cancer in their lifetime. In 2007, this amounted to 218,890 men. Judging from death rates during previous recent years, approximately 12%–13% of these will die, and 71% of these deaths will be of men 75 years of age or older. As is also true for colon cancer, a very sensitive screening test for prostate cancer exists, namely, the prostate-specific antigen (PSA) test coupled with the digital rectal examination. Which one of the following choices describes the screening recommendation for prostate cancer as promulgated by the USPSTF in 2008 for men 75 years of age or older?

(A) The USPSTF recommends the service. There is high certainty that the net benefit is substantial.
(B) The USPSTF recommends the service. There is high certainty that the net benefit is moderate, or there is moderate certainty that the net benefit is moderate to substantial.
(C) The USPSTF recommends against routinely providing the service. There may be considerations that support providing the service in an individual patient. There is at least moderate certainty that the net benefit is small.
(D) The USPSTF recommends against the service. There is moderate or high certainty that the service has no net benefit or that the harms outweigh the benefits.
(E) The USPSTF concludes that the current evidence is insufficient to assess the balance of benefits and harms of the service. Evidence is lacking, of poor quality, or conflicting, and the balance of benefits and harms cannot be determined.

26 A 70-year-old woman was referred to an ophthalmologist by her primary care physician, whom she had been seeing for many years. Her complaint was that she had thought her vision was deteriorating. After his examination, the ophthalmologist determined she had an exudative form of age-related macular degeneration. He recommended laser photocoagulation. As a result of this treatment, the patient should expect which one of the following?

(A) Improvement in visual acuity within a week following the procedure
(B) Gradual improvement in visual acuity by the end of 6 months
(C) No change in visual acuity
(D) Worsening of visual acuity
(E) Loss of peripheral vision

27 A mother brings her 3-year-old son to the clinic with a history of recurrent blister formation after minor trauma. An interview with the mother reveals that this is a second marriage for both parents, and each parent brought two children into the union. The child in question is hers, and the stepfather is an alcoholic, a heavy smoker, and has temper tantrums. Which of the following is the most likely diagnosis?

(A) Ehlers-Danlos syndrome
(B) Systemic sclerosis
(C) Epidermolysis bullosa
(D) Osteogenesis imperfecta
(E) Child abuse

28 A large multicenter trial was conducted to test the efficacy of a new screening test to confirm exposure to a viral disease of Asian origin. There were two groups of adults: one group had been exposed to the disease and the other had not. There were 600 adult men and women in each group. The mean age for each group was 35. Given the standardized $2 \times 2$ table below, which of the following options reflects the study group in a cohort study design?

| | Disease Present (D+) | Disease Absent (D−) | Totals |
|---|---|---|---|
| Exposed (E+) | a | B | a + b |
| Non-exposed (E−) | c | D | c + d |
| Totals | a + c | b + d | |

(A) a + c
(B) c + b
(C) a + b
(D) c + d
(E) (a + c) + (c + d)

29 A 65-year-old man makes an emergency appointment to see his family physician because of sudden loss of vision in the right eye. In presenting a history, the patient states that he first noticed it when he closed his left eye while taking aim at target practice. He further reveals that he has no pain, and other than a history of coronary artery disease, which causes angina, he has no other medical problems. His only medication is nitroglycerin sublingual tablets on an as-needed basis. Physical examination reveals a patient who is not in pain and has normal vital signs. His eyelids are normal. There is no conjunctival or circumcorneal injection. In the affected eye, the anterior chamber appears normal. The pupil is moderately dilated and fails to react to direct light, but responds to consensual light reflex. Funduscopy reveals pallor of the optic disc, a cherry-red fovea, and bloodless arterioles. These findings are most consistent with which one of the following choices?

(A) Central retinal vein occlusion
(B) Acute angle-closure glaucoma
(C) Corneal abrasion
(D) Central retinal artery occlusion
(E) Optic neuritis
(F) Branch retinal vein occlusion

30 A 20-year-old African-American woman, gravida 3, para 2, has a history of a seizure disorder since 10 years of age. She is currently at 17 weeks' gestation and is being treated with phenytoin orally three times per day. A phenytoin level determined on a sample drawn a week ago is within the therapeutic range. First-trimester bleeding that spontaneously resolved with conservative management complicated her prenatal course. Blood for a maternal serum triple-marker screen was drawn 10 days ago, but the results are not yet available. A complete blood count (CBC) was obtained as part of her routine prenatal laboratory tests. On her first prenatal visit, she was given a prescription for prenatal vitamins. At this time, the following values are noted: hemoglobin (Hgb), 9.3; hematocrit (Hct), 29; mean corpuscular volume (MCV), 150 $\mu m^3$ (normal is 80–100 $\mu m^3$). Which of the following is the most likely diagnosis?

(A) Sickle cell trait
(B) Iron deficiency
(C) Physiologic anemia
(D) Folate deficiency
(E) Thalassemia

**31** A 17-year-old woman presents to the emergency department with sudden onset of abdominal pain. She was playing in the school band when it began. She describes the pain as starting 30 minutes ago in the left lower quadrant without any radiation. The pain is 7 on a scale of 1 to 10 and not associated with nausea, vomiting, or diarrhea. Onset of menarche was age 13. Although initially her menses were irregular, she has had regular menstrual periods for the past 6 months. She has no fever, and her vital signs are stable. She is sexually active and is on combination oral contraceptive pills. She denies taking other medications. Physical examination reveals a flat abdomen with normal peristalsis. Pelvic examination reveals a normal vagina with a normal-appearing cervix. There is no mucopurulent cervical discharge. Bimanual examination is remarkable with a tender 5-cm mass in the left adnexa. A pregnancy test result is negative. A pelvic sonogram exhibits a normal intrauterine pregnancy and a 5 × 6 cm complex mass of the left ovary, with focal areas of calcification. Which of the following is the most likely diagnosis?

(A) Follicular cyst
(B) Mucinous cystadenoma
(C) Cystic teratoma
(D) Brenner tumor
(E) Serous cystadenoma

**32** A 26-year-old female flight attendant presents with a history of palpitations and difficulty breathing. She denies a history of allergies, long-term medications, or previous medical problems. She does not smoke but is a social drinker. Physical examination reveals a tall, medium-build female who appears anxious. Her vital signs are as follows: pulse, 88/min regular; blood pressure, 130/90 mm Hg; and, temperature, 37°C (98.6°F). Cyanosis, clubbing of the fingers, and pedal edema are absent. Which of the following is the most likely diagnosis?

(A) Aortic stenosis
(B) Mitral stenosis
(C) Aortic regurgitation
(D) Mitral regurgitation
(E) Congestive cardiac failure

**33** A 27-year-old woman presents with a history of two episodes of agitation, pressured speech, grandiose delusions, and disorganized behavior. One episode occurred 4 years ago and lasted several weeks. The current episode has been present for 1 month. Between episodes, the woman is friendly, outgoing, and emotionally stable. Mental status examination reveals increased psychomotor activity and impaired judgment. Which of the following is the most likely diagnosis?

(A) Bipolar disorder, manic phase
(B) Brief psychotic disorder
(C) Delusional disorder, erotomanic type
(D) Major depressive disorder with mood congruent psychosis
(E) Schizophrenia

**34** A 75-year-old man presents with puffiness of the face, arms, and shoulders associated with a bluish to purple discoloration of the skin. In addition, he complains of dizziness, shortness of breath, and cough. He has a 35 pack-year history of smoking. Physical examination reveals clubbing of the fingernails, emphysematous chest, and distended neck veins. The pathogenesis for this patient's findings most likely results from which one of the following disorders?

(A) Primary lung cancer
(B) Pericardial effusion
(C) Sclerosing mediastinitis
(D) Polycythemia rubra vera
(E) Right ventricular failure

**35** A 35-year-old man involved in an automobile accident is rushed to the nearest emergency room. The patient is conscious and in acute pain. He has tachypnea and sinus tachycardia, and his blood pressure is 90/60 mm Hg. He has bruising over the left lower rib cage, and point tenderness is noted here. Air entry is normal in both lungs. These findings are most likely secondary to which one of the following?

(A) Pulmonary contusion with hemorrhage into the pleural cavity
(B) Rupture of the spleen
(C) Rupture of the colon
(D) Transection of the abdominal aorta
(E) Rupture of the kidney

**36** A 7-month-old infant is brought to the emergency department. The mother states that the patient previously had been well but fell from a sofa onto the carpeted floor while taking a nap. The infant cried immediately according to the mother. However, on physical examination the child is noted to be lethargic. He is also noted to have retinal hemorrhages. Computed tomography of the head is performed and shows a subdural hematoma. After initial stabilization of this patient, which of the following is the most appropriate next step in management?

(A) Administer a pain reliever.
(B) Notify the patient's primary care provider.
(C) Contact the state agency that deals with child abuse.
(D) Obtain consent from the mother to admit the infant to the hospital.
(E) Tell the parents that you suspect that the child has been abused.

**37** At a routine prenatal visit, a 28-year-old woman, gravida 5, para 4, at 28 weeks' gestation, reports that she has not felt the baby move for 2 days. She first felt fetal movement at 17 weeks' gestation. She denies any vaginal bleeding or fluid leakage. Her pregnancy has been complicated by chronic hypertension, for which she is being treated with twice-daily tablets of methyldopa. She is afebrile and her vital signs are stable. On physical examination, you measure the fundal height at an appropriate 30 cm. Four weeks ago, the fundus measured 26 cm. Leopold's maneuvers reveal the fetus to be in transverse lie. Her blood pressure is 145/85 mm Hg. A urine dipstick test result is negative for albumin. You are unable to obtain fetal heart tones with a Doppler fetoscope. Which of the following is the most appropriate next step in the management of this patient?

(A) Perform a nonstress test.
(B) Perform an amniocentesis.
(C) Obtain a real-time ultrasound assessment for cardiac motion.
(D) Obtain a maternal abdominal x-ray assessment of the fetus.
(E) Perform a quantitative β-human chorionic gonadotropin (β-hCG) assay.

**38** As a teenager, a 46-year-old man secretly set several major fires that caused much property damage. He was never caught and says that he rarely thinks about what he now calls "dead history." Although he is married and works as an accountant, he spends many weekends planting trees in parklands and volunteering as a firefighter. Which of the following defense mechanism is most strongly suggested by this behavior?

(A) Denial
(B) Dissociation
(C) Intellectualization
(D) Sublimation
(E) Undoing

**39** A 31-year-old woman seeks medical assessment for an overwhelming number of physical complaints involving practically every organ system. She has seen numerous physicians over the last 10 years and describes them all as "quacks." A complete medical assessment yields unremarkable findings. Which of the following is the most appropriate next step in the management of this patient?

(A) Refuse to see her again
(B) Warn her to use medical resources sparingly
(C) Refer her, to another clinician
(D) Arrange, scheduled medical visits
(E) Try of various medications

**40** A 65-year-old male high school teacher who had a long history of smoking cigarettes and chronic obstructive airway disease saw his physician for increasing difficulty with breathing. Recently, he noticed that he could get some relief if he pursed his lips while exhaling. This caused a slight whistling sound, and his students had even nicknamed him "Mr. Whistler." He informed the physician that he had episodes of early morning cough with expectoration on some occasions, which was yellowish or greenish in color. He confessed that he did not like to go to see a doctor unnecessarily, but this time his wife forced him to do so since he seemed confused at times; this worried her, as she thought he was getting Alzheimer disease since his father had died from it. The physician's recommendation would have been which one of the following?

(A) A course of corticosteroids
(B) A course of corticosteroids and antibiotics
(C) A course of antibiotics
(D) Oxygen
(E) Donepezil

*Directions for Matching Questions (41 through 50): Each set of matching questions is preceded by a list of 4 to 26 lettered options followed by a brief explanation of the required task and then by a series of numbered statements. For each lettered statement, you are to select ONE lettered option that best fulfills the task as it relates to that statement. Remember, each of the listed options might be correctly selected once, more than once, or not at all.*

## Questions 41–50 Medicine

(A) Acetaminophen with codeine

(B) Rofecoxib

(C) Oseltamivir

(D) Alendronate

(E) Fluoxetine

(F) Allopurinol

(G) Cyclosporine ophthalmic emulsion

(H) Ibuprofen

(I) Zoledronic acid

(J) Adalimumab

*Select the ONE most appropriate drug to prescribe for each patient and/or condition described below.*

**41** A nonsteroidal anti-inflammatory drug (NSAID) was withdrawn from the market because of alleged negative effects on the cardiovascular system.

**42** A 62-year-old woman who wished to work until she was 65 years old, so that she could retire with full Social Security benefits, was forced to retire because of muscle pains and allodynia.

**43** A 45-year-old woman has had extremely itchy dry eyes and mouth for the past 6 months was prescribed this medication.

**44** A 74-year-old former football player takes 400 mg of this medication daily because of sore knees.

**45** This medication is prescribed for a 109-lb, 74-year-old woman of Chinese descent who has no obvious medical problems other than a pronounced buffalo hump.

**46** A 74-year-old mentally challenged, 114-pound Caucasian woman who recently broke her left wrist with minimal trauma is prescribed this medication.

**47** This medication is prescribed for a 45-year-old woman stricken with a severe case of arthritis in both legs and hands. She tests positive for the rheumatoid factor.

**48** This medication is prescribed for a 35-year-old man by his dentist after performing a root canal procedure.

**49** This medication is prescribed for a 62-year-old man who suddenly comes down with a fever of 104°F (40°C), headache, and muscle pain. He presently is confined to a rehabilitation facility while recovering from a broken leg.

**50** This medication is prescribed for a 55-year-old man who is overweight, has an inflamed big toe on his right foot, and a higher than normal serum uric acid level.

# Answer Key

| | | | | | | | | |
|---|---|---|---|---|---|---|---|---|---|
| **1** A | | **11** A | | **21** A | | **31** C | | **41** B |
| **2** C | | **12** A | | **22** D | | **32** D | | **42** E |
| **3** C | | **13** C | | **23** E | | **33** A | | **43** G |
| **4** D | | **14** C | | **24** A | | **34** A | | **44** H |
| **5** D | | **15** E | | **25** D | | **35** B | | **45** D |
| **6** E | | **16** C | | **26** D | | **36** C | | **46** I |
| **7** B | | **17** D | | **27** C | | **37** C | | **47** J |
| **8** C | | **18** D | | **28** C | | **38** E | | **48** A |
| **9** E | | **19** C | | **29** D | | **39** D | | **49** C |
| **10** A | | **20** E | | **30** D | | **40** D | | **50** F |

# Answers and Explanations

**1** **The answer is A** *Obstetrics and Gynecology*

Placenta previa is bleeding arising from a placenta abnormally implanted in the lower uterine segment. The bleeding is typically painless and is mediated by normal stretching of the lower uterine segment, which avulses the anchoring placental villi (choice **A**). This is seen in 0.5% of pregnancies at term.

Abruptio placenta (choice **B**) usually involves painful bleeding from a normally implanted placenta. Risk factors include severe preeclampsia, blunt abdominal trauma, and cocaine use. This is seen in 1% of pregnancies at term. Bleeding from vasa previa (choice **C**) is of fetal origin, mediated by either spontaneous or artificial rupture of a fetal vessel traversing the membranes overlying the cervix. This is a rare finding. While the mother's vital signs remain stable, the bleeding from the fetoplacental circulation usually results in exsanguination of the fetus. The normal fetal heart rate with no decelerations rules this diagnosis out. A bloody show (choice **D**) is usually blood-tinged mucus from early cervical dilation and would not have significant clots. Uterine rupture (choice **E**), although rare, is often a catastrophic event for both mother and fetus and is never painless.

**2** **The answer is C** *Pediatrics*

The specific antidote for nicotinic manifestations of organophosphate toxicity is pralidoxime (choice **C**). It restores the activity of acetylcholinesterase. Nicotinic effects for organophosphates include fasciculations, twitching, weakness, areflexia, tachycardia, and hypertension.

Atropine (choice **A**) is an antidote for the muscarinic effects of organophosphate toxicity. Some muscarinic effects include salivation, lacrimation, urination, defecation, and abdominal cramps. British antilewisite (BAL; choice **B**) and calcium disodium ethylenediaminetetraacetate (Ca-EDTA; choice **D**) are used for the treatment of lead toxicity. These therapies are used in patients with a venous blood lead level concentration of 70 µg/dL or above. Ca-EDTA and BAL are used in combination for children with encephalopathy or evidence of encephalopathy. Naloxone (choice **E**) is used as an antidote for opioid poisoning.

**3** **The answer is C** *Preventive Medicine and Public Health*

The index case is most likely suffering from influenza A. Because the infected patient is ambulatory and sociable and living in a closed community, the risk of spreading the disease among the other residents is very high. In addition, the mortality rate and the incidence of serious complications are increased in the elderly. Therefore, the nursing home medical staff should take advantage of every preventive measure available. Assuming a vaccine is prepared from viruses similar to those responsible for the epidemic (which it was, in this case), prophylactic vaccination has been demonstrated to reduce the number of infected individuals by 50%–80%. Moreover, the severity of complications among those who still get infected is, in general, reduced. However, it takes approximately 2–4 weeks after vaccination for antibody levels to build up to an effective level, so the vaccination received 6 days ago will be ineffective. Therefore, other prophylactic measures should be considered (choice **A** is wrong). Administration of either amantadine or rimantadine has been shown to be an effective prophylactic measure in the prevention of influenza A, which has little or no effect on the immune response to the virus or vaccine. Therefore, all residents should be treated with one of these drugs (choice **C**).

Treatment with ampicillin or any other antibiotic would be ineffective against a viral infection (choice **B**). Isolation of contacts would be a difficult and likely futile exercise (choice **D**). The residents were just immunized, so administration of a booster shot would not be appropriate (choice **E**).

**4** **The answer is D** *Medicine*

Creatine phosphokinase (CPK) is a dimeric protein predominately found in skeletal muscle, brain, and heart. The subunits of the skeletal muscle isozyme are called M-type and the intact dimer is called CPK-MM or CPK-3; the brain isozyme is composed of two B-type subunits and is called CPK-BB or CPK-1, whereas the heart isozyme is formed from one B-type subunit and one M-type subunit and is called CPK-MB or CPK-2. Since the myocardium is the only tissue that expresses the MB hybrid at a significant concentration, an increase in the circulating level of the MB isozyme specifically signifies damage to heart muscle. After a myocardial infarct (MI), the MB starts to rise within 3–8 hours, peaks in 12–24 hours, and returns to normal in 12–48 hours. Thus, its presence 4 days after the initial infarct signifies reinfarction (choice **D**).

Recurrent pain (choice **A**) could be due to reinfarction, gastroesophageal reflux, or a vivid imagination. A third heart sound (choice **B**) is usually a low-pitched sound that is apical in location. It is physiologic in children. However, after the age of 30, it signifies volume overload or left ventricular failure. Bibasilar rales (choice **C**) usually occur in congestive cardiac failure. The patient would be dyspneic and may have cyanosis and distended jugular veins. In patients with extensive myocardial infarction, bibasilar rales and a third heart sound could result from the reasons elaborated above.

Lactate dehydrogenase (LDH) isoenzymes are composed of tetramers of H and M polypeptides. These polypeptides form five distinct isoenzymes, which are numbered from 1 to 5. These isoenzymes are tissue specific. $LDH_1$ and $LDH_2$ are primarily located in the red blood cells, cardiac muscle, and the kidneys. $LDH_3$ is located primarily in the lungs, whereas $LDH_4$ and $LDH_5$ are found in the skeletal muscles, skin, and liver. The wide distribution of these enzymes therefore limits their usefulness in testing. However, in myocardial infarction, they are useful in ruling out other causes of chest pain. The proportion of these polypeptides varies from tissue to tissue. In normal serum, $LDH_2$ is in greatest concentration and that of $LDH_1$ exceeds $LDH_3$; the concentrations of $LDH_3$ and $LDH_4$, on the other hand, are almost equal to one another. The proportional concentrations of $LDH_1$ and $LDH_2$ in red blood cells and myocardial tissue are as follows:

| Location | Activity of $LDH_1$ | Activity of $LDH_2$ |
| --- | --- | --- |
| Red blood cell | Low | High |
| Cardiac muscle | High | Low |

Therefore, in normal situations, the concentration $LDH_1$ in the serum will remain low, and that of $LDH_2$ high, because there is no myocardial damage, and even though there is no hemolysis, more of the enzyme leaks out of erythrocytes. Following myocardial tissue damage, $LDH_1$ will spill into the blood. As a result, the concentration of $LDH_1$ in the serum will exceed that of $LDH_2$, resulting in the flip. The $LDH_1/LDH_2$ flip has a sensitivity of 80% and a specificity of 95%. However, it is first evident 14 hours post-MI, peaks in 2–3 days, and disappears in 7 days. Therefore, in this patient, who is 4 days post-MI, one would expect to find an $LDH_1/LDH_2$ flip even in the absence of reinfarction, as the flip remains for up to 7 days. Therefore, in this case it does not contribute to the diagnosis of reinfarction (choice **E** is not correct).

**5** **The answer is D** *Pediatrics*

The Arnold-Chiari syndrome type II consists of progressive hydrocephalus and myelomeningocele. The hydrocephalus is a noncommunicating one (choice **D**). The fourth ventricle is elongated, there is kinking of the brainstem, and portions of the brainstem and cerebellum are displaced into the cervical spinal canal, causing obstruction of flow of cerebrospinal fluid (CSF). Skull films show a small posterior fossa and widened cervical canal (platybasia). Type I Chiari malformation is usually not associated with hydrocephalus and is first noted during adolescence or adult life.

A leptomeningeal cyst (choice **E**) is a rare and late complication of a linear skull fracture and appears as an expanding pulsatile mass on the surface of the skull. Chronic subdural hematomas (choice **B**) are characterized by headache, personality change, and loss of consciousness. Classically, patients with epidural hematoma (choice **A**) experience a brief period of unconsciousness followed by a variable lucid interval and are unconsciousness thereafter. Expansion of the hematoma also leads to headache, vomiting, and focal neurologic signs. Children who are victims of shaken baby syndrome have acute subdural hematomas. In addition, retinal hemorrhages are present, and there may be additional clinical evidence to support child abuse (choice **C**).

**6** **The answer is E** *Psychiatry*

This patient's worrying suggests hypochondriasis, which is characterized by misinterpretation of the meaning of a physical symptom. Moreover, this patient does not respond to physician reassurance after an adequate workup. Hypochondriacal symptoms usually become evident during periods of psychologic stress. Resolution of the stressor through brief psychotherapy that includes exploration of current life problems (choice **E**) often results in symptom resolution.

By definition, reassurance (choice **A**) and explanations (choice **C**) are ineffective, and suggesting she have frequent follow-ups will only reinforce her fear that something is wrong. Benzodiazepines (choice **B**) may be used to help reduce anxiety; however, they cannot be considered central to treatment because they will not alleviate the psychologic stressors that presumptively cause the condition, and they carry a risk of creating drug dependency if used over a long period. Placebo (choice **D**) response is usually temporary, at best.

**7** **The answer is B** *Surgery*

Boerhaave syndrome (choice **B**) refers to a full-thickness rupture of the distal thoracic esophagus or stomach and is associated with vomiting or retching. In most cases, this syndrome is associated with alcoholics who have forceful vomiting or retching. However, it is also the most serious complication of bulimia nervosa, an eating disorder associated with binging on excessive amounts of food followed by self-induced vomiting.

Gastroesophageal reflux (choice **A**), tension pneumothorax (choice **C**), gastric ulcer disease (choice **D**), and esophageal cancer (choice **E**) all may cause retrosternal pain but are not associated with vomiting and bulimia.

**8** **The answer is C** *Medicine*

This lady has hyperparathyroidism (choice **C**). Hypercalcemia is tantamount to a diagnosis for hyperparathyroidism, since few other conditions raise serum calcium levels beyond normal levels; consequently, about 98% of the time, a total calcium value greater than normal is diagnostic of hyperparathyroidism. In the case illustrated, the value reported shows the total serum calcium concentration at 10.4 mg/dL (2.6 mmol/L), just within the normal range. This may tempt the physician to believed that this patient does not have hypercalcemia and consequently does not have hyperparathyroidism; however, it is easy to forget that this value includes all forms of calcium: protein bound (~45%), bound to small diffusable molecules (citrate, bicarbonate, lactate, and phosphate; ~10%), and the critical and metabolically active free ion (~45%). The best thing is to measure calcium ion, but this determination is not always available. A convenient empirical test is to add 0.8 mg for each mg albumin less than 4 (i.e., the less of total calcium concentration bound, the greater the amount of free ion). In this case, that equals 1, so true effective total calcium concentration is 10.4 plus 1 or 11.4 mg/dL indicating that, in reality, this patient has hypercalcemia and consequently very likely hyperparathyroidism. This diagnosis is further confirmed by the other symptoms shown; the most evident is a kidney stone, but muscle weakness, inability to concentrate, and increased depression all are signs of hypercalcemia. In addition, her arthritic pain and relatively high alkaline phosphates level may be due to a high degree of bone remodeling. If her bone density was measured, she likely would show signs of osteoporosis or at least osteopenia. It is useful to remember the ancient mnemonic "painful bones, renal stones, abdominal groans, and psychic moans," which describe typical symptoms of hyperparathyroidism.

Primary hyperthyroidism is a relatively common and probably somewhat underdiagnosed disease. It has been reported to affect 1 in 500 females and 1 in 2,000 males, usually after the age of 40 years, with increasing frequency with age. It almost always is due to a benign adenoma in one of the four glands and almost never to a malignancy (in less than 0.5% of patients). Nephrolithiasis that occurs in about 20% of patients with hyperparathyroidism is difficult to overlook; however, other symptoms of hypercalcemia are generally more subtle and, as noted above, total serum calcium measurements can be misleading. Although the introduction of a newer immunoradiometric assay for parathyroid hormone that only detects the fully intact molecule may improve the accuracy of measuring serum levels of the hormone, this determination also can provide ambiguous results. Because of these uncertainties, there is a diversity of opinions concerning the best treatment of seemingly asymptomatic persons with borderline high total calcium levels; recommended treatments vary from watchful waiting to immediate surgery to remove the suspected offending gland. In making such a judgment, one should remember that the seemingly asymptomatic, often elderly person may be fatiguing more readily than her or his optimal potential, and/or may be suffering from cognitive fogginess not readily observed in your office or, conversely, too easily ascribed to early signs of dementia.

Sarcoidosis (choice **A**) is an autoimmune disease that causes granulomas to form on various organs. Remission may occur within 10 years, or conversely, the disease may worsen. This disease is relevant to the diagnosis of hyperparathyroidism in that it is one of the few not rare conditions inducing hypercalcemia. Production of parathyroid hormone by ectopic tumors (choice **B**) will lead to symptoms of hyperparathyroidism, but such tumors are rare and the tumors will likely cause additional symptoms. Familial hypocalciuric hypercalcemia (FHH; aka, familial benign hypercalcemia; choice **D**) is a rare, essentially innocuous genetic condition almost always inherited as an autosomal loss of function mutation in the calcium sensor receptor (CASR) gene. This gene codes for a CASR normally found in many tissues, including the parathyroid gland and the kidneys. In the presence of a functionally challenged CASR receptor, the parathyroid gland does not respond as readily to feedback inhibition by $Ca^{++}$. Hence, calcemia occurs, the degree of which is related to how badly the receptor is damaged. Because of the hypercalcemia, this condition is easily confused with primary hyperparathyroidism. Basically, it is diagnosed genetically and by family history. A careful family history and genetic testing for an FHH-associated mutation can avoid inappropriate surgery. Milk-alkali syndrome (choice **E**) is one more condition that can result in hypercalcemia. Presently, it usually results from the ingestion of large quantities of calcium as calcium carbonate along with milk or yogurt. The relative frequency of the milk-alkali syndrome as a cause of hypercalcemia has been estimated to range from about 1% to over 10%. No matter how common or uncommon, clearly, it may cause profound kidney damage.

### **9** The answer is E  *Surgery*

Sinus tachycardia, which will increase the pulse rate (choice **E**), is the most common presentation of a pulmonary embolus. In a patient such as this, who is at risk for pulmonary embolus, unexplained tachycardia should always lead one to suspect the possibility of pulmonary embolus and should be investigated more thoroughly.

Swelling of the calf (choice **A**) indicates the presence of a possible deep venous thrombus, which can lead to a pulmonary embolus if it is not preempted from doing so. Calf tenderness (choice **B**), also known as Homan's sign, is an indicator of deep venous thrombosis but it is not very reliable. It is important to note that choices **A** and **B** are features of deep venous thrombosis and not primary features of pulmonary embolus per se, which this question is all about. Chest pain on deep inspiration (choice **C**) is pleuritic in origin. It is certainly seen in pulmonary embolus, but may well be absent. However, it is not the earliest feature, nor is tachypnea and cough with hemoptysis, which also can be present. Fever (choice **D**) develops later and may be low-grade.

### **10** The answer is A  *Pediatrics*

The most common cause of blood in the stool of a newborn is swallowed maternal blood. The Apt test (choice **A**) helps distinguish adult hemoglobin (Hb) from fetal Hb. It is easier and less expensive than electrophoresis (choice **B**). If adult Hb is detected, the blood swallowed is maternal blood. If fetal Hb is found, a search begins for the cause of the bleeding.

A barium enema (choice **C**) is both diagnostic and therapeutic for intussusception, which is rare before 3 months of age. The Clinitest (choice **D**) is used to quantify the urinary level of reducing sugars. The presence of leukocytes in the stool is determined by the methylene blue stain (choice **E**).

### **11** The answer is A  *Obstetrics and Gynecology*

This case scenario is characteristic of primary dysmenorrhea, which is classically associated with normal pelvic examination findings. Onset is typically within 2 years of menarche, when ovulatory cycles begin. When progesterone withdrawal bleeding occurs, there is prostaglandin-induced spiral arteriolar spasm resulting in excessive myometrial contractions (choice **A**), which cause uterine ischemia and pain.

Myometrial irritation from ectopic endometrial glands (choice **B**) is known as *adenomyosis*. This is a cause of secondary dysmenorrhea and is associated with an enlarged, soft, tender uterus. Pelvic congestion from dilated spiral arterioles (choice **C**) is also associated with a tender, enlarged uterus. Excessive endometrial proliferation from unopposed estrogen (choice **D**) is found with chronic anovulatory syndromes but does not result in pain. Bleeding into rapidly growing uterine leiomyomas or fibroids (choice **E**) is known as *red* or *carneous degeneration*. This occurs with high-estrogen states, such as pregnancy, when fibroid proliferation occurs so rapidly that the fibroid outgrows its own blood supply resulting in ischemia and severe pain. This is not a cause of primary dysmenorrhea.

#### 12 The answer is A *Medicine*

The disease described is cutaneous sporotrichosis, caused by the fungus *Sporothrix schenckii*. This fungus is found on plants and in the soil in many areas and can cause infection when minor trauma inoculates the fungus into subcutaneous tissue. Spread of the infection along lymphangitic channels is common and accounts for ascending erythematous streaks up the right arm with several draining pustules along their course, as described in the case history. However, extracutaneous forms of infection are rare. Pain is unusual. Diagnosis is confirmed by culture of a skin biopsy or, when present, pus from a draining pustule. Without treatment, the infection becomes chronic and usually does not heal. Itraconazole (choice **A**) has become the drug of choice for cutaneous and most other types of infection with *S. schenckii*.

Historically, a saturated solution of potassium iodide (SSKI; choice **B**) had been the preferred treatment. Although it remains relatively inexpensive, most clinicians prefer itraconazole because SSKI is poorly tolerated by many patients and although controlled comparative studies apparently have not been conducted, it may not be as effective as itraconazole or other available oral azole antifungals. Amphotericin B (choice **C**) is primarily used as initial treatment for extracutaneous forms of *S. schenckii* infection. Erythromycin (choice **D**), dicloxacillin (choice **E**), and cephalexin (choice **F**) are antibiotics used to treat bacterial, not fungal, infections.

#### 13 The answer is C *Pediatrics*

A strong association exists between galactosemia and *Escherichia coli* (choice **C**) sepsis, which may be a presenting feature in infants with galactosemia. Classic galactosemia results from a deficiency of galactose-1-phosphate uridyltransferase. Galactose, derived from lactose (milk sugar), is not metabolized past galactose-1-phosphate, which then accumulates and damages the liver, kidney, and brain. Galactitol, a polyol byproduct of galactose, also can accumulate, causing cataracts. Among other manifestations are jaundice, hepatomegaly, hypoglycemia, vomiting, aminoaciduria, and failure to thrive. Early diagnosis is important, and dietary management contributes to a good prognosis.

Although group B streptococcus (choice **A**), *Listeria monocytogenes* (choice **B**), *Staphylococcus aureus* (choice **D**), and pneumococcus (*Streptococcus pneumoniae*; choice **E**) are also pathogens seen in neonatal sepsis, only *E. coli* has a strong association with galactosemia.

#### 14 The answer is C *Medicine*

The diagnosis of syphilis is usually made by serology. This patient has latent syphilis because he has no physical findings that point to the disease, but has a positive result for a screening test that is highly sensitive. The highly sensitive nontreponemal tests (aka, reagin tests), namely the Venereal Disease Research Laboratory test (VDRL) and the similar Rapid Plasmin Reagin test (RPR), are used for initial screening and to monitor treatment; they usually become nonreactive after 1 year of treatment (choice **C**). They are called *nontreponemal* because they are directed against a cardiolipin–lecithin–cholesterol antibody and not against the spirochete itself. False-positive VDRL and RPR test results occur in many conditions, but the titers rarely exceed 1:8. In those who are suspected of having the disease, titers above 1:8 have a false-positive incidence of 1%–3%. Patients with human immunodeficiency virus (HIV) infection and IV drug users may have concomitant syphilis. Treponemal tests, those that target the spirochete itself, such as the fluorescent treponemal antibody absorbed test (FTA-ABS) and microhemagglutination-*Treponema pallidum* test (MHA-TP) are highly specific. They confirm syphilis when nontreponemal tests are positive, identify false-positive VDRL and RPR results, and, unlike the nontreponemal tests, remain positive even after therapy. Evaluation for neurosyphilis by examining the cerebrospinal fluid obtained via lumbar puncture is recommended for those with neurologic symptoms and signs. Other indications include untreated syphilis, failed therapy, disease for more than 1 year, or a serum VDRL or RPR titer above 1:32. Cerebrospinal fluid examination should also be done in patients with a positive VDRL or RPR result after 1 year of treatment.

Choice **A** is incorrect. Because of the organism's unusually slow rate of multiplication, a long exposure to medication is required. Therefore, short-acting penicillins, such as procaine penicillin, will be ineffectual. The treatment of choice for primary, secondary, or early latent syphilis is penicillin G benzathine. For neurosyphilis, the treatment is aqueous penicillin G or aqueous penicillin G procaine with oral probenecid. Tetracycline is approved for treatment of patients who are allergic to penicillin. Treatment should be monitored by determining quantitative VDRL or RPR titers repeated in the first, third, sixth, and twelfth month. If the titer rises, or it fails to fall fourfold, or if the symptoms recur, the patient should be retreated and cerebrospinal fluid examined to exclude the presence of neurosyphilis. Choice **B** is incorrect because RPR is not a specific test but a sensitive one. Choice **D** is incorrect because the disease is communicable, and sexual partners should be tested. Choice **E** is incorrect; treponemal test results remain positive even after treatment.

## 15 The answer is E *Pediatrics*

Specific evidence of child abuse includes old healed fractures, belt marks, bruises on the buttocks or lower back (areas where children are unlikely to harm themselves), subdural hematomas, and rupture of internal organs. Hot-water-dunking burns occur when a parent holds the child's thigh against the abdomen and places the buttocks and perineum in scalding water. This causes a circular type of burn restricted to the buttocks (choice **E**). The hands and feet are spared, which is not compatible with falling into a tub. Evidence of sexual abuse includes genital or anal trauma, sexually transmitted disease, and urinary tract infection.

Coin rubbing (choice **A**) is a nonabusive healing practice of the Vietnamese that involves vigorous stroking of the skin of a febrile child, producing a peculiar bruising pattern. A blue, nontender lesion in the presacral area (choice **B**) is a "Mongolian spot" often seen in African American, Oriental, and East Indian infants. Unlike a bruise, the Mongolian spot does not change color. Although caloric insufficiency from child abuse may explain weight below the fifth percentile for age (choice **C**), it is not the sole reason for failure to thrive. Bruised knees (choice **D**) are commonly seen in children of this age because of falls and are not specific evidence of child abuse.

## 16 The answer is C *Medicine*

The symptoms of fever, myalgias, periorbital edema, hemorrhages, and eosinophilia are suggestive of trichinosis, especially in a patient with a history of eating potentially infected meat. The most common cause is ingestion of infected, undercooked pork products, but it can also be found in a variety of carnivorous and omnivorous animals, including walrus. Diagnosis is made by a muscle biopsy in which histologic examination (choice **C**) shows larvae of *Trichinella spiralis* encysted in the muscle. Currently available antihelminthic drugs are ineffective against the larvae in muscle, and therapy is primarily supportive.

Because the cysts are in muscle, they will not be found in blood (choice **A**) or stool (choice **B**). An echocardiogram (choice **D**) will not identify them in heart muscle. There is no specific serologic test for febrile agglutinins (choice **E**).

## 17 The answer is D *Psychiatry*

His symptoms of becoming increasingly withdrawn and apathetic are strongly suggestive of a depressive episode. There is a relationship between hypertension and depression. Studies show that hypertensive patients run a higher risk of undergoing a depressive episode than do normotensive individuals, and vice versa. Several different mechanisms have been postulated. One is that certain drugs used to treat hypertension promote depression, and some drugs used to treat depression affect blood pressure; in the latter case this effect is, not surprisingly, most strongly demonstrated by the monoamine oxidase inhibitors. Although one can still read articles that implicate hypertensive agents in general as potential causes of depression, a high risk appears to be limited to reserpine and methyldopa (choice **D**). Methyldopa is a centrally acting $\alpha_2$ agonist, whereas reserpine depletes the brain of norepinephrine and serotonin (possibly accounting for its action as a depressant) and the peripheral store of norepinephrine in the sympathetic nerve terminal. Although some studies also implicate the $\beta$-blocker propranolol as potentially having a risk of causing depression, others do not; in this case, competition for cytochrome P450 isozymes is the cited mechanism, implying that this effect is only seen if the patient is already being treated with an antidepressant.

The antihypertensives clonidine, guanethidine, prazosin, and hydralazine, and thiazide diuretics, such as hydrochlorothiazide (choice **A**) all may have some, but if so only low, risk of causing depression. Other agents used to combat hypertension, including angiotensin-converting enzyme (ACE) inhibitors, calcium channel blockers, and nonthiazide diuretics, have not been implicated in causing depression. Neither have oral hypoglycemic agents such as metformin (choice **B**) or the analgesic acetaminophen (choice **C**).

## 18 The answer is D *Medicine*

The most distressing symptom is photophobia. Flashing lights (choice **D**) tend to zigzag within the visual field. Patients have a hard time keeping their eyes open, as even the available light tends to distress them.

Headache (choice **A**), although severe and throbbing, is not as distressing. It can be relieved by medication. Likewise, nausea (choice **B**) and vomiting (choice **C**) can be relieved and are not as distressing as photophobia. Although there is certainly increased sensitivity to sound (choice **E**), it is not as distressing as photophobia.

**19** **The answer is C** *Pediatrics*

Osgood-Schlatter disease (choice **C**) is an overuse injury that is more common in physically active boys around puberty. It is characterized by pain and swelling of the tibial tubercle. The treatment is focused on reduction of the activity. Anti-inflammatory medications are usually not helpful. The condition is usually self-limiting and resolves in 12–24 months.

Legg-Calvé-Perthes (choice **A**) presents with a gradual limp, stiffness, and pain in the groin, hip, thigh, or knee. This avascular necrosis of the femoral head usually occurs between the ages of 2 and 12 years (mean 7 years). Slipped capital femoral epiphysis (choice **B**) typically occurs in adolescents who are overweight and have delayed skeletal maturity, or in those who are tall and thin and have had a recent growth spurt. The chronic condition is associated with endocrine abnormalities such as hypothyroidism. Septic arthritis (choice **D**) is an infection within a joint space causing pain and limitation of motion. Analysis of the joint fluid is mandatory for diagnosis. Patients with idiopathic adolescent anterior knee pain syndrome (choice **E**), formally known as chondromalacia patellae, develop knee pain of unknown cause in early adolescence. Strenuous physical activity, such as running, may cause knee pain in these adolescents. However, there are no other associated findings.

**20** **The answer is E** *Medicine*

This patient is suffering from giardiasis, a widespread protozoal disease that causes diarrhea, abdominal pain, bloating, belching, flatus, nausea, and vomiting. Surface waters, such as mountain streams, are at risk for contamination. Treatment with metronidazole (choice **E**) or quinacrine is effective, with cure rates over 80%. Infections are caused by ingestion of the hardy cysts, which exist in the duodenum and live and multiply in the small intestine. Acute giardiasis usually lasts for more than a week, but untreated infections can become chronic and last for years. Therefore, reassurance (choice **A**) is not the appropriate treatment. Humoral responses appear to be important for development of immunity because patients with hypogammaglobulinemia commonly suffer from prolonged, severe infections that are resistant to treatment.

Penicillin (choice **B**) and tetracycline (choice **C**) are effective against bacteria but have no effect on protozoa. Azidothymidine (AZT; choice **D**) is used to combat human immunodeficiency virus (HIV) infections and has no antiprotozoal activity.

**21** **The answer is A** *Obstetrics and Gynecology*

Cervical cancer is the third most common female reproductive malignancy; it is responsible for 20% of all gynecologic cancers. The prevalence of cervical cancer has been markedly decreased over the past decades because of the widespread use of the Pap smear for cytologic screening. The most common tumor type is squamous cell carcinoma. This is the only gynecologic cancer that is not surgically staged. Although staging is clinical, an intravenous pyelogram (choice **A**) can be used. The primary staging is based on the depth of invasion through the basement membrane established by the histology of the cervical biopsy. The degree of spread to the broad ligament and pelvis is established by bimanual pelvic exam.

Laparoscopy (choice **B**) is not used for surgical staging of any gynecologic cancer because adequate visualization cannot be achieved. Exploratory laparotomy (choice **C**) is used for staging of ovarian and endometrial carcinoma. Lymphangiogram (choice **D**) and lymphadenectomy (choice **E**) may be helpful in assessing spread of vulvar cancer but are not used for cervical cancer staging.

**22** **The answer is D** *Medicine*

This patient has gonococcal urethritis (GCU), which is caused by *Neisseria gonorrhoeae*. GCU is more common among homosexual men and those of the lower socioeconomic strata. Nongonococcal urethritis (NGU) on the other hand, is more commonly encountered in heterosexual males and those of higher socioeconomic class. NGU is twice as common as gonococcal urethritis in the United States; it is the most common sexually transmitted disease (STD) in men and is usually due to *Chlamydia trachomatis*. However, *Trichomonas vaginalis* or herpes simplex virus (HSV) can also cause NGU. At one time, the standard treatment would have been penicillin (choice **C**). However, because of increasing resistance, penicillin is no longer recommended for gonorrhea. Ceftriaxone (choice **A**) and cefixime are drugs that inhibit cell wall synthesis and are not susceptible to β-lactase hydrolysis; therefore, they are recommended replacements for penicillin in the treatment of gonorrhea. The quinolones, ciprofloxacin (choice **B**) and ofloxacin, inhibit bacterial DNA gyrase and have a relatively broad spectrum of activity. They too are effective against gonorrhea. However, because chlamydial infections so often accompany gonococcal infections, the Centers for Disease Control (CDC) recommends that all patients with suspected or proved gonococcal urethritis also be treated as if they had chlamydial NGU. Although the quinolones have antichlamydial activity in vitro, they have not been recommended for clinical infections. *C. trachomatis* is susceptible to tetracyclines such as doxycycline (choice **E**), but strains of tetracycline-resistant *N. gonorrhoeae* have also become too common to recommend its use. Therefore, combined therapy, such as ceftriaxone and doxycycline (choice **D**), is required to treat both infections. Alternatively, because both organisms are still susceptible to the relatively new drug azithromycin, it can be used alone.

## 23 The answer is E *Pediatrics*

Associated characteristics of fragile X syndrome (choice **E**) include mental deficiency, prominent jaw, large ears with soft cartilage, and macroorchidism in postpubertal males. Fragile X syndrome is the most common form of inherited mental retardation, affecting approximately 1 in 1,250 males and 1 in 2,000 females. Although inheritance is X-linked, inheritance does not follow classic Mendelian patterns. Most males who carry the mutation are retarded and show the typical phenotypic pattern, whereas about 20% have no obvious symptoms but nonetheless are obligate carriers. Conversely, about 33% of heterozygous females show phenotypic effects, but mental retardation only occurs if the mutation is inherited from the mother. Moreover, the risk of clinical symptoms and the degree of mental retardation increases in succeeding generations. The explanation lies in the fact that a CGG triplet repeat is found in the first untranslated exon; in affected individuals, this repeat is expanded to hundreds or even thousands of repeats. Above a certain critical number, the gene becomes hypermethylated and is shut off. Further variability is built into the condition by the fact that the expanded repeat is unstable during mitosis, causing extensive somatic mosaicism with respect to the number of repeats in various cell types. The diagnosis of fragile X syndrome should be considered in any child with undiagnosed developmental and/or mental retardation. This can now be done using molecular methodologies that are more efficient and easier to do than the classic cytogenetic analyses.

Clinical features of trisomy 18 (choice **B**) are a prominent occiput and low-set, posteriorly rotated, malformed auricles; clenched hand with overlapping fingers; and rocker-bottom feet. Physical manifestations of trisomy 21 (choice **D**) include epicanthal folds, Brushfield's spots, and simian crease, a wide space between the first and second toes, a short fifth finger, and small ears. In patients with Klinefelter syndrome (choice **A**), hypogonadism, long extremities, decreased intelligence, and behavioral problems can be seen. The physical features associated with Prader-Willi syndrome (choice **C**) include a narrow face, almond-shaped eyes, a thin upper lip, hypoplastic gonads, small hands and small feet, and truncal obesity after 1–4 years of age. These patients also have slow motor development, delayed puberty, mental retardation, and behavioral problems.

## 24 The answer is A *Medicine*

The patient has a stress fracture of the tibia (choice **A**). It is caused by repetitive overload to the bone, usually from a change in training habits. The junction of the middle and distal thirds of the tibia is a common site.

Chronic exertional compartment syndrome (choice **B**) is caused by elevated pressure within an enclosed leg fascial compartment. There is no localized bony tenderness on examination. In overuse myositis (choice **C**), there is tenderness over the muscle–tendon units instead of along the tibia. Acute compartment syndrome (choice **D**) is caused by a short-term increase in tissue pressure within a fascial compartment. Patients have severe pain, weakness of muscles in the compartment, and elevated compartment pressures. Patients with anterior tibialis tendinitis (choice **E**) have pain over the dorsum of the feet. There is tenderness, and sometimes swelling, over the anterior tibialis tendon.

## 25 The answer is D *Preventive Medicine and Public Health*

The U.S. Preventive Services Task Force (USPSTF) concludes that prostate cancer is a clinically heterogeneous disease. In some patients, the diseases follows an aggressive course, whereas in the majority, the course is indolent. Moreover, it typically is a disease of old age. Except in African Americans, the disease is very rarely found in men younger than 50 years old; in African Americans, rarely in men younger than 40 years of age. Conversely, it becomes quite common after the age of 70, and after the age of 80, estimates suggest as many as 90% of men have the disease. Few, however, have significant adverse symptoms and because of its typical slow rate of development these older men will typically die of something other than prostate cancer before serious symptoms become evident. It follows that a large fraction of cases detected by screening will receive no benefit from finding an incipient cancer and because biopsy is at the least inconvenient and treatment may cause harm, the USPSTF cautions about screening older men. Quoting the 2008 report: "The USPSTF found convincing evidence that treatment for prostate cancer detected by screening causes moderate to substantial harms, such as erectile dysfunction, urinary incontinence, bowel dysfunction, and death. These harms are especially important because some men with prostate cancer who are treated would never have developed symptoms related to cancer during their lifetime. . . . There is also adequate evidence that the screening process produces at least small harms, including pain and discomfort associated with prostate biopsy and psychological effects of false-positive test results."

The report continue: "In men age 75 years or older, the USPSTF found adequate evidence that the incremental benefits of treatment for prostate cancer detected by screening are small to none." Consequently, they recommend against the service because there is moderate or high certainty that the service has no net benefit or that the harms outweigh the benefits (choice **D**).

Even in men younger than 75 years old, the USPSTF found: "inadequate evidence to determine whether treatment for prostate cancer detected by screening improves health outcomes compared with treatment after clinical detection." Hence, their cautious recommendation, namely: "The USPSTF concludes that the current evidence is insufficient to assess the balance of benefits and harms of the service. Evidence is lacking, of poor quality, or conflicting, and the balance of benefits and harms cannot be determined" (choice **E**). This recommendation continues: "If the service is offered, patients should understand the uncertainty about the balance of benefits and harms." Choices **A**, **B**, and **C** are irrelevant to this problem.

## 26 The answer is D *Surgery*

The correct answer is **D**. The macula has the highest density of cones. Laser photocoagulation targeted at drusen may inadvertently damage cones. Unfortunately, this is not preventable. For this reason, it is important to advise the patient that deterioration in visual acuity would follow the procedure, and that the reason for recommending it is to slow progression of the disease, which if left unchecked, would soon leave her legally blind.

Choices **A**, **B**, and **C** are incorrect, since choice **D** is correct. Choice **E** is incorrect because peripheral vision remains relatively intact in macular degeneration, since drusen—tiny, yellow or white hyaline bodies that are one of the most common precursor signs of age-related macular degeneration—tend to accumulate in the macular area and a few are present elsewhere.

## 27 The answer is C *Medicine*

This patient has epidermolysis bullosa (choice **C**). This is an inherited condition that affects 1 in 50,000 individuals in the United States. The skin breaks down and forms blisters, usually after minor trauma. Even stretching the skin can cause the lesion, and this is done to confirm the diagnosis. Treatment is symptomatic.

Ehlers-Danlos syndrome (choice **A**), of which there are 11 types, is an inherited condition in which there is hyperelasticity of the skin and hypermobility of the joints. The skin does not break down. The incidence for all types collectively is approximately 1 in 5,000 births and is higher in African Americans. The symptomatology varies depending on the type of disease and ranges from mild to life-threatening. The skin may be very thin, and the subjacent blood vessels may be seen. On the other hand, the skin may look like velvet and have extreme stretchability ("rubber man" syndrome). Scars may look like cigarette paper, and hyperpigmentation over the joints is not uncommon. The pattern of inheritance varies with the type of disease, and in most forms, the biochemical defect has to do with collagen synthesis. Osteogenesis imperfecta (choice **D**) also exists in multiple forms, having in common osteopenia (decreased bone mass). The simplest functional classification is: type I, mild; type II, lethal; and type III, moderately severe. Type I commonly is found over several generations in families and is characterized by a triad of blue sclera, brittle bones, and deafness. Joint laxity can also be a problem. Multiple fractures are most common before puberty and in association with premature osteoporosis in the elderly. Fractures are minimally displaced, and soft-tissue swelling is minimal. Deafness of the conductance type generally starts in the third or fourth decade. Penetrance of the blue sclera approaches 98%, whereas bone fractures and deafness are expressed less often. Some families with type I (type Ib) osteogenesis imperfecta also have dental abnormalities. Patients with type II osteogenesis imperfecta who do not die in utero or shortly after birth become progressively worse. Some of the subtypes of type III osteogenesis imperfecta do not have blue sclera. The diagnosis is clinical, and x-ray films reveal decreased bone density. This can be confirmed by photon or x-ray absorptiometry. Type I procollagen defects have been noted in most patients.

Systemic sclerosis (choice **B**), also known as scleroderma, is a multisystem disorder of unknown etiology in which there is progressive fibrosis of the skin, blood vessels, and visceral organs in the chest and abdomen. The condition may predominantly involve the skin, in which there is rapid symmetric thickening of the skin of the proximal and distal extremities, face, and trunk. The tightness of the skin across the face may make a patient appear as if is constantly grinning. In other cases, the patient may have localized sclerosis—CREST syndrome, which is an acronym for calcinosis, Raynaud's phenomenon, esophageal dysfunction, sclerodactyly, and telangiectasia. Child abuse (choice **E**), although a possibility, is usually associated with fractures in different stages of healing and retinal hemorrhages seen on ophthalmoscopy. Fractures involving the posterior aspect of the ribs, spiral fractures of the extremities, and bucket-handle fractures of the metaphysis are pathognomonic of child abuse. Skin lesions include bruises; circular burns from cigarettes, especially in the gluteal region; and symmetric scalds involving the lower extremities and gluteal area as a result of immersion in hot water. Distinguishing osteogenesis imperfecta from child abuse is important.

### 28 The answer is C *Preventive Medicine and Public Health*

Summation of $a + b$ represents the cohort involved in a prospective study group. In cohort designs, the investigator first identifies a study group of individuals who have common characteristics (cohort). Some of these will be exposed to a proposed risk agent for disease, while another group will not. The two are observed forward in time for the development of disease. The investigator then establishes the extent to which the disease develops in the two groups. The group $a + b$ (choice **C**) represents the cohort (i.e., the study group), while $c + d$ (choice **D**) represents the control.

The sum $a + c$ (choice **A**) represents the retrospective study group, which is studied backward in time—from the point of disease to the point of exposure. Note that in a prospective study, one can determine the incidence of the disease, but this is not possible in the case of a retrospective study. The sums $c + b$ (choice **B**) and $(a + c) + (c + d)$ (choice **E**) have no statistical value, because they represent two diverse groups. The cohort who are disease free after exposure are represented by $b$, while $c$ represents the control (nonexposed) group who develops disease.

### 29 The answer is D *Surgery*

The patient has central retinal artery occlusion (choice **D**). Retinal artery occlusion could be central or peripheral. The disorder is characterized by a sudden, complete, painless loss of vision in one eye. The patient often notices it when he or she closes one eye. Potential causes include atherosclerotic carotid disease, giant cell arteritis, lipid emboli from trauma, intravenous drug abuse, sickle cell anemia, and hypercoagulable states. Funduscopy reveals pallor of the optic disc, edema of the retina, and a cherry-red spot. The cherry-red spot represents ischemia and edema of the posterior retina, and occurs within hours following the occlusion. The red color is due to perfusion of the choroid through the thinner retinal tissue. Segmentation of retinal vessels giving a boxcar appearance is a feature as well. Initial management is massaging the eyeball. Thereafter, the patient is asked to breathe into a paper bag to increase $P_{CO_2}$. Doing so will induce vasodilatation of the artery and (one hopes) dislodge the embolus. Definitive treatment involves anterior chamber paracentesis under slit lamp examination. It is the best method to lower intraocular pressure and dislodge the embolus.

Central retinal vein occlusion (choice **A**) is characterized by a sudden, painful, unilateral loss of vision in patients with hypercoagulable states and thrombotic disorders such as deep venous thrombosis. Branch retinal vein occlusion (choice **F**) is most commonly seen in systemic hypertension. Funduscopy reveals a "blood and thunder" fundus, i.e.: dilated tortuous veins, flame-shaped hemorrhages, macular edema, cotton wool spots, and exudates. Neovascularization of the retina or iris can occur and result in secondary glaucoma. Treatment is laser photocoagulation. Acute angle-closure glaucoma (choice **B**) also is usually unilateral, but clinical features include intense ocular pain associated with nausea and vomiting and diminished vision with colored halos around lights. The pupil is mid-dilated and fixed, and perilimbal injection may be present. The anterior chamber is shallow, and this can be confirmed by gonioscopy. Failure to diagnose this condition and treat it in a timely manner will lead to blindness. Treatment involves decreasing intraocular pressure with β-blockers such as timolol, and carbonic anhydrase inhibitors as adjuncts. Miotics such as pilocarpine or cholinesterase inhibitors are also used. Corneal abrasion (choice **C**) is associated with pain and lacrimation (epiphora) and blepharospasm. Diagnosis is made by fluorescein staining of the cornea and observing it under a slit lamp. Treatment involves removal of the foreign body if present, and topical antibiotics. Optic neuritis (choice **E**) presents with unilateral central visual loss associated with painful eye movements. It is usually seen in patients with demyelinating disease such as multiple sclerosis. Most patients recover spontaneously over time. Funduscopy reveals a normal disc in most patients. Some patient may have edema.

**30 The answer is D** *Obstetrics and Gynecology*

Anemia in pregnancy is a common medical complication. Maternal megaloblastic anemia in pregnancy is most commonly caused by folate deficiency (choice **D**). Vitamin $B_{12}$ deficiency, also a cause of megaloblastic anemia, is associated with infertility and thus is seldom seen with pregnancy. Anticonvulsants are known to decrease folic acid absorption, so folate deficiency is associated with their use even when supplemented in the typical multivitamin pill. Fetal congenital malformations due to folic acid deficiency can occur as rare complications of anticonvulsant therapy, specifically treatment with phenytoin. However, phenytoin can diminish absorption of folate, resulting in macrocytosis, as seen in this patient.

All of the other options listed—sickle cell trait (choice **A**), iron deficiency (choice **B**), physiologic anemia (choice **C**), and thalassemia (choice **E**)—are associated with either normal or low mean corpuscular volume (MCV).

**31 The answer is C** *Obstetrics and Gynecology*

The human ovary can develop a wide variety of tumors. These tumors can be functional, inflammatory, metaplastic, or neoplastic, but most are benign. Benign cystic teratoma (choice **C**), also known as a dermoid cyst, is the most common benign complex ovarian tumor in young women. This can coexist with a normal pregnancy. The scenario describes a probable torsion of this enlarged ovary. Urgent surgical exploration is essential.

A follicular cyst (choice **A**) is probably the most common reason for ovarian enlargement. This is the dominant follicle found in all women prior to ovulation. However, these are always simple fluid-filled cysts and never have calcifications. A mucinous cystadenoma (choice **B**) is a benign epithelial ovarian tumor and is frequently multiloculated. They can attain a huge size, often filling the entire pelvis. If they rupture, they can cause pseudomyxoma peritonei. However, calcifications are not usually seen. A Brenner tumor (choice **D**) is also a benign epithelial ovarian tumor but it is solid, occurring most often in women over 50 years of age. A serous cystadenoma (choice **E**), another epithelial ovarian tumor, tends to be unilocular but does not show calcifications.

**32 The answer is D** *Medicine*

Mitral regurgitation (choice **D**) can occur because of a tear of papillary muscle, in which the mitral valve prolapses. This is usually seen in young women between the ages of 14 and 30. Mitral valve prolapse is usually asymptomatic, but in a small number of cases can become symptomatic. This condition may actually encompass a wide spectrum of features ranging from a systolic click, murmur, and mild prolapse of the posterior leaflet of the mitral valve to severe mitral regurgitation due to rupture of the chorda tendineae with massive prolapse of both leaflets of the mitral valve. The condition usually develops slowly over a number of years. Mitral valve prolapse is the most common cause of isolated severe mitral regurgitation. Most often, patients have arrhythmias, dizziness, and syncope. Auscultation most often reveals a middle or late nonejection systolic click. This may or may not be associated with a high-pitched, late, crescendo–decrescendo murmur. Mitral valve prolapse is believed to be autosomal dominant. Causes include heritable connective tissue disorders, such as Marfan syndrome, osteogenesis imperfecta, and Ehlers-Danlos syndrome; however, in most cases the cause is unknown. The pathology is believed to be due to decreased production of type III collagen.

Mitral stenosis (choice **A**) is most commonly seen in females. The most common cause is rheumatic fever, and it may rarely be congenital. Cough, paroxysmal nocturnal dyspnea, dyspnea on exertion, and cardiac failure can occur as the stenosis gets more severe. Atrial fibrillation is commonly seen in patients with mitral stenosis. This could result in recurrent pulmonary emboli. Aortic stenosis (choice **B**) can be congenital, may occur following rheumatic endocarditis, or may be due to idiopathic calcification usually noted in the elderly. Most cases of aortic stenosis occur in males. Physical examination reveals displacement of the apical pulse because of left ventricular hypertrophy, associated with a thrill, and an ejection systolic murmur conducted to the carotids. The volume of the pulse is decreased, and if the stenosis is severe, there may be evidence of left ventricular failure. Aortic regurgitation (choice **C**) is primarily seen in males, although aortic regurgitation with mitral regurgitation is more common in women. Most of the cases occur after rheumatic fever. Other causes of aortic regurgitation include syphilis, Marfan syndrome, and rheumatoid ankylosing spondylitis. Ventricular septal defects may be associated with aortic regurgitation. The most common and earliest complaint is an awareness of the heartbeat while lying down. Dyspnea, chest pains, and excessive sweating develop later. Physical examination reveals a displaced, forceful apex beat; diastolic thrill; and a high-pitched, decrescendo diastolic murmur; and an ejection click. The pulse is bounding (Corrigan's pulse).

Left ventricular failure could follow. Congestive cardiac failure (choice **E**) usually follows cardiac or pulmonary disease. There is a history of dyspnea, fatigue, and swelling of the ankles. Cyanosis may be present. Auscultation will reveal basal rales. Congestive hepatomegaly, pleural effusion, and ascites may also be features. Pulsus alternans, if present, signifies severe heart failure. This is a condition in which a regular cardiac rhythm results in alternate strong and weak pulses. A third heart sound is usually seen in left ventricular failure or left ventricular overload. A fourth heart sound is often heard in normal individuals. It is also heard in patients with aortic stenosis, hypertension, cardiomyopathy, hyperthyroidism, and anemia. The last two are associated with hyperdynamic circulation.

### 33 The answer is A *Psychiatry*

The presentation is most suggestive of bipolar disorder (choice **A**), which is characterized by periods of mania with relatively normal function between episodes. A manic episode is suggested by the presence of agitation, pressured speech, grandiose delusions, disorganized behavior, increased psychomotor activity, and decreased judgment. Periods of decreased sleep may be present as well.

Brief psychotic disorder (choice **B**) lasts less than 1 month and is usually not preceded by similar episodes. Delusional disorder, erotomanic type (choice **C**), is characterized by delusions about special relationships with relative strangers and minimum thought disorganization. Major depressive disorder with mood-congruent psychosis (choice **D**) is characterized by episodes of severe depression with hallucinations or delusions involving worthlessness, sickness, guilt, death, or other depressive themes. Schizophrenia (choice **E**) is characterized by the presence of residual symptoms such as affect blunting, lack of motivation, and social withdrawal between psychotic episodes.

### 34 The answer is A *Surgery*

The patient has superior vena cava syndrome, which is most commonly secondary to extension of a primary lung cancer (choice **A**; usually a small-cell carcinoma) into the neck, with obstruction of superior vena caval blood flow. Clinical findings consist of puffiness and bluish discoloration of the face, arms, and shoulders, along with distention of the jugular veins. Collateral venous circulation results, as evidenced by dilated and tortuous veins over the anterior chest. In addition, there are central nervous system signs of dizziness, visual disturbances, and convulsions. Prompt administration of diuretics, fluid restriction, and radiation therapy are useful in restoring blood flow. Surgery is rarely indicated. The mean survival is 6–8 months.

Pericardial effusion (choice **B**) distends the neck veins but would not be associated with the degree of venous engorgement noted in this case. Sclerosing mediastinitis (choice **C**) is uncommon and usually results from histoplasmosis. Polycythemia rubra vera (choice **D**) is associated with increased plasma volume and red blood cell mass, and a tendency for venous thrombosis. However, thrombosis of the superior vena cava is very unlikely. Right ventricular failure (choice **E**) is not associated with the degree of venous engorgement noted in this patient.

### 35 The answer is B *Surgery*

Blunt trauma to the upper left abdomen or lower left chest is frequently complicated by a ruptured spleen, especially in the presence of fractures of the lower ribs (choice **B**). This can be diagnosed by computed tomography or peritoneal lavage if the diagnosis is equivocal. However, the presence of shock in this patient is an indication for immediate surgical intervention—control of hemorrhage followed by splenorrhaphy. Splenectomy is no longer performed. Loss of the spleen would result in inability to opsonize encapsulated bacteria such as pneumococcus.

Pulmonary contusion with hemorrhage into the pleural cavity (choice **A**) is unlikely in the presence of normal breath sounds. The location of the injury and the presence of hypovolemic shock would argue against rupture of the colon (choice **C**) or transection of the abdominal aorta (choice **D**). Hematuria would be present with a ruptured kidney (choice **E**).

### 36 The answer is C *Pediatrics*

Subdural hematoma and retinal hemorrhages are common signs of fatal child abuse. In this case, they are signs of *shaken baby syndrome*, in which a child is shaken to stop him or her from crying. Initially, the patient must be medically stabilized using the ABCs (airway, breathing, circulation) of resuscitation. The next step, if abuse is suspected, is to consult social services and the state agency that deals with this problem (choice **C**).

Ongoing medical care (choice **A**) and notification of the patient's primary care provider (choice **B**) can be carried out after the state agency has been contacted. In cases of suspected child abuse, the physician neither has to inform the parents that child abuse is suspected (choice **E**) nor obtain consent from the parent to admit the child to the hospital (choice **D**).

**37** **The answer is C** *Obstetrics and Gynecology*

The case is strongly suggestive of intrauterine fetal death (IUFD). From a medical standpoint, once the embryo completes formation of all the organs at 10 menstrual weeks, it is referred to as a fetus. However, legally and technically, the definition of IUFD is fetal demise on or after 20 weeks' gestation. Prior to 20 weeks, it is legally referred to as a *spontaneous abortion*. IUFD complicates approximately 3 per 1,000 pregnancies. Real-time ultrasound examination for cardiac motion (choice **C**) is the method of choice for ascertaining fetal death. Failure to visualize cardiac motion is diagnostic. Other signs are overlapping of the skull bones. Maternal assessment of fetal movement (kicking) is not accurate in sensitivity or specificity.

The pregnancy test remains positive for a considerable time because the placenta continues to produce β-human chorionic gonadotropin (β-hCG), thus choice **E** is not appropriate. Amniocentesis (choice **B**) is an invasive test that relies on the finding of dark, turbid fluid, which is a late development. It is not appropriate to diagnose IUFD. Exposure of a possibly live fetus to x-rays is not recommended (choice **D**). A nonstress test (choice **A**) is the appropriate next step in management with maternal report of decreased fetal movement but would not be helpful in this case.

**38** **The answer is E** *Psychiatry*

Undoing (choice **E**) refers to the performance of an activity that symbolically reverses some previous behavior or thought. This defense mechanism is commonly present in individuals who feel either conscious or unconscious guilt.

The other choices are defense mechanisms that do not apply as well to this patient. Denial (choice **A**) is a failure to acknowledge a disturbing aspect of external reality. Dissociation (choice **B**) involves sealing off disturbing thoughts or emotions from consciousness. Intellectualization (choice **C**) is the transformation of an emotionally disturbing event into a purely cognitive problem. Sublimation (choice **D**) occurs when unacceptable impulses are channeled into more acceptable activities.

**39** **The answer is D** *Psychiatry*

This patient's symptoms suggest somatization disorder. Numerous studies have demonstrated that morbidity from this illness is significantly decreased with regularly scheduled follow-up medical appointments (choice **D**). The focus of such visits is general, and the physician should avoid arguments about the veracity of symptoms. Such an approach also decreases costs associated with overuse of emergency services without a verbal warning to the patient (choice **B**).

Refusal to see the patient again (choice **A**) or simply referring her to another clinician (choice **C**) is unlikely to benefit this patient. Trial of various medications (choice **E**) carry the risk of causing iatrogenic problems and are unlikely to be productive in light of the previous history.

**40** **The answer is D** *Medicine*

This patient has advanced chronic obstructive airway disease (COPD). His episodes of confusion are most likely manifestations of periods of hypoxia. Supplemental oxygen therapy (choice **D**) is the mainstay of treatment in patients who have COPD and hypoxemia.

A course of corticosteroids (choice **A**) alone would not abolish the hypoxemia. Corticosteroids and antibiotics (choice **B**) are indicated in exacerbations of COPD. There is nothing in the history that he currently suffers from cough with expectoration. Antibiotics (choice **C**) would certainly be indicated if he had an active chest infection, which he does not. His main problem is the advancing disease and hypoxia. Donepezil (choice **E**) is a centrally acting acetylcholine inhibitor used to treat Alzheimer disease. He does not have Alzheimer disease. In Alzheimer disease, there is a progressive loss of short-term memory and not episodic confusion. He could be at risk for it if there was a genetic predisposition, given that his father died from it.

**41** **The answer is B** *Medicine*

Rofecoxib (choice **B**) is a nonsteroidal anti-inflammatory drug (NSAID) that was touted as a wonder drug because it was a specific inhibitor of a cyclo-oxygenase (COX) isozyme present in connective tissue but not found in high concentration in the stomach. As a consequence, it was thought that Rofecoxib and other COX-2 inhibitors could be used to treat osteoarthritis and other conditions involving inflammation as well as pain with less concern about developing gastritis. Unfortunately, Vioxx was shown to adversely affect the cardio-vascular system and was withdrawn from the market; the other COX-2 inhibitors currently are under scrutiny.

**42** **The answer is E** *Medicine*

This unfortunate woman suffers from fibromyalgia. Fluoxetine (choice **E**) is a selective serotonin reuptake inhibitor that is most often prescribed as an antidepressant. It, however, is sometimes used for other conditions, such as fibromyalgia.

**43** **The answer is G** *Medicine*

Cyclosporine ophthalmic emulsion (choice **G**) is used to promote tear secretion in patients with Sjögren syndrome and other cases of severe dry eye (xerophthalmia).

**44** **The answer is H** *Medicine*

Ibuprofen (choice **H**) is a traditional nonsteroidal anti-inflammatory drug (NSAID) that inhibits both the COX-1 and COX-2 enzymes. Thus, despite its analgesic and anti-inflammatory action, it must be used with caution to avoid occult blood loss, peptic ulceration, and acute renal failure.

**45** **The answer is D** *Medicine*

This woman almost certainly has osteoporosis. Her sex (female), age (postmenopausal), ethnicity (Asian), and weight (less than 127 lb) all are risk factors for osteoporosis. Moreover, a common symptom is compression fractures of the spine, which result in shortened stature and a buffalo hump. It seems probable that she is soon headed for a major fracture unless treated. Alendronate (choice **D**) in a 70 mg is dose generally taken by mouth once a week. Several other bisphosphates are clinically available at this time. The bisphosphonates work by inhibiting osteoclastic activity and tip the balance during bone remodeling toward laying down bone rather than the net loss of bone that leads to osteoporoses among the aged.

**46** **The answer is I** *Medicine*

This lady very likely also has osteoporosis. Zoledronic acid (choice **I**) is another bisphosphate, it, however, is taken by infusion once per year rather than orally daily or weekly. This assures compliance, which otherwise may be a problem with a mentally challenged person. It is also used to treat persons who cannot tolerate an oral bisphosphate.

**47** **The answer is J** *Medicine*

This lady obviously has rheumatoid arthritis, a disease that most often affect women between the ages of 40 and 50. It is an autoimmune disease, which, if untreated, is disabling and deforming. Adalimumab (choice **J**) is one of a group of new drugs called *disease-modifying antirheumatic drugs* (DMARDs). Adalimumab is a tumor-necrosis factor blocker that serves to inhibit the progress of the disease. It or some other DMARD is now given early in the course of the disease, before irreversible changes occur.

**48** **The answer is A** *Medicine*

An analgesic is commonly prescribed as a sequel to a root canal procedure. Two analgesics are listed, ibuprofen and acetaminophen with codeine. Of these, acetaminophen with codeine (choice **A**) is a more effective pain modulator, and even though it contains the narcotic codeine, it can safely be prescribed for short-term use such as treating pain after a dental procedure. Moreover, the anti-inflammatory properties of ibuprofen are rarely relevant with respect to the root canal procedure.

**49** **The answer is C**  *Medicine*

This man appears to have developed influenza which should be treated as soon as possible to avoid an epidemic in this closed environment. If oseltamivir (Tamiflu; choice **C**) is administered within 48 hours after the appearance of initial symptoms, it may inhibit the further development of the disease.

**50** **The answer is F**  *Medicine*

This man suffers from gout. Most of the symptoms associated with gout are caused by hyperuricemia and the limited solubility of uric acid, which causes it to precipitate in joints and within the kidney. Allopurinol is a completive inhibitor of xanthine oxidase, the enzyme that catalyzes the conversion of xanthine to uric acid. Thus, as long as the hyperuricemia is caused by overproduction (not by limited excretion), allopurinol increases the concentration of the more-soluble intermediates xanthine and hypoxanthine and decreases the level of poorly soluble uric acid, thereby decreasing the possibility of precipitation. The xanthine and hypoxanthine is then salvaged to form xanthylic acid (XMP) and inosinic acid (IMP). These salvage reactions require phosphoribosyl pyrophosphate (PRPP), which is also used for the de novo synthesis of purines. As a consequence, allopurinol also inhibits purine synthesis, further enhancing its effectiveness.

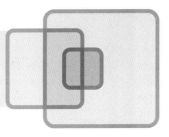

# test 9

# Questions

**Single Best Choice Directions:** *This section consists of numbered statements or questions followed by a list of potential answers; you are to select the ONE best answer.*

**1** A 21-year-old man presents with auditory hallucinations and the delusion that federal narcotics agents are monitoring his telephone calls. He was dealing methamphetamine and using large amounts of the substance daily until about 1 week ago, when he exhausted his supply and was too frightened to leave his home to get more. Mental status examination reveals an alert and anxious individual who is oriented and coherent. Urine toxicology testing result for methamphetamine is negative. Which of the following is the most likely fundamental diagnosis?

(A) Methamphetamine-induced anxiety disorder
(B) Methamphetamine-induced delirium
(C) Methamphetamine-induced psychotic disorder
(D) Methamphetamine intoxication
(E) Schizophrenia, paranoid type

**2** A patient with myasthenia gravis that has been well controlled with pyridostigmine for 2 years comes to the emergency department complaining of progressive muscle weakening during the last 24 hours. He has trouble swallowing and suffers from double vision. The patient has had flu-like symptoms for the past week. Which of the following is the most appropriate immediate course of action?

(A) Increase the dose of pyridostigmine.
(B) Replace pyridostigmine with physostigmine.
(C) Give a small dose of edrophonium.
(D) Decrease the dose of pyridostigmine.
(E) Administer succinylcholine.

**3** A 30-year-old Caucasian woman who claims to never have smoked presents with bilateral puffiness and swelling of the fingers with joint pains. Cold exposure and stress cause episodes of blanching or cyanosis of the fingers. She is not on any medications. The mechanism for this patient's disease is most likely the result of which one of the following?

(A) Vasospasm and thickening of the digital arteries
(B) Hyperviscosity due to an increase in immunoglobulin M (IgM) antibodies
(C) An immune complex vasculitis
(D) Thrombosis of the digital vessels
(E) An embolism to the digital vessels

**4** A 65-year-old woman presents to the emergency department with diffuse abdominal pain and vomiting. She has not had a bowel movement in the past 3 days. Physical examination reveals hyperstasis, tympany to percussion, and no rebound tenderness. Her temperature is 38°C (100.4°F). An abdominal x-ray film reveals distended loops of small bowel with a stepladder pattern of differential air–fluid levels. Which of the following is the mechanism that most likely produced these findings?

(A) Diverticulosis
(B) Adhesions from previous surgery
(C) Torsion of the bowel around the mesenteric root
(D) Intussusception of the terminal ileum into the cecum
(E) Ischemia secondary to thrombosis of the superior mesenteric artery

**5** A 62-year-old woman with a history of diabetes and hypertension presents to the emergency department with the right eye deviated outward and an obvious ptosis. She has a slight headache. The pupils are normal size. Which of the following is the most likely diagnosis?

(A) Cavernous sinus thrombosis
(B) Superior oblique palsy
(C) Posterior cerebral artery aneurysm with third-nerve impingement
(D) Vasculopathic (noncompressive) third-nerve palsy
(E) Internuclear ophthalmoplegia

**6** A 3-year-old Caucasian boy of Scandinavian descent, who had been developing normally, contracted otitis media. Because he had not felt well, he missed two meals. Suddenly, he became lethargic, started vomiting, had a violent seizure, and became comatose. His parents called 911, and he was put on a saline IV drip and taken to the emergency department. There, his physician immediately ordered a complete blood count, a liver panel, a chemistry panel, and a urinalysis. A finger prick test showed that the child was hypoglycemic but not ketonic. In taking a history from the mother, the attending physician finds that an older sibling died mysteriously in her sleep as an infant. He immediately orders the saline IV drip to be changed to a 10% glucose solution, and shortly thereafter, the patient starts to recover. Several hours later, when the laboratory results become available, it is determined that the boy's serum glucose value had been 35 mg/dL and that he had slightly elevated serum blood urea nitrogen (BUN), ammonia, and uric acid levels; an anion gap metabolic acidosis; and his liver enzyme values were also elevated. However, both his serum and urine ketone levels were zero. The child most likely has which one of the following?

(A) Glucose 6-phosphatase deficiency
(B) Medium chain acyl-CoA deficiency
(C) Carnitine acyltransferase deficiency
(D) Primary hyperinsulinemia
(E) Acute intermittent porphyria

**7** A worried father brings his 17-year-old daughter to the emergency department in Stockton, California, at 11:15 PM. He informs the triage nurse that his daughter has been experiencing headaches for about 2 days, and today she has been extremely fatigued. He is particularly concerned because she rarely experiences headaches and has always been very active. When seen by the doctor, the daughter tries to make light of her condition. She blames the drowsiness on taking too many acetaminophen/codeine pills prescribed several weeks ago by her dentist. She admits, however, that she took the pills because she has the "mother of all headaches"; she does not recall ever having one of such intensity. She further suggests that her fatigue may also be a consequence of the fact that she has been losing sleep because her headaches wake her up, being particularly intense at night. When asked if her neck is stiff, she gives an ambiguous answer. She is slightly nauseous, but has not vomited. She has never had any major illnesses, has been active in high school athletics, and does not know of anyone sick with whom she has been in contact.

Physical examination reveals the following: temperature, 40°C (100°F); blood pressure, 140/70 mm Hg; pulse, 120/min and regular. The cardiovascular, respiratory, gastrointestinal, and genitourinary systems are all normal. The central nervous system examination, including funduscopy, seems normal. She is oriented with respect to time and space; however, she is unduly sensitive to bright lights. There is a very slight resistance to the forward flexion of the neck. Neuromuscular tone and reflexes are normal.

The laboratory profile reveals the following: serum white blood cell (WBC) count of 10,500 cells/mm$^3$ (normal 4,800–10,800 cells/mm$^3$), erythrocyte sedimentation rate (ESR) of 20 mm/h (normal female <15 mm/h); electrolyte profile blood sugar level, serum amylase level, and chest x-ray film are all within normal limits.

On the basis of these data, a lumbar puncture is performed. The following results are obtained: cell count, 28 cells/mm$^3$, 95% mononuclear lymphocytes (normal is 0–5 cells/mm$^3$, lymphocytes); glucose, 48 mg/dL (normal is 48–85 mg/dL); protein, 85 mg/dL (normal is 15-45 mg/dL); and chloride, 120 mEq/L (normal is 118–132 mEq/L). Which of the following is the most likely diagnosis?

(A) Bacterial meningitis
(B) Cryptococcal meningitis
(C) *Coccidia immitis* meningitis
(D) Aseptic meningitis
(E) Actinomyces meningitis

**8** A 53-year-old man comes to his primary care physician. After some hesitation, he tells him that recently he has not been able to maintain an erection while trying to make love to his wife of 30 years. His medical history is significant for diabetes mellitus, which was first diagnosed a decade ago. Which one of the following choices is most likely to be true about this patient?

(A) He is maintaining optimum blood sugar levels.
(B) Erection is normal, but orgasm and ejaculatory problems are present.
(C) He has no penile nerve damage.
(D) Ejaculation is normal, but erectile problems are present.
(E) He has no vascular changes in the penis.

**9** A 35-year-old man with a long history of dyspepsia experiences sudden onset of severe epigastric distress with associated pain in the right shoulder. Physical examination reveals a patient who appears ill and who has a rigid, quiet abdomen with rebound tenderness. Which of the following is the most appropriate first step in the management of this patient?

(A) Order a barium study of the upper gastrointestinal system.
(B) Order upright and supine abdominal films.
(C) Perform a peritoneal lavage.
(D) Administer antacids.
(E) Do an exploratory laparotomy.

10 A 2-year-old child attends day care at a local neighborhood nursery. The parents report that one of his favorite activities at day care is to play in the sandbox. The parents tell you that the child especially enjoys this activity when the owner's puppies are in the sandbox too. According to the parents, until recently, the patient has been in his usual state of good health; in addition, he has no significant past medical history and his immunizations are up to date. However, at this office visit, the patient has wheezing, hepatosplenomegaly, and prominent peripheral blood eosinophilia. Which of the following diagnoses is most likely in this child?

(A) Enterobius vermicularis infestation
(B) Eosinophilic lung disease
(C) Ascariasis
(D) Visceral larva migrans
(E) Strongyloidiasis

11 A 16-year-old male distance runner presents with complaints of worsening athletic performance and increasing cough and sputum production after running. He is very concerned because the state track meet is only 2 weeks away. Findings of the physical examination are normal. Which of the following is the most appropriate next step in the management of this patient?

(A) Prescribe a $\beta_2$-agonist inhaler to be used 5 minutes before activity.
(B) Prescribe theophylline to be taken orally.
(C) Prescribe a cromolyn sodium inhaler to be used 15 minutes before activity.
(D) Prescribe erythromycin to be taken orally for 10 days.
(E) Explain that he has asthma and should refrain from strenuous activities from now on.

12 A 55-year-old Caucasian woman, who has a chronic cough from a 30 pack-year history of smoking, complains of pelvic pressure symptoms. The problem began gradually over the last 2 years. She states that when she increases intraabdominal pressure in having a bowel movement, a mass appears at her vaginal opening. It has been 3 years since her last menstrual period. She is not taking estrogen replacement therapy. She does complain of constipation and has difficulty in stool evacuation, having to press her fingers on her vagina to evacuate her stool. She had three vaginal deliveries, the largest infant weighing 4,500 g (9 lb 15 oz). Her postvoiding residual is 60 mL. Which one of the following physical findings would be most likely on pelvic examination?

(A) Rectocele
(B) Cystocele
(C) Enterocele
(D) Urethrocele
(E) Vaginocele

13 An obese 18-year-old presents at an emergency clinic in labor and asks for help in delivering her first child. The triage nurse takes a history and determines that the patient has had no prenatal care and cannot recall when her last menstrual cycle was, as she has always had irregular cycles. She further reveals that she first realized that she might be pregnant about 4 months ago; she denies the usage of drugs, alcohol, or tobacco and also denies having any sexually transmitted diseases. The baby was quickly delivered with no untoward incidences. At delivery, the infant is noted to be large for gestational age and has cracked, peeling skin. The infant's fingernails are long and its fingers are stained green. There is absence of lanugo. Which of the following is the most likely gestational age of this infant?

(A) 34 weeks
(B) 36 weeks
(C) 38 weeks
(D) 40 weeks
(E) 42 weeks

14 A 40-year-old woman develops an unmanageable fear of snakes while being courted by an avid hiking enthusiast. She has never been married or had any other intimate relationships with men. Prior to being courted by this man, she enjoyed mountain walks and was never concerned with such fears. Although she knows that no poisonous snakes inhabit her area, she can no longer make herself hike. Which of the following is the most commonly postulated psychodynamic defense mechanism in such situations?

(A) Dissociation
(B) Projection
(C) Displacement
(D) Conversion
(E) Resistance

**15** A 20-year-old man is stabbed in the left side of his chest, medial to the nipple. Upon examination, his blood pressure is 90/60 mm Hg and his pulse is 130/min. His jugular venous pulse increases on inspiration, whereas his peripheral pulse and blood pressure decrease on inspiration. Breath sounds are normal bilaterally. The patient's chest x-ray film is unremarkable. After receiving 2 L of isotonic saline, his blood pressure remains low, whereas his central venous pressure rises to 32 cm $H_2O$. Which of the following is the most appropriate next step in the management of this patient?

(A) Insert a chest tube into the left pleural cavity.
(B) Increase parenteral fluids until the blood pressure increases.
(C) Order an echocardiogram.
(D) Decrease venous pressure by administering a venodilator.
(E) Decrease venous pressure by administering a loop diuretic.

**16** A 59-year-old woman has gradual onset of emotional lability, loss of memory (particularly of recent events), forgetfulness (absent mindedness), impulsiveness, and, as a consequence, difficulty organizing her finances and appointments. Physical examination reveals a bilateral Babinski sign. Which one of the following dietary deficiencies most likely causes her symptoms?

(A) Vitamin $B_{12}$
(B) Vitamin C
(C) Iron
(D) Magnesium
(E) Lecithin

**17** A 5-year-old girl with severe mental retardation is brought to the pediatrician for immunizations. According to the history, the patient appeared to be developing normally until 18 months of age, when she acquired dementia and her head circumference plateaued, resulting in microcephaly. She wrings her hands, and sighs. She is noted to have ataxia and marked loss of gross motor skills. In addition, she has loss of language milestones. Which of the following is the most likely diagnosis?

(A) Autism
(B) William syndrome
(C) Rett syndrome
(D) Turner syndrome
(E) Russell-Silver syndrome

**18** A 27-year-old woman, gravida 3, para 0, abortus 2, comes to the outpatient office at 15 weeks' gestation by dates with complaints of exquisite vulvar pain and blisters. The onset of the symptoms was 48 hours ago, and she experienced numbness and tingling in her perineum before any lesions appeared. She states she has had similar episodes prior to the pregnancy for the past 5 years. Her vital signs are as follows: temperature, 37°C (98.6°F); pulse, 95/min; respiration, 20/min; blood pressure, 128/74 mm Hg. On examination, you find exquisitely painful vesicles on her left labia minora. Inguinal nodes are negative bilaterally. She has a past history of a right Bartholin's abscess, which was marsupialized. She had a positive cervical chlamydial culture on her first prenatal visit, which was treated with a single dose of oral azithromycin. Which one of the following statements is true?

(A) She should undergo a cesarean section to protect her infant from infection.
(B) Her fetus has an increased risk of congenital malformations.
(C) Transplacental transmission to her fetus is a significant concern.
(D) Breastfeeding of her infant is probably unsafe and should be avoided.
(E) Decisions regarding route of delivery are best made at the onset of labor.

**19** A 71-inch tall (1.8 m), 57-year-old man weighs 208 pounds (94.3 kg), feels healthy, and wants to take out life insurance. Consequently, he is subjected to a physical examination with subsequent laboratory analyses. The following data are obtained: blood pressure, 155/84; fasting blood glucose, 115 mg/dL; total cholesterol, 265 mg/dL; triglycerides, 157 mg/dL; high-density lipoprotein (HDL), 39 mg/dL; low-density lipoprotein (LDL), 125 mg/dL. Which one of the following is also most likely true regarding this man?

(A) His plasminogen activator inhibitor-1 (PAI-1) is lower than normal.
(B) His insulin levels are higher than normal.
(C) Glucose uptake into his muscles is inhibited.
(D) Glucose uptake into his adipose tissue is inhibited.
(E) His uric acid level is lower than normal.

**20** A 55-year-old Caucasian man visits his family physician because he is concerned that he may have a "heart problem." The patient states that he has had twinges of chest pain when he walks up the stairs or runs for a short distance. The pain lasts for a few minutes, and he becomes winded as well. He smokes approximately three or four cigarettes a day, and had been doing so for several years. His mother died at the age of 72, and she had diabetes mellitus for years. Upon examination, the physician noted normal vital signs, but he also observed that the patient had reddish yellow lesions over the gluteal area. This physical finding would most likely be due to which one of the following?

(A) A markedly elevated very-low-density lipoprotein level
(B) A markedly elevated high-density lipoprotein level
(C) A markedly elevated free triglyceride level
(D) A markedly elevated free cholesterol level
(E) Xanthomatosis
(F) Xanthelasma
(G) Markedly elevated low-density lipoprotein levels

**21** A 62-year-old, obese African American man was seen in the emergency room. He was sweating profusely and was also nauseous and complaining of an acute crushing substernal chest pain. He also has had a prior history of recurrent attacks of angina, was on medication for diabetes mellitus, and smoked one pack of cigarettes per day. The most likely immediate cause for his presenting problem is which one of the following?

(A) Cigarette smoking
(B) Atherosclerosis
(C) A dislodged plaque
(D) Increased weight
(E) Narrowing and closure of a coronary artery or arteries

**22** A 52-year-old woman claims that her landlord is pumping poisonous gas into her apartment. Mental status examination reveals anxiety, perseveration, and persecutory ideation. She refuses to cooperate with mental status testing. Which of the following is the most likely diagnosis?

(A) Dementia
(B) Obsessive-compulsive disorder
(C) Panic disorder
(D) Posttraumatic stress disorder
(E) Generalized anxiety disorder

**23** A 33-year-old woman, gravida 3, para 2, is at 25 weeks' gestation. Her gestational age was confirmed by a 10-week sonogram performed because of early pregnancy spotting. A 20-week sonogram revealed a normal-appearing single male fetus, appropriate size for dates, without any gross congenital anomalies. On examination in the office today, her fundal height measures 31 cm. A repeat obstetrical ultrasound examination today reveals a single fetus in transverse lie with no part of the fetus touching the uterine wall or placenta. It was determined that there was a 4-quadrant amniotic fluid index (AFI) of 30 cm with the deepest single amniotic fluid pocket measuring 9 cm. Which one of the following maternal conditions does this patient most likely have?

(A) Asthma
(B) Diabetes mellitus
(C) Hypothyroidism
(D) Seizure disorder
(E) Sickle cell anemia

**24** Forty-eight hours after a total hysterectomy for low-staged endometrial carcinoma, a 35-year-old woman, with a 20 pack-year history of smoking, presents with the sudden onset of tachypnea, dyspnea, cough, and right-sided pleuritic chest pain. She has a low-grade fever, sinus tachycardia, and a blood pressure of 100/70 mm Hg. Examination of the chest shows scattered, bilateral expiratory wheezes and dullness to percussion at the right lung base. No calf tenderness is present. A chest radiograph shows a small pleural effusion at the right lung base, as well as a wedge-shaped area of hypovascularity and atelectasis in the right lower lobe. An electrocardiogram (ECG) shows nonspecific ST and T-wave abnormalities. An arterial blood gas (ABG) sample drawn with the patient breathing room air reveals a pH of 7.50 (normal is 7.35–7.45), a $PaCO_2$ of 29 mm Hg (normal is 33–44 mm Hg), a $PaO_2$ of 70 mm Hg (normal is 75–105 mm Hg), and a bicarbonate level of 21 mEq/L (normal is 22–28 mEq/L). Which of the following is the most appropriate first step in the management of this patient?

(A) Perform a pleural tap.
(B) Order a perfusion scan of the lungs.
(C) Order a sputum analysis for Gram's stain, culture, and sensitivity.
(D) Order pulmonary function tests.
(E) Order a consultation for bronchoscopy.

[25] A 62-year-old man who had a myocardial infarction (MI) is taking an 81 mg aspirin tablet daily, plus a maintenance dose of warfarin, which is adjusted to give a prothrombin time (PT) of 11–15 seconds. While on vacation, he starts using over-the-counter cimetidine for acid indigestion. A day or two before returning home, he develops a urinary tract infection for which trimethoprim-sulfamethoxazole is prescribed by a local physician. When he returns home, his PT is 27 seconds. Which of the following statements about this situation is most accurate?

(A) The dose of warfarin should be increased to ensure adequate anticoagulation.
(B) The antibiotics have increased the activity of liver enzymes that metabolize warfarin.
(C) The antiplatelet action of aspirin has blocked the effects of warfarin.
(D) Cimetidine has inhibited the hepatic metabolism of warfarin.
(E) Warfarin should not have been prescribed because it is not used prophylactically after an MI.

[26] An 80-year-old man with a history of coronary artery disease (CAD) and prostate cancer presents with weakness of both legs that has lasted for a week. Starting yesterday, he developed pain in his lower abdomen and had great difficulty emptying his bladder. Examination shows that he has sensory loss from T10 downward and is barely able to move his legs. Which one of the following is the proper treatment strategy?

(A) Admit the patient and schedule a magnetic resonance imaging (MRI) study the next day.
(B) Order an emergency MRI study after administering an intravenous (IV) bolus of steroids.
(C) Schedule plasmapheresis for Guillain-Barré syndrome.
(D) Order electromyography (EMG).
(E) Order radiation therapy over lumbar and sacral levels.

[27] A 22-year-old woman, gravida 5, para 2, abortus 3, has a history of prenatal substance abuse. Because she had delayed onset of prenatal care (with her first visit in the third trimester), she was too late for maternal serum triple-marker screening for fetal anomalies. She is unsure who is the father of this pregnancy. Late ultrasound examination of the fetus showed intrauterine growth restriction (IUGR) but

normal amniotic fluid volume. At 37 weeks' gestation, she underwent a spontaneous vaginal delivery of a small-for-gestational-age male neonate with short palpebral fissures, epicanthal folds, flat midface, hypoplastic philtrum, and thin vermillion border. These findings are characteristic in offspring born to mothers who prenatally abused which one of the following substances?

(A) Tobacco
(B) Alcohol
(C) Marijuana
(D) Amphetamines
(E) Narcotics

[28] A 46-year-old man reports for a preemployment physical. He recently moved to California to take up employment as a research scientist at a prestigious university. He had had a distinguished career in biochemistry while he lived in Cleveland, Ohio, his place of birth. He did not smoke, drank wine on social occasions, never used recreational drugs, and had led a healthy lifestyle. He did not have a history of diabetes, hypertension, or coronary artery disease, nor did he have a history of chest pains, shortness of breath, cough, expectoration, or recent weight loss. He was not on any medications. There was no significant history of medical illness on either side of his family. Physical examination revealed a fit man, whose vital signs were normal. He had no pallor, icterus, or cyanosis. No clubbing of the fingers was noted. Cardiovascular examination revealed normal heart sounds, with sinus rhythm and no murmurs or carotid bruits. He did not have distended jugular veins. Examination of the respiratory system revealed a mild right shift of the trachea, good symmetric chest expansion, and absence of adventitious sounds. Examination of the abdomen was unremarkable, and a neurologic examination was normal as well. His Seibert purified protein derivative of tuberculin (PPD) test result was negative, and a routine chest radiograph revealed a 0.5 cm concentrically calcified coin lesion in the upper left lobe of the lung. Which of the following is the most likely cause of the lesion?

(A) A primary lung cancer
(B) A bronchial hamartoma
(C) Metastatic cancer
(D) A granuloma
(E) A calcified tuberculosis lesion

**29** A 3-year-old child is evaluated in the emergency department for a lump on his head, which his mother says appeared after he accidentally hit his head while jumping on the bed. According to the mother, the patient fell from the bed onto a noncarpeted wooden floor. The child did not lose consciousness, and did not have emesis, visual changes, or changes in behavior. Examination reveals a tense swelling over the right parietal area and no neurologic deficits. Which of the following is the most likely diagnosis?

(A) Epidural hematoma
(B) Subdural hematoma
(C) Intraventricular hemorrhage
(D) Subgaleal hematoma
(E) Lipoma

**30** The data in the following table were obtained from five inhalational anesthetics. Which of the following agents will provide the most rapid rate of recovery?

| | Anesthetic | Blood: Gas Partition Coefficient | Minimum Alveolar Concentration (%) |
|---|---|---|---|
| (A) | Nitrous oxide | 0.5 | >100 |
| (B) | Desflurane | 0.4 | 7 |
| (C) | Sevoflurane | 0.7 | 3 |
| (D) | Isoflurane | 1.4 | 1.4 |
| (E) | Halothane | 2.3 | 0.8 |

**31** A 28-year-old man has rapid onset of insomnia, pressured speech, and hypersexuality. He had a similar episode at age 21, and also had a period of depression and suicide attempts at age 23. Between these episodes, his behavior seems to have been unremarkable. There is no history of substance abuse. Which of the following statements about the pathophysiology of his likely diagnosis is most accurate?

(A) Pathognomonic abnormalities in ion transportation occur at the cellular membrane.
(B) Mood-stabilizing medications are used as treatment because they lock central α-adrenergic receptors.
(C) The etiologic lesion does not appear to be heritable.
(D) Abnormal levels of neurotransmitters have been reported during manic episodes.
(E) Chromosomal abnormalities are often detected.

**32** A 24-year-old man was admitted to the hospital with a history of fatigue and confusion. A few days previously, he developed an infection in his foot, which has become worse. The patient is a diabetic who takes insulin. His temperature is 38.5°C (101.3°F); pulse, 96/min regular; respirations 20/min; and blood pressure, 90/60 mm Hg. His tongue is dry, and he has poor skin turgor. Apart from confusion, his neurologic examination is nonfocal. Cardiovascular examination is normal except for a sinus tachycardia. Respiratory system examination is unremarkable with the exception of a fruity odor in his breath. He has diffuse abdominal tenderness, but no masses or organomegaly are noted. Bowel sounds are present. He has cellulitis of his right leg, as a result of the infection in his foot. Serum glucose level is 700 mg/dL. The appropriate diagnosis was made, and he received intravenous fluids, antibiotics, and human insulin. During therapy, the patient develops respiratory paralysis requiring intubation and assisted ventilation. Which one of the following is the cause for the patient's respiratory failure?

(A) An anaphylactic reaction due to insulin
(B) Glucose toxicity
(C) Ketoacidosis
(D) Hypophosphatemia
(E) Hyperkalemia
(F) Bacteremia

**33** A 20-year-old man presents with a history of delayed developmental milestones, problems with impulse control, and an IQ of 65. He was in special education classes during his schooling. There was no history of substance abuse by his mother during the prenatal period, and all his first-degree relatives have IQ values above 100. Which of the following is most likely to be revealed by a complete assessment?

(A) Genetic or chromosomal abnormalities
(B) Perinatal insults
(C) Sociocultural deprivation
(D) Maternal substance abuse
(E) Mild mental retardation

**34** A mother brings her 12-month-old child to the emergency department because he is having painless rectal bleeding. She tells this physician, new to her, that approximately 2 months ago the patient was evaluated for anemia by his primary care pediatrician and was prescribed supplemental iron for presumed iron deficiency anemia. However, the iron deficiency anemia has been refractory to iron therapy. On physical examination, the child's stool is repeatedly positive for occult blood. Which of the following is the most likely diagnosis?

(A) Intussusception
(B) Duodenal ulcer
(C) Adhesions
(D) Meckel's diverticulum
(E) Ulcerative colitis

**35** A 17-year-old girl has not had a menstrual period for 4 months. She underwent menarche at age 11. She has been sexually active for the past year, but states she has only occasional intercourse. She states that she uses a diaphragm for contraception, but she does not always remember to use it. Her boyfriend occasionally uses a condom. A qualitative serum β-human chorionic gonadotropin test is reported back as a negative result. She is given medroxyprogesterone acetate (MPA) orally for 7 days, and she has a normal withdrawal bleed of 5 days of menstrual flow. Which one of the following statements is correct in respect to this diagnostic modality?

(A) It can assess whether the patient is pregnant.
(B) It will indicate whether the endometrium is estrogen primed.
(C) It differentiates primary from secondary amenorrhea.
(D) It can rule out a pituitary adenoma.
(E) It provides no help if the response is only spotting.

**36** A 55-year-old man came to see his physician for recurring attacks of headache. He stated that the headaches were mainly in the occipital area, and occurred at different times. He worked as a manager in a local office supply store and would get an exacerbation of headaches when he was under stress. There was no nausea or vomiting. At times, he would become dizzy and would have to sit down. A few hours ago, he experienced left-sided chest pains that lasted about 2 minutes, then went away. He denied head trauma, difficulty in breathing, and swelling of his legs. Over the past few months, he had to get up at night to urinate, and this had been getting worse. He did not smoke, used wine on social occasions, and had no family history of medical disease.

Upon examination, the physician found him to be a well-built Caucasian male, who was not in distress, had no pallor or cyanosis. His blood pressure was 150/100 mm Hg and was the same when repeated later. The pulse was 80/min regular, respirations 16/min, and his temperature was 37°C (98.6°F). He weighed 75 kilograms (165.3 pounds). Funduscopy revealed some arteriolar narrowing with A-V nipping. There were no hemorrhages or exudates, and the disc margins were sharp. There were no carotid bruits. The second heart sound was loud. There were no murmurs, gallops, or rubs. The chest was clear to auscultation bilaterally, and examination of the abdomen and extremities was normal. No peripheral edema was noted. Which one of the following medications was prescribed by the physician?

(A) Atenolol
(B) Furosemide

(C) Hydrochlorothiazide
(D) Diltiazem
(E) Doxazosin

**37** A 72-year-old man with a history of uninterrupted employment as an accountant has insidious onset of difficulty concentrating on tasks and remembering recent events. Physical examination reveals no hypertension, cardiac findings, or focal neurologic signs. Routine laboratory examination is unremarkable. Mental status examination reveals emotional lability, difficulty naming common objects, and recall of only one object of three after 5 minutes. Which of the following is the most likely cause of his symptoms?

(A) Alcoholic dementia
(B) Alzheimer disease
(C) Cerebrovascular disease
(D) Depression
(E) Normal aging

**38** A 34-year-old Hispanic woman, gravida 3, para 2 initiated prenatal care at 14 weeks' gestation. Her two previous pregnancies were 5 and 8 years ago. They resulted in spontaneous vaginal deliveries at term of a 9 lb (4,082 g) daughter and a 9 lb 8 oz (4,309 g) son. Her weight is 180 lb (82 kg). She is 62 inches (157 cm) tall. She underwent a 1 hour 50 g glucose screen at 26 weeks' gestation with a resulting value of 165 mg/dL. After 3 days of carbohydrate loading, she then proceeded to have a 3 hour 100 g oral glucose tolerance test. The resulting values are as follows: fasting, 92; 1 hour, 194; 2 hours, 170; 3 hours, 135. In White's classification of diabetes in pregnancy, she meets the criteria for which of the following categories?

(A) Class A1
(B) Class A2
(C) Class B
(D) Class C
(E) Class D

**39** A 51-year-old obese woman was admitted to the hospital for recurrent pain in the right upper quadrant of her abdomen that radiated to the back. She also complained of occasional nausea and vomiting, but revealed no other relevant medical history. At that time, her vital signs were normal, and she had no icterus, pallor, or cyanosis. Tenderness was present to palpation in the right upper abdominal quadrant; there was no guarding or rigidity. No organomegaly was noted, and no masses were felt. Bowel sounds were normal. Findings of examinations of the cardiovascular and respiratory systems were normal. Her electrolytes and serum chemistries were normal except for a mild leukocytosis. Ultrasound confirmed cholelithiasis, for which she underwent laparoscopic cholecystectomy under general anesthesia. She now has an IV line in place, together with an indwelling urinary catheter and a nasogastric tube. Twenty-four hours after the procedure, she develops fever, tachycardia, sudden difficulty breathing, and pain in the chest. The most likely cause for this patient's current condition is which of the following?

(A) Pulmonary embolus
(B) Postoperative wound infection
(C) Atelectasis
(D) IV catheter–related sepsis
(E) Spontaneous pneumothorax
(F) Aspiration pneumonitis

**40** A 4-month-old infant is brought to the emergency department with sudden onset of lethargy and poor feeding. The mother reports that the infant had been in her usual state of good health until recently, when she developed constipation. The mother also states that she has recently stopped breastfeeding and has changed to formula feeding. According to the mother, the infant does not like the formula unless it is sweetened; hence, she adds a teaspoonful of honey. On physical examination, the infant is noted to be afebrile and have generalized hypotonia and weakness, as well as ophthalmoplegia. Which of the following is the most likely diagnosis?

(A) Guillain-Barré syndrome
(B) Hypothyroidism
(C) Werdnig-Hoffmann disease
(D) Infant botulism
(E) Hypomagnesemia

*Directions for Matching Questions (41 through 50): Each set of matching questions is preceded by a list of 4 to 26 lettered options followed by a brief explanation of the required task and then by a series of numbered statements. For each lettered statement you are to select ONE lettered option that best fulfills the task as it relates to that statement. Remember, each of the listed options might be correctly selected once, more than once, or not at all.*

## Questions 41–50

(A) Cross-over study
(B) Single-blind study
(C) Double-blind study
(D) Meta-analysis
(E) Nonconcurrent prospective study
(F) Cross-sectional study
(G) Case report
(H) Case series report
(I) Case-control study

*For each description, select the ONE appropriate investigative method used.*

**41** A physician reports an unusual clinical presentation in a 50-year-old man with carcinoma of the lung.

**42** A physician reports several cases of abdominal pain, neuropathy, and optic neuritis in a coastal population after consumption of fish.

**43** An international multicenter trial was conducted on a new antihypertensive drug to reach a definite conclusion about its efficacy. This involved more than 2,000 patients in several hospitals in the United States, Mexico, Canada, Britain, and France.

**44** A researcher interested in establishing the risk factors for a rare collagen disease retraces the illness from its end point to its origin.

**45** An experimental study design was developed to assess differences between two groups of women receiving different treatment for carcinoma of the breast. Neither the investigator nor the participants are aware of the group to which they have been assigned

**46** An investigator conducts a survey to establish the prevalence of bronchial asthma in Los Angeles, California.

**47** An investigator wants to establish the efficacy of a new analgesic. He administers the drug to group A, and a placebo to group B. Thereafter, group B receives the drug, while group A receives the placebo. The results after both studies are recorded.

**48** A clinical trial is conducted for a new drug to treat rheumatoid arthritis. The goal is to observe if the patients improved, became worse, or showed no change with the new medication. Participants and the investigator are oblivious of allocation to the control and treatment group.

**49** An epidemiologist discovers that several workers in a chemical factory became ill after exposure to a chemical. He wants to establish the effect of this exposure, and looks back at the health records of workers exposed to the same chemical 30 years earlier.

**50** An investigator wants to establish the effect of a recent radiation leak from a nuclear plant, within a specific cohort.

# *Answer Key*

| | | | | | | | | | |
|---|---|---|---|---|---|---|---|---|---|
| **1** C | | **11** A | | **21** C | | **31** D | | **41** G | |
| **2** C | | **12** A | | **22** A | | **32** D | | **42** H | |
| **3** A | | **13** E | | **23** B | | **33** E | | **43** D | |
| **4** B | | **14** C | | **24** B | | **34** D | | **44** I | |
| **5** D | | **15** C | | **25** D | | **35** B | | **45** C | |
| **6** B | | **16** A | | **26** B | | **36** E | | **46** F | |
| **7** D | | **17** C | | **27** B | | **37** B | | **47** A | |
| **8** D | | **18** E | | **28** D | | **38** A | | **48** C | |
| **9** B | | **19** B | | **29** D | | **39** C | | **49** E | |
| **10** D | | **20** A | | **30** B | | **40** D | | **50** I | |

# Answers and Explanations

**1** **The answer is C** *Psychiatry*

This presentation is most suggestive of methamphetamine-induced psychotic disorder (choice **C**), characterized by hallucinations and delusions caused by methamphetamine use. Methamphetamine-induced psychosis often starts during a binge of methamphetamine use and persists for 1–2 weeks after cessation of methamphetamine use.

The presence of psychosis explains his anxiety (choice **A**), but the anxiety doesn't cause the psychosis. Delirium (choice **B**) is unlikely because he is alert and oriented. Methamphetamine intoxication (choice **D**) is unlikely because he last used the substance 1 week ago, and his urine toxicology testing result is negative. Schizophrenia (choice **E**) might present with similar symptoms, but the diagnosis is less likely because of the patient's history of methamphetamine use.

**2** **The answer is C** *Medicine*

The patient may be experiencing a cholinergic crisis from taking an overdose of pyridostigmine or a myasthenic crisis from not taking an adequate dose. Infections in myasthenic patients may alter drug dosage requirements, and because gastrointestinal (GI) upsets are common in "flu," the physician cannot reliably use changes in bowel activity to aid in diagnosis. To determine whether his crisis is due to too much or too little pyridostigmine, a small dose of edrophonium (usually 2 mg, 1 hour after the last oral dose of pyridostigmine) should be given (choice **C**). This will inhibit acetylcholine esterase and increase acetylcholine levels. It should be followed by careful observation to see whether muscle strength improves (indicating an inadequate dose of pyridostigmine) or worsens (indicating an excessive dose). In the former case, the dose of pyridostigmine should be increased (choice **A**). In the latter case, the worsening effect is quite brief, lasting only a few minutes. Subsequently, the dose of pyridostigmine should be decreased (choice **D**). Equipment for intubation should be at hand should this be required.

Physostigmine (choice **B**) is a tertiary amine cholinesterase inhibitor that readily enters the central nervous system and the eyes. It is a specific antidote for tricyclic antidepressant and anticholinergic poisoning. It competitively blocks the hydrolysis of acetylcholine by cholinesterase, allowing acetylcholine to accumulate and counter the muscarinic effects of tricyclic overdose. In the case of the eye, it promotes contraction of the ciliary muscle, with resultant miosis and increased outflow of aqueous humor from the posterior chamber into the canal of Schlemm. The net effect is lowering intraocular pressure. Hence, it is used in open-angle glaucoma. It has no role in the treatment of myasthenia gravis. Neither is succinylcholine (choice **E**) of any value in the treatment of myasthenia gravis. Succinylcholine is a depolarizing agent that causes neuromuscular blockade, with resultant skeletal muscle paralysis. It is an agonist at the nicotinic end-plate receptor.

**3** **The answer is A** *Medicine*

Two forms of scleroderma exist, limited (in 80% of cases) and diffuse also known as systemic sclerosis (in 20%). The limited form is usually restricted to the hands and feet and includes CREST syndrome (characterized by **c**alcinosis of the digits, **R**aynaud's phenomenon, **e**sophageal motility dysfunction, **s**clerodactyly of the fingers, and **t**elangiectasia over the digits and under the nails), and pulmonary hypertension. The limited form of the disease has a better prognosis than the diffuse one. Both systemic sclerosis and localized scleroderma present with Raynaud's phenomenon in almost all patients, often antedating other manifestations of the disease by years. Cold temperatures and stress are stimuli that produce color changes of the fingers (sometimes toes), which first blanch, then become cyanotic, and then red. Vasospasm and thickened digital arteries (choice **A**) are responsible for these changes. CREST syndrome is characterized by calcinosis of the digits, Raynaud's phenomenon, esophageal motility dysfunction, sclerodactyly of the fingers, and telangiectasia over the digits and under the nails; the anticentromere antibody is positive in about 50% of cases.

Systemic sclerosis is a more generalized disorder of connective tissue, characterized by degenerative and inflammatory changes that result in the subsequent increase of collagen tissue deposition in various tissues. Tightening of the skin of the face and extremities is a universal finding. Esophageal motility problems, with dysphagia for solids and liquids, occur in 80% of patients. Other problems include arthritis (80%), renal involvement with concomitant thickening of the interlobular arterial intima followed by concentric onion skin hypertrophy during the healing stage (60%), pericardial effusions (20%–50%), pulmonary fibrosis with restrictive lung disease (35%), and subsequent pulmonary hypertension and renal crisis (15%). The antinuclear antibody test result is positive in 70%–90% of cases. The anti-Scl-70 antibody is specific for systemic sclerosis and is noted in 20%–33% of cases. D-Penicillamine may improve long-term survival, as it may improve skin sclerosis. Cryoglobulinemia caused by proteins that precipitate in cold temperatures, cold agglutinins with immunoglobulin M (IgM) antibodies that clump red blood cells in the digital vessels (choice **B**), and immune complexes causing vasculitis (choice **C**) are not present. Other causes of Raynaud's phenomenon are thromboangiitis obliterans (Buerger disease), which is an inflammatory vasculitis producing thrombosis of the digital vessels (choice **D**) in male smokers and in ergotamine poisoning. Embolism to digital vessels in the hand is uncommon (choice **E**).

### 4 The answer is B *Surgery*

The patient has a small bowel obstruction, which is most commonly caused by adhesions from a previous surgery (choice **B**). Characteristic physical findings in small bowel obstruction are vomiting, colicky midabdominal pain, abdominal distention, hyperperistalsis, obstipation (i.e., absence of stool and flatus), and a lack of rebound tenderness. Abdominal x-ray films show distended loops of bowel with a "stepladder" pattern of differential air–fluid levels. In some cases, intestinal intubation relieves the entrapped gas and fluids, causing the obstruction to subside. Other cases require surgical intervention.

Diverticulosis (choice **A**) usually causes no symptoms, and noninflamed diverticula are generally discovered by chance during an ancillary examination such as a colonoscopy for cancer screening. Torsion of the bowel around the mesenteric root (choice **C**) is a volvulus. It produces obstruction and strangulation of bowel. Intussusception (choice **D**) is uncommon in adults and produces a combination of obstruction and infarction. Generally, a small bowel infarction resulting from thrombosis over an atherosclerotic plaque in the proximal superior mesenteric artery causes bloody diarrhea (choice **A**). "Thumbprinting" from submucosal edema is noted in barium studies.

### 5 The answer is D *Medicine*

Vasculopathic third-nerve palsy due to third-nerve deficit (choice **D**) is the correct diagnosis. This causes rotation outward from medial rectus weakness and ptosis from levator palpebrae weakness and is associated with a normal pupillary size.

A compressive lesion, such as an aneurysm (choice **C**) or a tumor, would compress the dorsomedial portion of the third nerve and cause a dilated, unreactive pupil. This distinction is important because a third-nerve lesion that spares the pupil is generally nonemergent, whereas lesions that involve the pupil are best considered medical emergencies. Cavernous sinus thrombosis (choice **A**), although possible, is less likely because it would generally involve other cranial nerves as well. A superior oblique palsy (choice **B**) from fourth cranial nerve damage can be congenital, but acquired cases are usually caused by trauma. Isolated fourth-nerve damage causes upward deviation of the eye and inability of depression on adduction, and often first becomes apparent while descending the stairs. Internuclear ophthalmoplegia (choice **E**) is due to interruption of the signal from the sixth-nerve nucleus contralateral to the medial rectus nucleus of the third cranial nerve that is conveyed via the medial longitudinal fasciculus. This results in the inability of the medial rectus to contract in a synchronous manner when the lateral rectus does, resulting in diplopia on conjugate lateral gaze. The condition could result from vascular or demyelinating disease.

### 6 The answer is B *Pediatrics*

This child almost certainly has medium chain acyl-CoA deficiency (MCAD; choice **B**). The first step in the β-oxidation of fatty acids is catalyzed by acyl-CoA dehydrogenases. There are at least four classes of acyl-CoA dehydrogenases: those that act on very-long-chain fatty acids (e.g., the 20-carbon arachidonic acid); those that act on long-chain fatty acids, C12 to C18; those that act on medium-chain fatty acids, C6 to C12; and, those acting on shorter-chain fatty acids, less than C6. Inborn errors inhibiting the activity of each of these dehydrogenases have been reported; these all are inherited as autosomal recessive traits, and all but medium-chain acyl-CoA dehydrogenase (MCAD) deficiency (choice **B**) are extremely rare. MCAD deficiency has a reported incidence of 1 per 6,500 births among North European Caucasians, and from 1 per 9,000 to 1 per 17,000 births in the general U.S. population. Among certain ethnic groups, the presence of a mutant gene has been reported to be as high as 1 per 40 individuals. The prevalence of the disease is as at least as high as that of phenylketonuria, yet newborn screening is only required in a few states. The high prevalence rate has provoked a debate in many states concerning the need to require newborn screening. This has been inhibited by the unavailability of an inexpensive or readily available methodology: the classic method, tandem mass spectrophotometry requires a large investment in instrumentation, while molecular DNA probes are not yet available for such sizeable studies. Moreover, genetic analysis will only recognize the presence of the more prevalent *K304E* mutation. This MCAD gene is located on chromosome 1p31, and 26 different mutant forms have been characterized. However, studies conducted to date suggest the K304E *MCAD* mutation accounts for 90% of cases; 81% of these cases are homozygous for this gene, and 18% are compound heterozygotes.

As in the case described, typically, the deficiency is characterized by sudden attacks after an infection and/or after fasting for 8–16 hours. The pathophysiology results from an inability to accomplish the first step in β-oxidation of mid-chain fatty acids, either those ingested (minor contribution) or longer-chain fatty acids that have been partially metabolized to 10–12 carbons and thus become the normal substrates for MCAD. Attacks are provoked by any situation that normally requires increased fatty acid oxidation, such as fasting or an illness. Since increased fat metabolism is not possible, continued existence in MCAD patients depends entirely upon glucose metabolism; consequently, hypoglycemia results. To make matters worse, gluconeogenesis is inhibited because acetyl-CoA cannot be formed but is required for the activity of pyruvate carboxylase to produce oxaloacetate from pyruvate; thus, amino acids cannot be used as a fuel. Furthermore, since acetyl-CoA cannot be formed, ketone bodies also cannot be synthesized and the brain is also deprived of this alternate fuel. The final insult is provided by the cell's attempt to metabolize the accumulated fatty acids by an endoplasmic reticular detoxifying P450 cytochrome mixed oxidase system that converts them into shorter-chain dicarboxylic acids by sequentially oxidizing and then removing the ω-carbon by ω-oxidation. This results in the accumulation of several unusual and abnormal mono- and dicarboxylic acids and causes an anion-gap metabolic acidosis that will increase as more of these acids accumulate. Octanoic acid is one of these abnormal acids; it is a mitochondrial toxin suspected of inhibiting the urea cycle, causing an elevated blood urea nitrogen (BUN) level and hyperammonemia; the latter may induce an encephalopathy.

About 25% of babies succumb to respiratory or cardiac arrest during the first attack, which usually occurs between the ages of 6–24 months. Subsequent attacks are seldom fatal but are characterized by vomiting, seizures, lethargy, and sometimes coma and encephalopathy. Over the long term, the majority of individuals with identified symptoms have developmental and behavioral problems, often with chronic muscle weakness, attention deficit disorder, and/or cerebral palsy; however, others may seem normal. The penetrance is unknown, and it is believed that an unknown number of homozygous individuals never develop symptoms. Because infants who die during the first attack generate few physical clues relating to the cause of death, it was postulated that such cases are a common cause of the sudden infant death syndrome (SIDS). However, subsequent studies have shown that only 0.01% of SIDS cases are due to MCAD.

Glucose 6-phosphatase deficiency (choice **A**), also known as type I glycogen storage disease or Von Gierke disease, also causes a severe fasting hypoglycemia and hepatomegaly, but the latter is due to accumulated glycogen, whereas in MCAT all carbohydrate stores are depleted. Carnitine acyltransferases I and II are required to shuttle fatty acids in and out of the mitochondria. As a consequence, carnitine acyltransferase deficiency (choice **C**) results in an inability to use long-chain fatty acids as fuel, causing myoglobinemia and weakness following exercise. Although hypoglycemia occurs in hyperinsulinemia (choice **D**), a metabolic sequence similar to that described is not caused by fasting or illness. Acute intermittent porphyria (choice **E**) is characterized by unexplained abdominal crises, acute peripheral or central nervous system dysfunctions, recurrent psychiatric illness, hyponatremia, and porphobilinogen in the urine during an attack.

**7** **The answer is D** *Medicine*

Upon even slight suspicion of meningitis, it is wise to perform a spinal tap, provided of course that there is no evidence of raised intracranial pressure. Features common to most cases of meningitis include headache (often the predominant presenting symptom, and unlike most headaches, it is generally more severe when lying down and resting); photophobia; vomiting; giddiness; fever; and stiffness of the neck, spinal muscles, and hamstrings. This patient presents with sufficient symptoms to suggest that she has meningitis. The analysis of the spinal fluid indicates that she suffers from aseptic meningitis (choice **D**), most typically induced by a viral infection. In viral meningitis, at most there are only few more white blood cells than normal, and as in a normal sample, these primarily are mononuclear lymphocytes. In aseptic meningitis, the spinal fluid glucose level is usually in the low-normal range, and protein levels tend to be elevated, as in the case described.

Although the patient presented with sufficient symptoms to diagnose a case of meningitis, many symptoms were marginal, suggesting that it was not a fulminating case, as is often seen in bacterial meningitis (choice **A**). Bacterial meningitis is characterized by a greater number of leukocytes (from 200 to 20,000), which are primarily polymorphonuclear neutrophils. The spinal fluid glucose level is generally significantly lower than normal, and protein levels are elevated to a greater degree than in aseptic meningitis (often above 100 mg/mL). Cryptococcal meningitis (choice **B**) is almost always an opportunistic infection in an immuno-compromised host. The patient's history strongly suggests that this is not a relevant factor. Although human immunodeficiency virus (HIV) and herpes simplex virus type 2 infections may cause chronic viral meningitis, her history tends to rule these out as causative agents. Actinomyces meningitis (choice **E**), although uncommon, might be suspected in this case because the patient had recent dental work, a significant risk factor for infection by this anaerobic class of bacteria. However, as discussed above, the laboratory results are not characteristic of a bacterial infection. *Coccidia immitis* meningitis (choice **C**), although relatively rare, might also be suspected because the patient comes from the San Joaquin Valley in California. However, to make this diagnosis, the glucose level in the spinal fluid should be well below normal. Other pointers to it in the cerebrospinal fluid would be increased cell count, lymphocytosis, the presence of complement-fixing antibodies, and, a positive culture in approximately 30% of cases.

It is critically important to distinguish between bacterial and viral meningitis. If bacterial meningitis is not properly managed, the consequences are severe, often resulting in death, whereas viral meningitis is generally self-limited. Viral meningitis caused by herpes or human immunodeficiency virus (HIV) is a major exception to this rule.

### 8 The answer is D *Medicine*

One-fourth to one-half of diabetic men suffer from erectile dysfunction; generally, ejaculation is normal, but erectile problems are present (choice **D**).

Obviously, if choice **D** is correct, choice **B** (orgasm and ejaculation are less likely to be affected than erection) is incorrect. Microscopic nerve damage (choice **C**) and vascular changes (choice **E**), as well as psychologic factors, influence the erectile problems associated with diabetes. Poor metabolic control of diabetes is associated with increased incidence of sexual problems; therefore, this patient is most likely not maintaining optimum blood sugar levels (choice **A**).

### 9 The answer is B *Surgery*

About 5% of ulcer patients develop perforations, most commonly on the anterior wall of the stomach or duodenum, and more commonly in males than in females. The incidence of perforations is increasing; it has been hypothesized that this is due to increased use of nonsteroidal anti-inflammatory drugs (NSAIDs) and/or crack cocaine. Perforation of a peptic ulcer is characterized by the sudden onset of epigastric pain with radiation of the pain into the right shoulder, which results from irritation of the phrenic nerve (C4) from air underneath the diaphragm. Abdominal rigidity, rebound tenderness, and ileus occur as a result of chemical peritonitis. The first step in management is to obtain an upright and supine film (choice **B**) of the abdomen, which shows air beneath the diaphragm in 75%–85% of cases; the presence of air establishes a diagnosis. Intravenous cefazolin is given as prophylaxis against infection. Surgical intervention is necessary. Modern, minimally invasive laparotomy techniques coupled to postoperative treatment of possible *Helicobacter pylori* infection has reduced the overall mortality to about 5%.

One cannot conclude that there is no perforation if air is not present beneath the diaphragm; as a consequence, a follow-up upper gastrointestinal series should be done. However, barium studies (choice **A**) should not be performed in patients with suspect perforation. Peritoneal lavage (choice **C**) is usually indicated in the workup of intraabdominal bleeding. Antacids (choice **D**) are not indicated in the treatment of peptic ulcer perforation. Exploratory surgery (choice **E**) is not the initial step in management of abdominal pain.

### 10 The answer is D *Pediatrics*

Visceral larva migrans (choice **D**) is caused by infection with *Toxocara* larvae. It is most common in children 1–4 years of age, especially if they have pica or have a tendency to place their fingers in their mouth and have close contact with dogs or cats, because *Toxocara* are common parasites of both. Sandboxes are common areas for both pets and children. Symptoms include fever, hepatomegaly, wheezing, pulmonary disease, and eosinophilia.

Eosinophilic lung disease (choice **B**), sometimes called Löffler syndrome, is a group of disorders not commonly found in children in the United States; they are linked by the common findings of eosinophilia and pulmonary infiltrates. Anal pruritus and insomia are the presenting complaints in Enterobius vermicularis infestation (choice **A**). Eosinophilia does not occur in most cases as tissue invasion is absent. Ascariasis (choice **C**) may cause fever, urticaria, allergic symptoms, and granulomatous disease. Vomiting, abdominal distention, and abdominal pain may also be present. Pulmonary infections with *Strongyloides stercoralis* (strongyloidiasis; choice **E**) are usually mild and may pass unnoticed. However, in immunosuppressed and malnourished children, massive parasite invasion with *S. stercoralis* may cause generalized abdominal pain, fever, and shock due to gram-negative sepsis.

## 11 **The answer is A** *Medicine*

The athlete is suffering from exercise-induced asthma. Common symptoms include postexercise cough, dyspnea out of proportion to the level of exertion, poorer performance than expected, wheezing, chest tightness, and sputum production. The treatment of choice is $\beta_2$-agonists, usually two puffs to be inhaled 5 minutes prior to exercise (choice **A**).

Cromolyn sodium (choice **C**) is a second-line agent. It is given in the form of two sprays, 1 hour prior to exercise. It is used in combination with $\beta_2$-agonists in the treatment of severe recurrent bronchial asthma. Other uses include the prevention of allergic rhinitis and allergic ocular disorders. A rare but serious complication is angioedema. Theophylline (choice **B**) is usually indicated for rapid relief of symptoms in acute asthma or as a prophylaxis for bronchial asthma and bronchospasm induced by chronic bronchitis and emphysema. It has potentially serious side effects, including seizures, hypotension, cardiac arrhythmias, and even respiratory arrest. Erythromycin (choice **D**) should not be part of the treatment plan because there are no signs of an infection. Lifelong abstinence from strenuous activity (choice **E**) would be a gross overreaction.

## 12 **The answer is A** *Obstetrics and Gynecology*

The patient in this scenario has many risk factors for pelvic relaxation: she is white, postmenopausal without estrogen replacement; multiparous and has delivered at least one large infant; and, she has a long history of smoking. However, her symptom of difficulty in stool evacuation is more referable to lower posterior vaginal relaxation due to a rectocele (choice **A**) that contains the rectum. The diagnosis is made on the basis of inspection at the time of pelvic examination, when the patient is asked to cough or perform the Valsalva maneuver (increasing intraabdominal pressure). Management is posterior vaginal repair (colporrhaphy).

Incorrect options include a cystocele (choice **B**) (an upper anterior vaginal relaxation that contains the bladder). This is the most common finding with vaginal wall relaxation and may be associated with urinary stress incontinence. An enterocele (choice **C**) (an upper posterior vaginal relaxation that contains the small bowel), is a more uncommon finding and is associated with rather nonspecific symptoms. A urethrocele (choice **D**) (a lower anterior vaginal relaxation that contains the urethra) may also be associated with urinary incontinence but does not cause defecation symptoms. Vaginocele (choice **E**) is a spurious distracter.

## 13 **The answer is E** *Pediatrics*

Infants born before 37 weeks' gestation (choices **A** and **B**) are preterm. Preterm infants may have lanugo hair; smooth, pink skin with visible veins; faint plantar creases; and ears that are soft with slow recoil. Term infants are defined as those who are born between 37 and 42 weeks' gestation (choices **C** and **D**). Term infants have a small amount of lanugo and some bald areas; smooth, slightly thickened skin; ears that have good recoil; and indentations over more than the anterior third of the plantar area. Postterm babies are born after 42 weeks' gestation (choice **E**). They tend to be large for gestational age and hyperalert. Lanugo is absent, and the skin is cracked and peeling. Fingernails are long. They are at increased risk for meconium aspiration.

## 14 **The answer is C** *Psychiatry*

The woman's most likely diagnosis is specific phobia, defined as fear of a discrete object or situation. In this case, the object is snakes. The defense mechanism most closely associated with specific phobias is displacement (choice **C**). Displacement occurs when the emotions associated with a psychologically unacceptable object, idea, or activity is transferred to another object or situation, which is often symbolically related to the original one. A psychodynamic explanation for onset of the specific phobia in this case would be the symbolic association between a snake and a penis.

The other choices are defense mechanisms that are not so closely associated with simple phobias. Dissociation (choice **A**) is the fragmentation or separation of aspects of consciousness, including memory, identity, and perception. To some degree such dissociation is normal and may even be a useful defense mechanism; we all have a tendency to forget unpleasant events, and this helps reduce chronic anxiety. However, if a person's consciousness becomes too fragmented, it becomes pathologic. Examples are dissociative amnesia, fugue, identity disorder, and depersonalization disorder. Projection (choice **B**) is the transfer of uncomfortable inner feelings, such as guilt or anger, to others; such persons often seem bitter and suspicious. Conversion (choice **D**) is the transfer of emotional conflicts into physical symptoms. Resistance (choice **E**) is the active opposition to bringing unconscious feelings to the conscious level.

### 15 The answer is C  *Surgery*

Cardiac tamponade is characterized by decreased cardiac output and increased central venous pressure owing to restriction of blood flow into and out of the heart as fluid in the pericardial sac restricts filling of all the cardiac chambers. An echocardiogram (choice **C**) is the most sensitive and specific noninvasive test to establish the presence of fluid in the pericardial sac. After the diagnosis is established, pericardiocentesis should be performed to immediately reduce intrapericardial sac pressure. Surgery follows to locate the source of the tamponade in those cases that are associated with trauma. Distention of the neck veins on inspiration is called *Kussmaul's sign*. Normally, the increase in negative intrathoracic pressure on inspiration sucks blood from the jugular venous system into the right side of the heart. However, if the right side of the heart is restricted by fluid in the pericardial sac, the blood regurgitates into the jugular veins on inspiration.

A drop in the pulse or the blood pressure of more than 10 mm Hg on inspiration is called *pulsus paradoxus*. It reflects the drop in inflow of blood into the right side of the heart, which automatically decreases the outflow of blood from the left ventricle. An increase in central venous pressure without an increase in blood pressure further documents the inability of the heart to receive fluid and pump it out into the systemic circulation; therefore, giving additional fluid (choice **B**) would exacerbate the condition. Inserting a chest tube into the left pleural cavity (choice **A**), decreasing venous pressure by administering a venodilator (choice **D**), and decreasing venous pressure by administering a loop diuretic (choice **E**) would be incorrect steps in management, at least at this time.

### 16 The answer is A  *Psychiatry*

This woman's symptoms are suggestive of dementia and neuromotor degeneration secondary to subacute combined degeneration of the cord as a result of vitamin B$_{12}$ deficiency (choice **A**). Causes of vitamin B$_{12}$ deficiency include strict vegetarianism (vegans), alcoholism, or pernicious anemia. It is relatively more common in older adults and should be investigated as part of any workup for dementia, particularly since it is treatable. Although the classic feature of vitamin B$_{12}$ deficiency is a macrocytic, hypochromic anemia, this may be masked by ingestion of adequate folate.

The other choices are not commonly associated with dementia. Vitamin C deficiency (choice **B**) presents with hemorrhagic, not mental, symptoms. Clinically significant magnesium deficiency (choice **D**) may present with cognitive changes and weakness but is rare, since magnesium is found in a wide variety of foods. Iron deficiency (choice **C**) presents with lassitude, weakness, and microcytic, hypochromic anemia but not with dementia and neuromotor degeneration. Diet-related deficiencies of lecithin (choice **E**) or its metabolic products are rare. Hereditary absence of the enzyme lecithin-cholesterol acyltransferase prevents the conversion of lecithin to lysolecithin and produces anemia and renal failure.

### 17 The answer is C  *Pediatrics*

Rett syndrome (choice **C**) occurs only in females. Girls with Rett syndrome appear to be developing normally until 6–18 months of age, when they manifest dementia, develop microcephaly, and lose purposeful movements of their hands (i.e., hand-wringing). They may also have ataxia, seizures, scoliosis, and loss of gross motor skills. They may have sighing respirations associated with apnea and cyanosis.

Autism (choice **A**) may manifest with great variability in severity and range of symptoms. The usual presenting complaint is regression of language and play without loss of motor skills. Characterizations of William syndrome (choice **B**) include a depressed nasal bridge, epicanthal folds, prominent thick lips with open mouth, and short stature. Short stature, webbed posterior neck, broad chest with widely spaced nipples, and an increased carrying angle of the arms characterize Turner syndrome (choice **D**). Key features of Russell-Silver syndrome (choice **E**) are short stature, triangular facies with down-turned corners of the mouth, clinodactyly, and a head that appears disproportionately large.

### 18 The answer is E *Obstetrics and Gynecology*

The description in this case is that of recurrent genital herpes. The herpes simplex virus has potential for significant adverse impact on the fetus, neonate, or both. Although the herpes simplex virus does not increase the risk of congenital malformations (choice **B**), infectious sequela are possible. The decision about route of delivery cannot be made until the onset of labor (choice **E**). If no lesions are present at the start of labor, this woman can safely undergo labor and vaginal delivery. If lesions are present at the start of labor, cesarean delivery is indicated (choice **A**). Because she has protective antibodies against herpes, she does not experience viremia; therefore, there is no risk of transplacental viral passage (choice **C**). If she has no breast lesions after delivery, she can safely breastfeed (choice **D**).

### 19 The answer is B *Medicine*

The metabolic syndrome (once called syndrome X, insulin resistance syndrome, or the deadly quartet) is a prediabetic condition in which there is hyperglycemia (but not to the level that diabetes can be diagnosed), hypertension, dyslipidemia, and hyperinsulinemia. Three of the parameters of this "deadly quartet" are attributed to this patient in the clinical vignette; these are:

- *Hyperglycemia.* The normal fasting serum glucose value is defined as less than 110 mg/dL; thus, his value of 115 mg/dL is hyperglycemic. Such values that fall between 110 and 125 mg/dL are characteristic of impaired glucose tolerance, generally indicate prediabetes, and probably should be treated, at least by appropriate dietary changes. Frank diabetes is indicated by repeated fasting values of greater than 125 mg/dL.
- *Hypertension.* The table illustrated below summarizes the characterization of blood pressure values. As demonstrated in the following table, the patient's blood pressure of 155/84 mm Hg is classified being stage 1 hypertensive. This is a second member of the "deadly quartet" and is also a risk factor for eventual congestive heart failure, as well as for stroke, myocardial infarcts, and other long-term anomalies, thus it should be treated immediately.

| Classification | Systolic Pressure (mm Hg) | Diastolic Pressure (mm Hg) |
|---|---|---|
| Normal | 90–119 | 60–79 |
| Prehypertension | 120–139 | 80–89 |
| Stage 1 | 140–159 | 90–99 |
| Stage 2 | ≥160 | ≥100 |
| Isolated systolic hypertension | ≥140 | <90 |

- *Dyslipidemia.* The following table summarizes the desirable levels for the various lipoproteins. Clearly, his total cholesterol value of 265 mg/dL; his low-density lipoprotein (LDL) value of 125 mg/dL, and his triglyceride value of 157 mg/dL are above acceptable normal values. Conversely, his good cholesterol, the high-density lipoprotein (HDL) value of 39 mg/dL, is way below that recommended. Clearly, he also has dyslipidemia—a third member of the "deadly quartet."

**Lipoproteins (Measured after an overnight fast, concentrations expressed as mg/dL)**

| | Total Cholesterol | LDL-Cholesterol | HDL-Cholesterol | Triglycerides |
|---|---|---|---|---|
| Desirable (Optimal) | <200 | <100 | ≥60 | <150 |
| Near optimal/ above optimal | N/A | 100–129 | N/A | N/A |
| Borderline high | 200–239 | 130–159 | N/A | 150–199 |
| High | ≥240 | 160–189 | N/A | 200–499 |
| Very high | ≥190 | N/A | N/A | ≥500 |
| Undesirable | N/A | N/A | <40 | N/A |

In so much as this man has been demonstrated to have three of the four characteristics that define metabolic syndrome, it is highly probable he also has the fourth one, namely:

- *Hyperinsulinemia* (choice **B**). Also, this man's height and weight correspond to a body mass index (BMI) of 29 kg/m², which is classified as overweight, borderline obese. Obesity is anything above 30 kg/m²; it is an additional important factor in the development of the syndrome, but is of itself not an intrinsic component, as shown by the fact that many obese individuals do not develop the syndrome.

The complex of abnormalities making up the syndrome often precedes type 2 diabetes, sometimes as much as by 9–10 years, and during this time some of the vascular complications, such as retinopathy and nephropathy, may begin. Thus, the condition should be treated before frank diabetes manifests. The first line of treatment is usually diet and exercise. As little as a 15-lb weight loss can make remarkable changes and even prevent the development of diabetes.

Although the four factors described are those usually associated with the syndrome, there are others. One is an increase in plasminogen activator inhibitor-1 (PAI-1) (it is not lower than normal, choice **A**). This inhibits fibrinolysis, and along with hypertension and dyslipidemia, further promotes development of coronary and other artery disease. Although muscle and adipose tissues become resistant to insulin, glucose uptake into muscle (choice **C**) or adipose cells (choice **D**) is not decreased, because the resistance to insulin is compensated for by an increase in its concentration, thus leading to a minimal hyperglycemia. That uptake of glucose into adipose cells is not inhibited is clearly demonstrated by the fact that pre–type 2 diabetics gain weight. Not all cells become insulin resistant; thus, the hyperinsulinemia causes a metabolic imbalance that is related to the symptoms associated with the syndrome. This state of affairs continues until the ability of the pancreas to compensate becomes limited; when it does, the circulating glucose levels increase until frank diabetes occurs. An increase in serum uric acid levels, not a decrease (choice **E**), also occurs in this prediabetic state.

**20** **The answer is A** *Medicine*

This patient has a history suggestive of angina pectoris and has risk factors for this, including being a smoker, a family history of diabetes mellitus, and now, a hyperlipidemia demonstrated by xanthomas (the reddish yellow lesions) over the gluteal area. These papules are filled with lipid that can erupt (eruptive xanthoma). They may be located under the skin or even on some tendons. They may be present in normal populations but generally are increased in patients with diabetes mellitus and lipid disorders such as hypertriglyceridemia, hypercholesterolemia, lipoprotein lipase deficiency, and abetalipoproteinemia. They signify a markedly elevated very-low-density lipoprotein (VLDL) level (choice **A**). Separated xanthomata such as these should be distinguished from xanthomatosis (choice **E**), a generalized increase in xanthomata that may be seen in malignancies such as lymphomas and multiple myeloma or in familial hypercholesterolemia syndrome and Wolman disease. (Wolman disease is an autosomal recessive cholesterol ester storage disease that is due to a defect in lysosomal sterol esterase. It results in the accumulation of triglycerides and cholesterol esters. It usually occurs in consanguineous cohorts. These patients have hepatomegaly, adrenal calcification, steatorrhea, and anemia in addition to xanthomatosis). Xanthelasma (choice **F**) on the other hand are yellowish that which contain lipid-laden histiocytes that surround blood vessels. They are usually located over the medial aspect of the eyelid. They are not due to hyperlipidemia in the elderly, but they certainly are in younger people.

An elevated high-density lipoprotein (HDL) level (choice **B**) is not a risk factor for hyperlipidemia; in contrast this, the "good cholesterol" fraction, is beneficial in keeping the other lipoprotein levels in check. Although an elevated triglyceride level greater than 1,000 mg/dL is usually seen in patients with eruptive xanthomas, they are mainly increased due to an elevated VLDL level, not to free triglyceride (choice **C**). Most of the serum triglyceride is carried in the VLDL fraction.

The predominant lipids carried in the blood are cholesterol and triglycerides; both are carried on specific "apoproteins," which, when complexed with their appropriate lipoidal component, form the various lipoproteins. They are not carried as the free lipids (choice **D**).

Lipoproteins are classified according to their density as originally determined by ultracentrifugation; the more lipid, the less dense it is. Markedly elevated low-density lipoprotein (LDL) levels (choice **G**) are associated with tendinous xanthomata; this represents a genetic triglyceridemia. Such a dyslipidemia, which is inherited in a classic Mendelian pattern, is called a primary dyslipidemia, as distinguished from the more common secondary dyslipidemias that may be influenced by genetics but are primarily caused by life style. The xanthomata due to tendinous xanthomata are deposited in certain tendons such as the Achilles, quadriceps, and extensor tendons of the hand. In such cases, serum triglyceride levels may be above 2,000 mg/dL (extremely high levels) and cream-colored retinal blood vessels may be seen in the fundus, a condition known as lipemia retinalis.

### 21 The answer is C *Medicine*

This patient is demonstrating the classical signs of a myocardial infarct. A ruptured atherosclerotic plaque (choice **C**) followed by thrombosis is believed to be responsible for most myocardial infarctions (MI). The rupture is believed to be triggered by inflammation and metalloproteinase activity. Matrix metalloproteinases are a family of enzymes that remodel the extracellular matrix of the cardiac blood vessels. On the positive side, they may act to help stabilize rupture-prone plaques; conversely, the imbalanced action of some specific isoforms may promote failure of the remodeling process, causing the fibrous cap covering the lipid core to break down. This disperses lipoidal material distally, leading to vascular occlusion and subsequent infarction of the myocardium and perhaps even causing sudden death. Factors that increase the vulnerability of plaques to rupture include greater lipid content and an increase in the number of macrophages resulting in a thin fibrous seal, which can give way easily.

Cigarette smoking is the most important preventable risk factor for cardiovascular disease. However, it is not the immediate cause of MI (choice **A** is incorrect); it is believed that smoking contributes to the atherosclerotic process and plaque instability, in part by increasing the adherence of macrophages to the vessel wall and inducing the release of proteolytic enzymes (metalloprotein isoforms?). Approximately 20% of women and 25% of men smoke in the United States. Those who quit smoking will have a 50% drop in the risk for cardiovascular disease after just 1 year. Hence, it is important to encourage and help patients to quit smoking altogether. Atherosclerosis is not an immediate cause for a myocardial infarct (choice **B** is incorrect). Atherosclerosis results from hyperlipidemia, which is a risk factor for coronary artery disease. Initially, fat is deposited in the subendothelial space. This is known as a fatty streak. Macrophages enter this area and take up the lipids, giving them the appearance of foam cells. Further progression leads to the migration of myocytes. If there is no further accumulation of lipids and migration of macrophages, fibrosis is followed by calcification. The vessel wall undergoes remodeling at the cost of a decreased lumen and impaired blood flow, which could result in myocardial ischemia (angina pectoris). Obesity is a risk factor for coronary artery disease and not the cause for the MI that has occurred (choice **D** is incorrect). Narrowing and closure of a coronary artery or arteries is gradual, and is not an acute event (choice **E** is incorrect).

### 22 The answer is A *Psychiatry*

The patient presents with the psychotic symptom of persecutory delusions. Of the disorders listed, only dementia (choice **A**) commonly presents with psychotic symptoms. Delusions, mood changes (e.g., anxiety, depression), and other thought disturbances (e.g., perseveration) often accompany significant cognitive impairment in dementia, and are sometimes the presenting problem. Other disorders with similar psychotic symptoms include schizophrenia and delusional disorder. However, in these disorders, obvious cognitive impairment would be absent.

Obsessive-compulsive disorder (choice **B**) may present with anxiety about bizarre ideas, but the individual usually recognizes the irrational nature of the thoughts. Panic disorder (choice **C**), posttraumatic stress disorder (choice **D**), and generalized anxiety disorder (choice **E**) may all present with anxiety but do not explain the presence of psychosis.

### 23 The answer is B *Obstetrics and Gynecology*

The case scenario describes polyhydramnios. The amount of amniotic fluid can be quantified using the four-quadrant amniotic fluid index (AFI), which is the sum of the measurements of the deepest amniotic fluid pockets in the four abdominal quadrants, measured by sonography. Polyhydramnios is present when the AFI exceeds 25 cm or the deepest single amniotic fluid pocket exceeds 8 cm. Excessive amniotic fluid is a result of imbalance of secretion and absorption. The only option listed that is associated with polyhydramnios is diabetes mellitus (choice **B**), in which polyhydramnios appears to be related to a lack of glucose control.

Asthma (choice **A**), hyperthyroidism (choice **C**), seizure disorder (choice **D**), and sickle cell anemia (choice **E**) are not associated with polyhydramnios.

### 24 The answer is B *Surgery*

This woman has a pulmonary embolus with infarction, a condition most commonly seen in the setting of postoperative recovery associated with stasis of the venous circulation in the proximal (femoral) veins of the leg, the most common location (90%) for thromboembolism. Signs and symptoms depend on the size of the embolus. Large saddle emboli that block four of the five pulmonary artery orifices result in sudden death because of acute strain on the right side of the heart. Small emboli lodge peripherally, where they produce an infarction in fewer than 10% of patients. Infarction is more likely in patients with preexisting lung disease, such as seen in heart failure or in chronic obstructive lung disease. Pulmonary angiography is the gold standard test for diagnosing a pulmonary embolus, particularly when other studies give conflicting results. However, most clinicians begin with a perfusion scan of the lungs (choice **B**), which has a high probability of indicating an infarction if a lobar perfusion defect accompanies ventilation mismatch, the latter demonstrated by a ventilation scan. Perfusion defects last 7–14 days.

A pleural tap (choice **A**), Gram's stain with culture and sensitivity of sputum (choice **C**), pulmonary function studies (choice **D**), and a bronchoscopy (choice **E**) are noncontributory in the initial workup of a pulmonary embolus.

## 25 The answer is D  *Medicine*

The anticoagulant drug warfarin has been implicated in numerous drug interaction scenarios. Warfarin is documented to exert prophylactic actions after a myocardial infarction (MI) (choice **E** is incorrect), and the dosage regimen was appropriately adjusted in this patient (choice **A**) to result in an approximate 50% increase in prothrombin time (PT) (normal range is 11–15 seconds). The further increase in PT described is likely to result in a bleeding episode, and reflects increased activity of warfarin at the established dose. The histamine ($H_2$)-blocking drug cimetidine is known to be a potent inhibitor of liver drug-metabolizing enzymes, including those forms of cytochrome P450 that are responsible for the metabolic inactivation of warfarin. Thus, concomitant administration of cimetidine is anticipated to increase PT; by inhibiting the hepatic metabolism of warfarin (choice **D**), it increases its circulating concentration. Other causes that can prolong PT include inadequate vitamin K in the diet; inadequate absorption, as in Crohn disease, and severe hepatic dysfunction.

Trimethoprim-sulfamethoxazole does not increase the activity of hepatic drug-metabolizing enzymes (rifampin does) and would result in a decreased PT if warfarin metabolism was increased (choice **B**). The antiplatelet action of aspirin does not antagonize the effects of warfarin and may lead to an increased bleeding tendency (choice **C**). Salicylates and sulfonamides may also increase PT by competition with warfarin for plasma protein binding, leading to an increase in the plasma-free fraction of warfarin. Note that many drugs capable of inducing the formation of liver drug-metabolizing enzymes (e.g., barbiturates, carbamazepine, and phenytoin) will decrease PT in patients on warfarin.

## 26 The answer is B  *Medicine*

This patient has neoplastic metastatic epidural cord compression that has arisen from carcinoma of the prostate. The compression has worsened over the past 24 hours but began a week earlier with weakness of his legs. The initial management would be to administer a bolus dose of dexamethasone intravenously (IV) and then perform a magnetic resonance imagining (MRI) study (choice **B**) of the spine with and without gadolinium contrast. The sensitivity of this test is greater than 90%. Thereafter, IV administration of dexamethasone should be continued every 6 hours to combat spinal cord edema. This is a neurosurgical emergency, and immediate decompression should be carried out to salvage neurologic function. The development of urinary bladder problems makes this an even greater reason to act as quickly as possible. Thereafter, the patient should be referred for radiotherapy of the appropriate region.

Waiting for 24 hours before doing an MRI (choice **A**) would only jeopardize neurologic recovery. The patient does not have Guillain-Barré syndrome. This is usually seen in a younger individual, in whom there is a prior history of upper respiratory tract or gastrointestinal infection, following which ascending motor paralysis results. There is no sensory or urinary bladder involvement. Hence, plasmapheresis (choice **C**), a treatment for Guillain-Barré syndrome, is not indicated. Ordering electromyography (choice **D**) would not contribute to diagnosis or management. It would only confirm what is known clinically—that the patient has weakness of his legs due to motor involvement. Even then, abnormalities will be noted approximately 3 weeks after the onset of weakness. Sending him for radiotherapy of the lumbar and sacral spine (choice **E**) is incorrect. Radiotherapy usually follows surgical decompression and has to be done along the extent of the tumor, as delineated by the MRI. In some cases, however, surgical decompression is not done, and radiotherapy is carried out under steroid cover following a radiologic diagnosis.

### 27 The answer is B *Obstetrics and Gynecology*

Substance use by an expectant mother can affect reproduction, from fertility through pregnancy and lactation. Research is difficult in this area because of the confounding effects of poor nutrition and exposure to multiple substances. The findings described in the case are consistent with fetal alcohol syndrome (FAS; choice **B**). In the United States, this is the most common preventable cause of mental retardation. Not all children with FAS have the distinctive physical findings, yet they are still at risk for lifelong neurological sequelae, such as attention-deficit disorder, hyperactivity, and memory and impulse control difficulties.

Prenatal tobacco exposure (choice **A**) is associated with sudden infant death syndrome and childhood behavioral problems but not with any specific syndrome. Prenatal marijuana exposure (choice **C**) is linked to premature births, small birth size, difficult or long labor, and an increase in newborn jitteriness but not to birth defects. Prenatal amphetamine (choice **D**) and narcotics (choice **E**) are associated with neonatal abstinence syndrome, which refers to the constellation of signs and symptoms exhibited by infants with drug dependencies, but only alcohol has a clearly defined syndrome with intrauterine growth restriction, central nervous system effects, and facial anomalies.

### 28 The answer is D *Surgery*

About 60% of the solitary coin lesions in the lung are benign. Of the benign causes, granulomas (choice **D**) account for 95%, while the remaining 5% are due to hamartomas or mixed tumors. The patient's midwestern origins strongly suggest histoplasmosis as the cause for the calcified granuloma. Calcification of a coin lesion is more commonly seen in granulomas than in cancer. Absence of growth within 2 years noted on serial radiography of the chest, target or popcorn calcifications, or concentric calcifications strongly favors a benign process. A malignancy would be suggested by indistinct margins, increased growth rate compared with previous films, flecks of calcium in the mass, and sizes greater than 3 cm in diameter. A history of living in an endemic granuloma area and not smoking, in conjunction with no cough, chest pain, weight loss, rhonchi, or hemoptysis all suggest that the lesion is not cancer. Its benign nature also is strongly supported by the fact that it is concentric, calcified, and less than 1 cm in diameter. However, follow-up radiography should be conducted (first yearly, then less regularly) for at least 10 years to make sure the lesion is not growing.

Mixed tumors, also known as bronchial hamartomas (choice **B**), are so called because they are pleomorphic and contain epithelial cells, cartilage, and mesenchymal cells. Malignant change is rare in them. Hamartomas are the result of faulty development that results in tissue overgrowth. Indeed, the word *hamartoma* in Greek means fault and was the term used when spear throwers missed their mark. The remaining 40% of the causes of solitary coin lesions in the lung are primary lung cancer (35%; choice **A**) and metastatic lung cancer (5%; choice **C**). A negative tuberculosis skin test result proves that it is not a calcified tuberculosis lesion (choice **E**).

### 29 The answer is D *Pediatrics*

This patient has a subgaleal hematoma (choice **D**), which is a result of blood collecting subadjacent to the galea. It is seen after minor injury and can be very alarming. It is not associated with loss of consciousness. The best treatment for this condition is to leave it alone. Aspirating the hematoma would only introduce infection, which could be disastrous. The parent should be reassured that no treatment is necessary.

An epidural hematoma (choice **A**) results from blood collecting within the cranial cavity, and is usually seen after a tear of the middle meningeal artery as it courses on the inner aspect of the temporal bone, in which a fracture line is seen. It is associated with a lucid interval and signs of raised intracranial pressure (i.e., headache, vomiting, loss of consciousness, enlarging pupil on the ipsilateral side, and hemiplegia on the contralateral side). A subdural hematoma (choice **B**) results from intracranial hemorrhage within the subdural space. It may be acute or chronic. A fracture may be absent. The patient is comatose from the time of injury and has evidence of cerebral injury. The prognosis is poor. Intraventricular hemorrhage (choice **C**) is associated with coma and may result from trauma. However, it is more commonly seen after hypertensive intracranial hemorrhage, in which the bleeding spreads to the ventricular system. A lipoma (choice **E**) is a benign soft-tissue tumor and does not develop suddenly.

**30** **The answer is B** *Surgery*

With an inhalational anesthetic, both rate of onset and rate of recovery depend on the physiochemical properties of the agent, which are reflected in its blood:gas partition coefficient. Anesthetics with low blood:gas partition coefficients are advantageous because they act rapidly, and the time to recover from their effects is short. As can be seen from the table in the vignette, desflurane (choice **B**) has the lowest blood:gas ratio of all the choices provided. Thus, recovery from the anesthetic effects of desflurane occurs more rapidly than with nitrous oxide (choice **A**), sevoflurane (choice **C**), isoflurane (choice **D**), and halothane (choice **E**). The minimum alveolar concentration is the percentage of anesthetic in the inspired gas that results in immobility in 50% of a patient population exposed to a noxious stimulus. Minimum alveolar concentration is inversely related to the potency of an anesthetic agent and does not influence the kinetics of anesthetic onset or recovery.

**31** **The answer is D** *Psychiatry*

The case is most suggestive of bipolar I disorder; the incident at 23 years of age shows a depressive phase and at 28 years a manic phase. This disorder is characterized by one or more episodes of mania, without known biologic cause and without persisting psychosis between episodes. Evidence of elevated levels of several central nervous system (CNS) neurotransmitters (choice **D**) has been reported during manic episodes in bipolar I disorder. The reasons for the antimanic properties of mood-stabilizing medications are unknown.

Family histories of individuals with bipolar I disorder suggest that the lesion is heritable (choice **C**), but consistent chromosomal abnormalities have not been detected (choice **E**). Although genetic variations occur in several ion transport mechanisms, no particular abnormality has been clearly identified as a marker for bipolar I disorder (choice **A**). The mechanisms of action for mood-stabilizing medications, which include lithium, various anticonvulsants, and newer antipsychotic drugs, are not known. α-Adrenergic blockade is not known to be the reason for their therapeutic effects (choice **B**).

**32** **The answer is D** *Medicine*

This patient has diabetic ketoacidosis (DKA), most likely due to the increased insulin requirement generated by the infection, a common problem. In DKA, glucosuria results in the loss of significant amounts of sodium, potassium, and phosphorus in the urine. When insulin is used in the treatment of DKA, phosphate is normally transported along with glucose into muscle and adipose cells; this permits phosphorylation of glucose, allowing further metabolism. Insulin treatment also enhances glycolysis, which further depletes the already decreased concentration of phosphate in the blood, leading to hypophosphatemia (choice **D**). Depletion of phosphate results in a corresponding decrease in adenosine triphosphate (ATP) within the muscle, leading to paralysis of the respiratory muscles and respiratory failure in the patient. This sequence of events is the rationale for providing phosphate supplementation in the treatment of DKA when phosphate levels begin to decline during insulin therapy.

Human insulin does not produce anaphylactic reactions (choice **A**). Glucose toxicity (choice **B**) refers to the effect of hyperglycemia in reducing the sensitivity of tissues to insulin therapy in both type 1 and type 2 diabetes mellitus. Ketoacidosis (choice **C**) is not a cause of muscle weakness resulting in respiratory problems. Although hyperkalemia (choice **E**) is commonly seen in the setting of DKA, it is not due to an excess of potassium stores, but is the result of a transcellular shift of potassium out of cells as excess hydrogen ions in ketoacidosis are buffered intracellularly. This transcellular shift often disguises the marked deficits in total body potassium that these patients have because of urinary potassium loss due to the osmotic effect of glucosuria. Severe hypokalemia can also cause muscle paralysis by preventing muscle repolarization. Therefore, potassium supplementation is extremely important in the treatment of DKA and can be given as potassium phosphate rather than potassium chloride. Bacteremia (choice **F**) is a feature of septic shock, in which the cardiovascular system is the target. Endotoxins, especially those due to gram-negative sepsis, lead to hypotension, tachycardia, and tachypnea but not to paralysis of the respiratory muscles.

**33** **The answer is E** *Psychiatry*

The symptoms suggest a diagnosis of mild mental retardation (choice **E**), defined as mental retardation associated with an IQ of between 50 and 70. Degrees of mental retardation are denoted by IQ: mild (50–70), moderate (35–50), severe (20–35), and profound (<20). The cause of mild mental retardation is usually idiopathic, with no clear physical or social pathology (e.g., maternal substance abuse [choice **D**], perinatal insults [choice **B**], and sociocultural deprivation [choice **C**]). More severe mental retardation results from known physiologic lesions (e.g., genetic or chromosomal abnormalities [choice **A**]).

### 34 The answer is D *Pediatrics*

Meckel's diverticulum (choice **D**) usually presents as painless rectal bleeding. The condition is best remembered as the disease of twos; it affects 2% of the population, occurs in the first 2 years of life, and is a sacculation 2 feet proximal to the ileocecal junction. Iron deficiency anemia can result from chronic blood loss. The diverticulum usually consists of ectopic gastric tissue. Diagnosis is made by Meckel radionuclide scan, which is performed after intravenous infusion of technetium$^{99m}$ pertechnetate. Surgical excision is the treatment of choice.

Intussusception (choice **A**) presents as an acute abdomen with currant-jelly stool. Patients with duodenal ulcers (choice **B**) have pain. Adhesions (choice **C**) are fibrous bands that may cause bowel obstruction after abdominal surgery, causing abdominal pain, nausea, and vomiting. They are not associated with rectal bleeding. Ulcerative colitis (choice **E**) typically presents with bloody diarrhea with mucus.

### 35 The answer is B *Obstetrics and Gynecology*

This patient meets the criteria for secondary amenorrhea, which are absence of menses for 3 months if previously menses were regular or an absence of menses for 6 months if menses were previously irregular. A negative serum β-human chorionic gonadotropin (β-hCG) test result virtually rules out pregnancy, the most common cause of secondary amenorrhea. The β-subunit is produced by only placental tissue with pregnancy or with an ovarian tumor (choriocarcinoma). The second most common cause of secondary amenorrhea is anovulation. A positive progesterone challenge test result indicates only that the patient has an adequate amount of estrogen to prepare her endometrium for ripening and shedding by progesterone (choice **B**). The patient can be assumed to be anovulatory.

Medroxyprogesterone acetate (MPA) orally is not helpful as a pregnancy test (choice **A**). The only definitive way to rule out pregnancy is a negative urine or serum β-hCG test result. It also cannot rule out a pituitary adenoma (choice **D**), which requires a screening test with a serum prolactin level followed by a central nervous system (CNS) imaging study of the sella turcica. Even a spotting response is adequate to be a positive result (choice **E**). Primary and secondary amenorrhea can be differentiated from a good history, not from a progesterone challenge test (choice **C**).

### 36 The answer is E *Medicine*

This patient has two problems: hypertension and prostatic hypertrophy (which most often is benign). The latter diagnosis is based on the history of frequency of urination at night. Patients with both prostatic hypertrophy and hypertension are best treated with an α-1 selective antagonist such as doxazosin (choice **E**). This medication relaxes smooth muscles in the prostate, enabling better egress of urine, as well as those in the arterioles, thus lowering blood pressure. The half-life of doxazosin is about 24 hours. There are several α-1 selective antagonists. Prazosin relaxes the smooth muscles not only in the prostate, but in the arterioles and venules as well, thus enabling efficacious treatment for both conditions. The drawback is that, when taken orally, only 50% of the drug is utilized, shortening its half-life to approximately 3 hours. Another medication, tamsulosin, has a far greater effect on prostatic smooth muscle than it does on arterioles and hence has very little effect in lowering blood pressure. An alternative to doxazosin is terazosin, which also is efficacious in treating both benign prostatic hypertrophy and hypertension. However, terazosin has a half-life of slightly less than 12 hours.

Atenolol (choice **A**) is a β blocker. It is utilized in the treatment of hypertension associated with angina and supraventricular tachycardia. In patients with angina, β blockers decrease oxygen demand by the myocardium. In patients with hypertension and supraventricular tachycardia, β blockers prolong the refractory period in the AV node thereby delaying AV conduction. Furosemide (choice **B**) is a loop diuretic that is very useful in patients with congestive cardiac failure and/or peripheral edema. Although loop diuretics have been used in patients with mild to moderate hypertension, thiazide diuretics are usually the first choice in treating early hypertension. Given this patient's urinary outflow problems, a loop diuretic could lead to acute urinary retention due to outflow obstruction. Hydrochlorothiazide (choice **C**) is a thiazide diuretic that is usually given initially in the treatment of mild hypertension and as an adjunct for higher grades. It probably acts by inducing arteriolar dilatation. Once again, administering a diuretic to a patient who has problems with urination due to prostatic hypertrophy could lead to acute urinary retention due to outflow obstruction. Diltiazem (choice D) is a calcium channel blocker. Other calcium channel blockers include nifedipine and verapamil. Although calcium channel blockers will lower the blood pressure, they will not relax prostatic smooth muscle. They relax the smooth muscles in arterioles and arteries, causing blood pressure to drop, thus making them useful for managing hypertension. They also delay conduction in the AV node, slowing the ventricular rate in patients with atrial fibrillation and reversing supraventricular tachycardia.

### 37 The answer is B *Psychiatry*

This man's symptoms are most suggestive of dementia. The most common cause of dementia in this age group is Alzheimer disease (choice **B**), which is often characterized by a gradual onset of memory impairment and an absence of focal neurologic disease.

Alcoholic dementia (choice **A**) is less likely in the absence of any suggestion of alcohol-related work impairment. Cerebrovascular disease (choice **C**) is less common than Alzheimer disease and often has a more sudden onset and evidence of focal neurologic impairments or other vascular disease. Depression (choice **D**) may cause difficulty concentrating but is unlikely to interfere with objective testing for agnosia or short-term memory. Aging alone (choice **E**) does not cause significant difficulties with everyday cognitive function.

### 38 The answer is A *Obstetrics and Gynecology*

Gestational diabetes is a common medical complication of pregnancy with a prevalence of 3%–5%. Common risk factors include ethnic background (Hispanic, African American, American Indian, and Pacific Islander), elevated body mass index, and age over 25 years. The patient in this case has many risk factors. The incidence of overt diabetes mellitus in pregnancy is less than 0.5%. If present, it can adversely affect both mother and fetus. The levels in White's classification of diabetes in pregnancy describe increasing perinatal risks as the alphabet letters increase. Class A diabetes is the lowest risk with onset during the pregnancy. The case presentation describes a normal fasting, but abnormal 1- and 2-hour glucose values. This description meets the criteria for class A1 (choice **A**); therefore, the disorder can be treated with diet alone.

Class A2 (choice **B**) is gestational diabetes requiring insulin. Class B (choice **C**) diabetes describes overt diabetes with onset after age 20 and duration less than 10 years. Class C (choice **D**) diabetes describes overt diabetes with onset between ages 10 and 19 years, with duration between 10 and 19 years. Class D (choice **E**) diabetes describes overt diabetes with onset before age 10 years and duration over 20 years. All classes beyond Class A1 require additional insulin therapy.

### 39 The answer is C *Surgery*

The word *atelectasis* (choice **C**) implies that there has been no expansion of the lung tissue. Nevertheless, it is the term used to describe the postoperative condition in which small airways and alveoli lose their patency and collapse. It is the most common complication following general anesthesia. Patients with nasogastric tubes are at higher risk to develop this. Under normal circumstances, alveoli do collapse but expand thereafter because of release of surfactant. Taking deep breaths stimulates release of surfactant in the normal individual. As a result of pain following surgery, the patient cannot take deep breaths, and the tidal volumes are also low. This inhibits the release of surfactant, leading to collapse of the alveoli. If the patient has tenacious sputum, this in turn will aggravate the situation further. Clinically, rales, diminished breath sounds, tachycardia, and fever all point to this diagnosis. Pain may or may not be a feature. Chest radiography may demonstrate atelectasis even in the absence of clinical signs. Most often, atelectasis is patchy and does not involve large segments of the lung. Treatment involves clearing the secretions and promoting expansion of the lungs. Physiotherapy, nebulized mucolytic agents, deep breathing exercises, incentive spirometry, and early ambulation are helpful.

Pulmonary embolus (choice **A**) is a sudden event that usually occurs several days after surgery and is usually due to venous stasis in the calf secondary to deep venous thrombosis. Breakage of the clot leads to a shower of emboli that commonly enter the pulmonary circulation. A massive embolus could be fatal immediately. It has even been known to happen so rapidly that a patient stops talking in midsentence. In other cases, the patient will complain of sudden chest pain and shortness of breath and have hemoptysis. Tachycardia and hypotension also occur. Dyspnea and tachycardia are the most frequent clinical features, and there will be an audible split pulmonary second sound on auscultation. Some patients will have gallop rhythm and cyanosis. Postoperative wound infections (choice **B**) are more common in the 5- to 10-day postsurgical period. Intravenous (IV) catheter-related sepsis (choice **D**) usually results in thrombophlebitis at the site of cannulation. Its frequency is much greater if it is done in the lower extremities. Hence this route is reserved only if no venous access is available elsewhere. Fever due to phlebitis usually occurs on the third postoperative day. The local area is inflamed and tender. If it leads to a suppurative phlebitis, the patient looks very ill. Tachycardia and hypotension may ensue together with tachypnea. Chest pain is unusual. Removing and relocating the intravenous catheter is essential. Blood samples should be drawn and sent for culture and sensitivity together with the tip of the catheter, and antibiotics started. A spontaneous pneumothorax (choice **E**) is a cause of atelectasis. It is associated with chest pain, difficulty breathing, and tachycardia. Fever is not a feature. Aspiration pneumonitis (choice **F**) is associated with dyspnea, cyanosis, and tachycardia. It usually occurs within half an hour after aspiration. Clinical examination will reveal wheezes and rales. Respiratory failure could ensue.

### 40 The answer is D *Pediatrics*

Infant botulism (choice **D**) usually occurs in infants younger than 1 year of age, particularly between 2 and 6 months. It occurs after the ingestion of *Clostridium botulinum* spores, which can be found in honey and corn syrup, as well as in soil and house dust. The course of the disease varies but progresses quickly. Typically, the child is afebrile and has been previously healthy. The infant becomes constipated and feeds poorly. A weak cry, hypotonia, and loss of head control are then seen. Descending paralysis progresses over hours to days. Ventilatory support may be necessary.

Guillain-Barré syndrome (choice **A**) consists of weakness that begins in the lower extremities and spreads to the trunk, the upper extremities, and the bulbar muscles. This pattern is known as Landry ascending paralysis, and respiratory failure may result. Although hypothyroidism (choice **B**) and Werdnig-Hoffmann disease (choice **C**) present with hypotonia, it is seen earlier in life, and progression of symptoms occurs more slowly. Hypomagnesemia (choice **E**) usually presents in conjunction with hypocalcemia and manifests as tetany.

### 41 The answer is G *Preventive Medicine and Public Health*

A case report (choice **G**) is a brief objective report of a clinical feature or outcome from a single patient or event. It is studied retrospectively. Because it pertains to only one case, no statistical analysis or comparison can be made; however, it can form the basis for hypothesis testing. Thus, one can report drug interaction or adverse reaction or even an unusual clinical feature or presentation.

### 42 The answer is H *Preventive Medicine and Public Health*

A case series report (choice **H**) is an objective report of a number of cases that present with similar features. Its main benefit is in defining the symptoms and signs of a specific disease. A case series report can be a retrospective or a prospective study. The problems in a case series report are the inherent bias built into it and the lack of controls, which prevents generalization of the information.

### 43 The answer is D *Preventive Medicine and Public Health*

One of the problems faced with clinical studies investigating the same phenomenon is the absence of concurrence in terms of conclusion. To obtain a definite conclusion, meta-analysis (choice **D**) is used, wherein the total results of all the studies are pooled so that a single conclusion can be established. To ensure that the meta-analysis is correct, it is analyzed by meta-meta-analysis.

### 44 The answer is I *Preventive Medicine and Public Health*

This is a retrospective study that is also a case-control study (choice **I**). Case-control studies can be retrospective or prospective. A retrospective study follows the group backward in time, from the time of manifestation of disease to the point of initial exposure. Cases with disease and the control group are randomly selected. Interviews are conducted by chart audit; namely, use of questionnaires. A 2 × 2 table is constructed to ascertain whether exposure caused the disease. Thus, a retrospective study compares the frequency of exposure between the two groups—those exposed to the suspected risk factor and those who were not exposed. There are several advantages to conducting a retrospective study: it can be used to establish risk factors for rare diseases, it is relatively inexpensive (does not require long follow-ups), and volunteers are not required.

### 45 The answer is C *Preventive Medicine and Public Health*

This is a clinical trial. These are prospective studies, but are slightly different from observational prospective studies in which the investigator is a passive observer who only records the effect of a factor in a group of individuals exposed to it and in a group who were not exposed (e.g., cigarette smoking). In a clinical trial, the investigator intervenes by withholding intervention in the control group while allowing it in another; thus, the investigator is actively involved. To eliminate bias, which could be introduced by the investigator, the participant, or both, blinding techniques are used. A double-blind study (choice **C**) is used, so that neither the investigator nor the participants are aware of whether they have been assigned to the treatment or the control group.

**46** **The answer is F** *Preventive Medicine and Public Health*

This is a cross-sectional study (choice **F**), which is used to determine prevalence or to establish etiology. It is most commonly used in surveys designed to establish the distribution pattern of a disease. For example, if one wanted to establish the prevalence of bronchial asthma in a population in Los Angeles, variables such as age, sex, ethnicity, occupation, and place of residence can be incorporated into the study to determine how these influence the disease.

**47** **The answer is A** *Preventive Medicine and Public Health*

This is a cross-over study (choice **A**), which is a variation of the double-blind study. In a cross-over study, the two groups have an equal opportunity to receive the intervention and the placebo, so that each group can act as its own control.

**48** **The answer is C** *Preventive Medicine and Public Health*

This is another example of a double-blind study (choice **C**). In double blinding, neither the investigator nor the participants are aware of to which group they will be assigned (i.e., the control or the treatment group). This is useful if one wants to ascertain the end point of intervention—is there improvement, no change, or does the condition become worse? Double-blinding techniques are used in clinical trials; however, there is no cross-over.

**49** **The answer is E** *Preventive Medicine and Public Health*

This is a nonconcurrent prospective study (choice **E**), also known as a historical cohort. This study is carried out entirely or partially from existing records. In this type of study, events of interest that include exposure and disease have already occurred. The problem is that bias can enter into the study because one may not be sure in some instances whether the exposure resulted in the disease or whether it occurred de novo.

**50** **The answer is I** *Preventive Medicine and Public Health*

This is a case-control study (choice **I**), which differs from the one presented in question 44 in that it is a prospective study (i.e., it is carried forward in time). A prospective study enables one to ascertain the incidence of a disease. It usually involves a cohort, which is a group that shares a common characteristic or experience within a given time frame (e.g., those who survived a stroke). Sometimes, individuals in a prospective study have to be singled out and studied. Such studies are called *longitudinal studies*. A prospective study involves two groups of individuals: those who have been exposed to the factor and those who have not been exposed (i.e., the control group). The groups are followed until it is possible to establish the number of individuals in the two groups who develop the disease. Bias is low because neither the participants nor the investigator are aware of who will develop the disease and who will not. A prospective study is therefore an observational prospective study, because the investigator is a passive observer and does not manipulate the groups, as he or she would in the case of clinical trials. Disadvantages include attrition (people may not come to follow-up), cost (requires a long period of study), and the need for volunteers (the sample size should be large).

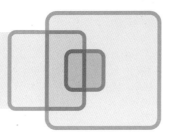

# test **10**

# *Questions*

***Single Best Choice Directions:*** *This section consists of numbered statements or questions followed by a list of potential answers; you are to select the ONE best answer.*

**1** A 2-year-old boy presents to the pediatrician with a 12-hour history of recurrent and severe paroxysmal colicky pain. The pain is accompanied by straining efforts, loud cries, and vomiting. Abdominal distention and tenderness are present on physical examination, and an oblong mass is palpated in the midepigastrium. Bloody mucus is noted on the examiner's finger as it is withdrawn after rectal examination. Which of the following is the most likely diagnosis?

(A) Meckel's diverticulum
(B) Congenital pyloric stenosis
(C) An intussusception
(D) Meconium ileus
(E) Necrotizing enterocolitis

**2** An institute for female felons conducted the following study to confirm that sodium restriction lowered systolic blood pressure in their mix of patients. They divided 300 prisoners into two 150-person groups that are matched with respect to age, ethnicity, and approximate blood pressure values; all were in the prehypertensive range (systolic pressure between 130 and 139 mm Hg, diastolic pressure between 80 and 89 mm Hg), none is diabetic, and none is taking any relevant medication. One group was put on a sodium-restricted diet permitting 2,000 mg of sodium daily. The other group was permitted to consume the usual prison fare, which provided an average of 5 g of sodium daily. (The typical daily consumption in the United States is between 4 and 6 g [175–260 mEq] daily). After 2 months on these diets, the difference in mean diastolic blood pressure among the 150 subjects in the low-salt diet group and the 150 subjects in the nonrestricted-salt group is 5 mm Hg, a difference significant at a *P* value of .04851. Which one of the following statements about the two groups is true?

(A) The blood pressure difference is clinically significant.
(B) The chance that an individual would benefit from a low-salt diet is less than 0.05%.
(C) It is unlikely that random variation accounted for the difference in diastolic blood pressure between the two groups.
(D) Increasing the number of subjects would tend to change the *P* value from significant to nonsignificant.
(E) To show a statistically significant difference, the sodium-restricted group should have been limited to an intake of less than 1,000 mg of sodium per day.

**3** A 16-year-old boy tells his gym instructor that he just isn't strong enough to do more than one push-up, and he isn't able to run a lap without being left breathless. The instructor suspects malingering but nonetheless sends him to the school physician for evaluation. Physical examination reveals a tall, gangly young man who is 5 ft 10 in (1.8 m) tall and weighs 155 lb (70.3 kg). His has a strikingly narrow face, an arm span of 6 ft 4 in (1.9 m), long legs, long thin fingers, pectus excavatum, and is myopic. His heart sounds reveal a pansystolic murmur near the apex of the atrium, with a prominent third heart sound. Which one of the following connective tissue components is most likely abnormal in this young man?

(A) Fibrillin-1
(B) Keratin 5 or 14
(C) Type IV collagen
(D) Type I collagen
(E) Type XI collagen
(F) Fibroblast growth factor receptor

**4** A 62-year-old man with Parkinson disease but no previous psychiatric history is admitted to the hospital with a 1-week history of emotional lability, disinterest in personal appearance, intermittent inattention and confusion, peculiar beliefs about his wife poisoning his food, and intermittent visual hallucinations concerning insects in the house. He is currently taking carbidopa-levodopa and trihexyphenidyl. He reportedly has a history of alcohol abuse and has been drinking more lately. Mental status examination reveals that the patient is oriented to the year but not the month. Which of the following is the most likely diagnosis?

(A) Alcohol-induced dementia
(B) Alcohol-induced psychotic disorder
(C) Delirium of unknown cause
(D) Dementia due to Parkinson disease
(E) Mood disorder due to Parkinson disease

**5** A 69-year-old man with a history of coronary artery disease and hypertension presents with acute onset of right facial weakness and numbness. On examination, his speech and extremity strength are normal, but he has significant weakness of the right side of the face, including the orbicularis oculi. In addition, he complains of roaring in the right ear, and his taste sensation is absent on the right side of the anterior tongue. Sensation is normal to pinprick. Which of the following would best explain these findings?

(A) Bell's palsy
(B) Brainstem glioma
(C) A stroke due to occlusion of the left middle cerebral artery
(D) Lacunar stroke of the left internal capsule
(E) Parotid tumor

**6** A 33-year-old woman complains of being unable to leave her home unless others accompany her. Whenever she is faced with the necessity of traveling beyond her front fence, she calls her friend to help her. She feels discouraged and angry about her condition. Mental examination reveals a normally alert and attentive woman with mild depressive symptoms but no evidence of disorganized thinking or delusions. Which of the following is the most likely disorder associated with this patient's phobia?

(A) Major depressive disorder
(B) Obsessive-compulsive disorder
(C) Panic disorder
(D) Schizophrenia
(E) Somatization disorder

**7** An 8-year-old boy is taken to a family physician by his mother who tells the physician that she is worried that her child may have sugar diabetes because he urinates frequently and is almost always thirsty. The mother says she knows that these are signs of diabetes because her 58-year-old husband developed type 2 diabetes earlier this year, and her 76-year-old mother was diagnosed with diabetes only 5 years ago. She asks, "How can my child escape diabetes with such a family history?" During the physical examination, the physician notes that the boy is grossly underweight, there is a fruity smell on his breath, and he seems lethargic. His blood pressure is 105/55 mm Hg. The nurse conducts a finger-prick blood glucose determination and the resultant value is 325 mg/dL. Which one of the following statements concerning this boy and his condition is true?

(A) The boy should be placed on an insulin regime as soon as possible.
(B) It cannot be concluded that the boy has diabetes until a fasting blood glucose value is obtained.
(C) The mother was right to suspect the boy inherited diabetes from either his father or grandmother.
(D) A metabolic syndrome associated with diabetes is liable to make the boy obese as he ages.
(E) The boy can be best treated with oral antihyperglycemic agents.

**8** The star quarterback for a university football team presents to the school physician 2 weeks after the onset of symptoms of infectious mononucleosis. He wants to return to playing football and is requesting medical clearance. He states that he feels fine; his muscle aches and fatigue have resolved. Upon examination, his heart and lungs are normal, his spleen is not enlarged, he has no temperature, and his liver enzyme values are normal. Which one of the following statements is correct regarding when he may return to playing football?

(A) Since he seems fine, he may return to football immediately.
(B) He should return for another check-up next week and possible clearance to play.
(C) He should return for another check-up in 2 weeks and possible clearance to play.
(D) He may return to football when the mono-spot test result is negative.
(E) He may return to football when the lymphocyte count returns to normal.
(F) He is out for the remainder of the season (3 months) but may play again next season.

**9** A laboratory test has a reference mean value of 20 mg/dL and a standard deviation of 2. Which of the following is the range in which 95% of repeated laboratory determinations would be expected to fall?

(A) 20–22
(B) 18–22
(C) 16–24
(D) 14–26
(E) 19–21

**10** A 26-year-old woman planned to go biking. As she was dressing, she noticed her period had just started, so she inserted a tampon. While biking, a car turned right immediately in front of her; she crashed into it and catapulted over the hood. She was unable to get up, and when she looked at her right leg, she found that her knee had traveled more than half way up her thigh. The paramedics approximately realigned the femur, splinted it, and transported her to a local hospital, where they set the fracture by implanting a metal rod down the shaft of the bone. Because of her blood loss she was administered two units of blood, after which her hemoglobin level was 7 g/dL. After 2 days in the hospital, the surgical wound continued to seep blood, but she seemed on the road to recovery and was transferred to a neighboring rehabilitation facility. Because of everything else going on, nobody thought of replacing the tampon. The morning after arriving at the rehabilitation facility, she complains of dizziness and a feeling of weakness and seems somewhat disoriented. She has a temperature of 103°F (39.4°C) and has a generalized rash that even covers her hands and the soles of her feet. Her skin is warm to the touch, and her blood pressure is 150/90 mm Hg. The duty nurse calls in a physician, who arrives 45 minutes later. By the time the physician gets there, the patient's skin appears gray and is cold and clammy, she has tachycardia and the heart sounds are weak, she has a shallow and rapid rate of breathing, her blood pressure is 74/49 mm Hg, her eyes are lusterless, and she is staring without showing signs of recognizing anything. At this time, which of the following choices represents the most probable diagnosis?

(A) Hypovolemic shock
(B) Toxic shock syndrome
(C) Cardiogenic shock
(D) Anaphylactic shock
(E) Shock cause by a gram-negative organism

**11** A 20-year-old woman, gravida 2, para 0, abortus 1, is at 25 weeks' gestation with a twin pregnancy. An obstetric ultrasound examination notes 30% discordance between the estimated fetal weights of the two fetuses. In addition, the largest single vertical amniotic fluid pocket is 9 cm in the sac of the larger twin, but only 1 cm in the sac of the smaller twin. Assessment of fetal anatomy is normal in both fetuses, and bladders are seen in both twins. Which of the following statements is most likely to be true?

(A) The donor twin is more likely to develop hyperbilirubinemia than the recipient twin.
(B) The type of placentation is dichorionic and diamniotic.
(C) The recipient twin often develops signs of volume overload.
(D) The pregnancy was the result of ovulation induction agents.
(E) The fetuses are of opposite gender.

**12** A 27-year-old woman was first diagnosed with schizophrenia at age 18 and has a history of epilepsy that started at about age 5. Her epilepsy is stabilized on divalproex. She was started on clozapine for her schizophrenia 1 week ago, and now complains of sedation and sialorrhea. Which one of the following laboratory examinations should be performed immediately?

(A) Clozapine level
(B) Prolactin level
(C) Thyroid function
(D) Divalproex level
(E) White blood cell count

13. A patient has Alzheimer disease, which has advanced to the extent that he can no longer make rational decisions but still enjoys walking in the neighborhood with his caretaker. However, he now has difficulty ambulating because of a problem with his knee. His physician believes his knee problem is due to a cartilage injury and wants to conduct a magnetic resonance imaging study to determine if surgery is needed and, assuming it is, to follow up with appropriate surgery. Which of the following represents the procedure that takes precedence prior to starting treatment of the knee?

(A) Follow directions the patient expressed in a living will.
(B) Obtain written permission from a person named in a durable power of attorney.
(C) Obtain written permission from the director of the patient's managed care organization.
(D) Invoke the state's involuntary treatment law.
(E) Have the patient sign an informed consent form.

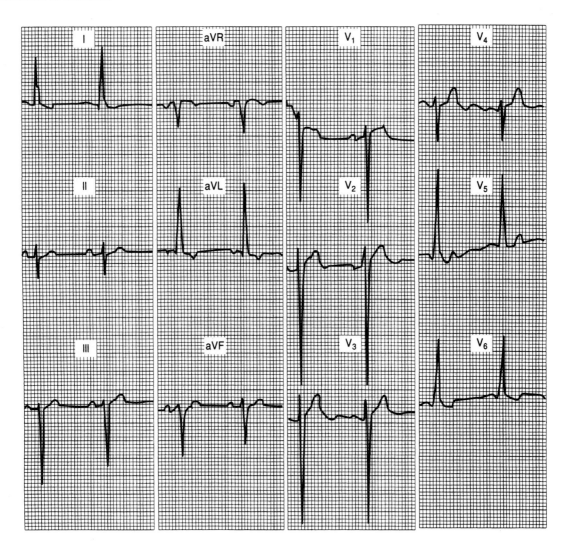

14. A 65-year-old man with multiple myeloma presents with confusion, severe depression, vomiting, constipation, and polyuria. His electrocardiogram is shown above. Which of the following is the most appropriate first step in the management of this patient?

(A) Give calcium gluconate.
(B) Infuse saline.
(C) Administer sodium bicarbonate.
(D) Infuse furosemide.
(E) Initiate mithramycin therapy.

**15** A 76-year-old woman sees her physician with complaints of muscle pain around the neck, a headache particularly intense in the temporal area, a tender scalp, and jaw pain when chewing. She says that these symptoms started about 3–4 weeks earlier and seem to be getting progressively worse. In addition, she has felt tired, lost her appetite, and as a result lost 5 lb. A more recent problem that she finds worrisome is blurred vision, in which a single object appears as two. Upon examination, she was found to weigh 140 lb (63.5 kg), to be 5 ft 5 in tall (1.65 m), have a temperature of 100.9°F (38.3°C), and a blood pressure of 125/82 mm Hg. Her heart rate and rhythms were regular, her lungs clear to auscultation, her abdomen was soft and nontender, the liver and spleen were of normal size, her temporal region was tender to touch, and she had small retinal hemorrhages. Which one of the following laboratory test or procedures will provide the most significant clue regarding the diagnosis?

(A) A complete blood count
(B) A computed tomography study of her head
(C) An erythrocyte sedimentation rate determination
(D) A carotid ultrasound
(E) A lumbar puncture with subsequent culture

**16** A 36-year-old woman has a 20-year history of social withdrawal and lack of motivation that began insidiously during high school. She has had several episodes of hallucinations and delusions; however, there have been no clear-cut episodes of depression or mania. There is a history of significant excessive alcohol use from age 20 to 30. Compared with the general population, which one of the following would most likely be found with studies of cerebral morphology and/or functional neuroimaging?

(A) Abnormalities of dopaminergic transmission
(B) Decreased metabolic activity in the prefrontal cortex
(C) Decreased size of the lateral ventricles
(D) Increased cerebral asymmetry
(E) Increased thickness of the corpus callosum

**17** A mother presents to the emergency department with her 2-month-old daughter. The child appears lethargic and dehydrated. The mother reports that the patient has not been feeding well for the past few days. She adds that she recently changed the infant's feedings from formula to cow's milk because the infant does not care for the taste of formula. Which nutrient normally in high concentration in cow's milk could cause the symptoms seen in this infant?

(A) Linoleic acid
(B) Linolenic acid
(C) Calcium
(D) Protein
(E) B-complex vitamins

**18** A 22-year-old woman has had undiagnosed acute intermittent gastrointestinal pains since the age of 17. However, today she presents at an emergency clinic with such severe abdominal pain that the resident on duty seriously considered recommending an emergency laparotomy to find out what is wrong. However, he reconsidered after she complains about pain in both feet, becomes semi-incoherent, and starts to act abnormally. Despite her semi-incoherent state, he elicited the fact that she recently started having sexual relations with her first serious boyfriend, and as a consequence, started taking an estrogen-based contraceptive. In addition, to make sure she remained attractive to this, "her one and only love of her life," last week she started a 1,200-calorie/day diet. Further questioning disclosed that her father had been bothered by intermittent stomach pains for many years, and although these annoyed him, they never were severe enough to require medical attention. Otherwise, both parents, now in their mid-50s, seemed healthy. A physical examination was unremarkable except for borderline hypertension; the resident suspected that the pain in her feet was due to peripheral neuropathy. A blood panel indicated that she suffered from hyponatremia. On the basis of the foregoing information, the resident made a tentative diagnosis. To confirm his suspicion, he asked the laboratory to run a urine analysis for which one of the following compounds?

(A) Porphobilinogen
(B) Uroporphyrin
(C) Uroporphyrinogen I
(D) Coproporphyrinogen I
(E) Coproporphyrinogen III
(F) Lead

**19** A 59-year-old man made an appointment to see his physician because he had noticed blood in his urine for the past week. Otherwise, he felt healthy, and he had no problem voiding his urine. His primary care physician found no other unusual signs or symptoms and referred him to a urologist, who conducted a cystoscopic examination of his bladder. A small sample of the bladder wall was removed and examined microscopically. The view obtained is illustrated below.

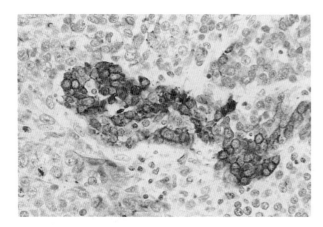

The lesion was evaluated as being a stage T1 papillary carcinoma, which has invaded the lamina propria but has not invaded the superficial layer of the muscularis propria. The lesion was completely excised by transurethral resection. Which one of the following is true concerning this condition?

(A) The prevalence of the types of bladder cancer is equally common throughout the world.

(B) The type of carcinogen having the greatest potential of causing this condition is found in smoked foods.

(C) Removal of the growth by transurethral resection usually is not followed by recurrence of the condition.

(D) Usually, the condition described is treated by radical cystectomy.

(E) Pelvic pain and difficulty in voiding urine are the earliest signs of bladder cancer.

(F) Women and men have an equal chance of developing bladder cancer.

(G) In the United States, most primary bladder cancers are transitional cell carcinomas.

(H) Bladder cancer is primarily a disease of the middle aged, 40 to 55 years old.

**20** After leaving a bar in a five-star hotel, a 38-year-old man trips and falls while descending a flight of stairs. Subsequently, he feigns severe back pain, seeks medical attention, and then initiates legal action against the hotel in a bid to receive compensation for pain,

suffering, and lost wages. Which of the following is the most likely diagnosis?

(A) Conversion disorder
(B) Factitious disorder
(C) Malingering
(D) Pain disorder
(E) Somatization disorder

**21** A child is referred to a pediatric endocrinologist for further management of hypophosphatemia. On review of the family history, she notes that the patient's mother has fasting hypophosphatemia. Laboratory results show that the patient has a slightly reduced serum calcium level, a moderately reduced serum phosphate level, elevated alkaline phosphatase activity, and no evidence of secondary hyperparathyroidism. On physical examination, the child is noted to have smooth bowing of the lower extremities, coxa vera, genu varum, genu valgum, and short stature. Which of the following is another characteristic seen on physical examination in patients with familial hypophosphatemia?

(A) Tetany
(B) Rachitic rosary
(C) Harrison's groove (pectus deformity)
(D) Myopathy
(E) Waddling gait

**22** An 8-year-old boy is brought to his pediatrician by his mother, who disclosed that the patient had been in his usual state of good health until this morning, when he awoke covered with bruises and purple dots. The patient has no history of trauma, and there is no history of bleeding disorders in the patient or family. The past medical history is only significant for a mild upper respiratory infection 1 week ago. The pediatrician notes that the boy has petechiae and purpura over his entire body. A complete blood count (CBC) is obtained. The platelet count is 20,000 platelets/μL (normal is 150–450 × $10^3$/μL), but the rest of the CBC results are normal. No hepatosplenomegaly is present. A bone marrow aspirate exhibits normal megakaryocytes, but platelet budding is poor. Which of the following is the most appropriate approach to the management of this patient?

(A) Platelet concentrates should be given prophylactically to prevent bleeding.

(B) Whole blood should be administered to prevent bleeding.

(C) γ-Globulin and/or corticosteroid should be administered.

(D) Vitamin C should be administered.

(E) Vitamin K should be administered.

(F) Splenectomy should be performed.

**23** A 16-year-old boy died yesterday. His father died from cancer before he was born, and his mother died from cancer a week ago, leaving the boy in a depressed state. He confessed to his school psychologist that he wasn't sure life was worth living. However, even prior to his mother's death, he engaged in several antisocial activities. He was a member of a street gang that had recently been conducting a violent turf war with a rival gang; he smoked marijuana, snorted free-base cocaine, and loved to drag race while high. Judging by public health statistics among adolescents and young adults between the ages of 15 and 24 years, his death yesterday most probably resulted from which one of the following?

(A) Suicide
(B) Homicide
(C) Drug overdose
(D) Automobile accident
(E) Cancer

**24** A young mother left her 3-year-old daughter alone in the kitchen while she answered the phone in an adjacent room. In the few minutes, she was out of the room the child grabbed a hot frying pan sitting on the stove. The child started to wail and run in a circle waving her hand; the mother panicked, smeared butter on the burned hand, and rushed the child to a nearby walk-in clinic. The physician in attendance examined the child and found that the child's thumb, index finger, and the palm of her right hand were red. There was also a 0.5 $\times$ 0.25 in (1.27 $\times$ 0.64 cm) blister at the base of her thumb and a smaller one on the tip of her index finger. No other injury could be ascertained. Which of the following is the most appropriate first course of action?

(A) Cool the burn site by immediately immersing the hand in ice-cold water.
(B) Clean the area and dress it with gauze.
(C) Aspirate the fluid underneath the blister.
(D) Débride the wound, aspirate the fluid, and apply an antibiotic cream.
(E) Provide tetanus prophylaxis.

**25** A 4-month-old infant is brought to the pediatrician by his mother because he has not been feeding well. The patient has been in his usual state of good health until 1 day earlier. The patient has not had fever and does not attend day care. There are no ill contacts, pets, or recent travel. Physical examination of the mouth reveals curd-like plaques on the tongue and buccal mucosa that do not scrape off easily. Which one of the following is the bodily area most likely to also be affected?

(A) Eyes
(B) Ears
(C) Nose
(D) Scalp
(E) Perineum

**26** A 6-year-old girl is brought to the pediatrician because of severe dysuria. The history is unremarkable except for the patient having a sore throat. There is no history of hematuria, fever, use of bubble bath, pinworms, tight clothing, nylon underwear, or recent medication. Inspection of the perineum reveals an intense erysipelas-like erythema of the vulva, distal vagina, and perineal area. A serosanguineous vaginal discharge is present. Which of the following is the most likely cause?

(A) *Haemophilus influenzae*
(B) *Neisseria gonorrhea*
(C) *Chlamydia trachomatis*
(D) Group A β-hemolytic streptococcus
(E) *Streptococcus pneumoniae*

**27** Prospective parents seek counseling about the risk of having a child with schizophrenia. There is no history of the disease in her family, but an uncle and his son in the potential father's family have been diagnosed with the disease. Which one of the following statements should be shared with these prospective parents?

(A) There is no evidence of a familial basis for the disease.
(B) The disease appears to be more prevalent in families that share certain patterns of interpersonal communication.
(C) Climate and season of birth will have no effect on the child's risk of developing the disease.
(D) The child's risk of developing the disease will be less than 10% that of the prevalence rate among first-degree relatives, but greater than 1% that of the general population.
(E) The mother should avoid eating wheat gluten during pregnancy.

**28** A 27-year-old nulligravid woman and her 29-year-old husband come to the outpatient office with a 2-year history of infertility. They have been married for 4 years and have been trying for pregnancy for the past 2 years. Since she discontinued oral contraceptive pills 48 months ago, they engage in intercourse regularly, about twice weekly, without using any contraception. They have not undergone any formal medical evaluation but desperately desire children. The family history for both partners is negative for genetic diseases or congenital anomalies. Which one of the following causes of infertility would most likely be found in the workup?

(A) Ovulatory factor
(B) Uterine factor
(C) Tubal factor
(D) Male factor

**29** A 47-year-old man presents to a physician at a free clinic complaining of upper abdominal pain, severe heartburn, nausea, bloating, and vomiting of undigested food. He also states that he eats little because he feels full almost immediately upon eating; consequently, he has been losing weight. Upon taking a history, the physician finds that the patient was diagnosed with diabetes at the age of 6 years. The patient further admits that, although initially his parents made sure he kept his glucose levels under tight control, as he grew older he became careless, mainly because he could not afford health insurance. Consequently, he has been self-treating with insulin obtained illegally via the Internet. He believed that worked well since, until now, he had no real health problems except a need for glasses. He solved that problem by buying a cheap pair on display at a local drug store.

His physician arranged for hemoglobin A1c analysis; the value was 11.5%. Although the free clinic couldn't afford a sophisticated follow-up test, such as scintillation scanning, the physician believed the symptoms described were sufficient to prescribe treatment. Which one of the following drugs did the physician prescribe as the first step in treatment?

(A) Metoclopramide
(B) Adiponectin
(C) Sitagliptin
(D) Pramlintide acetate
(E) Exenatide

**30** A nonsmoking 42-year-old woman consults her physician after finding a lump in her right breast. Upon examination, the physician finds a painless, freely mobile, and well-circumscribed spherical growth with a rubbery consistency. On the basis of this examination, he tells her that he is over 99% sure that this lump is due to benign fibrocystic disease, but just to make sure he would recommend a needle biopsy. The woman breathes a sigh of relief; she was very worried because her mother died from metastatic breast cancer at the age of 38 years. This was particularly tragic because, as a girl and young woman, her mother had endured a life of hardship after her Jewish family escaped from eastern Poland when the Nazis invaded in 1939. She asks the doctor about her chances of developing breast cancer. Which of the following choices represents the most accurate assessment?

(A) Since she is an otherwise healthy non-Hispanic white woman, she has about a 13.3% chance of developing a mammary cancer.
(B) She has at least a 66.5% chance of developing breast cancer.
(C) Because she is older now than her mother was when she died, she has little risk of developing an inherited form of cancer.

(D) Since she has fibrocystic disease, the probability of ever developing a breast malignancy is reduced.
(E) Since she doesn't smoke, the probability of developing breast cancer is reduced.

**31** A 45-year-old woman has a history of many years of reclusiveness and peculiar fantasies about the lives of media celebrities. She does not have a history of hallucinations, delusions, or disorganized behavior. She refuses to interact with other people. There is a history of schizophrenia in two uncles. She has had a trial of antipsychotic medication that decreased her preoccupation with celebrities, but she refused to continue taking it. Which of the following is the most likely diagnosis?

(A) Avoidant personality disorder
(B) Obsessive-compulsive disorder
(C) Schizoid personality disorder
(D) Schizophrenia, residual type
(E) Schizotypal personality disorder

**32** A 24-year-old Caucasian female makes an appointment to see an ophthalmologist; she complains that her eyes seep "thick, viscous, yellowish sticky stuff" that tends to mat her eyelashes, making it difficult for her to open her eyes in the morning. In addition, she says her eyes feel gritty when she blinks, and they appear to her to be "bloodshot." The sclera are a "pink-red" color, but they do not hurt, and her vision seems normal, although sometimes she has to wipe "gunk" away from her eyeball. Examination reveals a mild photophobia, a normal pupillary reaction to light, and normal intraocular pressure. This woman most likely has which of the following disorders?

(A) Acute viral conjunctivitis
(B) Optic neuritis
(C) Acute bacterial conjunctivitis
(D) Uveitis
(E) Central retinal artery occlusion
(F) Anterior blepharitis

**33** A 3-year-old child with sickle cell disease presents to the emergency department with a temperature of 40°C (104°F). The mother states that the child had been in his usual state of relatively good health until 4 hours ago. Starting at that time, the mother states that the child became progressively listless. Upon physical examination, the physician notes that the child has nuchal rigidity. The patient has no known ill contacts and takes no medication. Immunizations are up to date. A spinal tap would most likely reveal which of the following pathogens?

(A) *Streptococcus pneumoniae*
(B) Group B streptococcus
(C) *Escherichia coli*
(D) *Listeria monocytogenes*
(E) Group A β-hemolytic streptococcus

**34** A 30-year-old woman recently back from a photographic safari trip to Tanzania presents with headache, fever with temperature spikes of 40.6°C (105°F), and scleral icterus. Physical examination reveals tender hepatosplenomegaly. Laboratory data show an increase in the liver transaminases. A complete blood cell count shows a normocytic anemia and an increased corrected reticulocyte count. A direct Coombs' test result is negative. Results of a urine dipstick test for blood are positive. A peripheral blood smear shows many red blood cells with one to three ringlike structures. Which of the following is the most likely diagnosis?

(A) Autoimmune hemolytic anemia
(B) Congenital spherocytosis
(C) Glucose 6-phosphate dehydrogenase (G6PD) deficiency
(D) Hemolytic anemia caused by pyruvate kinase deficiency
(E) *Plasmodium falciparum* malaria

**35** A 65-year-old white woman slipped and fell on an icy walkway. When seen in the emergency department, she complained of pain in the right hip, and had shortening and external rotation of the right leg. X-ray films confirmed a diagnosis of a fractured femur neck, for which she underwent arthroplasty. Two days after surgery, she complained of difficulty breathing. On clinical examination, her vital signs were as follows: pulse, 88/min; temperature, 36.9°C (98.4°F); respiration, 18/min; and blood pressure, 130/90 mm Hg. She had distended jugular neck veins. Auscultation of the heart revealed a third heart sound, while that of the chest revealed bibasilar inspiratory crackles. In addition, she had dependent pitting edema. Results of a complete blood cell count including platelet count were normal. Which of the following is the most likely diagnosis?

(A) Endotoxic shock
(B) Cardiogenic shock
(C) Overzealous fluid resuscitation
(D) Fat embolism syndrome
(E) Syndrome of inappropriate antidiuretic hormone

**36** A 29-year-old man with a 9-year history of alcoholism recently successfully completes an outpatient drug rehabilitation program. This was the second time he had "dried out." The previous time, he vowed he would never touch a drop again but within a month after completing this second program, he had "just one night out with the boys" and starting drinking again. He was arrested for disorderly conduct and ordered to enter an inpatient drug rehabilitation program. He seeks advice about the most effective way to maintain sobriety after discharge. Which of the following is the most accurate advice?

(A) Take disulfiram before participating in a social situation in which he might expect to consume alcohol.
(B) Take naltrexone before participating in a social situation, because one drink will make him nauseous.
(C) Do not try to totally abstain from alcohol consumption, but rather limit consumption to socially appropriate amounts because this will keep the urge to drink within tolerable limits.
(D) Have a definite number of drinks in mind before engaging in a social event involving alcohol.
(E) Join a local chapter of Alcoholics Anonymous.

*Directions for Matching Questions (37 through 50): Each set of matching questions is preceded by a list of 4 to 26 lettered options followed by a brief explanation of the required task and then by a series of numbered statements. For each lettered statement you are to select ONE lettered option that best fulfills the task as it relates to that statement. Remember that each of the listed options might be correctly selected once, more than once, or not at all.*

## Questions 37–43

(A) Cervical
(B) Ovarian
(C) Endometrial
(D) Vaginal
(E) Vulvar
(F) Oviduct

*For each of the following numbered staging descriptions below, select the ONE most appropriate lettered gynecologic malignancy from the list above. Each staging description may be used once or more than once.*

**37** This gynecologic cancer has no official staging criteria.

**38** This gynecologic cancer is clinically staged.

**39** This gynecologic cancer has a staging category of IA2.

**40** This gynecologic cancer has the highest 5-year survival rate for stage I disease.

**41** This gynecologic cancer is epidemiologically considered a sexually transmitted disease.

**42** This gynecologic cancer has staging categories of IC, IIC, and IIIC.

**43** This gynecologic cancer has the highest overall mortality rate among all gynecologic cancers.

## Questions 44–50

(A) Pramlintide acetate
(B) Glyburide
(C) Nateglinide
(D) Sitagliptin
(E) Acarbose
(F) Metformin
(G) Exenatide
(H) Rosiglitazone

*Select the ONE most appropriate lettered diabetic drug from the list above that matches the appropriate numbered description below. (Although generic names are used as the mainstay, the trade names are also provided in the answers because they are so commonly used.)*

**44** A second generation sulfonylurea

**45** An oral antidiabetic that does not enter into the body

**46** An oral antidiabetic medication whose mechanism of action involves activation of the intracellular peroxisome proliferator-activated receptor-γ

**47** An oral antidiabetic medication whose mechanism of action involves activating AMP-activated protein kinase.

**48** An oral antidiabetic medication whose mechanism of action involves inhibition of dipeptidyl peptidase-4

**49** An oral antidiabetic secretagogue that is normally taken between 1 and 30 minutes before a meal

**50** A nonamyloidogenic analogue of amylin

# Answer Key

| | | | | | | | | | |
|---|---|---|---|---|---|---|---|---|---|
| 1 | C | 11 | C | 21 | E | 31 | E | 41 | A |
| 2 | C | 12 | E | 22 | C | 32 | C | 42 | B |
| 3 | A | 13 | B | 23 | D | 33 | A | 43 | B |
| 4 | C | 14 | B | 24 | B | 34 | E | 44 | B |
| 5 | A | 15 | C | 25 | E | 35 | C | 45 | E |
| 6 | C | 16 | B | 26 | D | 36 | E | 46 | H |
| 7 | A | 17 | D | 27 | D | 37 | F | 47 | F |
| 8 | C | 18 | A | 28 | D | 38 | A | 48 | D |
| 9 | C | 19 | G | 29 | A | 39 | A | 49 | C |
| 10 | B | 20 | C | 30 | B | 40 | A | 50 | A |

# Answers and Explanations

### 1 The answer is C *Pediatrics*

Intussusception (choice **C**) is the most common cause of intestinal obstruction in children between 3 months and 6 years of age, but decreases in frequency after 3 years. The cause is unknown, but it has been associated with gastroenteritis, Meckel's diverticulum, polyps, and sarcoma. Patients have paroxysmal colicky abdominal pain. A sausage-shaped mass can usually be palpated in the right upper abdomen, and bloody, currant-jelly stools are passed. Barium enema reveals a coil-spring sign and may even be therapeutic. However, the use of "air" enemas in the diagnosis and treatment of intussusception has supplanted hydrostatic reduction. If enema reduction is unsuccessful, surgical reduction is necessary.

Pyloric stenosis (choice **B**) is characterized by nonbilious projectile vomiting in a 1- to 3-month-old. Meckel's diverticulum (choice **A**) usually presents as painless rectal bleeding, and symptoms usually arise within the first 2 years of life, but it is not uncommon for initial symptoms to be seen in the first decade. Meconium ileus (choice **D**) and necrotizing enterocolitis (choice **E**) both present in the neonatal period.

### 2 The answer is C *Preventive Medicine and Public Health*

In biologic systems, a *P* value of less than .05 (i.e., the probability that random variation accounted for the difference between the two groups is less than 5 times out of 100) is commonly considered statistically significant; thus, a value of .04851 is statistically significant, meaning that it is unlikely that random variation accounted for the difference in diastolic blood pressure between the two groups (choice **C**).

However, as important as this is, without further follow-up studies concerning the health of the participants, it does not prove that this effect is clinically significant (choice **A**). Choice **B** is incorrect for two reasons. First, clinical benefit cannot be determined on the basis of two sets of numbers that do not directly refer to a health-based parameter (e.g., Were there significantly fewer myocardial infarcts among the salt-restricted cohort?). Second, as the choice is worded, potential significance would decrease as the *P* value does; therefore, to make sense, it should say "the chance that an individual would benefit from a low-salt diet is more than 0.05%." If the number of subjects were increased (assuming that the means and the standard deviations of the groups remained the same), the *P* value would tend to be lower and would be more, rather than less, statistically significant (choice **D**). Since a 2,000 mg diet provided a statistically significant difference, it obviously is not necessary to further reduce sodium intake to prove a statistical difference (choice **E**). In fact, reducing sodium further is liable to be counterproductive because a diet providing 1,000 mg or less of sodium per day is difficult for most people to tolerate; thus, even in a prison population, compliance is apt to be low. In contrast, patients on a 2,000 mg daily intake for 2–3 months often adapt to this diet, may actually find excess salt to be unpleasant, and often continue to voluntarily restrict salt intake.

### 3 The answer is A *Medicine*

The features described in the clinical vignette suggest that this boy has Marfan syndrome, a trait that is inherited as an autosomal dominant mutation in the fibrillin-1 gene and results in an aberrant fibrillin-1 protein (choice **A**). Marfan's syndrome is one of the most common connective tissue disorders, with an incidence of about 1 in 5,000 births, and about 25% of these cases are due to new mutations. Fibrillin-1 is a major constituent in the elastic fibrillin microfilaments that provide both support and elasticity to connective tissue throughout the body. Persons with Marfan syndrome may show a wide range of symptoms. Typically, they are tall, with abnormally long arms (arm span is greater than height), long legs and fingers (arachnodactyly), and a rather long thin face. (Many believe that Abraham Lincoln expressed the typical phenotype.) In addition to this typical phenotype, affected individuals may show a wide variety of other symptoms, some of which lead to physical weakness and lack of stamina, as in the case described. These symptoms may include mitral valve prolapse, aortic root dilation, pectus excavation, scoliosis, joint dislocations, pneumothorax (due to the collapse of a lung), and ectopic lentis. Mitral valve prolapse is the most common symptom (85% of cases); it may eventually contribute to early heart failure and is likely responsible for the unusual heart sounds heard in the patient described. Although heart failure may be responsible for the early demise of Marfan patients, aortic root dilation resulting in eventual dissection is the most common fatal consequence of Marfan syndrome. Prophylactic administration of a β blocker to slow the heart rate and lower blood pressure is used to help delay expansions of the aorta, and expansion is screened for by annual or even biannual echocardiograms. Once the aortic diameter expands beyond a certain critical diameter, prophylactic surgery can be performed. Similarly, the mitral valve can be surgically replaced if needed. As a consequence, life expectancy of treated Marfan patients is now similar to that of the general population. The major reason for the great variation in symptoms among Marfan patients is that, at the molecular level, Marfan syndrome is many diseases. The fibril-1 gene is large, with 65 exons, and a 1997 study found 85 different mutations among 94 unrelated patients. To add further variety to the mix, even in a given family there can be major differences in the degree to which different tissues are affected, presumably because of the nature of other structural connective tissue proteins.

Epidermolysis bullosa (EB) is a constellation of conditions resulting in skin that blisters with minimal trauma. EB is relatively rare; the reported incidence varies from 1 case per $10^6$ births in the United States to 54 cases per $10^6$ births in Norway. On the physiologic level, the common feature of the various forms of EB is a weak connection between the upper and deeper layers of the skin due to aberrant supportive proteins. The worst cases result in death during infancy due to sepsis caused by bacterial invasion. Three major types are recognized: EB simplex (92% of cases), junctional EB (1%), and dystrophic EB (5%); the remaining 2% of cases are unclassified. EB simplex is due to mutations in either keratin 5 or 14 (choice **B**) proteins that form intermediate filaments in basal keratinocytes. A deficiency of, or defects in, these proteins make these cells prone to cytolysis.

Alport syndrome causes inherited kidney disease coupled to extrarenal complications, including sensorial deafness and eye abnormalities. It is due to mutations in one of the several genes coding for type IV collagen (choice **C**). Type IV collagen is the major structural component of basement membranes, where it provides a framework for the binding of other basement membrane components and is a substratum for cells. Type IV collagen has the typical collagen triple-stranded structure, and the individual strands are coded for by one or more of six different genes, *COL4A1* through *COL4A6*. About 85% of the cases of Alport syndrome are due to mutations in *COL4A5* located on the X-chromosome. Males with mutations in this gene present with hematuria in infancy, which then progresses to uremic syndrome and end-stage renal disease by the second or third decade. Females are also affected, causing the disease to be classified as X-linked dominant; however, the course of the disease is less severe, and they often die at a normal age without developing end-stage renal disease. *COL4A6* is also located on the X-chromosome, but mutations are less common and are associated with leiomyomatosis in epidermal cells. *COL4A3* and *COL4A4* are located on chromosome 2, and mutations in these genes cause an autosomal recessive form of Alport syndrome. *COL4A1* and *COL4A2* are located on chromosome 13; mutations in these genes cause less than 1% of cases of Alport syndrome, and these are inherited as autosomal dominant traits.

Type I collagen (choice **D**) is composed of two α1 and one α2 peptides wound in the typical triple-stranded helix. It is the most abundant of the collagens; it provides tensile strength to bone and tendons and also contributes to a lesser degree in other tissues. Any of a number of mutations in either *COL1A1* or *COL1A2* causes osteogenesis imperfecta, a heterogeneous group of conditions generally clinically characterized by easily broken bones, loose and easily torn tendons, and in most cases (about 98%), blue sclera caused by a thin translucent cornea. Although at a molecular level one can describe scores of mutations, clinically they are classified into three or four subtypes. The three major clinical variants are: type I, the most common and least severe form; type II, generally fatal in utero or during the neonatal period; and type III, with severe consequences resulting in deformed limbs and dwarfism. Type I is inherited as an autosomal dominant trait, whereas types II and III are almost always either new mutations (which, if affected individuals were to reproduce, would be transmitted in an autosomal dominant manner) or are inherited as recessive traits; the latter likely result from mutations in enzymes that catalyze posttranslational modifications of procollagen. Some investigators also recognize type Ib or IV. Type IV is an uncommon variant similar to type I but in which the sclera are not affected. Others group these cases together with type I. Type Ib is a variant in which teeth are prominently affected.

Stickler syndrome is caused by aberrant type XI collagen (choice **E**) or type II collagen due to mutations in *COL11A1, COL11A2,* or *COL2A1*. It can be inherited as an autosomal dominant trait. Affected individuals demonstrate a wide variety of symptoms ranging from subtle to severe. Type XI and type II collagens have a similar tissue distribution and primarily are found in joints, including the temporomandibular, and in the spinal column, inner ear, and vitreous fluid of the eye. Persons with Stickler syndrome are generally characterized by a flattened facial appearance caused by underdevelopment of the bones of the mid face, including the cheekbones and the bridge of the nose. The syndrome may also include cleft palate, myopia, glaucoma, retinal detachment, hearing loss, hypermobile joints, and early-onset osteoarthritis.

Mutations in *FGFR1* or *FGFR2*, the genes that code for the fibroblast growth factor receptor (choice **F**) cause Pfeiffer syndrome, an autosomal dominant condition characterized by premature fusion of skull bones (craniosynostosis), brachydactyly (flat broad thumbs and big toes facing away from the other digits), and syndactyly (webbing between digits). Type I Pfeiffer syndrome may be caused by mutations in either *FGFR1* or *FGFR2*. These mutations cause early maturation of osteoclasts during embryogenesis, resulting in premature fusion of bones in the skull, hands, and feet. Although the craniosynostosis causes an unusual facies with bulging wide-set eyes, an underdeveloped upper jaw, and a peaked nose, most individuals with type I Pfeiffer syndrome have normal intelligence and normal lifespan. However, persons with type II or III Pfeiffer syndrome, always due to mutations in *FGFR2*, suffer more severe symptoms, often involving the nervous system.

### 4 The answer is C  *Psychiatry*

The symptoms are most suggestive of delirium, which is characterized by disturbances of awareness or attention, cognitive problems, rapid onset, and fluctuations in severity. Associated findings, such as hallucinations and persecutory ideation, are common. Although possible physiologic causes include L-dopa toxicity from carbidopa-levodopa, anticholinergic toxicity from trihexyphenidyl, and alcohol withdrawal, no definitive information suggesting a cause is provided. As a consequence, the most specific diagnosis possible is delirium of unknown cause (choice **C**). Patients who are elderly or who have preexisting dementia are much more likely to develop delirium.

Dementias, such as alcohol-induced dementia (choice **A**) or dementia due to Parkinson disease (choice **D**), would usually present with a history of increasing cognitive problems; however, this patient has no previous history of psychiatric problems. Alcohol-induced psychotic disorder (choice **B**) or mood disorder due to Parkinson disease (choice **E**) would not be diagnosed in the presence of cognitive problems such as inattention, confusion, and disorientation.

### 5 The answer is A  *Medicine*

Bell's palsy (choice **A**) is idiopathic and nearly always acute. All the patient's deficits are referable to the peripheral nervous system, including the loss of taste (chorda tympani branch of the facial nerve) and hyperacusis (branch of the stapedius muscle of the ear).

The strokes (choices **C** and **D**) are unlikely, because of sparing of the rest of the right side of the body and no other central signs. Although brainstem glioma (choice **B**) and parotid tumor (choice **E**) commonly present with facial nerve weakness, they are unlikely choices considering the sudden onset of the event.

### 6 The answer is C  *Psychiatry*

This patient's symptoms are most suggestive of agoraphobia, which is characterized by a fear of experiencing panic attacks in a place where help would be unavailable. Agoraphobic symptoms are almost always associated with panic disorder (choice **C**), and rarely occur without a history of panic attacks.

Patients with panic disorder often have moderate depressive symptoms (not major depressive symptoms [choice **A**]) as a result of frustration with their condition. Obsessive-compulsive disorder (choice **B**) is characterized by irrational thoughts and urges. Schizophrenia (choice **D**) may present with social withdrawal but also includes psychotic symptoms. Somatization disorder (choice **E**) is characterized by multiple physical complaints.

### 7 The answer is A  *Medicine*

The high blood glucose value, coupled to the boy's age, the fruity breath smell (ketosis), lethargic behavior, and thin physique all point to type 1 diabetes mellitus. That he seems ketotic and lethargic suggests that treatment should be started as soon as possible, and insulin injection is the required treatment for type 1 diabetes (choice **A**). (Recently, pramlintide acetate an injectable was approved for use by type 1 diabetics; it is the only noninsulin anti-type 1 diabetic drug developed since insulin was developed in 1922; it is an amylin analogue that permits type 1 patients to use less insulin.) Naturally, a decision should first be made concerning dosage and type of insulin to use, and arrangements must be made to ensure that the possibility of any adverse reaction will be rapidly monitored and addressed.

The American Diabetes Association (ADA) criteria for diagnosing diabetes are any one of the following: (1) one fasting blood value exceeding 125 mg/dL, (2) one random plasma glucose value exceeding 199 mg/dL in the presence of symptoms, or (3) a 2-hour plasma value exceeding 199 mg/dL in an oral glucose tolerance test. Thus, choice **B** is incorrect because he meets the ADA diagnostic criterion 2. That the mother was right to suspect the boy inherited diabetes from either his father or grandmother is not correct (choice **C**) because the ages of onset indicate that both these relatives most likely have type 2 diabetes. Whereas the risk of contracting type 2 diabetes increases if first-degree family members have the disease, the pathophysiologic mechanisms responsible for type 1 are entirely different, and in terms of inheritance, it is an entirely different disease. Type 2 diabetes is typically part of the so-called metabolic syndrome characterized by abdominal obesity, hypertension, hyperlipidemia, insulin resistance, and only eventually hyperglycemia. Insulin resistance appears in some way related to the influence of obesity on the *peroxisome proliferator active receptor* (PPARγ); this is indicated by the facts that some degree of obesity is almost always a precursor event and that the drug thiazolidine lowers blood glucose levels by decreasing insulin resistance via a mechanism involving its interaction with PPARγ. However, this boy has type 1 diabetes, which typically is associated with a thin not an obese physique (choice **D**). (PPAR was first discovered as a factor that enhanced peroxisome proliferation. It has since been discovered that there is a super-family of different PPARs, all acting as transcription factors when they interact with the proper ligand. PPARγ is the family member implicated as a player in metabolic syndrome.) Type I diabetes results from an immunologic reaction that makes the pancreatic β cells incapable of synthesizing insulin; as a consequence, endogenous levels fall to zero. The oral antihyperglycemics either increase the ability of the pancreas to secrete insulin more effectively or increase the ability of peripheral cells to use circulating insulin more efficiently. As a consequence, for these oral agents to work, the pancreas must retain the ability to synthesize and secrete some insulin. Since this ability is lost in type I diabetes, oral antihyperglycemic agents cannot be used to treat patients with this disease (choice **E**).

### 8 The answer is C *Medicine*

Assuming a general state of good health, the present return-to-play recommendation for athletes participating in contact sports who are recovering from infectious mononucleosis is that if the athlete has no splenomegaly or fever, results of liver function tests are normal, and all complications have resolved, he or she may return to contact sports 4 weeks after the onset of symptoms. Since, in the case described, symptoms started only 2 weeks ago, he needs to wait an additional 2 weeks and return for another check-up (choice **C**). Assuming he still is symptom free, he then will be cleared to play.

He cannot return to football immediately simply because he feels fine 2 weeks after symptoms began (choice **A**); a possible complication of premature return to play is splenic rupture, which ensues in 0.1%–0.2% of cases; the rupture can be spontaneous or trauma-related. Rupture only occurs in enlarged spleens, and spleen enlargement may occur between days 4 and 21 after the onset of symptomatic illness. Thus, a final physical examination is essential no earlier than 4 weeks after the first symptoms. He should return next week for another check-up and possible clearance to play (choice **B**) is incorrect since at this time only 3 weeks will have passed since symptom onset. Had he been participating in a noncontact sport, this would have been a permissible time interval. Approximately 10% of individuals with infectious mononucleosis will not develop a negative mono-spot test result (which tests for heterophile antibodies); therefore, a negative result should not be grounds for sending him back to play football (choice **D**). In those with a positive test result, it can take anywhere from 1 to 52 weeks before mono titers are undetectable. A normal lymphocyte count is not assurance that all complications have resolved or that splenomegaly is not present (choice **E**). Provided he passes the 4-week physical, there is no reason to keep him from playing football for the remainder of the season (choice **F**).

### 9 The answer is C *Preventive Medicine and Public Health*

Assuming a normal distribution, the mean ± 2 standard deviations describes the range in which it can be expected that 95% of repeated observations or determinations would fall. In the scenario described (with a mean of 20 and a standard deviation of 2), the normal range would be 20 ± 4, or 16 to 24 (choice **C**).

Choices **A**, **B**, **D**, and **E** are incorrect ranges.

### 10 The answer is B *Surgery*

Shock is a condition in which peripheral blood flow is compromised, depriving cells of adequate oxygen supply. Several different conditions can cause shock, but there is commonality in the symptoms produced. By the time she is seen by the physician, the patient described is suffering from toxic shock syndrome (TSS; choice **B**) due to failure to remove the tampon over the course of 4 days. The early phase, including high temperature, rash, hypertension, and warm skin, reflects the inflammatory effects of toxins caused by bacteria growing in the tampon. In TSS, this phase generally lasts about 30 minutes and is then followed by the more typical symptoms of shock due to a toxin-induced shutdown of the vascular system. These typical shock symptoms include pale or gray skin that is cold and clammy to the touch; tachycardia with weak heart sounds; shallow, rapid breathing; hypotension; lack of focus with confusion; and possibly delirium. In the 1980s, a small epidemic of TSS was associated with a specific brand of "super-absorbant" tampons that allegedly could be left in place for an extended period. Since that brand was removed from the market, the condition has become much less common. TSS more often occurs in response to factors other than tampon use in menstruating women. The hypothesis regarding tampon-induced TSS is that, when women leave tampons in place for a long time, they may become infected with *Staphylococcus aureus*. This bacteria breeds in the tampons and produces toxins that induce septic shock. The tampons are a perfect growth medium, the environment is warm and moist, and the blood is a rich source of nutrients. Moreover, while in the tampon, the bacteria cannot be affected by normal physiologic defense mechanisms and are largely immune even to the influence of antibiotics.

Hypovolemic shock (choice **A**) can be caused by loss of blood (either externally as by a wound or internally as in gastrointestinal bleeding or a fractured femur) or by dehydration from loss of fluid from extravascular compartments (as in vomiting or diarrhea). The symptoms are the same as those described for this patient, but the onset of shock would not be preceded by the early reaction to toxins. Cardiogenic shock (choice **C**) occurs when the supply of blood to peripheral tissues falls below a critical level because of inadequate pumping ability of the heart. The symptoms again are as those described, and the condition may be caused by a myocardial infarct, heart failure, cardiac arrhythmias, or cardiac tamponade. Anaphylactic shock (choice **D**) is caused by an allergic reaction to any of a host of potential allergins. As in TSS, shock is preceded by a brief inflammatory period. However, there is no reason to suspect an allergic reaction in the case presented. Shock caused by a gram-negative organism (choice **E**) would represent classic septic shock, likely caused by an ingested pathogen or infection from gastrointestinal or urinary tract pathogens. As in TSS and anaphylactic shock, the onset of shock is preceded by a brief inflammatory period. However, gram-negative bacteria are rarely, if ever, associated with tampon-induced shock.

### 11 The answer is C *Obstetrics and Gynecology*

The scenario describes the clinical findings frequently noted with twin–twin transfusion syndrome (TTTS). It is diagnosed by polyhydramnios (single amniotic fluid [AF] pocket >8 cm) in one sac along with oligohydramnios (single AF pocket >2 cm) in the other sac. TTTS occurs with a shared placenta when an artery from one twin delivers blood to the vein of the other. The recipient twin receives much more blood, and because of the increased volume, the recipient twin can develop volume overload (choice **C**). This may result in heart failure and hydropic changes.

Because the recipient twin receives much more blood and becomes polycythemic and plethoric, the recipient twin, not the donor twin (choice **A**), is at higher risk for hyperbilirubinemia. Such placental vascular anastomoses occur with high frequency only in monochorionic (monozygotic) twins, thus are not the result of dizygotic (dichorionic; choice **B**) pregnancies or from ovulation induction (choice **D**). Twins of opposite genders (choice **E**) always are found with dichorionic, diamniotic placentation; consequently, TTTS virtually always occurs in twins of the same gender.

### 12 The answer is E *Psychiatry*

Clozapine monitoring requires weekly white blood cell counts (choice **E**) because of an associated 1% risk of agranulocytosis. Sedation and sialorrhea (drooling) are common untoward effects of clozapine treatment.

Clozapine and divalproex levels (choices **A** and **D**) may have clinical significance but are not as immediately required in this patient's treatment. There are no short-term indications in this case for prolactin level determinations (choice **B**) or thyroid function tests (choice **C**).

### 13 The answer is B *Preventive Medicine and Public Health*

Individuals commonly wish to assure they will have a voice in determining what medical treatment they are to receive if they become mentally incapacitated. To do this, they create a legal document called an advanced directive. There are two not mutually exclusive types of advanced directives: living wills and durable powers of attorney for health care. In the latter case, a person while demonstrably of sound mind draws up a legal document in which another person is named to make medical decisions for the patient should he or she become mentally incompetent. The person named in such a durable power of attorney (choice **B**) becomes the legal surrogate for a mentally incapacitated patient, and the physician must turn to him or her for permission to perform any medical procedure.

A living will (choice **A**), the other type of advanced directive, is a legal document that persons, while still of sound mind, have drawn up to express their wishes for medical treatment should they become mentally incapacitated. Since nobody can predict if they will become mentally incapacitated and what medical problems they will have if they do, such a document needs to be drawn up in general terms (e.g., "I wish to have every conceivable life support measure available used to keep me alive before I am declared dead"). Specifics, such as a knee operation, have to be dealt with as they arise, by a rational being—namely, the person named in the durable power of attorney. The director of the patient's managed care organization (choice **C**) may have some practical input in determining the cost–benefit ratio in providing health care, but has no legal right to determine whether or not a patient receives any particular treatment. A state's involuntary treatment law (choice **D**) could only be invoked when a patient is a danger to self or others. For a patient's signature on an informed consent form (choice **E**) to have a legal impact, he or she must be of sound mind. If the patient is mentally incapacitated, the person named in a durable power of attorney has the right and obligation to sign, or not sign, the informed consent form. In the absence of a durable power of attorney, a close relative or, in extreme cases, a state representative may sign the informed consent form. However, it is not unheard of for persons to quarrel over who has that right and what should be done, particularly if money is involved in the outcome.

### 14 The answer is B *Medicine*

This patient has clinical and electrocardiographic (ECG) evidence of hypercalcemia. The hypercalcemia is due to the production of osteoclast-activating factor by myeloma cells in the bone marrow. The illustrated ECG shows shortening of the QT interval (0.28–0.3), which is the characteristic finding in hypercalcemia. Neuropsychiatric findings in hypercalcemia involve personality changes, confusion, depression, acute psychosis, or coma. Cardiovascular changes include hypertension, potentiation of cardiac glycosides, and shortening of the QT interval. Gastrointestinal signs and symptoms consist of nausea, constipation, peptic ulcer disease (calcium stimulates gastrin release), and acute pancreatitis. Pseudogout can occur in the joints. Metastatic calcification in the kidney produces nephrocalcinosis (calcification in the basement membranes of the tubules), which produces polyuria, natriuresis (leading to volume contraction), and problems with urine concentration. Saline infusion (choice **B**) is the first step in management of hypercalcemia because it corrects volume contraction, which is a stimulus for further calcium reabsorption, and it enhances kaliuresis.

Once hydration is achieved, a loop diuretic (e.g., furosemide [choice **D**]) is added to potentiate the kaliuresis. If saline administration and furosemide are ineffective, or if chronic hypercalcemia is anticipated, a number of other options are available. Bisphosphonates are particularly useful in malignancy-induced hypercalcemia because they inhibit bone resorption. Corticosteroids are recommended in hypercalcemia associated with hypervitaminosis D, sarcoidosis, hematologic malignancies, and breast cancer. Mithramycin (choice **E**), an antineoplastic antibiotic, is generally effective but requires close monitoring because of its toxicity. Calcitonin is only effective for 1 or 2 weeks; then, hypercalcemia reappears. Sodium bicarbonate (choice **C**) and calcium gluconate (choice **A**) are useful in the treatment of hyperkalemia, not hypercalcemia.

### 15 The answer is C *Medicine*

The symptoms described suggest giant-cell arteritis, also known as temporal arthritis. This is a systemic condition affecting medium-sized and large arteries throughout the body, but having the greatest propensity to involve the temporal artery. It is a disease of the aged, with a mean onset in the 70s, and it affects women more often than men. The symptoms are as those described; however, up to 40% of patients have additional symptoms, including cardiac irregularities, thoracic aorta aneurysms, and respiratory problems. The nature of these symptoms depends upon which other arteries are involved; in fact, classic polymyalgia rheumatica and classic temporal arteritis are believed to be the opposite extremes of a continuum of conditions due to the same underlying cause, with many patients showing symptoms of both entities. In both conditions, an exceedingly high erythrocyte sedimentation rate (ESR; choice **C**) is almost diagnostic. In temporal arteritis, ESR values are over 50 mm/h in more than 90% of patients and often exceed 100 mm/h (although the exact value is laboratory-specific, the normal rates are usually considered to be less than 10 mm/h for males and less than 15 mm/h for females). Although the ESR is increased in most inflammatory conditions, the magnitude of the increase is rarely this great; thus, the sensitivity is good but not perfect since about 5% of affected individuals provide false-negative values with ESR values below 40 mm/h. C-reactive protein and interleukine-6, other sensitive markers of inflammation, are also increased, and particularly the latter may prove to be even more sensitive than the ESR. However, the test is more expensive and not widely obtainable, and available data are limited. The definitive diagnosis is made by temporal artery biopsy. Treatment with a corticosteroid must be started immediately to prevent blindness, even before laboratory of biopsy results are available.

A complete blood count (choice **A**) is of limited value. The most significant finding will be a normal white cell count, which will rule out infection and some other inflammatory conditions. A computed tomography study of her head (choice **B**), a carotid ultrasound study (choice **D**), or a lumbar puncture with subsequent culture (choice **E**) will contribute little to the diagnosis.

### 16 The answer is B *Psychiatry*

The symptoms are most suggestive of schizophrenia. Sophisticated studies of cerebral morphology and functional neuroimaging in schizophrenia have yielded some fairly consistent findings, including decreased metabolic activity in the prefrontal cortex (choice **B**).

Such studies of individuals with schizophrenia have also found decreased cerebral asymmetry (not increased, choice **D**), decreased size of the corpus callosum (not increased, choice **E**), and increased size of the lateral ventricles (not decreased, choice **C**). Abnormalities of dopaminergic transmission (choice **A**) are not currently measurable with functional neuroimaging. Although several abnormalities of dopamine metabolism in schizophrenia have been reported using other experimental techniques, none is found consistently.

### 17 The answer is D *Pediatrics*

Cow's milk is not recommended for children until they are 1 year of age because the high level of protein (choice **D**) causes an increased solute load to the kidneys. It is this overload that led to the lethargic, dehydrated state of the 2-month-old infant.

Linoleic acid (choice **A**), linolenic acid (choice **B**), calcium (choice **C**), and B-complex vitamins (choice **E**) are not present in high concentrations in cow's milk and would not be expected to cause the symptoms noted in this patient.

### 18 The answer is A *Medicine*

A deficiency of uroporphyrinogen I synthetase activity (aka, porphobilinogen deaminase) is inherited as an autosomal dominant trait and is responsible for a disease known as *acute intermittent proporphyria*. This disease is characterized by intermittent bouts of acute gastrointestinal attacks causing extreme pain; occasionally, during one of these sessions (which in some patients may last for an extended period), there is also constipation, urinary retention, hypertension, and neurologic symptoms that may include neuropathies, seizures, and psychotic episodes. The neural problems are likely caused by hyponatremia, which is in part caused by inappropriate release of antidiuretic hormone and in part due to gastrointestinal loss. After standing, the urine voided during an attack turns dark to a color sometimes described as muddy reddish or purplish. Uroporphyrinogen I synthetase catalyzes the condensation of four molecules of porphobilinogen to form uroporphyrinogen III, the first ring product in heme synthesis. Because uroporphyrinogen I synthetase activity is inadequate during an attack, the substrate, porphobilinogen, accumulates and is excreted in the urine (choice **A**), a finding considered to provide the definitive diagnosis. Although this disease is autosomal dominant, its penetrance is low and the disease may appear to skip generations. Clinical symptoms are most commonly reported by women beginning in their teens or 20s. Presumably, the intermittent nature of the condition reflects the fact that the uroporphyrinogen I synthetase activity inherited from the nonaffected parent is borderline sufficient, and attacks only occur when triggered by some factor that causes a need for greater activity. Such known precipitating factors include a long list of drugs, most, if not all, of which share the property of being metabolized by the P450 cytochrome (heme) system. The implied mechanism is that activation of the P450 enzymes reduces the availability of free heme, a feedback inhibitor of heme synthesis; this releases the heme synthesis sequence of reactions from partial inhibition and produces porphobilinogen at an accelerated rate, faster than the limited activity of the remaining uroporphyrinogen I synthetase activity can use it. Among the drugs that induce an attack are barbiturates, commonly used in test questions as an example, and the estrogens, used as an example in the case presented. However, in addition to being triggered by drugs, attacks are also induced by infections and caloric deprivation (used as an ancillary precipitating factor in the vignette). An acute attack can be life-threatening, and emergency treatment by intravenous hematin (an inhibitor of the first step in heme synthesis) and glucose coupled with administration of an analgesic that is not metabolized by the P450 system is often used as the first line of treatment. Long-term treatment is avoidance of known precipitating factors and maintenance on a high-carbohydrate diet, at least 300 g of carbohydrate per day.

Uroporphyrin (choice **B**) accumulates in porphyria cutanea tarda, a condition caused by an inherited deficiency of uroporphyrin decarboxylase; this is the most common of the porphyrias. Uroporphyrinogen I (choice **C**) and coproporphyrinogen I (choice **D**) accumulate in the urine of patients with congenital erythropoietic porphyria, a disease in which uroporphyrinogen III cosynthetase activity is lacking. Coproporphyrinogen III (choice **E**) accumulates in hereditary coproporphyria because of a deficiency of coproporphyrinogen oxidase. Congenital erythropoietic porphyria is inherited as an autosomal recessive trait, the rest of the porphyrias as autosomal dominant conditions. In each of the diseases described with respect to choices **B**, **C**, **D**, and **E**, the intermediates that accumulate have the heme-like tetrapyrrole structure, and consequently, patients are photosensitive. This sensitivity is thought to be due to superoxide free radicals produced via the reaction of the tetrapyrrole compound with oxygen in a reaction catalyzed by ultraviolet light. Note that acute intermittent proporphyria is the only porphyria that is not light sensitive, because a tetrapyrrole compound does not accumulate. Lead (choice **F**) is an extremely toxic heavy metal with an affinity for SH groups. As a consequence, it inhibits several enzymes, two of which are involved in heme synthesis—δ-aminolevulinic synthase, the first and rate-limiting enzyme in heme synthesis, and ferrochelatase, the last enzyme. Consequently, lead poisoning, among other effects, causes a microcytic anemia.

### 19 The answer is G *Surgery*

Bladder cancer is the sixth most common cancer diagnosed in the U.S. Approximately 65,000 cases are diagnosed annually; these cause around 12,000–14,000 deaths. Of these cases, about 98% are due to epithelial malignancies, and 90% of these are transitional cell carcinomas (choice **G**). (The transitional cell layer of the bladder epithelium is sometimes also called the urothelium because it continues throughout the urinary tract, from the area of the kidney where urine collects through the top of the ureters where they connect to the kidney, down into the bladder, and throughout the majority of the urethra. Carcinomas arising from this layer are known as transitional cell carcinomas.) In the U.S., adenocarcinomas account for about 2% of the epithelial malignancies, and squamous cell cancers constitute about 7%. However, squamous cell carcinomas are far more common in countries such as Egypt and Sudan, where urinary schistosomiasis due to infestation with *Schistosoma hematobium* is endemic. Consequently, choice **A** is incorrect; the prevalence of the types of bladder cancer is not equally common throughout the world.

About half of all transitional cell carcinomas in the United States are believed to be caused by smoking tobacco; longstanding exposure to paints or aniline-based dyes, organic solvents, and similar compounds are estimated to cause as much as another one-fourth of the cases. The bladder is particularly susceptible to such toxins because, although the kidney is exposed briefly to toxins as it filters them out of the bloodstream, these toxins tend to accumulate and linger in the bladder until eliminated by urinating. However, there is little evidence suggesting that carcinogens found in smoked foods (choice **B**) causes bladder cancer to a significant degree.

Cancers that have not invaded deeply into the bladder wall, such as the one described in this case, are removed by cystoscopic resection. However, without further treatment 50%–75% of patients will suffer a recurrence of the condition within 3 years (choice **C** is incorrect). As a consequence immuno- and/or chemotherapeutic agents are delivered directly into the bladder by catheter after resection. Since the condition described has not invaded deeper layers of the bladder wall, it is unlikely to be treated by radical cystectomy (choice **D**). Such a procedure involves removal of the prostate as well as the bladder in men, and removal of the ovaries, uterus, and a portion of the vagina in women. Pelvic pain, hematuria, and difficulty in voiding urine are signs generally associated with more advanced cases of bladder cancer but are usually not the earliest signs (choice **E** is wrong). Hematuria, pelvic pain, and voiding difficulties are also common signs of cystitis and the passing of stones; therefore, these conditions must be carefully considered in making a diagnosis. Bladder cancer is about four times more prevalent in men than in women (choice **F**), and the mean age at the time of diagnosis is 65 years (choice **H**), thus choices F and H are incorrect.

### 20 The answer is C *Psychiatry*

In malingering (choice **C**), the patient deliberately produces complaints in the presence of external incentives, such as money. These external incentives are sometimes referred to as secondary gains.

Symptoms in factitious disorder (choice **B**) also are deliberately produced (i.e., made up, self-inflicted, dramatically exaggerated); however, the motivation is not external but internal, so that the patient can assume the sick role, which is sometimes referred to as a primary gain. Symptoms in conversion disorder (choice **A**) are not voluntarily produced and involve a loss of sensory or motor function. A person who has pain disorder (choice **D**) experiences actual pain that is largely mediated by psychologic factors. In somatization disorder (choice **E**), multiple somatic complaints are present. Individuals with somatization disorder do not deliberately produce their symptoms for external incentives or to assume the sick role.

**21** **The answer is E** *Pediatrics*

Familial hypophosphatemia (also know as X-linked or as vitamin D–resistant rickets) is the most common nonnutritional form of rickets. It is X-linked dominant, so some mothers as well as fathers may have clinical manifestations of the disease. Hypophosphatemia occurs because of defects in the proximal renal tubular reabsorption of phosphate caused by failure in the conversion of 25-(OH)-vitamin D to 1,25-(OH)$_2$-vitamin D. Bowing of the legs is a common presentation. In addition, these children may have a waddling gait (choice **E**) and short stature. Calcium levels in the serum are normal, and thus there is no associated tetany, myopathy, or secondary hyperparathyroidism. Treatment consists of supplementation with phosphate and calcitriol. Two syndromes often confused with X-linked hypophosphatemia are vitamin D–dependent rickets type I and receptor-deficient rickets (formally known as vitamin D–deficient rickets type II). Neither consistently causes hypophosphatemia, and they are autosomal recessive conditions.

Tetany (choice **A**), rachitic rosary (choice **B**), Harrison's groove (pectus deformity; choice **C**), and myopathy (choice **D**) are present in calcium-deficient rickets. Classic vitamin D–deficiency rickets has become rare in the U.S. because of food supplementation and styles that bare much of the body to the sun.

**22** **The answer is C** *Pediatrics*

This patient has idiopathic (autoimmune) thrombocytopenic purpura (ITP). ITP is the most common thrombocytopenic purpura of childhood. The disease usually follows a viral infection. The infection seems to trigger an immune mechanism that starts platelet destruction. This destruction is manifested as sudden onset of bruising and petechiae. Other than this condition, the patient looks well, but bleeding into tissues can occur. Platelet counts are depressed and bleeding time is prolonged, but the white blood cell (WBC) count is normal. Platelet antibodies are commonly seen. Bone marrow examination reveals normal megakaryocytes. The disease is self-limited, with resolution of the petechiae over 1 or 2 weeks; although thrombocytopenia may persist longer. The prognosis for ITP is excellent. Most patients recover within 2 or 3 months. Approximately 90% of children regain normal platelet counts within 9–12 months. In cases of mild thrombocytopenic purpura, with no hemorrhages of the retina or mucous membranes, therapy may not be appropriate. However, therapy with intravenous (IV) γ-globulin infusions and/or corticosteroid therapy (choice **C**) can be beneficial. IV γ-globulin infusions induce a sustained rise in platelet counts, while corticosteroid therapy reduces the severity and shortens the duration of the initial phase.

In the context of thrombocytopenia, splenectomy (choice **F**) should be reserved for those patients with chronic thrombocytopenic purpura or severe cases not responding to therapy. Platelet concentrates (choice **A**) are recommended only in life-threatening situations because their short lifespan is reflected by the temporary nature of the rise in platelet count. Vitamins C (choice **D**) and K (choice **E**) will not ameliorate the disease. The patient's complete blood count (CBC) is normal except for the platelet count. Therefore, it is not necessary to administer whole blood (choice **B**), which should only be used emergently for hypovolemia due to blood loss.

**23** **The answer is D** *Preventive Medicine and Public Health*

Accidents are the most common cause of death in youth between the ages of 15 and 24 years, and 75% of these accidents occur in automobiles (choice **D**). Further increasing the odds he would die in a motor accident is the fact that he loved to drag race while high.

Generally speaking, suicide (choice **A**) and homicide (choice **B**) are the second and third leading causes of death among such youth. Although suicide is a major factor in early death in this age group, and suicidal thoughts are common, actual suicides are uncommon because the overall death rate in this group is so low. In some surveys, homicide is second, and suicide is third; this appears to reflect the demographics of the group surveyed. In most middle- and upper-class neighborhoods, adolescent homicide is almost unheard of; in contrast, homicide is all too common in neighborhoods permeated by gangs. Drug overdose (choice **C**) is a less common cause of death in youth than accidents, suicide, and homicide, although use of drugs—alcohol in particular—is a major contributor to deaths in automobile accidents. In this age group, death from any disease, including cancer (choice **E**), is rare.

**24** **The answer is B** *Surgery*

This child suffered first- and second-degree burns on her hand and fingers. The first-degree burns are indicated by the reddened area, second-degree burns by the blisters. The primary treatment should be gently cleaning the burned area with a cool, not cold, antiseptic solution, applying a topical antibiotic, and dressing the injured area with a nonadherent dressing (choice **B**). Following that, a conforming protective material should be applied. The mother suffered from shock at seeing her child suffer and guilt at leaving her unattended and needs to be reassured that, luckily, the child's burns are minor and should heal without scarring in the course of a couple of weeks. She should also be informed that application of butter or any other greasy substance is not suitable treatment because it traps the heat of the burn, possibly making it worse. She ought to also be advised that a better course of action in the event of any serious accident is to call 911 rather than rush off to a walk-in clinic.

Cooling the burn site by immediately immersing the hand in ice cold water (choice **A**) introduces a risk of compromising circulation to marginally surviving areas of the burn and should not be done for any burn more serious than a first-degree one. In addition, for burns covering an extensive area such cooling also creates a risk of hypothermia. On the other hand, washing relatively nonextensive first- or second-degree burns with cool water, about 60–80°F (15–25°C), eases the pain. Most authorities believe the blister should be left intact as long as possible because the skin of a blister may act as a natural dressing, protecting the wound against infection and reducing the amount of pain; consequently, choice **C** (aspirate the fluid underneath the blister) and choice **D** (débride the wound, aspirate the fluid, and apply an antibiotic cream) are incorrect. In addition to cooling to reduce pain, an oral analgesia such as acetaminophen (not aspirin) should be provided. Tetanus prophylaxis (choice **E**) is important in all patients with burns in whom the skin is or may be broken. Thus, if this child's tetanus immunization is not up to date, it should be brought up to date. The best course of action in this particular case would be to contact and inform the child's regular physician of the accident and treatment, to determine the child's immunization status, and to arrange for a follow-up appointment either at the walk-in clinic or better yet with the child's usual physician. In any case, the child should be seen again within 48 hours to make sure that there is no secondary infection.

**25** **The answer is E** *Pediatrics*

*Candida* species are common causes of oral thrush and diaper dermatitis in infants. Thrush consists of white, curd-like plaques on the tongue, gums, and buccal mucosa that are difficult to remove. The skin manifestations include a beefy-red maculopapular rash that may coalesce and form satellite lesions. Intertriginous areas, especially in the diaper area (perineum), also are usually involved (choice **E**).

*Candida* infections of the eyes (choice **A**), ears (choice **B**), nose (choice **C**), and scalp (choice **D**) are not usually associated with thrush. Disseminated *Candida* infection is most commonly associated with an immunocompromised host.

**26** **The answer is D** *Pediatrics*

Nonvenereal infectious vulvovaginitis is not uncommon in prepubertal patients. Poor perineal hygiene is the most common cause of nonspecific vulvovaginitis and accounts for 70% of all pediatric vulvovaginitis cases. Most of these cases are secondary to fecal contamination. Bacterial vulvovaginitis due to a primary respiratory or skin pathogen may also be found. Group A β-hemolytic streptococcus may be associated with streptococcal nasopharyngitis or scarlet fever, or may occur alone. Vulvovaginal symptoms of group A β-hemolytic streptococcal (choice **D**) infection include severe perineal burning, dysuria, and erythema similar in appearance to erysipelas in the perineal area. Most patients will have a serosanguineous or grayish white vaginal discharge.

*Streptococcus pneumoniae* (choice **E**) and *Haemophilus influenzae* (choice **A**) may cause a purulent vaginal discharge causing vulvovaginitis following, or in conjunction with, an upper respiratory infection. Sexual abuse should be suspected when *Neisseria gonorrhea* (choice **B**) or *Chlamydia trachomatis* (choice **C**) are found in a prepubertal child. In this case, there is no history of bubble bath, pinworms, tight clothing, nylon underwear, or recent medications, all of which have been implicated in vulvovaginitis. Likewise, although there is severe dysuria, there is no history of hematuria or fever, which makes a urinary tract infection less likely.

**27 The answer is D** *Psychiatry*

Because the potential father's uncle and cousin are second-degree relatives who have been diagnosed with schizophrenia, the risk of the child developing the disease is greater than 1% the lifetime risk in the general population, but less than 10% of the prevalence rate among first-degree relatives (choice **D**).

Choice **A** is incorrect because there is clear evidence of a familial basis for this disease; namely, there is a 10% chance of a first-degree relative getting the disease, and a greater than 50% concordance rate between monozygous twins. However, no particular family communication style appears to cause schizophrenia (choice **B**). For unknown reasons, the risk of developing schizophrenia is higher for individuals born in winter months in temperate regions (choice **C**). Gluten intolerance (celiac disease) has been associated with higher risks for schizophrenia, but no data suggest that prenatal exposure plays any role (choice **E**).

**28 The answer is D** *Obstetrics and Gynecology*

Up to 15% of couples experience infertility, defined as inability to conceive within 12 months of regular unprotected intercourse. This patient has primary infertility, since she has never successfully conceived. In 40% of couples, multiple causes may be present. The etiology of infertility may involve both partners simultaneously in 20% of cases, and in another 30%–35% of the cases, a male factor alone; consequently, of the factors listed, the most common is male factor (choice **D**). This is diagnosed with semen analysis, which may show inadequate ejaculate volume, too few sperm, no sperm, immobile sperm, or morphologically aberrant sperm.

Other causes of infertility are ovulatory factor (choice **A**), seen in 15%–20% of couples and characterized by chronic anovulation, which may be result of hypothyroidism, hyperprolactinemia, or polycystic ovarian syndrome. Uterine factor (choice **B**) occurs in 5% of couples and involves anatomic defects of the uterine cavity. Tubal factor (choice **D**) is seen in 15%–25% of cases and is diagnosed by hysterosalpingogram revealing anatomic tubal pathology.

**29 The answer is A** *Medicine*

This man undoubtably is suffering from type 1 diabetes and has developed diabetic gastroparesis, a condition reported to occur in at least 12% of individuals who have had diabetes for 10 or more years. The underlying problem is that he has poorly controlled diabetes; the American Diabetes Association recommends that all diabetics keep their A1c values below 7%, whereas the American Association of Clinical Endocrinologist recommend maintaining it below 6.5%; this man's was 11.5%. Obviously, such exposure to too-high glucose levels is damaging his nervous system and blood vessels. Gastroparesis is caused by damage to the vagus nerve and often accompanies other diabetic complications such as nephropathy, retinopathy, and peripheral neuropathy. The vagus normally transmits signals to the digestive system, causing the stomach and intestines to contract in a synchronous fashion, maneuvering food undergoing digestion from the stomach into and then through the intestines. The neuropathy underlying diabetic gastroparesis interrupts these signals, and food backs up in the stomach. In addition to the symptoms described, this makes production of glucose after a meal erratic and contributes to problems with the regulation of glucose levels. Over an extended period, bacterial growth may occur in the undigested food, and the food may form hard lumps, called *bezoars,* which might eventually block a person's digestive system. As the first course in treatment, his physician would most likely recommend eating smaller meals more often and would write a prescription for an agent that stimulates gastric emptying and increases intestinal contractions, thus helping to move the food out of the stomach and along the intestines. At present, few medications are available to treat gastroparesis. Those most commonly employed are metoclopramide (choice **A**), erythromycin, domperidone, and cisapride. In addition to stimulating gastric emptying, its action in the brain helps control the vomiting reflex; thus it acts as both a prokinetic agent and an antiemetic. Unfortunately, it should not be used longer than 3 months because it has a risk of causing irreversible tardive dyskinesia. (As of September 2009, the U.S. Food and Drug Administration required this drug to carry a boxed warning alerting physicians to this potential problem.) Getting his diabetes under control is, of course, advisable but this would be a long-term project, made even more difficult because of the patient's limited resources.

Adiponectin (choice **B**) is a hormone produced by adipocytes that helps regulate glucose and lipoprotein levels. Studies to date have largely been limited to mice; therefore, no physician could write a prescription for it. Sitagliptin, pramlintide acetate, and exenatide (choices **C**, **D**, and **E**) are all drugs used to treat type 2 diabetes and could have no function in cases involving type 1 diabetes. In addition, pramlintide acetate and exenatide also can delay food from moving out of the stomach—not a good property for treating gastroparesis.

**30** **The answer is B** *Preventative Medicine and Public Health*

Excluding skin cancers, breast cancer is the most common neoplasm in females, although more females now die from lung cancer. The American Cancer Society reported that, in 2008, the lifetime chance of non-Hispanic white women developing breast cancer was 13.3%; thus, 1 in 7.5 women in this cohort developed the cancer (choice **A**). However, this woman has at least one additional risk factor: her mother—a first-degree relative—also developed breast cancer. Having a first-degree relative with breast cancer increases the risk another five-fold. Thus, this patient's minimal risk is 13.3 × 5 or 66.5% (choice **B**). Since she is an Ashkenazi Jew (her Jewish family comes from Eastern Europe), her risk might even be greater since this ethnic group has a high incidence of *BRCA1* and *BRCA2* gene mutations, which can increase the lifetime risk to almost inevitable. In fact, since her mother died relatively young from breast cancer, the chances she had one of these cancer-causing mutations is high, and the physician might well recommend that this patient undergo genetic screening.

Because she is older now than her mother was when she died, choice **C** (she has little risk of developing an inherited form of cancer) is not true. In fact, the risk of cancer increases with age; the incidence increases particularly rapidly between the ages of 40 and 55 years, after which the risk rate remains constant. Choice **D** (having fibrocystic disease reduces the probability of ever developing a breast malignancy) is not true; in fact, it increases the risk slightly. Breast cancer is one of the few cancers that doesn't seem to be increased by smoking, thus the fact that she is a nonsmoker doesn't reduce her chance of developing cancer (choice **E**).

**31** **The answer is E** *Psychiatry*

Schizotypal personality disorder (choice **E**) is characterized by social withdrawal, peculiar ideation, and the absence of any history of psychosis. Antipsychotic medication sometimes decreases the peculiar ideation seen in this disorder. Schizotypal personality disorder is associated with a family history of schizophrenia.

Schizophrenia, residual type (choice **D**), would have a very similar presentation, but a history of at least one episode of psychosis is necessary to make this diagnosis. Avoidant personality disorder (choice **A**) is often characterized by reclusiveness, but individuals with this disorder have a desire for human interaction and a fear of rejection. Obsessive-compulsive personality disorder (choice **B**) is characterized by behavioral inflexibility and a preoccupation with meaningless details. Schizoid personality disorder (choice **C**) is characterized by social aloofness without any bizarre ideation.

**32** **The answer is C** *Surgery*

This woman has conjunctivitis. All forms of conjunctivitis share certain features, including a pink or red coloration of the cornea ("pink eye"), a feeling of fine grit in the eye upon blinking, and production of a yellow-tinted exudate. The observation that the exudate is sticky and viscous indicates it caused by a bacterial infection (choice **C**). The three most common infectious agents are *Staphylococcus aureus, Streptococcus pneumoniae,* and *Haemophilus* species. The latter two are more common in children; *S. aureus* is most common in adults. Infections are termed *acute* because, as a rule, they clear up spontaneously within 2 weeks; however, a topical antibiotic can be used to typically cure the infection within a few days.

Acute viral conjunctivitis (choice **A**) can be distinguished from bacterial conjunctivitis by the observation that the discharge is copious and watery with scant exudate; it too resolves spontaneously, but antibiotic treatment does not accelerate recovery. Children most commonly get viral conjunctivitis. The most common infective agent is adenovirus type 3; it is highly infectious, and rapid dissemination to a full classroom is not unknown.

Optic neuritis (choice **B**) refers to inflammation of the optic nerve, which may be secondary to multiple sclerosis, glaucoma, or infection, as in tuberculosis or syphilis. There is a sudden unilateral loss of vision and pain on eye movements. The optic disc frequently appears swollen and associated with flame-shaped pericapillary hemorrhages. Intravenous and oral steroid therapies are used for treatment.

Uveitis (choice **D**) is an inflammation of the uveal tract, a space formed by the iris, ciliary body, and choroid. Central retinal artery occlusion (choice **E**) is characterized by a sudden, almost complete but painless loss of vision in one eye, most commonly in an elderly patient. Retinal examination reveals pallor of the optic disc, edema of the retina, a cherry-red fovea, and bloodless, constricted arterioles. Anterior blepharitis (choice **F**) is a commonly occurring inflammation of the eyelids, skin, eyelashes, and associated glands; it is easily recognized by red-rimmed eyes with scales hanging onto the lashes. The eyes tend to feel irritated and itchy. There may be small peripheral ulcers caused by staphylococci. Effective home therapy is often achieved by removing the scales from the lid margins on a daily basis with a damp cloth or cotton wad, using baby shampoo as an emulsifier, and by keeping the face and scalp exceptionally clean. In some cases, an antibacterial ointment is also used.

**33** **The answer is A** *Pediatrics*

Patients with sickle cell disease are at increased risk for developing severe pneumococcal disease because of impaired immunologic response to *Streptococcus pneumoniae* (choice **A**). Patients with sickle cell disease should be immunized with the polyvalent pneumococcal vaccine in addition to all other routine immunizations of childhood. The polyvalent pneumococcal vaccine should be administered to asplenic children 2 years of age and older. The pneumococcal vaccine may not be as effective in children under 5 years old as it is in older individuals. Even if patients with sickle cell disease are given prophylactic antibiotics, there is still a chance that they will develop pneumococcal meningitis before 5 years of age.

*Escherichia coli* (choice **C**), *Listeria monocytogenes* (choice **D**), and group B streptococcus (choice **B**) are more common pathogens in newborns. The most common sites of infection for group A β-hemolytic streptococci (choice **E**) are the upper respiratory tract, skin, soft tissues, and blood.

**34** **The answer is E** *Medicine*

Four *Plasmodium* species cause malaria: *P. falciparum, P. ovale, P. malariae,* and *P. vivax. P. falciparum* infection is generally the most dangerous. An estimated 30,000 travelers from developed counties to tropical areas are infected with malaria annually, and several hundred die. The patient described in the vignette has *P. falciparum* malaria (choice **E**), which is endemic in many east African countries including Tanzania. The peripheral blood findings in the vignette described multiple ring forms, a characteristic finding in *P. falciparum* infections. The tertian fever pattern (recurring every other day, with occasional fever spikes) correlates with intravascular hemolysis, which causes hemoglobinuria (positive dipstick test result for blood), and extravascular hemolysis leads to jaundice, as splenic macrophages remove parasitized red blood cells (RBCs) and degrade the hemoglobin into unconjugated bilirubin. This hemolytic anemia is associated with an increase in the corrected reticulocyte count. Hepatosplenomegaly is present after the fourth day in all of the malarias.

Malaria is transmitted to humans primarily by the bite of a female *Anopheles* mosquito. Because *P. falciparum* malaria produces a greater degree of parasitism of red blood cells resulting in cytoadherence of parasitized red cells in capillaries and postcapillary venules, it is the most severe form of malaria. Complications include central nervous system hemorrhage, disseminated intravascular coagulation, acute respiratory distress syndrome, and liver cell necrosis with an increase in transaminases.

The effectiveness of antimalarial drugs varies depending upon parasite species and stage of the parasite's life cycle. Tissue schizonticides, primarily primaquine, act in the liver to eliminate developing exoerythrocytic schizonts or latent hypnozoites. Blood schizonticides, such as chloroquine, amodiaquine, proguanil, pyrimethamine, mefloquine, quinine, quinidine, halofantrine, artemisinin, and atovaquone, suppress parasite development in the red blood cell and in gametocides; for *P. falciparum*, primaquine kills gametocytes in the blood. There are no true prophylactic drugs, but proguanil, chlorproguanil, atovaquone, and primaquine prevent maturation of early *P. falciparum*, whereas the blood schizonticides, when given weekly for a month after exposure, prevent development of *P. falciparum* as well as *P. malariae,* and thereby result in a cure. Resistant *P. falciparum* strains have developed worldwide, particularly to chloroquine in east Africa; otherwise, chloroquine is used for prevention of all types of malaria. It is safe during pregnancy, kills blood schizonts, and is gametocidal to all malaria species *except P. falciparum. P. vivax* and *P. ovale* infections are treated with chloroquine plus primaquine. Malarone, mefloquine, or quinine sulfate plus doxycycline or some other drug combination is used for prevention when there are chloroquine-resistant strains of *P. falciparum* present. The treatment of chloroquine-sensitive *P. falciparum* is chloroquine without primaquine.

When autoimmune hemolytic anemia (choice **A**) is suspected, a direct Coombs' test is ordered. It detects IgG and C3b on the surface of the RBCs. The negative Coombs' test result in this patient rules out an autoimmune hemolytic anemia. Congenital spherocytosis (choice **B**) is an autosomal dominant disorder that causes hemolytic anemia with jaundice and splenomegaly. It is not associated with a spiking fever or the intraerythrocytic ring forms that are present in this patient, and erythrocytes have a spherocytic or oval shape. Glucose-6-phosphate dehydrogenase (G6PD) deficiency (choice **C**) is an X-linked recessive disorder (patient is a woman) that causes a predominantly intravascular type of hemolytic anemia that presents with hemoglobinuria. The less predominant extravascular hemolytic component is responsible for producing jaundice. The RBCs do not have intraerythrocytic ring forms. Pyruvate kinase deficiency (choice **D**) is an autosomal recessive disorder associated with a hemolytic anemia. The peripheral blood shows shrunken and spiculated RBCs with no intraerythrocytic inclusions.

**35** **The answer is C** *Surgery*

The patient has volume overload due to overzealous fluid resuscitation (choice **C**) during and after surgery. Volume overload is the most common cause of congestive cardiac failure after surgery. A third heart sound is the first cardiac sign of left- or right-sided congestive heart failure. Bibasilar inspiratory crackles indicate left-sided heart failure, and jugular venous distention and peripheral pitting edema are features of right-sided heart failure. Volume overload can be corrected by administration of a loop diuretic and by restricting fluid volume. It is always important to monitor fluid intake and output carefully in patients to avoid inadvertent fluid overload.

Endotoxic shock and cardiogenic shock (choices **A** and **B**) are incorrect responses because the patient has a normal blood pressure. Fat embolism syndrome (choice **D**) is associated with tachycardia, dyspnea, thrombocytopenia, and petechiae over the chest. The latter two findings are not present in this patient. Syndrome of inappropriate secretion of antidiuretic hormone (SIADH; choice **E**) is not associated with peripheral pitting edema because it refers to retention of water without sodium. Serum sodium is usually less than 120 mEq/L; water restriction is the treatment of choice.

**36** **The answer is E** *Psychiatry*

For most adult alcoholics, active participation in Alcoholics Anonymous (AA) (choice **E**) offers the best chance of preventing relapses. In Alcoholics Anonymous, total abstinence is mandatory. Support is obtained via a "buddy" system.

Naltrexone is an opiate antagonist that may sometimes help prevent relapse by blunting the euphoric effect of alcohol. It can be used as an adjunct in the treatment of alcoholism, but would not be recommended in the absence of a supportive program; it would not make him nauseous after one drink (choice **B**). Disulfiram (choice **A**) is a drug known to reduce the chance of relapse by interfering with alcohol metabolism through inhibition of aldehyde dehydrogenase (ADH); this causes the plasma concentration of acetaldehyde to increase, inducing the "acetaldehyde syndrome" in which, within 5–10 minutes after ingestion of ethanol, rising levels of acetaldehyde cause physical discomfort, including flushing, due to the vasodilator effects of acetaldehyde. Many studies have demonstrated that individuals with alcoholism have extreme difficulty in limiting alcohol consumption once they have started drinking, and advice to do this is rarely useful (choices **C** and **D**).

**37** **The answer is F** *Obstetrics and Gynecology*

Fallopian tube or oviduct malignancies (choice **F**) are extremely rare and have no official International Federation of Gynecology and Obstetrics (FIGO) staging criteria. However, because they are intraperitoneal organs, intimately related to the ovaries, with a similar mode of metastasis, they are staged with criteria similar to those for ovarian carcinoma (choice **B**).

**38** **The answer is A** *Obstetrics and Gynecology*

Staging criteria use the best information from a variety of sources to assess the degree of cancer dissemination. All gynecologic cancers use surgical staging methods, with the exception of cervical cancer (choice **A**), which uses only clinical information from noninvasive methods such as pelvic examination, intravenous pyelography, cystoscopy, sigmoidoscopy, and imaging studies.

**39** **The answer is A** *Obstetrics and Gynecology*

Cervical carcinoma (choice **A**) has three subcategories in stage I (IA1, IA2, and IB), based on degree of invasion through the basement membrane as measured on histological examination of the cervical biopsy. Stage IA1 (minimally invasive) has <3 mm invasion; stage IA2 (microinvasion) has between 3 and 5 mm invasion, and stage IB (frank invasion) is >5 mm invasion. The likelihood of metastasis increases with the depth of invasion.

Endometrial (choice **C**) and ovarian (choice **B**) cancer also have three stage I subcategories (IA, IB, and IC). The subcategories were created because the treatment and prognosis is different for each one. Vulvar cancer (choice **E**) has no subdivisions of stage I.

**40** **The answer is A**  *Obstetrics and Gynecology*

Stage I cervical carcinoma (choice **A**) has the best 5-year survival rate (90%), largely because it usually is diagnosed in a minimally invasive or microinvasive early stage.

The survival rates for the other stage I malignancies are as follows: vaginal (85%) (choice **D**), endometrial (75%) (choice **C**), ovarian (70%) (choice **B**), and oviductal (60%) (choice **F**).

**41** **The answer is A**  *Obstetrics and Gynecology*

Cervical malignancy (choice **A**) of the squamous cell type is associated with human papillomavirus (HPV) subtypes 16 and 18, which are sexually transmitted. Therefore, it is considered epidemiologically to be a sexually transmitted disease.

**42** **The answer is B**  *Obstetrics and Gynecology*

Ovarian carcinoma (choice **B**) is the only gynecologic malignancy that has subcategories A, B, and C for stages I through III. Each of these subdivisions is necessary for directing specific treatment planning.

**43** **The answer is B**  *Obstetrics and Gynecology*

Cancer of the ovary is the second most common gynecologic malignancy, and the one associated with the highest mortality (choice **B**). Diagnosis is made by staging exploratory laparotomy with multiple biopsies. There are no early symptoms for ovarian cancer, and there is no screening test available. Therefore, by the time it is diagnosed, it has already spread throughout the peritoneal cavity, making it stage III. Fifty percent of women with stage III ovarian cancer will be dead in 18 months. Approximately 1% of all women will develop ovarian cancer. It accounts for more deaths than all other primary pelvic cancers combined.

**44** **The answer is B**  *Medicine*

The sulfonylurea antidiabetic drugs are a large group of oral drugs available to treat type 2 diabetes. They share the ability to increase the secretion of insulin by binding to an adenosine triphosphate (ATP)-dependent $K^+$ channel on the cell membrane of pancreatic β-cells. This opens voltage gated $Ca^{++}$ channels, increasing the intracellular $Ca^{++}$ concentration, which in turn leads to the fusion of insulin granules to the cell membrane, enhancing the secretion of pro-insulin. Consequently, like insulin itself, they promote weight gain and may cause hypoglycemia. The first-generation sulfonylureas introduced in 1955 were bound to serum proteins; this was a disadvantage because various factors could promote the release of this bound insulin, causing an unpredictable increase in the free drug and possibly inducing an unpredictable bout of hypoglycemia. Glyburide (choice **B**) is a second-generation sulfonylurea antidiabetic drug, which as a class does not bind to carrier proteins and therefore is less likely to cause acute problems with hypoglycemia. Glimepiride, approved in June 2009, is a third-generation sulfonylurea that seems to be less prone to induce hypoglycemia; it induces a mild reduction to insulin resistance.

**45** **The answer is E**  *Medicine*

Acarbose, miglitol, and the more newly introduced voglibose are α-glucosidase inhibitors that slow the digestion of carbohydrates other than monosaccharides; this decreases the degree of postprandial hyperglycemia. These drugs must be taken with the first bite of a carbohydrate-rich meal to have maximal effect. Acarbose (choice **E**) and voglibose are not systemically absorbed; although miglitol is systemically absorbed, it is not metabolized and is excreted by the kidneys. All three of these drugs leave undigested di- and/or polysaccharides in the large intestine; these are then metabolized by gut bacterial flora, resulting in flatulence and/or diarrhea. Monotherapy with these drugs will not cause hypoglycemia or weight gain. However, patients using one of these drugs in combination with an additional antidiabetic drug may become hypoglycemic; in the event this occurs, they should use glucose to restore serum glucose levels since di- or polysaccharides will not be rapidly digested.

**46** **The answer is H**  *Medicine*

As mentioned in question 7, the intracellular peroxisome proliferator-activated receptor-γ (PPARγ) is implicated as a player in metabolic syndrome, a major risk factor for type 2 diabetes. Although the thiazolidinediones rosiglitazone and pioglitazone have some ability to inhibit liver gluconeogenesis and to combat dyslipidemia, their primary mode of action is to activate insulin receptors on insulin-sensitive cells. They accomplish this by binding to the intracellular PPARγ receptors (choice **H**), which in turn attach to specific DNA base sequences, leading to synthesis of specific proteins that raise sensitivity to insulin. This permits the cells to absorb more glucose and thereby lower serum glucose levels. Unfortunately, as discussed in test 3, they also may promote weight gain, edema, heart failure, and macular degeneration. In 2007 the manufactuer stated that this medication increased the risk for axial skeletal fractures in female diabetics also on metformin or glyburide. Currently rosiglitazone is only recommended for use in patients in whom glycemic control is no longer achieved by other medications.

Pioglitazone is awaiting the outcome of an FDA safety review concerning reports of bladder carcinomas in patients taking this medication.

### 47 The answer is F  *Medicine*

Adenosine monophosphate (AMP)-activated protein kinase (AMPK)—not to be confused with cAMP-activated protein kinase—is an enzyme that plays a key central role in regulating energy metabolism in liver and other tissues. Activation of this enzyme by metformin (Glucophage; choice **F**) induces an inhibition of gluconeogenesis; this is the primary mechanism by which metformin reduces hyperglycemia. The rate of gluconeogenesis in the "typical" type 2 diabetic is about three times that of a normal person, and metformin treatment reduces this by more than a third. In addition to suppressing gluconeogenesis, metformin has several secondary effects, including enhancing sensitivity of peripheral cells to insulin, thereby increasing their uptake of glucose; decreasing the rate of absorption of glucose from the gut; and increasing fatty acid oxidation. Most of these properties are also suspected to result from the action of metformin on AMPK. Since metformin does not work by increasing secretion of insulin, when taken alone it does not cause hypoglycemia or weight gain. Moreover, it modestly reduces serum low-density lipoprotein and triglyceride levels, helping to protect against diabetic-induced cardiomyopathy. However, this drug is contraindicated for use with patients who have a risk of developing lactic acid acidosis; this includes patients with lung, liver, or kidney disorders (even those with only a creatinine level of 150 $\mu$mol/L or more). The reason that metformin may induce lactic acid acidosis is believed to be that it inhibits gluconeogenesis, the normal pathway through which lactate is normally removed from the circulation under semianaerobic conditions. Other adverse effects of metformin include gastrointestinal upset and malabsorption of vitamin $B_{12}$.

### 48 The answer is D  *Medicine*

Dipeptidyl peptidase-4 (DPP-4) is a proteolytic enzyme found on the surface of many cell types. It has a broad substrate specificity with at least 62 substrates; of particular relevance to this question is its degradation of the two known incretins, glucagon-like peptide-1 (GLP-1) and glucose-dependent insulinotropic peptide (GIP), formally known as gastric inhibitory peptide. These incretins lower circulating glucose levels via several modes of action, including causing an increased amount of insulin to be released after a meal, even before serum glucose levels are elevated; delaying gastric emptying, thus reducing the rate of glucose absorption into the body; inhibiting glucagon release from the pancreatic $\alpha$-cells, thereby signaling that gluconeogenesis should cease; and stimulating the satiety center, thus encouraging a person to stop eating. GIP seems also to play a role in regulating lipid metabolism. Normally, these actions of the incretins are down-regulated by DPP-4; consequently, inhibition of this enzyme results in increased insulin secretion, less glucagon secretion, and decreased absorption of glucose from the gastrointestinal tract. Sitagliptin (Januvia) is an oral antidiabetic that inhibits DPP-4 (choice **D**); thus, it lowers circulating glucose levels. However, on September 29, 2009, the U.S. Food and Drug Administration (FDA) revised the prescription information for sitagliptin and sitagliptin-metformin by announcing that 88 postmarketing cases of acute pancreatitis in patients using sitagliptin or sitagliptin-metformin had been reported to the FDA; 66% of these were hospitalized, four were admitted to an intensive care unit, and the condition resolved in only 53% of the cases after sitagliptin was discontinued. Consequently, physicians are recommended to carefully monitor patients for signs of pancreatis after initiation of or dose increases in these drugs.

### 49 The answer is C  *Medicine*

Nateglinide (Starlix) and repaglinide (Prandin) are the two meglitinides presently approved as oral antidiabetics. They should be taken shortly before the start of a meal—nateglinide between 1 and 30 minutes before (choice **C**), and repaglinide between 15 and 30 minutes before beginning to eat. Both have a short action time, peaking in about 1 hour and lasting only 3 hours; thus, they act only while glucose levels are raised after a meal and are usually used to reduce the postprandial rise in blood glucose levels. Their mode of action is similar to that of the sulfonylureas, but at a different binding site. Because of this similarity, they too tend to increase weight and have the potential of inducing hypoglycemia; however, the latter effect is minimized since their action is likely to be limited to a period of postprandial hyperglycemia. A meglitinide can be combined with a basal insulin to provide superior control in patients with residual β-cell insulin production; the basal insulin keeps the fasting blood sugar at a reduced level, while the meglitinide controls the after-meal glucose rise. Less common side effects include nausea, vomiting, diarrhea, muscle pain, flu- and cold-like symptoms, and head- and/or backache. Although of no use for type 1 diabetes and contradicted for patients with liver disease, they may be used in patients with kidney disease or allergies to sulfa drugs, such as the sulfonylureas.

### 50 The answer is A  *Medicine*

Pramlintide acetate (choice **A**) was approved by the U.S. Food and Drug Administration in 2005 as adjunct therapy to treat type 1 and type 2 diabetes. It is an injectable that cannot be mixed with insulin; thus, it must be injected at a separate time, usually before a meal providing at least 250 calories. It is a nonamyloidogenic analogue of amylin, a polypeptide hormone normally released in conjunction with insulin by pancreatic β-cells. Injection of pramlintide acetate inhibits gastric emptying, thus slowing the absorption of carbohydrates. It promotes a feeling of satiety via its influence on hypothalamic receptors (these differ from those receptors influenced by GLP-1) and inhibits the action of glucagon. Consequently, it permits type 1 patients to use less insulin, and for both type 1 and 2 patients, it reduces the unhealthy rise in glucose levels that occurs in diabetics after eating, thereby lowering HbA1c values.

### REMAINING INCORRECT CHOICE

Exenatide, first discovered in Gila monster saliva (hence the nickname lizard spit), is a synthetic 39-amino acid polypeptide analogue of the incretin hormone glucagon-like peptide -1 (GLP-1), which has a much longer half-life in vivo than does GLP. Basically, it is a more direct way of eliciting incretin action than that provided by DPP-4 inhibitors; consequently, it has very similar actions (see question 48 above). Although more direct, it must be injected twice a day. Presently, it and pramlintide acetate are the two injectable drugs approved to treat type 2 diabetes.

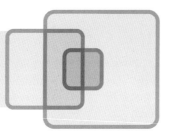

# test 11

# Questions

**Single Best Choice Directions:** *This section consists of numbered statements or questions followed by a list of potential answers; you are to select the ONE best answer.*

**1** A 36-year-old man with type 1 diabetes left for work one Friday morning in late September feeling fine, but by the time he came home at 6 PM, he was complaining of a headache and general malaise. His wife had him lie down before dinner; by dinner time, he felt worse and had also developed a cough, sore throat, aching muscles, and a temperature of 103°F (39.4°C). He suspected he had caught the flu from colleagues at work. He had no appetite, and his wife suggested he go directly to bed and try to get a good night's sleep. He did so, but by morning, he was no better. Because he was extremely thirsty but still had no appetite, his wife gave him an 8 ounce glass of orange juice in lieu of his usual breakfast. Usually, he checked his blood glucose level before going to bed and upon rising to estimate his optimal insulin therapy. However, because he felt so poorly, he neglected to take any insulin the previous night and only took a minimal dose in the morning, figuring that he ate very little. After drinking his orange juice and injecting the insulin, he fell back to sleep. Two hours later, he woke up because he had to urinate. In addition, he was uncomfortable because his mouth was very dry, he was extremely thirsty, his vision was blurred, he had a stomach ache, he expressed some difficulty with breathing, and he was nauseated and vomited. Which one of the following choices describes the most critical next step to take in the treatment of this individual?

(A) Check for elevated levels of urinary ketones.
(B) Check for hypoglycemia.
(C) Administer oseltamivir.
(D) Administer acetaminophen.
(E) Administer zolpidem.

**2** A 14-year-old boy constantly tests the limits of discipline with parents and teachers by speaking out of turn, flaunting rules about dressing and grooming, and staying out past his curfew. However, he gets along well with his peers, and he completes projects that he likes. He reached all developmental milestones at appropriate ages. He does not have a history of fighting, theft, or destruction of property. Mental status examination reveals an assertive child who tells the examiner that he does not wish to discuss his problems. Which of the following is the most likely diagnosis?

(A) Oppositional defiant disorder
(B) Mental retardation
(C) Conduct disorder
(D) Childhood disintegrative disorder
(E) Attention-deficit/hyperactivity disorder

**3** A 53-year-old woman presents with a history of a painless lump in the region of the right parotid gland. The lump has been present for about 6 years and has recently started growing in size. Her husband says that her speech has started to sound "funny." Examination reveals a firm, nontender mass with early evidence of peripheral facial nerve palsy. No lymphadenopathy is noted in the neck. Which of the following is the most likely diagnosis?

(A) Adenoid cystic carcinoma
(B) Adenolymphoma
(C) Pleomorphic adenoma
(D) Mucoepidermoid carcinoma
(E) Acinic cell carcinoma

**4** A 48-year-old man with postnecrotic cirrhosis due to chronic hepatitis B requires surgery to reduce portal veinous pressures. If the surgeon decides to use a shunt that reduces the risk for developing hepatic encephalopathy, the most likely shunt is which one of the following?

(A) Mesocaval
(B) Side-to-side portacaval
(C) End-to-side portacaval
(D) Distal splenorenal
(E) Mesosplenal

**5** A 54-year-old woman contracted a mild case of poliomyelitis in 1953, from which she completely recovered. In high school and during college, she participated in sports. After college, she participated in an annual local marathon until 1986, when she had to pull out of the race because of fatigue, which she attributed to a normal consequence of aging and not being in top physical shape. Since then, there has been a slow progressive weakening of her leg muscles not noticeable on a day-by-day basis. However, she is now consulting a physician because her calf muscles have begun to atrophy, and she has trouble straightening her back. The most probable diagnosis is which of the following?

(A) Postpolio syndrome
(B) Amyotrophic lateral sclerosis
(C) Osteoarthritis
(D) Tendinitis
(E) Guillain-Barré syndrome

**6** A 29-year-old man presents to the emergency room with a history of pain and swelling in the left side of the scrotum of 4 days' duration. There is no history of trauma. He did have sex recently with a woman whom he had met through the Internet, and he did not use a condom. The patient reported a burning sensation while passing urine, but no other problems. Physical examination revealed a young man in moderate distress, walking with a broad-based gait to avoid hurting his scrotum with his thighs. Examination of the genitalia revealed no penile abnormality or discharge through the urethra. Examination of the scrotum revealed dilated veins under the scrotal sac on the left side, which was tender to touch. Which of the following conditions is a possible diagnosis that must be excluded or confirmed?

(A) Torsion of the testis
(B) Incarcerated inguinal hernia
(C) Fournier's gangrene
(D) Epididymitis caused by chlamydia
(E) Renal carcinoma

**7** While surfing the Web, a 45-year-old man learned that, in 2009, the Centers for Disease Control and Prevention (CDC) reported that prostate cancer is the most common malignancy in men in the United States. In 2005, there were 142.4 new cases diagnosed per 100, 000 men, and 24.7 per 100,000 men died. He also read on the Internet that a simple blood test called the *prostate-specific antigen* (PSA) test will determine if a man does or does not have prostate cancer, and that, if a man were at risk to develop prostate cancer, a drug called finasteride can prevent cancer from developing. Consequently, he made an appointment to see his primary care physician and berated him, as well as all physicians in general, for not routinely screening all men for prostate cancer. He insisted that be tested. He also asked if he should be started on finasteride to prevent prostate cancer if the test results were negative, because he thought he might be at risk since his 68-year-old uncle was diagnosed with the disease last year. Which of the following choices is the most appropriate response?

(A) No health-related organization recommends prostate cancer screening before the age of 60.
(B) The PSA test needs to be used cautiously because false-positive results are a potential problem and he is at minimal risk; moreover, finasteride may cause its own problems.
(C) Finasteride is not recommended for use by the general male population because the lifetime risk of getting prostate cancer is only about 0.2%.
(D) Transrectal ultrasound is a simpler and better screening method than the PSA test and will soon replace it, so physicians hesitate to recommend the latter.
(E) Despite the endorsement of the PSA on the Internet, it is an inaccurate test.

**8** A 38-year-old man seeks treatment for a depressive episode. He complains of feelings of hopelessness and despair, with a marked lack of energy. He remarks that, on most days, he is too tired to get out of bed in the morning. He denies suicidal plans, stating, "There is really no point in suicide." At which of the following times is the patient most likely to commit suicide?

(A) When the patient admits his feelings of guilt
(B) When the patient completes a course of electroconvulsive therapy
(C) At the start of treatment
(D) When the patient develops untoward effects to antidepressants
(E) When the patient begins to respond to antidepressant medication

**9** A 27-year-old man is arrested after robbing a liquor store. He has multiple tattoos featuring slogans about racial supremacy. Mental status examination reveals an angry and belligerent individual without evidence of psychosis or cognitive impairment. Which of the following would most suggest a diagnosis of antisocial personality disorder?

(A) A belief that other people are unimportant, coupled with idealization of past tyrants like Hitler
(B) A childhood history of enuresis, fire-setting, and cruelty to animals
(C) A history of abuse during childhood and incarceration for substance-related crimes

(D) A long and pervasive pattern of disregard for and violation of the basic rights of others

(E) Membership in cults with destructive ideologies and plans for future warfare

**10** An 18-year-old man left the Amish community in Lancaster County, Pennsylvania, in a rebellious mood and joined the army. He passed the preinduction physical with no problems but subsequent postinduction studies raised questions. The following data were obtained: red blood cell count, 3.4 × 10⁶/μL (normal range, 4.7–6.1 × 10⁶/μL); hematocrit, 26% (normal range, 39%–49%); hemoglobin concentration, 9 g/dL (normal range, 13.6–17.5 g/dL); reticulocyte count, 8% (normal range, 1%–2%); white cell count, 5.0 × 10³/μL (normal range, 4.8–10.8 × 10³/μL), indirect bilirubin value, 2 mg/dL (normal range, 0.1–0.7 mg/dL). Additionally, the basic red cell morphology is normal with no Heinz bodies but a few crenated forms. Electrophoresis shows no abnormal hemoglobin (Hb), with a normal ratio of Hb A, Hb A₂, and Hb F. Results of the Coombs, Ham, and Donath-Landsteiner antibody tests were all negative, and no cold agglutinins were found. This young man most likely had which of the following conditions?

(A) Paroxysmal nocturnal hemoglobinuria
(B) Pyruvate kinase deficiency
(C) Hereditary spherocytosis
(D) Glucose 6-phosphate dehydrogenase deficiency
(E) Hemoglobin C disease
(F) Paroxysmal cold hemoglobinuria
(G) Autoimmune hemolytic anemia

**11** A 26-year-old woman is admitted to a psychiatric unit with a diagnosis of bipolar I disorder. Her medical history, physical examination, and laboratory studies are unremarkable. She is started on lithium 300 mg PO t.i.d. Her manic symptoms remit over 14 days. At discharge from the hospital, she complains of a slight resting tremor but otherwise feels well. Which of the following findings would most likely represent a toxic response to lithium if discovered during a follow-up clinic appointment 1 month later?

(A) Abnormal liver function
(B) Fever
(C) Hypothyroidism
(D) Leukopenia
(E) Urinary retention

**12** A 65-year-old woman comes to the office with a 2-day history of fever, chills, and a cough productive of purulent sputum. She has a history of smoking two packs of cigarettes a day for the last 45 years. A chest x-ray shows a right lower lobe consolidation. Which

of the following organisms is the most likely cause of her infection?

(A) *Mycoplasma pneumoniae*
(B) *Haemophilus influenzae*
(C) *Streptococcus pneumoniae*
(D) *Legionella pneumophila*
(E) *Coccidioides immitis*

**13** A 65-year-old man presents to the emergency department with sudden onset of left retroperitoneal pain. He is 5 ft 9 in tall (1.75 m) and weighs 190 lb (86.2 kg). Physical examination reveals his blood pressure to be 85/45 mm Hg, and a pulsatile mass in the abdomen is palpitated. The pathogenesis of this patient's disease is most closely related to which of the following?

(A) Hypertension
(B) Atherosclerosis
(C) Elastic tissue fragmentation
(D) Immune complex-mediated inflammation
(E) Vasculitis secondary to syphilis

**14** A 29-year-old man suffered from hepatitis, splenomegaly, a Coombs-negative hemolytic anemia, and portal hypertension during his adolescent and earlier adult years. Now, he is showing signs of behavioral and personality changes with emotional lability. In addition, he has a profound resting tremor, his speech has become slurred and difficult to understand, and he drools and has trouble swallowing. Physical examination shows a rim of brown pigment around the perimeter of the cornea. Which one of the following laboratory findings would most likely be reported?

(A) Decreased serum ceruloplasmin
(B) Increased serum ferritin
(C) Increased serum mitochondrial antibodies
(D) Increased total serum copper
(E) Normal serum prothrombin time

**15** A 28-year-old woman who is an Olympic cyclist is seen in the orthopedic clinic with complaints of numbness in her fingertips and pain in her left hand that occasionally radiates up her arm. She is often awakened by the symptoms. On physical examination, there is decreased sensation over the radial three and a half digits of the hand, and results of the Phalen's test are positive. Which of the following is the most likely diagnosis?

(A) Carpal tunnel syndrome
(B) Pronator syndrome
(C) Cubital tunnel syndrome
(D) Ulnar nerve entrapment at the wrist
(E) De Quervain disease

16. A 19-year-old man born and brought up in Brooklyn, New York, visited his grandfather who lived in western North Carolina. His grandfather, wanting to give him a taste of the life of his ancestors, took him hunting. The following week, after his return to Brooklyn, he presents with fever, lethargy, headache, and abdominal pain. Petechial lesions are noted on the palms of his hands and soles of his feet. Which of the following is the arthropod vector most likely responsible for this disease?

(A) Flea
(B) Louse
(C) Mite
(D) Chigger
(E) Tick

17. A 28-year-old woman who habitually fed feral cats is bitten on the hand by one in the neighborhood park. Twenty-four hours later, the hand is swollen, and there is swelling and warmth around the puncture sites of the bite. Which one of the following organisms is most likely responsible for these findings?

(A) *Bartonella henselae*
(B) *Pasteurella multocida*
(C) *Staphylococcus aureus*
(D) Group A streptococci
(E) *Pseudomonas aeruginosa*
(F) *Eikenella corrodens*

18. A 15-year-old girl who has had regular menstrual cycles since the age of 12 makes an appointment to see her primary care physician because of the development of sudden onset of abdominal pain. Physical examination reveals a tender mass in the left adnexa. A pregnancy test is negative. An ultrasound exhibits a mass lesion of the left ovary, with focal areas of calcification (increased density). Which of the following is the most likely diagnosis?

(A) Follicular cyst
(B) Mucinous cystadenoma
(C) Cystic teratoma
(D) Brenner's tumor
(E) Serous cystadenoma

19. A random sample of 100 female students is selected from the freshmen class of a large university. The women are followed prospectively over 4 years to see if use of oral contraceptive pills is associated with a decrease in ovarian cysts. Which of the following is the proper name of this study design?

(A) Cohort study
(B) Case-control study
(C) Randomized controlled clinical trial
(D) Cross-sectional study
(E) Cross-over study

20. A 25-year-old woman without any prior history of psychiatric problems has a 3-week episode of racing thoughts, insomnia, increased psychomotor activity, and impulsivity. There is no history of substance abuse or general medical conditions. Prior to this episode, she has worked steadily as a secretary. There have been no recent emotional stressors. She has no history of depressive episodes, and has always led an active social life. Physical examination and routine laboratory studies, including thyroid function tests, are unremarkable. Mental status examination reveals a well-oriented female with pressured speech and mood lability, but no psychotic symptoms. Which of the following most closely approximates her lifetime percentage chance of experiencing another similar episode?

(A) 5%
(B) 25%
(C) 50%
(D) 75%
(E) 90%

21. On the day after Thanksgiving, a young man brings his 50-year-old mother to the emergency department. Her son tells the triage nurse that, after consuming a hearty Thanksgiving meal, his mother felt ill. Her pain and symptoms grew worse during the night and early morning, so he thought he ought to bring her in. He also tells her that his mother has had two or three earlier episodes of gallbladder trouble but none so severe. The nurse notes the patient has a temperature of 102°F (38.9°C), blood pressure of 90/42 mm Hg, severe right-upper-quadrant (RUQ) pain, and jaundice. She also observes that she seems to have a problem with answering her questions and sometimes babbles incoherently. Upon examination by the attending physician, the patient is also found to have mild hepatomegaly. She has normal heart sounds, but a pulse rate of 125/min. Her white cell count is $13.6 \times 10^3/\mu L$ (normal range, $4.8–10.8 \times 10^3$), her total bilirubin level is 6.6 mg/mL (36.3 $\mu$mol/L; normal range, 0.1–1.2 mg/mL [2.0–21 $\mu$mol/L]); her γ-glutamyl transpeptidase (aka, γ-glutamyltransferase) activity value is 105 units/mL (normal, 9–85 units/mL), and her alkaline phosphatase value is 176 units/L (normal range 41–133 units/mL). Urine analysis was normal. Which of the following is the most likely diagnosis?

(A) Amebic liver abscess
(B) Acute hepatitis
(C) Acute pancreatitis
(D) Ascending cholangitis
(E) Sclerosing pericholangitis

**22** A 40-year-old nurse has been complaining for years about long work hours, poor pay, and lack of concern from her supervisors for her well-being. However, despite her constant complaining, she reports to work punctually and gets her work done in a yeoman-like fashion. She starts to also complain of recurrent episodes of forgetfulness, associated with bouts of sweating, palpitations, anxiety, tremulousness, and fainting. As a consequence, she asks for a medical leave with pay. Before granting her request, she is given a physical examination. Laboratory studies show a serum glucose level of 55 mg/dL (normal, 70–110 mg/dL), elevated serum insulin levels, and a suppressed level of serum C-peptide. Which of the following is the most likely cause of the hypoglycemia?

(A) Benign tumor of β islet cells
(B) Ectopic secretion of an insulin-like factor
(C) Malignant tumor of α islet cells
(D) Pancreatic carcinoma
(E) Injection of human insulin
(F) Factitious disorder

**23** A 42-year-old woman with a body metabolic index (BMI) of 42 kg/m², who does not smoke, presents with diastolic hypertension and menstrual irregularities. Pertinent findings upon physical examination are a full, plethoric-appearing face, increased facial hair, predominantly truncal obesity with purple stria around the abdomen, and scattered ecchymoses over the entire body. Laboratory studies indicate a hemoglobin (Hb) level of 18 g/dL (normal, 12–16 g/dL), a white blood cell (WBC) count of 18,000 cells/mm³ (normal, 4,500–11,000 cells/mm³), and a normal platelet count. The leukocyte differential shows an absolute neutrophilic leukocytosis and absolute lymphopenia and eosinopenia. Which of the following screening tests is most useful in the initial workup of this patient?

(A) Captopril-enhanced renal radionuclide test
(B) Plasma cortisol at 8 AM and 4 PM
(C) Clonidine suppression test
(D) Bone marrow aspiration and biopsy
(E) Low-dose dexamethasone suppression test

**24** A woman comes to the physician's office stating that she has never had a menstrual period, nor has she ever been sexually active or ever used contraceptive agents. She started breast development at age 10 years and started her growth spurt at age 11 years. She states she is not on any medications. She graduated from high school a year ago and is a nursing student at the local university. Physical examination reveals normal female breast development, but no uterus can be palpated on pelvic and rectovaginal examination. The cause of her amenorrhea can best be discovered by testing for the serum level of which one of the following substances?

(A) Follicle-stimulating hormone (FSH)
(B) Luteinizing hormone (LH)
(C) Prolactin
(D) Testosterone
(E) Progesterone

**25** A 19-year-old woman, gravida 2, para 0, abortus 1, comes to the outpatient office for a prenatal visit. She is currently at 30 weeks' gestation, confirmed by an 18-week sonogram that showed a single fetus with size appropriate for dates. She states that the fetus is moving well. Pregnancy weight gain to date is 20 lb. Her fundal height today measures 25 cm. Fetal heart tones are heard in the right upper quadrant. An obstetric ultrasound examination reveals essentially no amniotic fluid. Which of the following fetal conditions is most likely associated with this scenario?

(A) Duodenal atresia
(B) Open spina bifida
(C) Tracheoesophageal fistula
(D) Renal agenesis
(E) Atrial flutter

**26** A 7-year-old boy is referred from a school because of poor speaking and reading ability, failure to follow directions, and classroom disruptiveness. He appears to be alert and affectionate with others. He does not appear to be preoccupied with internal stimuli. IQ testing results are in the normal range. Which of the following is the most likely cause of his symptoms?

(A) Autistic disorder
(B) Food allergies
(C) Hearing impairment
(D) Schizophrenia
(E) Seizure disorder

**27** A 23-year-old woman requests reduction mammoplasty because she is convinced that her breasts are grossly large and misshapen. This perception started in her teens but until now she has been inhibited from doing anything about it because she still lived at home and her parents simply pooh-poohed the idea, making fun of her and calling her stupid to even think of such an option. She now dresses in elaborate clothing to hide her shape and avoids situations in which she might be expected to disrobe even partially. Physical examination reveals large well-formed breasts well within the normal range of size and shape. Which of the following is the most likely diagnosis?

(A) Body dysmorphic disorder
(B) Delusional disorder, somatic type
(C) Hypochondriasis
(D) Major depressive disorder, single episode
(E) Somatization disorder

**28** A 26-year-old woman, gravida 3, para 2, at 14 weeks' gestation by dates, complains of severe nausea and vomiting for the past 2 weeks. She has had vaginal bleeding and states that she passed what looked like grapes from her vagina. Her two previous pregnancies were unremarkable prenatally, resulting in term vaginal deliveries of grossly normal neonates who are developing normally. She states that all three of her pregnancies were fathered by her husband. On examination, her uterine fundus is palpable at her umbilicus. No fetal heart tones can be heard with a Doppler stethoscope. Cytogenetic studies performed on this pregnancy tissue would most likely show which of the following karyotypes?

(A) 46, XX
(B) 69, XXX
(C) 46, XY
(D) 45, X
(E) 69, XXY

**29** A 67-year old man bought an old home near Shreveport, Louisiana, and decided to clean out an adjacent shed that was dark and dank and obviously had not been disturbed for a long time. While working, he feels a slight sting-like burning sensation on his arm, but thinks nothing of it. Later that day, while washing up after his days work, he notices a reddish spot with a clear center, like a bull's eye, on the underside of his forearm. The following morning, the spot has formed a pustule filled with blood, which breaks 3 days later, forming a necrotic crater-like lesion. He then develops generalized symptoms including malaise, an itchy rash, headache, nausea with vomiting, and low-grade fever, inducing him to consult a physician. The physician makes a diagnosis and prescribes dapsone and rest. The doctor further tells him the systemic symptoms should clear up shortly, but if they don't, to make another appointment. He also recommends icing the arm to reduce pain and tells the patient that the sore on his arm will continue to fester for a while but should heal spontaneously in 6–8 weeks; in the meantime, it is best to simply keep it clean and leave it alone. Which of the following is the most probable diagnosis?

(A) A red fire ant bite
(B) A black widow spider bite
(C) A bite by the deer tick, *Ixodes scapularis*
(D) A brown recluse spider bite
(E) A scorpion sting

**30** A 20-year-old man, a recent immigrant from Eastern Europe, comes to his family physician with a history of chest pain and difficulty in breathing. He also complained of becoming dizzy when he tries to lift boxes at work. He had never been to a physician before. His family history was positive for hyperten-

sion. On examination, his blood pressure was 130/100 mm Hg, pulse 82/min with a distinct double peak, respirations 18/min and regular, and his temperature was normal. Oxygen saturation on room air was 98%. The apical pulse was prolonged, and a loud S4 sound and an ejection systolic murmur was heard over the left sternal area. An electrocardiogram (ECG) showed left ventricular hypertrophy with some Q waves. An echocardiogram showed decreased left ventricular space due to asymmetric left ventricular hypertrophy. The best medication for this patient would be which one of the following?

(A) Digoxin
(B) Atenolol
(C) Diltiazem
(D) Furosemide
(E) Angiotensin-converting enzyme inhibitors

**31** Ever since she was a toddler, a girl has been nagged by her mother to stand up straight. As she became older, she had little interest in sports because of shortness of breath. She also constantly complained that the shorts and slacks her mother purchased for her were shorter in one leg than the other. In the sixth grade, at the age of 12 years, a school nurse asked her to strip to the waist and bend forward at a 90-degree angle while she looked at her back. On the basis of this examination, the nurse called in her parents to recommend that the girl see an orthopedic surgeon. Which of the following is the most likely diagnosis suspected by the nurse?

(A) Ankylosing spondylitis
(B) Pott's disease of the spine
(C) Idiopathic scoliosis
(D) Osteomyelitis
(E) Neurofibromatosis

**32** Which of the following statistical tests would be most appropriate for assessing whether there are significant differences in 1-minute Apgar scores between infants born by emergency cesarean section and those born by spontaneous vaginal delivery?

(A) Student's *t*-test
(B) Analysis of variance
(C) Correlation coefficient
(D) Chi-squared test
(E) Logistic regression

**33** A 51-year-old woman, gravida 4, para 4, presents to the outpatient office complaining of painless, continuous leakage of clear fluid through her vagina. She had initially come to the clinic for an annual examination, at which time a Pap smear was obtained for cervical cancer screening. The report came back "consistent with cancer." Colposcopy was performed, showing a lesion on the anterior cervix with abnormal vessels. A cervical biopsy was performed, with the histology report stating "squamous cell carcinoma with invasion of 6 mm but no vascular or lymphatic involvement." Bimanual pelvic examination did not reveal any vaginal lesions or broad ligament masses. She underwent a radical hysterectomy 3 weeks ago. Which of the following tests would best assess the cause of the complaint?

(A) Cystometric studies
(B) Urine culture
(C) Intravenous (IV) indigo carmine
(D) Pelvic ultrasonography
(E) Urethral pressure measurements

**34** A 60-year-old man complains of pain and numbness in the left leg when walking. The pain is relieved by resting. He also complains of impotence. Physical examination reveals atrophy of the left leg muscles, normal reflexes, and a bruit over the femoral artery. Which of the following is the most likely diagnosis?

(A) Leriche syndrome
(B) A herniated lumbar disc
(C) Osteoarthritis of the hip
(D) Phlegmasia alba dolens
(E) A peripheral neuropathy

**35** A 21-year-old nulligravid woman comes to the outpatient office for her first prenatal visit at 12 weeks' gestation by dates. A home urine pregnancy test result was positive 6 weeks ago. A pelvic examination performed today was unremarkable, with uterine size consistent with her dates. Fetal heart tones were heard with a Doppler stethoscope at a rate of 130/min. A prenatal laboratory panel is ordered. Her rubella IgG antibody titer is found to be negative. Which one of the following recommendations would be most appropriate in managing this patient?

(A) Avoid exposure to known rubella infections.
(B) Avoid breastfeeding after postpartum vaccination.
(C) Avoid pregnancy for 3 months after postpartum vaccination.
(D) Offer genetic amniocentesis for amniotic fluid culture.
(E) Provide γ-globulin for prophylaxis now.

**36** A mother was driving her 5-year-old daughter home after the child had a good time at a birthday party. While making left turn, an SUV ran into the side of the car. The mother emerged with a few scratches, but the daughter was killed instantly. However, the mother seems oddly detached and unemotional when told of her child's death by the paramedics. Which one of the following mechanisms is this mother using?

(A) Isolation
(B) Depersonalization
(C) Disorientation
(D) Intellectualization
(E) Derealization

**37** Two 16-year-old boys who did not know each other were admitted to a metropolitan county hospital on the same day for a broken tibia and fibula. The one boy was handsome, had an outstanding physique, and was the star quarterback for his high school team; he broke his leg during a game. The other boy was smaller, looked like a nerd wearing horn-rimmed glasses, and broke his leg by slipping on the ice while walking his dog. After having their fractures reduced and casted, the two boys shared a room for a couple of days. The football player had several good-looking coeds visiting him, while the only visitor the other boy had was his mother; consequently, he was quite jealous. Six weeks later, the boys met again when it was time to have their casts removed. This occurred right after lunch; the football player ate a huge lunch, including a steak sandwich, while the other boy only had a salad. As the casts came off, the football player fainted dead away as soon as the cast was cracked open while the other boy simply got up on his crutches after the cast was removed and walked out. That he didn't faint while the tough football player did made him feel superior. Which one of the following choices was most probably responsible for the fainting incidence?

(A) The football player was a sissy.
(B) Orthostatic hypotension
(C) The football player had hypertropic cardiac myopathy.
(D) A vasovagal response
(E) A postprandial rush of blood to the digestive system

**38** An article published in the April 2009 *Public Library of Science (PloS) Medicine* listed the ten most important avoidable risk factors contributing to U.S. deaths in 2005 (the last year for which sufficient data were available). The article points out that just the first two of these risk factors accounted for a little over one-third of the deaths in the U.S. during 2005. The ranking of these 10 factors differs in several respects for men and women. Which pair of the following risk factors are more than 10% greater for women than for men?

(A) Excess weight and high blood sugar
(B) Low intake of omega-3 fats and smoking
(C) High blood pressure and physical inactivity
(D) High intake of trans fats and low intake of fruits and vegetables
(E) High salt intake and high blood sugar

**39** A married, 22-year-old fourth-year medical student from southern California was accepted into an externship at the Mayo Clinic in Rochester, Minnesota. Not being used to Minnesota's weather, he walked to work coatless on a fall morning. By the time he left to go home, night had fallen and an early storm had come in, dropping the temperature into the freezing range with a cold wind bringing rain and sleet. Trying to hurry and to keep warm, he slipped stepping off of a curb and lay stunned with a twisted ankle for some time before being found by a nurse who got him on his feet and took him to her home, which was only a few yards away. Although he felt half frozen and his ankle hurt, once he warmed up he felt fine and, in fact, he and the nurse entered into a sexual relationship. As it happened, this nurse had rheumatoid arthritis. About a month later, by the time he got back to California, he was suffering from a variety of symptoms including pain in his legs and feet, including acute tendinitis in his Achillis tendons; spondylitis and sacroiliitis; and pink eye with irritation and pain. Blood tests showed he was positive for HLA-B27 but negative for rheumatoid factor and antinuclear antibodies, and he had an elevated erythrocyte sedimentation rate. The student most likely suffered from which one of the following conditions?

(A) Rheumatoid arthritis caught from the nurse
(B) Rheumatoid arthritis that developed because of his exposure to the cold
(C) Reactive arthritis
(D) Ankylosing arthritis
(E) Psoriatic arthritis

**40** During a routine update appointment an 81-year-old male type 2 diabetic hesitantly mentions to his family practice physician that lately he has been having problems with voiding urine. His major problems are that, under certain conditions, he cannot stop his bladder from emptying and also that the head of his penis had become irritated. With regards to the latter, he adds that the reddish color of the head of his penis reminded him of the diaper rash his son had; consequently, he thought it might help if he wiped his penis after urinating, and it did. In further describing his inability to inhibit voiding at will, he noted some typical conditions that caused him problems: Often, when he approached the toilet to void he would start to urinate before he could get his penis fully out of his pants, wetting his clothing and sometimes even onto the floor. He also found that certain external factors sometimes triggered loss of urine at inappropriate times, as when stepping into a cold environment or simply upon hearing running water. Which one of the following choices best describes the type of urinary incontinence that this man suffers from?

(A) Stress incontinence
(B) Overactive bladder
(C) Overflow incontinence
(D) Functional incontinence
(E) Structural incontinence

---

**Directions for Matching Questions (41 through 50):** *Each set of matching questions is preceded by a list of 4 to 26 lettered options, followed by a brief explanation of the required task and then by a series of numbered statements. For each lettered statement you are to select ONE lettered option that best fulfills the task as it relates to that statement. Remember that each of the listed options might be correctly selected once, more than once, or not at all.*

## Questions 41–50 Pediatrics

(A) Deferoxamine mesylate
(B) Atropine sulfate
(C) Oxygen
(D) Fomepizole
(E) Pyridoxine
(F) Methylene blue
(G) Naloxone hydrochloride
(H) *N*-Acetylcysteine
(I) Pralidoxime
(J) Fab antibody fragments

*Match the indicated antidote listed above with the description of the ONE appropriate poisoning/toxic sign listed below.*

**41** A 3-year-old is brought to the emergency center by ambulance. The parents state that the child's adolescent baby-sitter found him with an empty bottle of prenatal vitamins earlier in the day. The baby-sitter says that the child thought they were candy, and because they were vitamins, she wasn't concerned. However, 4 hours after the ingestion, the child developed vomiting and bloody diarrhea, and appears listless.

**42** A 5-year-old has an ulnar fracture that needs to be reduced. The orthopedic surgeon decides that this can be done in the emergency department with sedation. Consent is obtained, and the patient is prepped for the procedure. The nurse rapidly injects the medication and the patient develops chest wall rigidity.

**43** A 16-year old is brought to the emergency department via ambulance. The family states that the patient was found with an empty bottle of her father's tuberculosis medicine after getting into a verbal altercation with him about her boyfriend. On arrival, the patient complains of nausea. She is tachycardic and seems somewhat somnolent. Paramedics report that she had an unsteady gait at the scene. The patient begins to convulse in the emergency department, and a benzodiazepine is administered.

**44** A father brings his 34-month-old son to the emergency department for treatment. The father says that he had been in the family garage changing the radiator fluid when his wife called him into the house to answer the telephone. His son stayed behind and continued "helping." The father states that he couldn't have been on the phone more than 5 minutes, but when he returned to the garage he found his son playing with a spilled bottle of radiator fluid. He is uncertain if the child ingested any. In the emergency center, the child's urine is examined; it tests positive for crystals and fluoresces when viewed under a Wood's lamp.

**45** A 1-month old infant with severe cyanosis is brought to the emergency department of a local hospital. The mother states that the baby is her firstborn, a term infant born by spontaneous vaginal delivery without complications. The infant had been exclusively breastfed until 1 week ago, when the mother began supplementing breastfeeding with powdered formula feedings. The family lives on a farm and uses well water.

Although 100% oxygen is delivered via a non-rebreather, the child's oxygen saturation remained in the 80s. In addition, the infant was noted to be tachycardic and tachypneic. The lungs were clear to auscultation bilaterally, and no heart murmur was detected. Abdominal examination showed no hepatomegaly, splenomegaly, or tenderness. Neurologic examination did not reveal any deficiency, and the anterior fontanel was normal. The infant's height, weight, and head circumference were at 25% for age. Radiography and electrocardiography findings were normal. Laboratory tests were ordered, and the nurse tells you that when she drew the blood it looked chocolate brown.

**46** A 16-year-old girl decided that life was too difficult and too filled with sorrow after her boyfriend told her that he no longer wanted to date her. She "just wanted to die." The patient was found in her bedroom, unresponsive, with a note that told her family and ex-boyfriend that she loved them. With the note was an empty bottle of her mother's digoxin tablets. The teenager was taken to the emergency center by ambulance, where it was determined that she had atrioventricular block with extreme bradycardia. An external pacemaker was applied, but the patient developed intractable hyperkalemia (serum potassium of 8.5 mEq/L) with increasing pacing threshold and progressive intraventricular conduction delay.

**47** A 10-year-old child comes to the emergency department after a major snowstorm that resulted in power outages. The parents state that, for the last few hours, they have been using a barbecue grill inside their home for heat and to cook food. Prior to the storm, the patient had been in his usual state of good health but now complains of nausea, vomiting, and headache. Others in the family also have had similar symptoms since the storm. In fact, the patient's 6-year-old cousin is presently in the emergency center being evaluated for a seizure.

**48** A 3-year-old ingested acetaminophen from his grandmother's medicine cabinet. They were not in a childproof container because the grandmother has arthritis, and she changed containers for ease of opening. The grandmother says that she has used two tablets of acetaminophen from this bottle. The bottle originally had 50 tablets. At present, there are five tablets left. The patient receives oral charcoal. Blood for an acetaminophen level is drawn 4 hours post ingestion.

**49** A 10-year-old child was accidently sprayed with an organophosphate insecticide. He showed signs of sympathetic overactivity and neuromuscular dysfunction, including tachycardia, hypertension, dilated pupils, and muscle fasciculation and muscle weakness. Which of the above choices represents a suitable antidote for these symptoms?

**50** The same child described in question 49 also demonstrated muscarinic symptoms, including **s**alivation, **l**acrimation, **u**rination, **d**efecation, **g**astrointestinal problems (abdominal pain and diarrhea), and **e**mesis. A mnemonic for these effects is "SLUDGE." Which of the above choices represents a suitable antidote for these symptoms?

# Answer Key

| | | | | | | | | | |
|---|---|---|---|---|---|---|---|---|---|
| **1** A | | **11** C | | **21** D | | **31** C | | **41** A | |
| **2** A | | **12** C | | **22** E | | **32** A | | **42** G | |
| **3** C | | **13** B | | **23** E | | **33** C | | **43** E | |
| **4** D | | **14** A | | **24** D | | **34** A | | **44** D | |
| **5** A | | **15** A | | **25** D | | **35** A | | **45** F | |
| **6** E | | **16** E | | **26** C | | **36** A | | **46** J | |
| **7** B | | **17** B | | **27** A | | **37** D | | **47** C | |
| **8** E | | **18** C | | **28** A | | **38** C | | **48** H | |
| **9** D | | **19** A | | **29** D | | **39** C | | **49** I | |
| **10** B | | **20** E | | **30** B | | **40** B | | **50** B | |

# *Answers and Explanations*

### 1 The answer is A *Medicine*

Diabetic ketoacidosis (DK) can develop quickly in a diabetic person (particularly in a type 1 diabetic) whenever insulin levels are permitted to decline below the required level. In the case described, the extremely dry mouth, extreme thirst, and blurred vision are typical signs of very high serum glucose levels, and the stomach ache, difficulty with breathing, nausea, and vomiting, although possibly caused by the flu itself, are more typically early signs of DK. Several clues suggest that the patient was grossly insulin deficient: (a) the presence of the aforementioned early signs of DK; (b) that he already missed his normal evening insulin dose; (c) the stress hormones generated by the flu would have increased his normal insulin dose requirement and acted to counteract the insulin remaining in his system; and (d) his minimal morning insulin dose was very likely too little to counteract the effects of the load of glucose provided by the 8 ounce glass of orange juice, let alone to have overcome the earlier deficiency. An insulin deficiency prevents glucose from entering muscle and adipose cells; instead, levels build up in the blood. Excess blood glucose spills into the urine, taking water with it and causing excess thirst. The excess circulating level induces excess glucose to enter into the lens of the eye, producing an osmotic imbalance resulting in blurred vision. Because muscle and adipose tissue cannot absorb glucose, these tissues begin to depend upon fat for energy, increasing the degradation of fatty acids into acetyl CoA, which can't be metabolized to carbon dioxide ($CO_2$) because pyruvate levels are too low; instead the excess acetyl CoA is converted to acetoacetate, $\beta$-hydroxybutyrate and acetone, collectively known as ketones. In addition, $H^+$ accumulates. This condition is known as *ketoacidosis*, which, if left untreated, will cause loss of consciousness and eventual death. Since untreated DK can be fatal, it is important to determine if a patient's ketone level is markedly elevated, making choice **A**, checking for elevated levels of urinary ketones, the most critical next step among those listed for treating this patient. This can be done at home using a commercially available dip stick.

Check for *hypoglycemia* (choice **B**) essentially is nonsense since all the data provided point to hyperglycemia. On the other hand, if this choice were check for *hyperglycemia* or even simply to check the serum glucose value, it would have been correct because the value would likely have been higher than 300 mg/dL (16.5 mmol/L); high enough to persuade the patient to inject another bolus of insulin and/or consult a physician. Administering oseltamivir (choice **C**), acetaminophen (choice **D**), or zolpidem (choice **E**) might help treat the flu and its symptoms but would not directly affect the course of DK.

### 2 The answer is A *Psychiatry*

Oppositional defiant disorder (choice **A**) involves problems in relating to authority figures. Generally, such children get along well with peers and have no other problems of conduct or development.

Mental retardation (choice **B**) is associated with delayed developmental milestones and other evidence of impaired intellectual abilities. Conduct disorder (choice **C**) is characterized by violation of age-appropriate social norms, fighting, runaway behavior, theft, and destruction of property, and often is a sequel to oppositional defiant disorder. Childhood disintegrative disorder (choice **D**) involves the development of severe disturbances in social, communicative, and cognitive functions after a period of normal development. Attention-deficit hyperactivity disorder (choice **E**) is characterized by inattention, impulsivity, and hyperactivity. Individuals with this disorder would be unlikely to complete projects even if they were interested.

### 3 The answer is C *Surgery*

This patient has a pleomorphic adenoma (also known as a mixed parotid tumor; choice **C**). It is the most common tumor affecting the salivary glands, accounting for approximately 70% of parotid tumors and 50% of all salivary gland tumors. Pleomorphic adenomas are essentially benign and, as in this patient, are often present for more than 6 years. Malignancy can develop and is heralded by a sudden increase in size, pain, and infiltration into the facial nerve, where it traverses the gland.

Adenolymphoma (choice **B**; also called Warthin's tumor) is the second most common benign tumor of the salivary glands, and it is almost always located in the parotid gland. It most often is cystic and usually affects middle-aged or elderly males. More than one tumor may be found in one or both parotid glands. Mucoepidermoid carcinoma (choice **D**) is the most common malignant tumor of the parotid glands. It has varying degrees of differentiation and growth; the greater the squamous component, the worse the prognosis. When mucoepidermoid carcinoma occurs in the parotid gland, it does not usually cause facial nerve paralysis, because local invasion is limited. Metastasis is also limited to the local lymph nodes. Adenoid cystic carcinoma (choice **A**) is the most common malignant tumor of minor salivary glands and has a tendency to invade perineural tissue. As a result, the patient presents with pain, paralysis of muscles, and areas of anesthesia over involved skin. The tumor may even invade bone, without evidence of it on initial radiography. Thus, like an iceberg, it is far more extensive than encountered on physical examination or perceived on radiography. Acinic cell carcinoma (choice **E**) is a rare malignant tumor that is more common in women than in men. It is most commonly located in the parotid gland. It is slow growing, tends to be soft, is locally invasive, and may metastasize.

## 4 **The answer is D** *Surgery*

The surgical treatment for portal hypertension encompasses a variety of shunt operations. Shunt types include a portocaval shunt, mesocaval shunt, and the distal splenorenal shunt. Since the portal vein is formed by the superior mesenteric vein and the splenic vein, a distal splenorenal shunt (choice **D**) reduces portal vein pressure (splenic vein blood is shunted into the renal vein) without bypassing the liver. Therefore, portal vein blood containing ammonia produced by colon bacteria is partially metabolized in the liver by the urea cycle; this reduces the risk for inducing hepatic encephalopathy. In contradistinction, portosystemic shunts reduce portal pressure but deprive the liver of portal blood flow, thus exacerbating hepatic encephalopathy by increasing serum ammonia levels.

The side-to-side (portal vein–inferior vena cava) (choice **B**) and the end-to-side (portal vein–inferior vena cava) (choice **C**) shunts decompress sinusoidal pressure in the liver and relieve ascites in most patients by redirecting portal vein blood into the vena cava. Mesocaval shunts (choice **A**) are anastomoses between the superior mesenteric vein and vena cava, the portal vein and vena cava, and the mesenteric vein and renal vein. These are most often performed as an emergency procedure for active esophageal bleeding that is resistant to therapy. In general, these shunts decompress esophageal veins, control ascites, and have a high rate of patency. A mesosplenal shunt (choice **E**) is sheer nonsense.

## 5 **The answer is A** *Medicine*

Poliomyelitis, also known as infantile paralysis, was the scourge of the first half of the 20th century. Ironically, its prevalence increased as sanitation improved, because prior to that, persons were first exposed to the virus as infants while still protected by antibodies in their mother's milk; consequently, the most severe aspects of infection were mitigated and they developed long-term immunity. By the 1920s through the 1950s, polio epidemics occurred annually until Salk developed an injectable killed vaccine first widely used in 1954 and 1955; this was followed by Sabin's attenuated virus oral vaccine in 1963. Consequently, there has not been a case of polio in a native American resident since 1979 (on occasion it has been observed in an immigrant), and routine vaccination in the United States is no longer required. However, the effects of poliomyelitis are still with us. Individuals tend to develop a condition known as postpolio syndrome (choice **A**) 10–40 years after having had paralytic polio. This condition is characterized by slowly developing but progressively worsening symptoms that include fatigue and muscle weakness; commonly, joint pains and scoliosis also occur. Although the condition can be debilitating, it is only life-threatening if it affects the muscles of respiration. It is thought that postpolio syndrome is caused by fatigue of motor neurons, which serve more muscle fibers than normal after their former partner neurons were killed by the virus; one line of thought is that the condition can be aggravated by excess use. No known treatment modality exists, and most experts recommend limited, nonfatiguing exercise.

Amyotrophic lateral sclerosis (choice **B**), sometimes called Lou Gehrig's disease, is also a disease of motor neurons, but usually of unknown cause. It starts somewhat innocuously with weakness in a hand, foot, or leg, but then progresses, causing degeneration of anterior horn cells throughout the brain and spinal cord. Usually within 2–10 years after diagnosis, death ensues. The drug riluzole tends to slow, but does not stop, progression of the disease. Although most cases have no known cause, a mutated *SOD1* gene has been implicated in 2% of the cases, and about 20% of the cases have a familial connection. Osteoarthritis (choice **C**) and tendinitis (choice **D**) are both conditions that can develop because of overuse but usually at an older age, and a history of polio is rarely present; neither are characterized by fatigue or muscle weakness of the kind associated with postpolio syndrome. Guillain-Barré disease (choice **E**), also known as acute idiopathic polyneuropathy, is characterized by weakness that usually begins in the legs and spreads upward, frequently to the arms and face. Typically, it is symmetric, and the extent of weakness varies from case to case. It primarily affects motor neurons, but distal paresthesias and dysstasias commonly occur. Onset of the disease frequently follows immunizations, surgical procedures, or infections; an association with *Campylobacter jejuni* enteritis has been particularly well documented. Most patients recover spontaneously over a period of months, but about 10%–20% retain some degree of disability.

### 6 The answer is E *Surgery*

This patient has a varicocele involving the pampiniform plexus of veins. The classic description of this is that it feels like a bag of worms. Varicoceles are benign conditions and may be associated with a small hydrocele. However, the main concern on the left side is the presence of a latent renal carcinoma that can herald itself by presenting as a varicocele. This is because, whereas the right testicular vein drains directly into the inferior vena cava, in contrast, the left testicular vein drains into the left renal vein. As a consequence, renal carcinoma (choice **E**) can infiltrate into the left renal vein and block the inflow of blood from the left testicular vein, leading to backup and dilated veins in the scrotum. In such instances, the varicocele will not decompress when the patient is lying supine. Hence, the presence of renal carcinoma should be excluded at the earliest, rather than just dealing with the varicocele itself.

Torsion of the testis (choice **A**) is an unlikely diagnosis. This is usually associated with severe lower abdominal pain, retching, and vomiting, and the testis will be exquisitely tender. Moreover, the testis will be lying in a horizontal position. This man also does not have an incarcerated inguinal hernia (choice **B**). An incarcerated inguinal hernia will usually extrude from the inguinal canal into the scrotum. The scrotum will be swollen and tender. Dilated veins will not be found. The hernia will be distinct from the testis and will fail to reduce. Furthermore, one will not be able to "get above the swelling." Fournier's gangrene (choice **C**), also known as idiopathic scrotal edema, is a rare condition. Scrotal inflammation occurs suddenly, followed by rapid onset of gangrene. This leads to sloughing of the scrotal skin. Patients usually have severe scrotal pain, fever, prostration, and pallor. Treatment involves antibiotics and analgesics. Epididymitis (choice **D**) in young men most commonly results from sexually transmitted disease. Chlamydia is the leading cause, followed by gonorrhea. The epididymis is tender to palpation; however, no dilated veins or scrotal swelling is noted. If it spreads to the testis, the resultant disorder is called epididymo-orchitis.

### 7 The answer is B *Preventive Medicine and Public Health*

Routine screening of all men for prostate cancer is not recommended because it is feared that increased screening will result in unneeded biopsies, which have their own risk of complications, as well as increased cost, inconvenience, and pain. Although a 2003 study concluded that finasteride reduced the risk of prostate cancer by 25%, it does create its own problems (choice **B**). Cancers that develop while a patient is on finasteride are more aggressive than usual; in addition, libido is reduced, ejaculate volume is decreased, and reports of erectile dysfunction are increased.

Controversy remains concerning who should or should not be screened and at what age. Most agencies recommend some screening before the age of 60 (choice **A** is incorrect). The 2005 Centers for Disease Control and Prevention (CDC) Internet statement addresses the status as follows: all men have the right to hear the pros and cons concerning routine screening and then to make an informed decision. For those who insist on routine screening, CDC guidelines recommend that screenings, in the form of prostate specific antigen (PSA) level testing and digital rectal examination (DRE), be performed annually starting at age 50 (earlier for African American men or if a brother or father had prostate cancer) if life expectancy is greater than 10 years. According to 2005 CDC figures, over a lifetime, one of every six males (16.6%) will develop prostate cancer, not 0.2% (choice **C**). However, only 1 of every 2,500 45-year-old men will have prostate cancer; at age 50, the odds increase to 1 in 476; at age 55, 1 in 200; at age 60, 1 in 43; at 65, 1 in 21; at 70, 1 in 13: and by 75 years of age, 1 in 9. In fact, autopsy data suggest that all men may eventually develop prostate cancer, provided they live long enough. Risk development rate is accelerated among African Americans and in men who have an affected brother or father. The good news is that most cases of prostate cancer develop at an indolent rate, and many cancers remain asymptomatic for years; thus, most men who are first diagnosed in their late 70s or 80s will die of some other disease before their prostatic cancer becomes truly troublesome.

At this time, there are basically three methods available to screen for prostate cancer: PSA, DRE, and transrectal ultrasound. Transrectal ultrasound is more expensive than the other two modalities, moreover it has a low specificity (consequently a high biopsy rate), and its sensitivity is no greater than that of the PSA and digital rectal examination. Thus, it is not likely to replace them (choice **D**).

PSA is more sensitive than the DRE (not vice versa, choice **E**). Using the standard cutoff of 4 ng/mL, the PSA test will find that 2% of men older than 50 have prostate cancer, whereas the DRE will find that 1.5% do. Although the combined use of DRE and PSA increases the accuracy of prostate cancer diagnosis, problems remain. The DRE is subjective, and even the best diagnosticians cannot detect early cancer. PSA is elevated in benign prostatic hypertrophy (BPH) and other benign conditions that can increase PSA values into the "gray" risk zone of 4–10 ng/mL or even higher, causing false-positive results that trigger biopsy and further studies. Conversely, treatment of BPH with finasteride lowers PSA values and causes false-negative results. Many clinicians believe that testing high-risk subjects (primarily older men) annually and looking for an increase in the PSA value is a more sensitive test than relying on one value. An annual increase of 0.75 ng/mL or more, even if the value remains below 4 ng/mL, denotes a high probability of cancer. Other investigators tout the measurement of free and protein-bound PSA rather than the standard total PSA; cancer patients have a lower percentage of free PSA. A free PSA value of 25% or above means the risk of cancer is low even if the total PSA value is over 4 ng/mL, whereas a free value below 10% means the risk is very high. However, once again, a zone of uncertainty exists between 10% and 25%, making biopsy inevitable in such cases. Still another approach to increase the sensitivity of a PSA test is by establishing age-related cutoff values rather than assuming a value of 4 ng/mL fits patients at all ages.

## 8  The answer is E  *Psychiatry*

In major depressive disorder, the greatest risk for suicide occurs after partial response to antidepressants (choice **E**). Usually, energy and motivation return before a subjective improvement in mood. A patient who has been too apathetic to act on suicidal rumination may attempt suicide at this point. Also, some antidepressants provide the means for a suicide attempt by overdose. Close assessment of patients during treatment with antidepressant medication is therefore essential.

Admission of feelings of guilt (choice **A**), completion of a course of electroconvulsive therapy (choice **B**), the start of treatment (choice **C**), and development of untoward effects to antidepressants (choice **D**) are all situations that are not closely associated with a risk for suicide.

## 9  The answer is D  *Psychiatry*

A neglect of the basic rights of others (choice **D**) is most characteristic of antisocial personality disorder.

Dismissal of most people and idealization of a few famous or infamous figures (choice **A**) are characteristic of narcissistic personality disorder. A history of earlier abuse during childhood (choice **C**) and other childhood psychopathology (e.g., fire setting, cruelty to animals [choice **B**]) are often found in individuals with several types of adult psychopathology, including antisocial personality disorder, borderline personality disorder, or dissociative identity disorder. However, these early childhood problems are sometimes absent. Although a history of incarceration (choice **C**) is common in individuals with antisocial personality disorder, there are many incarcerated individuals without this disorder and many individuals with the disorder who are never incarcerated. The mere belief in violence (choice **E**) does not necessarily indicate antisocial personality disorder.

## 10  The answer is B  *Medicine*

In the red blood cell, pyruvate kinase (PK) catalyzes the net adenosine triphosphate (ATP)-producing reaction, and the major function of this ATP is to maintain activity of the sodium-dependent ATPase that sustains the ionic equilibrium of the cell. As a consequence, when ATP levels fall cells tend to become hypoosmotic, crenate, and be hemolyzed in the spleen. Thus, the primary symptom of pyruvate kinase deficiency (PKD) is a chronic hemolytic anemia. Surprisingly, most individuals with PKD do well despite being very anemic, similar to the man described in the vignette. This is because a limitation in the rate of flux of intermediates at the level of PK causes the concentration of intermediates proximal to this block to increase. The resultant increase in 2,3-diphosphoglycerate concentration shifts the $O_2$:Hb saturation curve to the right, increasing the efficiency of $O_2$ transfer to tissues. Thus, even though less Hb is present, what is there is more efficient. In addition, some compensation is also provided by the increased circulating reticulocyte count. Consequently, most affected individuals are nearly symptom free for much of their lives.

However, more than 100 different mutant PK variants have been described, and symptoms vary with the type of mutation. Some mutations affect the $V_{max}$, some the $K_m$, some the affinity for activators, some sensitivity to product inhibition, and some stability. Moreover, PKD is inherited as an autosomal recessive trait, and most nonconsanguineous cases are in compound heterozygotes. In addition, symptoms generally are more severe during the neonatal period and early childhood. Consequently, neonates often present with anemia, an abnormally severe and prolonged jaundice, and a delayed growth pattern. Cholecystolithiasis may develop after the first decade, but relatively few adults suffer the fatigue and other symptoms that usually are associated with profound anemia.

PKD (choice **B**) has a relative high prevalence among the Amish in Lancaster County, a factoid pointing toward PKD in the case described; however, selecting this choice depends more logically upon eliminating the other choices by using the data provided in the vignette. Paroxysmal nocturnal hemoglobinuria (choice **A**) is a disorder that results in abnormal sensitivity of the red cell membrane to lysis by complement. The underlying disorder is a defect in the phosphatidylinositol class A gene, which results in an aberrant glycosyl-phosphatidylinositol anchor for cellular membrane proteins, particularly the CD55 and CD59 complement-binding ones. The negative Ham test result rules out this possibility.

Hereditary spherocytosis (choice **C**) is a dominant trait resulting in a hemolytic anemia, in which hemolysis is caused by destruction of the less supple spherocytic erythrocyte in the sinuses of the spleen. Clearly, the man described in the vignette did not suffer from hereditary spherocytosis because his red cell morphology is normal. Glucose 6-phosphate dehydrogenase (G6PD) deficiency (choice **D**) is the most common disease producing red blood cell (RBC) enzymopathy in the world; both the African ($A^-$) and the Mediterranean ($B^-$) varieties are inherited as X-linked recessive traits that impart partial resistance to falciparum malaria. Except for perinatal jaundice, males carrying the mutated gene are asymptomatic until subjected to an oxidative stress that will induce an acute hemolytic crisis, which is more severe in the Mediterranean form. Clearly, the man described in the vignette is not suffering from an acute episode of hemolysis. Hemoglobin C disease (Hb C; choice **E**) is a hemoglobinopathy analogous to sickle cell disease in which a lysine, rather than a valine, substitutes for the normal glutamate in position 6 of the β-globin chain. Although this causes a chronic mild hemolytic anemia and a low level of chronic jaundice, this disease is ruled out by the finding of a normal electrophoretic pattern; Hb C runs more slowly toward the anode than either Hb A or Hb S. Paroxysmal cold hemoglobinuria (PCH; choice **F**) is a rare condition that primarily affects children after a viral disease, although it sometimes occurs in adults with certain neoplastic conditions. At one time, it was more common, as it is also associated with congenital syphilis in neonates and in adults having stage 2 or 3 syphilis. The pathophysiology relates to the binding of biphasic IgG to the "P" antigen, a glycosphingolipid that normally binds early complement components. In PCH, the P antigen is defective, and a change in temperature (such as might occur in the hands or feet) causes release and activation of the complement sequence, causing hemolysis. In the case described in the vignette, there is no clue suggesting such a system could be active, and results of the Donath-Landsteiner antibody test, which can be used to confirm PCH, are negative. Autoimmune hemolytic anemia (choice **G**) is due to the formation and binding of an IgG autoantibody to RBC membranes. The Fc portion of the antibody is "bitten off" by macrophages, along with a piece of the membrane. The damaged RBC takes on a spheroid shape and is hemolyzed in the spleen. In addition, when large amounts of IgG are attached to the membrane, complement components become "fixed" to the cell and the C3b factor is recognized by C3b receptors on hepatic Kupffer cells, which also participate in the hemolytic process. Half the cases are idiopathic; the remaining cases are associated with systemic lupus erythematosus, chronic lymphocytic leucemia, or lymphomas. The negative Coombs test result rules out autoimmune hemolytic anemia as a possibility.

## 11 The answer is C *Psychiatry*

Lithium-induced hypothyroidism (choice **C**) occurs in approximately 5% of individuals on lithium maintenance therapy. Lithium maintenance therapy may also induce weight gain, acneform skin eruptions, tremor, leukocytosis, and polyuria. The latter reflects a low incidence of potential renal toxicity. Consequently, routine monitoring during lithium maintenance therapy includes plasma lithium levels, complete blood count (CBC), blood urea nitrogen (BUN) concentration, creatinine levels, and thyroid function testing.

In contrast to its potential effect on the thyroid, lithium has no reported hepatotoxicity, which would cause abnormal liver function test results (choice **A**). Fever (choice **B**), urinary retention (choice **E**), and leukopenia (choice **D**) are rarely associated with lithium treatment.

### 12 The answer is C  *Medicine*

Typical community-acquired pneumonia is most commonly caused by *Streptococcus pneumoniae*, a gram-positive diplococcus. Azithromycin is the treatment of choice. Other organisms, such as *Haemophilus influenzae* (choice **B**) or *Moraxella catarrhalis*, are commonly found in smokers with chronic bronchitis or those with underlying lung disease, but *S. pneumoniae* remains the most common. Concern is increasing about the rising percentage of *S. pneumoniae* strains that are resistant to penicillin. The best way to protect elderly patients and those with underlying lung disease from pneumonia is by use of the pneumococcal vaccine, which is recommended for all persons over age 65 and in those younger patients who have underlying lung disease or who are asplenic.

Infections caused by *Mycoplasma pneumoniae* (choice **A**), *Legionella pneumophila* (choice **D**), and *Coccidioides immitis* (choice **E**) are not associated with cough or signs of lung congestion.

### 13 The answer is B  *Surgery*

The patient has a classic triad for a ruptured abdominal aortic aneurysm: an abrupt onset of back pain, hypotension, and a pulsatile mass in the abdomen. An aneurysm is a localized dilatation of a vessel. It is usually caused by structural weakness in the wall of the vessel due to atherosclerosis (choice **B**). Abdominal aortic aneurysms are the most common type of aneurysm in the vascular system, located below the orifices of the renal arteries. Most occur in men over 55 years of age, who are asymptomatic. Each year, approximately 9,000 Americans die from a ruptured abdominal aortic aneurysm, and most of these are men over 65 years of age. Ultrasound is the most effective means of making the diagnosis of an aneurysm. In 2005, the U.S. Preventive Services Task Force (USPSTF) recommended this procedure for routine screening of men between the ages of 65 and 75 who have smoked at least 100 cigarettes during their lifetime. The evidence for non-smokers is less compelling, but the possibility of screening others is left open. Rupture of the aneurysm is the most common complication. The aorta's normal diameter is less than 3 cm; a value above that is diagnosed as an aneurysm, but the risk of rupture is not great until the diameter exceeds 5 cm. Other risk factors for rupture include hypertension and the presence of chronic obstructive pulmonary disease (COPD). Indications for surgery include any symptomatic aneurysm or any asymptomatic aneurysm larger than 5 cm, because rupture is inevitable with time, and after rupture, mortality rates exceed 90%.

Hypertension (choice **A**) and elastic tissue fragmentation (choice **C**) are associated with dissecting aortic aneurysms. Immune complex–mediated inflammation (immune complex vasculitis; choice **D**) is the primary pathogenesis of small vessel disease. Vasculitis secondary to syphilis (syphilitic aortitis; choice **E**) is a late symptom rarely observed since the advent of penicillin.

### 14 The answer is A  *Medicine*

The patient has Wilson disease, which is an autosomal recessive disease due to genetic aberration in the "Wilson" gene on chromosome 13; the worldwide prevalence is 30 cases per $10^6$ persons. More than 200 different mutations have been uncovered, leading to some variation in symptoms. However, typically, the disease first presents in adolescence with liver disease plus a variety of hemolytic and other symptoms, then progresses in early adulthood to neurologic problems similar to those described. Once the disease progresses to the neurologic state, a Kayser-Fleischer ring (brown pigment around the perimeter of the cornea) is essentially pathognomic for the condition. The genetic defect affects a copper-transporting ATPase (ATP7B) in the liver and leads to accumulation of copper in the hepatocytes and oxidative damage to hepatic mitochondria. The major physiologic effects are due to a defect in the hepatocyte transport system for copper secretion into bile, leading to increased copper deposition in liver, brain, cornea, and kidneys. In addition, copper cannot be incorporated into an $\alpha_2$-globulin to produce ceruloplasmin, which is the copper-binding protein. Normally, the total serum copper equals copper that is bound to ceruloplasmin (95% of the total) plus copper that is unbound (free). In Wilson disease, the total serum copper level is decreased (not increased [choice **D**]) because ceruloplasmin is decreased (choice **A**). However, the free copper level in the serum and urine is increased because of defective excretion in the bile and subsequent accumulation of copper in the serum. Excess copper is deposited in Descemet's membrane of the cornea of the eye (producing Kayser-Fleischer ring) and in the basal ganglia. In the latter location, it may cause parkinsonism, choreiform movements, and dystonia in the bulbar musculature. This latter effect can produce dysarthria (problems with speech and/or drooling) and/or dysphagia.

Increased serum ferritin (choice **B**) in the setting of chronic liver disease is associated with hemochromatosis, an autosomal recessive disease with unrestricted reabsorption of iron from the gastrointestinal tract.

Hemochromatosis is not associated with corneal abnormalities or a movement disorder. Increased serum mitochondrial antibodies (choice **C**) is a marker for primary biliary cirrhosis, an autoimmune disease characterized by destruction of bile ducts in the portal triads. It is not associated with corneal abnormalities or a movement disorder. Since the patient has chronic liver disease (chronic hepatitis or cirrhosis), the prothrombin time is most likely increased (not normal [choice **E**]) because of decreased synthesis of coagulation factors in the damaged liver.

### 15 The answer is A *Surgery*

Carpal tunnel syndrome (choice **A**) is caused by compression of the median nerve at the level of the wrist. The median nerve supplies sensation to the radial three and a half digits of the hand, as well as innervation of the thenar musculature. Symptoms include numbness and tingling in the fingertips and pain that can awaken the patient at night and that can travel proximally up the arm. Hyperextension of the hand or tapping over the nerve reproduces the findings. There can be sensory loss in the median nerve distribution and muscle weakness in the thumb.

Pronator syndrome (choice **B**) is a median nerve entrapment in the proximal forearm. It is a pure sensory syndrome. The cubital tunnel is a groove in the posteromedial aspect of the elbow that contains the ulnar nerve. Cubital tunnel syndrome (choice **C**) is an ulnar nerve neuropathy. Ulnar nerve entrapment (choice **D**) can occur at the wrist in Guyon's canal. In both of these conditions, patients may complain of numbness in the ulnar one and a half digits and have weakness of the intrinsic muscles. De Quervain disease (choice **E**) is usually caused by repetitive use of the thumb for some activity. Patients have pain and tenderness at the region of the radial styloid.

### 16 The answer is E *Medicine*

All of the insects listed are vectors of rash-producing diseases caused by microorganisms in the Rickettsiae family. The man in the case described has Rocky Mountain spotted fever, which is due to the bite of a hard tick (*Dermacentor andersoni*, choice **E**) a vector for *Rickettsia rickettsii*. A diagnostic triad for the disease is rash, fever, and history of exposure to a tick. The incubation period is approximately 2–12 days after exposure. Unlike the other rickettsial organisms, which cause a rash extending from the trunk to the extremities in centrifugal fashion, the rash of Rocky Mountain spotted fever begins on the palms and soles and spreads to the trunk. The rash is due to a vasculitis caused by the rickettsial organisms invading the endothelial cells of small vessels and producing petechial lesions. Oklahoma and North Carolina share the lead for the highest incidence of Rocky Mountain spotted fever. The diagnosis is best made serologically using indirect immunofluorescent techniques rather than the outdated Weil-Felix reaction, which has a positive *Proteus vulgaris* OX-2 and OX-19 reaction. Doxycycline is the treatment of choice. The mortality rate is 20% without treatment and 5% with treatment.

The vector for murine typhus and the plague is the flea (choice **A**), and the disease-causing agent for typhus is *R. typhi*. The typical hosts are mice and rats, but the disease has also been transmitted by cats and opossums. In the United States, approximately 100 cases are recorded each year, primarily in southern California and Texas. The disease-causing agent for the plague is *Yersinia pestis*. The typical host is the rat, but it is also carried by other rodents, including the ground squirrel. Historically, plague epidemics killed millions, but since 1950, outbreaks have been sporadic and isolated due to modern sanitation, rodent control, and use of antibiotics. The typical vector for epidemic typhus is the human body louse (choice **B**). The disease-causing organism is *R. prowazekii*. Epidemic typhus is typically transmitted from human to human via the louse, under unsanitary conditions, and epidemics are often associated with wars. Mites (choice **C**) carry rickettsial pox. The primary host is the mouse, and the causative agent is *R. akari*. Mites also cause severe pruritic conditions, but directly by their bite, rather than serving as vectors. Scrub typhus is transmitted by mites (choice **D**). The disease-causing organism is *R. tsutsugamushi*, a distinct genus and species in the Rickettsiae family. Cases of scrub typhus primarily occur in Oceania and the Far East.

### 17 The answer is B *Medicine*

*Pasteurella multocida* (choice **B**) is the organism that most commonly infects the deep puncture wounds characteristic of cat bites. Signs of infection arise within 24 hours. There is also a potential for developing tendinitis and osteomyelitis. *P. multocida* responds to amoxicillin, penicillin G, or ampicillin.

*Staphylococcus aureus* (choice **C**), *Pseudomonas aeruginosa* (choice **E**), and group A streptococci (choice **D**) are not common pathogens in cat bites with symptoms presenting in the first 24 hours. *Bartonella henselae* (choice **A**) is the cause of cat-scratch fever. In this disease, there are granulomatous microabscesses in lymph nodes draining the infection site. In all bites (animal and human), the mainstay of therapy is proper cleansing of the wound with soap and water. All bites on the extremities should be treated aggressively because of the potential for septic arthritis and tenosynovitis. Antimicrobial amoxicillin prophylaxis is recommended for all human bites and most cat bites (due to *Eikenella corrodens*) (choice **F**). High-risk dog bites requiring antibiotic prophylaxis (e.g., amoxicillin) are those on the hand, those associated with puncture wounds, and wounds that are more than 6–12 hours old.

The risk of tetanus is always greater in contaminated wounds, puncture wounds, and wounds that come late to medical attention. In general, tetanus toxoid protects a person for 10 years. Tetanus immunoglobulin is reserved for dirty wounds in persons who have never been immunized (never received the primary series of three doses of tetanus toxoid) or whose status is unknown. If more than 5 years have elapsed since the last booster shot, a tetanus booster should be administered for a dirty wound (bite).

The decision for rabies prophylaxis in animal bites depends on the circumstance of the bite and the local prevalence of rabies. In this country, rabies is most commonly contracted from the bites of bats, skunks (most common), raccoons, and squirrels rather than dogs. In dogs or cats, a period of 10 days is sufficient to determine whether the animal is rabid. Strays or wild animals should be sacrificed and examined for rabies. If postexposure prophylaxis is required, washing the wound with soap and water is the first step in management. Half the dose of rabies immune globulin should be administered in the wound site and the other half in the gluteal region. Rabies vaccine is administered the same day and given at varying time intervals. Without treatment, there is a 100% fatality rate.

### 18 The answer is C   *Obstetrics & Gynecology*

Ovarian tumors are more likely to be benign than malignant in women younger than 45 years. They are classified into the following categories: surface-derived (65%–75% of tumors), germ cell (15%–20% of tumors), sex-cord stromal (3%–5% of tumors), and metastatic (5% of cases). Surface-derived cancers arise from coelomic epithelium and have the greatest number of malignant ovarian tumors. Germ cell tumors derive from primitive cells that differentiate along gonadal cell lines (e.g., dysgerminoma, most common malignant germ cell tumor), somatic cell lines (e.g., teratoma), and extraembryonic lines (e.g., yolk sac tumor, most common malignant germ cell tumor in children). Sex cord-stromal tumors derive from stromal cells and may be hormone-producing (e.g., estrogens, androgens). Breast cancer and stomach cancer are the most common cancers that metastasize to the ovaries. Risk factors for malignant tumors include nulliparity (increased number of ovulatory cycles increases the risk for surface-derived cancers), genetic factors (e.g., mutations of BRCA 1 and 2 suppressor genes), chromosomal aberrations (namely, Turner syndrome), and cigarette smoking. Oral contraceptives decrease the risk for surface-derived cancers by decreasing the number of ovulations.

There are varied clinical presentations for ovarian tumors. Malignant surface-derived tumors often spread by seeding and produce malignant ascites and increased abdominal girth. The ovaries of a postmenopausal woman are not usually palpable, because they undergo atrophy. Therefore, a palpable ovary in a postmenopausal woman is likely to be a primary ovarian cancer or an ovary with foci of metastatic cancer. Malignant pleural effusions are a common presentation of ovarian tumors. A number of ovarian tumors produce calcifications that are visible by x-ray; these include cystic teratomas (this case), gonadal-blastomas, and fibromas. Finally, ovarian tumors may present with signs of feminization (estrogen-secreting tumors, e.g., granulosa cell tumor) or masculinization (androgen-secreting tumors, e.g., Sertoli cell tumor). CA 125 is a tumor marker for surface-derived tumors.

The patient in this question has a cystic teratoma (choice **C**), which has undergone torsion, causing abdominal pain. Teratomas are the most common benign germ cell tumor. Common ectodermal derivatives include hair, sebaceous glands, teeth, and neuroepithelium. Examples of endodermal derivatives include gastrointestinal tissue and thyroid tissue. Common mesodermal derivatives include muscle, cartilage, and bone. Most of these derivatives are found in a nipple-like structure in the cyst wall called a Rokitansky tubercle. In rare cases, squamous epithelium in a teratoma may undergo malignant transformation and produce a squamous cell carcinoma. A struma ovarii type of teratoma has functioning thyroid tissue and is a rare cause of hyperthyroidism. The treatment for a cystic teratoma is surgical removal of the tumor.

A follicular cyst (choice **A**) is the most common ovarian mass in young women. It is due to an accumulation of fluid in a follicle or previously ruptured follicle. These may rupture and produce a sterile peritonitis with abdominal pain. An ultrasound is useful in identifying the cyst. There are no calcifications. A mucinous cystadenoma (choice **B**) is a benign surface-derived tumor that is lined by mucous-secreting cells (recapitulates endocervical epithelium). An ultrasound shows a large, multiloculated tumor without calcifications. A Brenner's tumor (choice **D**) is a benign surface-derived tumor that contains Walthard rests (transitional-like epithelium). It is commonly associated with benign mucinous cystadenomas. An ultrasound shows a solid ovarian mass without calcifications. A serous cystadenoma (choice **E**) is the most common benign tumor of the ovaries. It is a surface-derived tumor that is commonly bilateral. It is lined by ciliated cells (recapitulates fallopian tube epithelium). An ultrasound shows a cystic mass without calcifications.

**19** **The answer is A** *Preventive Medicine and Public Health*

This is a cohort study (choice **A**) because all subjects are free of illness at the start of the study.

In a case-control study (choice **B**), ill subjects (cases) and well subjects (controls) are compared with respect to a risk factor. In a randomized controlled clinical trial (choice **C**), some members of a cohort with a specific disorder are given one treatment and other members of the cohort are given a different treatment or a placebo. In a cross-sectional study (choice **D**), subjects are studied at a specific point in time. In a crossover study (choice **E**), some subjects receive the drug first while others receive the placebo first; later in the study, the groups switch treatments.

**20** **The answer is E** *Psychiatry*

This patient's presenting symptoms are most suggestive of a manic episode, which is characterized by an irritable, elevated, or euphoric mood, coupled with increased psychomotor activity, decreased need for sleep, grandiosity, and deterioration of judgment. Her most likely diagnosis is bipolar I disorder, manic phase, single episode. Bipolar I disorder is characterized by one or more episodes of mania that are not substance induced or due to a general medical condition. It is usually first evident in the third decade, but many exceptions exist. Its incidence is between 0.5% and 2%, and it is equally common in both sexes. There is no relationship to socioeconomic status. In bipolar I disorder, the lifetime chance of another episode is greater than 90% (choice **E**).

Therefore, choices **A** (5%), **B** (25%), **C** (50%), and **D** (75%) are incorrect. The chance of developing further episodes of other mental disorders varies. For example, the lifetime chance of another episode of depression following major depressive disorder, single episode, is approximately 50%. The chance of schizophrenia following the onset of schizophreniform disorder is between 33% and 50%.

**21** **The answer is D** *Surgery*

The patient has ascending cholangitis (choice **D**), which results from concurrent biliary tract infection and obstruction (e.g., by a stone, stricture, or neoplasm). Attacks are often precipitated by heavy fatty meals. The classic Charcot triad is colicky, right upper quadrant pain; fever; and jaundice to which, in cholangitis, can be added mental status change and sepsis. Laboratory studies reveal an absolute neutrophilic leukocytosis, direct hyperbilirubinemia, and elevation of alkaline phosphatase and γ-glutamyltransferase, which are increased in obstructive jaundice. Infection and subsequent sepsis may result from infection by *Escherichia coli*, *Klebsiella* species, enterobacteria, enterococci, and/or group D streptococci. Although 95% of the patients who present this way have common duct stone obstruction, only a small minority of patients with acute cholecystis present in this manner. This presentation is associated with infection, which often results from repeated attacks, as in the case described in the vignette. Septicemia frequently occurs as infected bile regurgitates into the liver and the liver sinusoids, and the tachycardia and hypotension are signs of septic shock. Ascending cholangitis is the most common cause of liver abscesses, because the infection extends into the portal triads. The initial treatment is with intravenous antibiotics. If the inflammation does not subside, then surgery is indicated to decompress the common bile duct and remove the source of obstruction. The mortality rate approaches 90% in untreated patients.

Acute hepatitis (choice **B**) is not associated with colicky pain and has a mixed indirect and direct hyperbilirubinemia. Acute pancreatitis (choice **C**) presents with a steady, boring, midepigastric pain, with radiation into the back or periumbilical area. Jaundice is unusual. An amebic liver abscess (choice **A**) does not present with colicky pain or jaundice. The organisms drain into the liver via the portal vein from a primary site of infection in the cecum. Sclerosing pericholangitis (choice **E**) is most commonly associated with ulcerative colitis.

**22** **The answer is E** *Medicine*

When preproinsulin in the β islet cell is delivered to the Golgi apparatus, proteolytic reactions generate insulin and a cleavage peptide called C-peptide. Therefore, C-peptide is a marker for endogenous synthesis of insulin. Injection of human insulin (choice **E**) increases serum insulin and produces hypoglycemia. Hypoglycemia suppresses β islet cells, causing a decrease in endogenous synthesis of insulin and a corresponding decrease in serum C-peptide. In this case, the nurse was titering her glucose level so that she would show clear symptoms of hypoglycemia without invoking serious central nervous consequences (serum levels below 50 mg/dL). Her motivation is to get time off with pay, an external motivation. Consequently, she is malingering. It is not a factitious disorder (choice **F**) because to be so the motivation must be internal, driven by a psychologic need.

Benign tumors of the β islet cells (choice **A**), or insulinomas, synthesize excess insulin, causing a severe fasting hypoglycemia. Both serum insulin and serum C-peptide levels are increased. Serum C-peptide is decreased in this patient. Ectopic secretion of an insulin-like factor (choice **B**) that causes hypoglycemia is most often produced by a hepatocellular carcinoma. Since the insulin-like factor is not measured in the serum as insulin, hypoglycemia suppresses β islet cells, resulting in a decrease in serum insulin and C-peptide. The patient has an increase in serum insulin and a decrease in C-peptide. Malignant tumors of α islet cells (choice **C**) secrete glucagon, which produces hyperglycemia by stimulating gluconeogenesis. The patient has hypoglycemia. Pancreatic carcinomas (choice **D**) usually develop in the head of the pancreas, causing obstruction of the common bile duct and an obstructive type of jaundice. The patient does not have jaundice. Furthermore, pancreatic carcinomas do not secrete insulin or insulin-like factors to produce hypoglycemia.

**23** **The answer is E** *Medicine*

The patient has Cushing syndrome, which is a state of hypercortisolism. There are several causes. Iatrogenic Cushing syndrome, which occurs most commonly in a patient taking corticosteroids, is the major non-pathologic cause. Pituitary Cushing syndrome is the most common pathologic cause of Cushing syndrome (~60% of cases). It is most often due to a benign pituitary adenoma secreting adrenocorticotropic hormone (ACTH). Adrenal Cushing syndrome and ectopic Cushing syndrome account for the remainder of causes of the syndrome. Adrenal Cushing syndrome is most often due to a benign adenoma secreting cortisol. The excess cortisol suppresses plasma ACTH. Ectopic Cushing syndrome is most often caused by a small-cell carcinoma of the lung with ectopic production of ACTH.

Clinical findings in Cushing syndrome are protean and parallel the excessive production of cortisol, weak mineralocorticoids (e.g., deoxycorticosterone), and 17-ketosteroids, which are weak androgens (e.g., dehydroepiandrosterone sulfate). Truncal obesity is a characteristic finding. Excess fat is distributed in the face ("moon face"), cervical area ("buffalo hump"), and abdomen, with sparing of the extremities. This peculiar distribution is due to the lipogenic effect of insulin, which is released in response to hyperglycemia caused by hypercortisolism (cortisol is a gluconeogenic hormone). Since most of the substrates for gluconeogenesis derive from amino acids, and amino acids are in abundance in muscle tissue, muscle catabolism is prominent in the arm and leg muscles. Wide purple striae are secondary to weak subcutaneous tissue and vessel instability, leading to ecchymoses and bleeding into the stretch marks. This tissue instability is the result of the inhibitory effect of cortisol on collagen synthesis. Hypertension in Cushing syndrome is associated with increased release of weak mineralocorticoids and subsequent retention of sodium. Hirsutism is due to an increased concentration of 17-ketosteroids, which are weak androgens. The plethoric face is due to vessel engorgement from secondary polycythemia induced by cortisol-enhanced erythropoiesis. Severe osteoporosis can result from cortisol's potentiation of the effects of parathyroid hormone and vitamin D on bone. Menstrual irregularities (usually amenorrhea) and mental aberrations round out the clinical picture. Hypercortisolism has an effect on the leukocyte count. Cortisol decreases neutrophil adhesion to endothelial cells, resulting in a neutrophilic leukocytosis; increases adhesion of lymphocytes in efferent lymphatics, which produces lymphopenia; and is cytotoxic to eosinophils, causing eosinopenia.

Laboratory testing for pathologic causes of Cushing syndrome involves the use of screening tests to establish the diagnosis and other tests to determine the type of Cushing syndrome. After documenting an increased level of serum cortisol, most clinicians screen for Cushing syndrome with a low-dose (1 mg) dexamethasone (an analogue of cortisol) suppression test (choice **E**) to see if the high-baseline cortisol can be suppressed to less than 5 μg/dL. Patients with pituitary, adrenal, and ectopic Cushing syndrome do not suppress cortisol below 5 μg/dL. False-positive results can occur in stressed patients and in obese patients. There is an increased false-positive loss of the normal diurnal rhythm of serum cortisol (high at 8 AM and low at

4 PM) in stressed or obese individuals; therefore, loss of a diurnal rhythm is not a useful screening test (choice **B**). Another excellent screening test is a 24-hour urine collection for free cortisol. This test, along with a low-dose dexamethasone suppression test, clearly confirms the presence of Cushing syndrome; however, they do not provide information as to the cause of the syndrome.

To determine the type of Cushing syndrome, the high-dose dexamethasone test (8 mg/day) has the highest specificity. Hypercortisolism in pituitary Cushing syndrome can be suppressed, whereas that associated with adrenal and ectopic Cushing syndrome cannot be suppressed. Plasma ACTH is also a useful study. Patients with adrenal Cushing syndrome have decreased levels, those with pituitary Cushing syndrome have normal to slightly increased levels, and patients with ectopic Cushing syndrome have extremely high concentrations.

A captopril-enhanced renal radionuclide test (choice **A**) is used to document renovascular hypertension, which is most commonly due to atherosclerosis of the renal artery in elderly men or fibromuscular hyperplasia of the renal artery in young to middle-aged women. Other than hypertension, renovascular hypertension has no other parallel signs and symptoms with Cushing syndrome. The clonidine suppression test (choice **C**) is used to confirm pheochromocytoma caused by a tumor secreting excess catecholamines. Clonidine is a centrally acting adrenergic drug that cannot suppress the excessive catecholamines associated with a pheochromocytoma. A pheochromocytoma presents with paroxysmal hypertension, drenching sweats, and excessive anxiety, findings that are not present in this patient. A bone marrow examination (choice **D**), ostensibly as a workup of polycythemia in this patient, is not indicated.

### 24 The answer is D *Obstetrics and Gynecology*

Primary amenorrhea is defined as absence of menses by age 14 without breast development, or by age 16 with breast development. It can be classified into four groups based on the presence or absence of normal breast development and the presence or absence of a palpable uterus. This woman, with normal breast development but without a uterus, has either complete androgen insensitivity or müllerian agenesis. In the former syndrome, a genetic male has a congenital lack of androgen receptors and so the normal male levels of testosterone are unrecognized. Development takes place in a female direction. Breast development is a response to normal testicular estrogen production. Normal female hormonal status is associated with congenital uterine absence, including normal low female levels of testosterone. Thus, measurement of serum testosterone (choice **D**) would be the most useful test for this patient.

Follicle-stimulating hormone (FSH) determination (choice **A**) is helpful for differentiating the cause of primary amenorrhea with absent breasts but uterus present. An elevated FSH level indicates absence of functional ovarian follicles, whereas a low FSH level indicates a hypothalamic–pituitary problem. Luteinizing hormone (LH) assay (choice **B**) is not helpful because it normally fluctuates significantly during a normal menstrual cycle. Prolactin (choice **C**) and progesterone (choice **E**) levels do not contribute to the workup of primary amenorrhea.

### 25 The answer is D *Obstetrics and Gynecology*

The case describes anhydramnios, or absent amniotic fluid. Marked deficiency in amniotic fluid volume may occur with decreased production or excessive removal of fluid. A serious consequence of oligohydramnios (amniotic fluid index <5 cm), regardless of cause, is umbilical cord compression leading to fetal hypoxia. The most serious consequence of anhydramnios is pulmonary hypoplasia, a lethal condition. The only option of the five provided that leads to anhydramnios is renal agenesis (choice **D**).

Polyhydramnios (amniotic fluid index of >25 cm) is found with each of the other options: duodenal atresia (choice **A**), more common with Down syndrome; open spina bifida (choice **B**), often diagnosed by an elevated maternal serum α-fetoprotein test; tracheoesophageal fistula (choice **C**), especially when the esophagus is a blind pouch; and atrial flutter (choice **E**), resulting in nonimmune hydrops.

### 26 The answer is C *Psychiatry*

Hearing impairment (choice **C**) is the most likely cause for this boy's poor communication ability and classroom problems. Sensory impairment is an important differential diagnosis for symptoms that suggest mental retardation, learning disorders, or communication disorders. Such children may appear to learn more slowly because they miss many cues. They may become frustrated and develop other behavioral disturbances.

Autistic disorder (choice **A**) is unlikely because the boy is affectionate and engaged with his environment. Food allergies (choice **B**) have not been clearly linked to behavioral problems. Schizophrenia (choice **D**) is very rare in children of this age and would often be manifested by a preoccupation with internal stimuli. Seizure disorder (choice **E**) might cause cognitive disturbances, but these should be detectable with IQ testing.

### 27 **The answer is A** *Psychiatry*

The symptoms are most suggestive of body dysmorphic disorder (choice **A**), a pathologic preoccupation with an imagined (or very minor) defect in appearance. The body parts most often involved are the nose, breasts, and thighs. The increased availability and effectiveness of reconstructive surgery have made diagnosis of this disorder more important. Surgical intervention is often ineffective in resolving it.

Delusional disorder, somatic type (choice **B**), is distinguished from body dysmorphic disorder by the presence of patently false beliefs about one's body. Delusional disorder may be associated with body dimorphic disorder. However, the onset of delusional disorder is generally in middle age or later, whereas body dysmorphic disorder generally starts in adolescence. Hypochondriasis (choice **C**) is characterized by misinterpretation of physical signs or symptoms. This patient shows no clear symptoms of depression (choice **D**). Somatization disorder (choice **E**) is characterized by the presence of many physical symptoms, especially pain.

### 28 **The answer is A** *Obstetrics and Gynecology*

The case scenario describes vaginal passage of grapelike vesicles, which are the markedly hydropic avascular villi found with a complete mole. Most hydatidiform moles are "complete," and have a 46, XX karyotype (choice **A**). All complete molar chromosomes are of paternal origin. Most complete moles arise from an anuclear ovum that is fertilized by a haploid sperm, which then duplicates its own chromosomes.

About 10% of complete moles have a 46, XY chromosomal pattern (choice **C**). This karyotype arises from fertilization of an anuclear ovum by two spermatozoa. While the chromosomes in the complete mole are entirely of paternal origin, the mitochondrial DNA is of maternal origin. A 45, X karyotype (choice **D**) is characteristic of gonadal dysgenesis, with the X chromosome maternally derived; the opposite of molar pregnancy. "Incomplete," or partial, moles often present with a coexistent fetus and have triploid karyotypes, most commonly 69, XXY (choice **E**) and less commonly 69, XXX (choice **B**).

### 29 **The answer is D** *Medicine*

The brown recluse spider (choice **D**), *Loxosceles reclusea*, is also known as the violin or fiddleback spider because of a dark violin-shaped design on its back. It has a habitat limited to the south-central part of the United States, centered near Shreveport, Louisiana. It is a shy creature that prefers dark, undisturbed areas, but it will bite if disturbed. Its bite is venomous, with symptoms varying from only an erythematous spot that clears up almost unnoticed to symptoms similar to those described, which may also include generalized pruritus, arthralgias, and, as it heals, severe pain; a death has never been reported. At one time, surgical débridement was recommended but was found to delay recovery. There is no antivenom or other recommended treatment other than oral administration of the antibiotic dapsone. Whereas the range of the true recluse spider *L. reclusea* is limited to an area roughly extending into eastern Texas to Alabama on the south and northward paralleling the Mississippi into Missouri, another 12 species of *Loxosceles* belong to the recluse family. The habitat of most of these spiders extends across the Southwest from Louisiana to the Pacific, mostly in desert areas; another species, the "Hobo spider," inhabits the Northwest, primarily Washington and Oregon. These spiders have habits similar to *L. reclusea*, but their bite usually is not as toxic, and the violin on their backs may be difficult, or even impossible, to see.

Red fire ants (*Solenopsis invecta*; choice **A**) were introduced into Mobile Bay in the ballast of ships coming from South America in the late 1920s or early 1930s and since have spread across the southern tier of states from the Atlantic to the Pacific. They are a very aggressive species, an expensive nuisance, and their bite is painful. It creates a red swollen area that will become a sterile pustule. Other than a remote chance of anaphylactic shock (<5%), the bite is not a health hazard. Six *Latrodectus* species of black widow spiders (choice **B**) live in the United States. In all species, the females have yellow to red markings on their abdomen. This clearly looks like an hourglass among the southern species, but is less so among the northern ones. All are shy, nocturnal, web-weaving animals in which the females inject neurotoxic venom that is 15 times more toxic than prairie rattlesnake venom. However, they inject so little that it is only mortally dangerous to the very young, old, and debilitated. Nonetheless, even healthy adults will develop severe abdominal pain, muscle pain, pain under the soles of their feet, alternating periods of dry mouth and excess salvation, perfuse sweat, swollen eyelids, and partial paralysis of the diaphragm. Typically, symptoms decrease in a day or so and clear up within several days. Antivenom is available.

A deer tick, *Ixodes scapularis*, bite (choice **D**) in and of itself does little harm but may transmit *Borrelia burgdorferi*, the organism that transmits Lyme disease. The habitat of this tick is in the northeast and north central states. In the far west, *Ixodes pacificus* serves as the vector spreading Lyme disease.

There are some 90 scorpion species in the United States, but only one, *Centruroides exilicauda*, has a venomous sting (choice **E**). *C. exilicauda*'s habitat is in the deserts of Arizona and eastern California, and its venom causes severe but rarely fatal symptoms. Antivenom is available.

### 30 The answer is B  *Medicine*

This patient has hypertrophic cardiomyopathy. The history of syncope, dyspnea, and chest pain are secondary to decreased outflow and obstruction. During systole, the left ventricular outflow is decreased due to decreased chamber volume and displacement of the anterior mitral valve leaflet forward. In addition, the aortic valve closes prematurely and reopens thereafter. All these factors play a role in the symptomatology. Patients with hypertrophic cardiomyopathy can die suddenly due to dangerous ventricular arrhythmias. Atenolol, a β blocker, will slow the heart and allow more time for diastolic filling, thereby enhancing the outflow volume and decreasing obstruction to some extent. In almost 50% of cases, symptoms of chest pain, dyspnea, and arrhythmias, if present, will be relieved.

Choice **A** is incorrect. Digoxin will increase cardiac contractility, which is not the problem here. It will further compromise the volume of blood being released into the greater circulation, and may lead to ventricular arrhythmias, with disastrous consequences. Choice **C**, diltiazem, is incorrect. Calcium channel blockers like diltiazem or verapamil can be administered to improve diastolic function, which accounts for initial improvement, but they also induce peripheral vasodilatation, which then increases outflow obstruction, leading to deterioration. The patient may feel better initially, only to feel worse later. Choice **D** is incorrect; furosemide or other diuretics are not indicated here because this patient does not have cardiac failure and fluid retention. Choice **E** is incorrect; an angiotensin-converting enzyme inhibitor (ACE inhibitor) is indicated in dilated cardiomyopathy.

### 31 The answer is C  *Surgery*

The nurse suspects that the patient has idiopathic scoliosis (choice **C**). The school screening test for this disorder is called the Adam's forward-bending test. By assuming this near 90-degree bent position, abnormal lateral curvature (S or C shape) of the spine is easy to observe. Confirmation is generally made by an imaging study in which the degree of curvature is determined by a geometrical process called the Cobb method. A curvature greater than 25 degrees is considered significant, greater than 45–50 degrees is considered severe. In the United States, the prevalence of scoliosis greater than 25 degrees is 1.5 cases per 1,000; most states have mandatory screening by a school nurse by the fifth or sixth grade. Scoliosis is most commonly idiopathic and often is first diagnosed in adolescent girls from 10 to 16 years of age. Scoliosis refers to lateral displacement of the spine, while kyphosis refers to forward displacement (e.g., hunchback) of the spine. A third type of unusual spinal shape is called lordosis (aka, sway back); this is not considered pathologic as long as the back remains flexible.

Pott's disease of the spine (choice **B**) refers to tuberculosis involving the vertebral column. Ankylosing spondylitis (choice **A**) is a human leukocyte antigen (HLA)-B27–positive arthropathy that is more common in men. Sacroiliitis and fusion of the spine (bamboo spine) are prominent features of this disease. Forward bending of the spinal column becomes increasingly more pronounced as the disease progresses. Osteomyelitis (choice **D**) does not typically produce spinal abnormalities. Neurofibromatosis (choice **E**) is associated with kyphoscoliosis; however, café au lait spots are likely to be present as well.

### 32 The answer is A  *Preventive Medicine and Public Health*

The question relates to assessing the statistic validity of differences in a continuous variable, which in this question are Apgar scores between two groups: babies born vaginally and those born by cesarean delivery. Statistical comparison of continuous variable data between two groups can best be assessed by Student's *t*-test (choice **A**), which, by the way, is named after a Dr. Student.

If the comparison were between two groups with a categorical variable, a chi-squared test (choice **D**) would be correct. If the comparison were among three groups with a continuous variable, analysis of variance (choice **B**) would be correct. A correlation coefficient (choice **C**) assesses the strength of association, not differences between groups. Logistic regression (choice **E**) is used to assess a categorical outcome for a continuous predictor.

### 33 The answer is C *Obstetrics and Gynecology*

The clear fluid leaking through the patient's vagina is probably urine. The history of painless, continuous vaginal leakage of urine with a recent pelvic surgery suggests the diagnosis of a fistula between the vagina and the urinary tract. Fistulas between the urinary tract and reproductive tract occur more frequently after radical pelvic surgery or pelvic radiation therapy. Intravenous (IV) indigo carmine (choice C), which is excreted in the urine and discolors a vaginal tampon, is the diagnostic modality of choice.

The other choices contribute nothing toward ruling out a fistula. Cystometry (choice A) assesses bladder pressure–volume relationships. Urine culture (choice B) identifies a urinary tract infection. Pelvic sonography (choice D) looks for pelvic masses. Urethral pressure measurements (choice E) are helpful in working up genuine stress incontinence.

### 34 The answer is A *Surgery*

The patient has Leriche syndrome (choice A). This is due to aortoiliac atherosclerotic disease and is characterized by claudication on walking, atrophy of the calf muscles, diminished or absent femoral pulses, and impotence from involvement of the hypogastric arteries.

A herniated lumbar disk (choice B) would not have a claudication history or problems with femoral pulses, and motor and sensory deficits would be present as well. Osteoarthritis in the hip (choice C) produces pain that is relieved by the use of a cane. It is not associated with vascular findings including impotence. Phlegmasia alba dolens (choice D) is a variant of femoral vein thrombosis in which femoral artery spasm occurs; this produces a pale, cool leg with increased pulses. A peripheral neuropathy (choice E) has both sensory and motor abnormalities. It does not disappear with rest.

### 35 The answer is A *Obstetrics and Gynecology*

Rubella is a highly contagious viral syndrome with potentially disastrous pregnancy impact. With the presence of rubella antibodies, there is lifelong immunity and a fetus in a subsequent pregnancy is protected. Without antibodies present, as in this scenario, the fetus is susceptible. The best answer is to avoid exposure to known rubella infections (choice A). The risk of rubella exposure is almost negligible since no cases of rubella originating in the United States have been documented since 2004.

Postpartum vaccination with the live attenuated virus vaccine is appropriate but there is no need to avoid breastfeeding (choice B). Pregnancy should be avoided for 1 month, not 3 months, as in choice C. Amniocentesis for amniotic fluid culture (choice D) is an unnecessary invasive procedure in an uninfected gravida. γ-Globulin (choice E) is not indicated for prophylaxis.

### 36 The answer is A *Psychiatry*

Isolation (choice A) describes the separation of a thought from its attached emotional tone, thereby making it tolerable. This defense mechanism is often used during highly stressful events. Depersonalization (choice B) and derealization (choice E) are other defenses that involve dissociation of mental functions, but both are more often accompanied by anxiety. Disorientation (choice C) and intellectualization (choice D) are not accompanied by odd calmness.

### 37 The answer is D *Medicine*

Syncope is caused by decreased blood flow to the brain. Passing out when blood flow to the brain is compromised for even a few seconds is a physiological defense mechanism; by assuming a prone position it becomes easier for the heart to pump blood to the head, and typically the person rapidly wakes from the faint. While the initiating factor may be something worrisome, as a rule a faint is triggered by something relatively innocuous, very often a vasovagal response to some emotional or physical factor. Vagus activation lowers blood pressure and slows the heart rate, momentarily limiting blood flow to the brain. In the case described, the triggering factors are a physical response to the sudden release of the pressure caused by splitting the cast plus the emotional response caused by first seeing the atrophied state of the lower limb being exposed (choice D). Common triggering factors include emotional stresses such as fear, having blood drawn, watching an operation or childbirth, loss of a loved one, a first kiss, etc.; or physical factors such as pain, having a difficult bowel movement, lifting weights, etc.

Although feeling that the football player was a sissy (choice A) may help the other boy's ego, it obviously has little to do with his fainting. Orthostatic hypotension (choice B) is a common cause of syncope, or at least of dizziness. When a person stands up, blood is drawn down into the legs by gravity; it has been estimated that this can result in as much as 20% of the total circulating volume being delivered to the legs, briefly depriving the heart, and consequently the brain, of that volume. Since the boy would be sitting while the cast was split, this could not be the mechanism responsible for his faint. A cardiac problem such as ventricular fibrillation, a defective valve, or hypertropic cardiac myopathy (choice **C**) could also cause a faint or even worse; however, such serious triggers are rare, particularly in a healthy young person. A postprandial rush of blood to the digestive system could also cause a faint (choice **E**) but in itself is an unlikely cause; however, it may have been a contributing factor in the case described since eating a heavy meal would have directed more blood to the digestive system prior to the stress of having his cast split.

### 38 The answer is C *Preventive Medicine and Public Health*

Whereas smoking ranks high for both sexes it was the most common avoidable cause among men, causing 248,000 deaths in 2005. For women, it was the second most common cause, responsible for 219,000 deaths. (A decade or so earlier, the influence of smoking on the death of women was much less.) In 2005, the factor causing the greatest number of deaths among women was hypertension, being responsible for 231,000 deaths; conversely, during this same year, high blood pressure killed 164,000 males. The difference has been speculated to reflect a societal belief that hypertension is more prevalent among males, thus resulting in less attention to blood pressure among females. Physical inactivity was the third most prevalent avoidable cause of death among women, responsible for 103,000 deaths; in men, it ranked fifth, causing 88,000 deaths. Thus, high blood pressure and physical inactivity (choice **C**) are two avoidable death-promoting factors that are greater than 10% more relevant for women than for men.

Excess weight and high blood sugar (choice A), low intake of omega-3 fats and smoking (choice **B**), and high intake of trans fats and low intake of fruits and vegetables (choice **D**) are all factors responsible for more deaths in men than in women. Although salt consumption among women is suspected of resulting in more deaths among women than among men (54,000 vs. 49,000), more men than women die from high blood sugar (choice **E**; 102,000 vs. 80,000).

### 39 The answer is C *Medicine*

Reactive arthritis (choice **C**), formerly known as Reiter's syndrome, commonly surfaces several weeks after a bacterial infection. In males, this is most commonly due to a venereal infection, most often with *Chlamydia trachoma*; however, it may be triggered by different organisms, and less often, in both sexes, by digestive tract infections. The name *reactive arthritis* was coined because the symptoms are a reaction to such an infection. Typically, large joints, such as the lower back, hips, knees, and ankles are affected, often with Achilles tendonitis and/or plantar fasciitis. Additionally, conjunctivitis or even uveitis frequently occurs. A small percentage of affected individuals develop small hard nodules on the soles of their feet and less often on their palms, as well as mouth ulcers. Approximately 20%–40% of affected men develop shallow ulcers on the head of the penis, as well as a penile discharge. To treat the arthritis, the infection must first be cured; initially, the pain is treated with analgesics. As a rule, the symptoms are self-limiting but those that linger on must be treated accordingly.

Rheumatoid arthritis is not contagious; thus, it could not have been caught from the nurse (choice **A** is incorrect); neither could it develop due to exposure to cold. Consequently, choice **B** also is incorrect. Ankylosing arthritis (choice **D**) and psoriatic arthritis (choice **E**) are classified as spondyloarthropathies, along with Crohn's disease, ulcerative colitis, and reactive arthritis because of similarities, but all have identifying distinctive clinical presentations.

### 40 The answer is B *Medicine*

The International Continence Society defines overactive bladder (OAB; choice **B**) as a syndrome of symptoms consisting of urgency with or without urgency urinary incontinence (UUI), often associated with urinary frequency and nocturia. Studies demonstrate that the prevalence rate for OAB ranges from 11.8% to 16.9%, increases dramatically with age, and is similar for both sexes. Despite the personal and societal costs, it remains underreported and undertreated; it has been estimated that only about 60% of cases are reported to physicians, and only about 27% are treated. Patients tend to avoid reporting incontinence problems because of embarrassment, a feeling that it is a normal consequence of aging, that there is no available treatment, and/or that no major morbidity is associated with it. Primary care physicians may avoid screening questions because they feel uncovering idiopathic incontinence will only reveal a nonvital condition to deal with in the short time allotted by Medicare standards. The initial goal in evaluating OAB is to determine whether it is idiopathic or if it is due to some specific underlying disease state that could be treated. However, once recognized, even idiopathic OAB is treatable. The first step is education and behavioral therapy; although this alone will not cure the condition, a patient may learn behaviors that will help keep his or her pants dry. Refractory cases are often treated with antimuscarinic drugs; however, long-term adherence is low because of uncomfortable side effects.

Stress incontinence (choice **A**) is the loss of urine due to extra pressure on the bladder caused by coughing, laughing, lifting something heavy—anything that creates extra pressure within the abdominal cavity, which then presses down upon the bladder. Normally, the sphincter muscles tighten up to prevent urine leakage when so stressed; however, if the muscles and ligaments of the pelvic floor are lax, the urethra has nothing to compress against as the bladder is pressed downward and leakage can occur. This condition is more common in women than in men as vaginal childbirth is a contributing factor. Overflow incontinence (choice **C**) occurs when the urethra is obstructed or if the bladder muscle contractions are weak, thus preventing complete voiding. As a result, the bladder becomes too full and eventually urine leaks out. This condition is most common in men because of an enlarged prostrate that blocks urine flow through the urethra. In women, this condition can occur in cases of prolapse of the uterus or bladder, creating a kink in the urethra. Patients with functional incontinence (choice **D**) have a normal urinary system but have mental or physical limitations that sometimes prevent them from getting to the toilet in time. Structural incontinence (choice **E**) relates to structural problems in the urinary system resulting in leakage. These are rare. Congenital anomalies are generally dealt with during infancy; structural problems arising in adulthood are generally due to accidents or wounds.

### 41 The answer is A  *Pediatrics*

This patient ingested prenatal vitamins (i.e., iron), one of the most common causes of childhood poisoning, and one that often causes death. The antidote for iron poisoning is deferoxamine mesylate (answer **A**), and it should be administered regardless of the serum iron level if the patient has moderate to severe symptoms (e.g., bloody diarrhea, hypotension, drowsiness) or if the patient's serum iron level exceeds 500 μg/dL, whether symptoms are present or not.

### 42 The answer is G  *Pediatrics*

This patient most likely received fentanyl, a synthetic opioid. Rapid IV administration can lead to a rigid chest wall and difficulty breathing. This effect may be reversed with naloxone hydrochloride (answer **G**) or may require a depolarizing muscle relaxant and mechanical ventilation until the patient recovers.

### 43 The answer is E  *Pediatrics*

This patient took isoniazid (INH). Initial manifestations may include nausea and vomiting, ataxia, tachycardia, mydriasis, and central nervous system depression, which may mimic an anticholinergic toxidrome. Acute INH overdose is associated with a triad consisting of seizures that are refractory to conventional therapy, severe metabolic acidosis, and coma.

When the diagnosis of INH overdose is established, or at the time it is strongly suspected, pyridoxine (vitamin $B_6$) (answer **E**) should be administered. INH is metabolized to hydrazines that, in overdose, cause a functional pyridoxine (vitamin $B_6$) deficiency. This occurs by inhibition of pyridoxine phosphokinase, the enzyme that converts pyridoxine to active $B_6$. Activated $B_6$ is required by glutamic acid decarboxylase to convert glutamic acid to γ-amino butyric acid (GABA), an inhibitory neurotransmitter. Decreased levels of GABA are thought to lead to seizures. Administration of pyridine alleviates seizures and may reverse coma and lactic acidosis.

### 44 The answer is D  *Pediatrics*

The fluorescence of the urine with a Wood's lamp confirms that the patient did ingest radiator fluid, or ethylene glycol. Many commercial antifreeze products have sodium fluorescein as an additive. Sodium fluorescein is renally excreted up to 6 hours after ingestion and may be detected when illuminated with a Wood's lamp. Fomepizole (answer **D**) is an effective competitive antagonist of alcohol dehydrogenase, inhibiting metabolism of ethylene glycol to toxic products. Its ease of dosing and lack of side effects are the major advantages of using fomepizole rather than ethanol. However, if fomepizole is not available, ethanol can still be used as an antidote. Both fomepizole and ethanol can also be used as an antidote for methanol poisoning.

## 45 The answer is F *Pediatrics*

This patient has methemoglobinemia, a blood disorder caused when nitrite interacts with the hemoglobin of the red blood cells. The nitrite can come from nitrate in drinking water, or from food (e.g., bacon, hot dogs), some drugs, or other sources. Blood samples appear chocolate brown and do not turn pink when exposed to air. A methemoglobin level can confirm the diagnosis. Methemoglobin can accumulate in red cells for three reasons: (1) a dominantly inherited abnormality in hemoglobin that prevents the reduction of methemoglobin to hemoglobin; (2) a recessively inherited deficiency in the enzyme methemoglobin reductase; or (3) exposure to hemoglobin-oxidizing chemicals or drugs, such as nitrates or nitrites contained in water and in some vegetables (such as carrots, spinach, zucchini, cauliflower, red beets), Xylocaine, or benzene derivatives. Infant methemoglobinemia, or *blue baby syndrome*, can be found in infants less than 6 months of age who are susceptible to methemoglobinemia because they have smaller amounts of the enzyme, NADH-cytochrome $B_5$ reductase, which converts methemoglobin back to hemoglobin. Nitrates in drinking water have been reported to be a primary cause of infantile methemoglobinemia. However, there have been reports of infantile methemoglobinemia in infants who became ill after being fed formula that was reconstituted with vegetable soup and nitrate-free water. The antidote for methemoglobinemia is methylene blue (answer **F**).

## 46 The answer is J *Pediatrics*

This patient has advanced digoxin toxicity and should receive purified digoxin-specific Fab antibody fragments (answer **J**) for rapid reversal. This antidote should be used for life-threatening digoxin toxicity and is indicated for life-threatening tachyarrhythmias, sinus bradyarrhythmias, severe AV blocks unresponsive to conventional therapy, and patients with serum potassium levels above 5 mEq/mL.

## 47 The answer is C *Pediatrics*

The patient has carbon monoxide poisoning as a result of indoor burning of charcoal briquettes. There are many reported cases of carbon monoxide poisoning secondary to indoor burning of charcoal briquettes for the purpose of either home heating or cooking. Most of these cases occur in the months of October through January, commonly during power outages or when electricity was intentionally disconnected.

Carbon monoxide toxicity occurs by displacing oxygen (it has an affinity for hemoglobin 250 times that of oxygen), impairing the ability of hemoglobin to release oxygen, and impeding oxygen use by binding cytochrome oxidase in tissues. These mechanisms cause tissue hypoxia. The antidote for carbon monoxide poisoning is 100% oxygen (answer **C**) via non-rebreather, or hyperbaric oxygen in severely poisoned patients. Early symptoms are nonspecific and can be confused with the flu, whereas higher concentrations can cause seizures, coma, respiratory instability, and death. Delayed therapy may cause permanent neurologic sequelae.

## 48 The answer is H *Pediatrics*

Acetaminophen overdose causes hepatic toxicity. Acetaminophen is rapidly absorbed from the gastrointestinal tract, with peak plasma levels usually occurring by 4 hours. Once absorbed, acetaminophen is metabolized by the liver by glucuronidation (60%) or sulfation (30%), and a small amount (4%–7%) is excreted unchanged in the urine. Approximately 4% of the ingested dose is metabolized by a hepatic cytochrome P450 mixed-function oxidase to an active toxic intermediate metabolite (NAPQI), which is normally detoxified by conjugation with glutathione. In cases of overdose, glutathione is rapidly depleted, and free unconjugated NAPQI can produce a centrilobular hepatic necrosis, which may progress to fulminant hepatic failure. There are four clinical stages of acetaminophen poisoning:

- Stage 1 occurs between 12 and 24 hours and is manifested by nausea, anorexia, vomiting, and diaphoresis.
- Stage 2 occurs between 24 and 48 hours and is characterized by resolution of above, right upper quadrant pain, and elevation of transaminases and the prothrombin time (PT). There may also be oliguria.
- Stage 3 occurs at 72–96 hours, and it is during this time that peak liver function abnormalities are seen, and nausea and vomiting may return.
- Stage 4 occurs at 4 days to 2 weeks, with either resolution of hepatic dysfunction or complete liver failure.

Although charcoal reduces the level of acetaminophen it will still be in the toxic range and *N*-acetylcysteine (answer **H**) is the antidote for acetaminophen toxicity. Indications for *N*-acetylcysteine include a toxic level on the Rumack-Matthew nomogram (a plot of the log of acetaminophen concentration versus hours after ingestion; a toxic level is one greater than the reference line); an ingested dose greater than 140 mg/kg with no level available within 8 hours; elevated liver function test results with a history of acetaminophen poisoning; and acetaminophen-induced hepatic injury.

**49** **The answer is I** *Pediatrics*

Pralidoxime (choice **I**) is administered as an antidote for the nicotinic effects of organophosphate poisoning, such as those described in question 49.

**50** **The answer is B** *Pediatrics*

Atropine (choice **B**) blocks the receptor site to decrease the stimulant effects produced by the muscarine-type poisons, but has no effect on nicotine receptors.

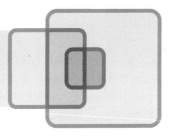

# test **12**

# Questions

**Single Best Choice Directions:** *This section consists of numbered statements or questions followed by a list of potential answers; you are to select the ONE best answer.*

**1** A 21-year-old nulligravid woman who has been married and sexually active for 2 years comes to the outpatient office complaining of pain with intercourse. She explains that the pain is worse with deep penetration. Although they have frequent sex and neither she nor her husband used any type of contraceptive since their marriage, she has not been able to get pregnant. The onset of her menarche was at age 11. Her menses were originally irregular but have been regular and predictable for the past 8 years. She has had pain with her menses, as well as pain with bowel movements, for the past 4 years. Laparoscopic examination shows diffuse involvement of her peritoneal surfaces with thickened, scarred, "powder-burn" implants of various sizes. Which one of the following statements concerning her probable diagnosis is correct?

(A) The most common site of lesions is the uterosacral ligaments.
(B) The most common site of lesions is the ovaries.
(C) The average age of onset is older than 35 years.
(D) The chance of malignant transformation is high.
(E) The relevant condition is associated with uterine leiomyomata.

**2** A 62-year-old woman recently was diagnosed with type 2 diabetes. She was told that her blood glucose levels should normally increase after a meal and decrease between meals. Consequently, she expected that her early morning serum glucose levels—obtained some 12 hours after her last meal—would naturally be lower than her bedtime level, obtained 2–3 hours after dinner. However, she observed that she typically had a higher serum level before breakfast than she had before bedtime the previous night. This made her worry that perhaps, in addition to being diabetic, she metabolized carbohydrates in some other abnormal fashion. As a result, she asked her physician to explain. Which of the following is a correct explanation?

(A) The livers of diabetic individuals are exposed to glucagon levels that are lower than normal and this decreases gluconeogenesis.
(B) Shortly before dawn, diabetics but not nondiabetics produce increased levels of cortisol and growth hormone.
(C) In both normal persons and diabetics, insulin resistance peaks shortly before dawn.
(D) Both normal individuals and diabetics produce increased levels of cortisol and growth hormone shortly before dawn.
(E) Eating dinner causes the liver to become loaded with glucose, which is suddenly released shortly before dawn in diabetics but not in nondiabetics.

**3** A 10-year-old child had an upper respiratory infection 5 days ago and was given aspirin for fever. She had seemingly recovered but now presents with fever, protracted vomiting, and lethargy. Physical examination reveals mild hepatomegaly. Total bilirubin, serum transaminases, and serum ammonia are increased. Cerebrospinal fluid (CSF) is obtained and is normal except for elevated pressure. Which of the following is the most likely diagnosis?

(A) Hepatitis A virus (HAV) infection
(B) Drug-induced hepatitis
(C) Reye syndrome
(D) Infectious mononucleosis
(E) Gilbert syndrome

**4** By 32 months of age, a male child had been unresponsive to normal stimuli since birth. He didn't smile or babble and was indifferent to his mother's attempts to kiss, hug, or socialize with him. He also had bizarre behavior patterns including repeating purposeless motions and banging on the floor or walls. Although able to talk, his choice of words and speech intonation was peculiar. However, he did like to play with his toy piano and could produce simple melodies. Physically, he seemed healthy. In which of the following ways does this developmental pattern trend typically describe diagnostic features of autistic disorder?

(A) It is a qualitative disturbance of normal development.

(B) It shows progressive deterioration of function over the developmental period.

(C) There is an absence of metabolic diseases.

(D) He showed evidence of a potential musical talent, presence of areas of brilliant accomplishment.

(E) Although noncommunicative, he seems of normal intelligence.

**5** A 26-day-old infant is brought to the emergency department with a temperature of 39.0°C (102.2°F). The mother is a 25-year-old gravida 2, para 2 who had good prenatal care. Culture of the cerebrospinal fluid (CSF), blood, and urine are sent for analysis. Prophylactic antibiotics are started. It is of paramount importance that the antibiotic treatment provides protection against which of the following pathogens?

(A) *Escherichia coli, Streptococcus pneumoniae,* and *Listeria monocytogenes*

(B) *Streptococcus pneumoniae, Neisseria meningitides,* and *Listeria monocytogenes*

(C) *Streptococcus agalactiae, Escherichia coli,* and *Listeria monocytogenes*

(D) *Streptococcus agalactiae, Escherichia coli,* and *Neisseria meningitides*

(E) *Neisseria meningitides, Streptococcus pneumoniae,* and *Streptococcus agalactiae*

**6** A 48-year-old Certified Public Accountant who gained 10 pounds during the recent busy tax preparation season celebrated the return of a less stressful work schedule by participating in a pickup basketball game with a group of men he met at lunch in a local tavern. As he made a jump shot, he felt a sharp pain in his left heel. The pain was accompanied by a popping noise. Although he could still walk, the ankle stiffened and he could no longer point with his toe or jump off. The injury this man suffered is most likely which one of the following choices?

(A) A repetitive strain injury

(B) An acute case of tendinitis

(C) A ruptured Achillis tendon

(D) An acute case of tendinosis

(E) A case of paratenonitis

**7** A pediatrician performs a physical examination on a newborn he is asked to evaluate. The pertinent findings he notes include severe hypotonia, generalized weakness, and absent tendon stretch reflexes. The baby lies flaccid with little movement, but there appears to be preservation of the extraocular muscle. The patient is also observed to have fasciculations of the tongue, and the nurse informs the pediatrician that the infant has had trouble feeding. Which of the following is the most likely diagnosis?

(A) Myotonic dystrophy

(B) Werdnig-Hoffmann disease

(C) Infant botulism

(D) Infantile myasthenia gravis

(E) Duchenne's muscular dystrophy

**8** A 48-year-old lady who worked as a coordinator for instructors preparing medical students for their board examinations paid a visit to her chiropractor because, during the past month, her wrists and fingers had become very stiff and painful. Moreover, she had a feeling of general malaise, fatigue, loss of energy, lack of appetite, low-grade fever, and also a generalized feeling of nonspecific aches, and stiffness. After two visits, the chiropractor referred her to a rheumatologist who told her he needed to get the results of several tests before he could make a definite diagnosis. Which one of the tests listed below would provide the most definitive diagnoses of the condition this lady was developing?

(A) Erythrocyte sedimentation rate

(B) C-reactive protein

(C) Anticyclic citrullinated peptide antibody

(D) Antinuclear antibody

(E) Rheumatoid factor

**9** A healthy 16-year-old girl moved with her family to Fairbanks, Alaska. Despite the fact that she dressed warmly and wore fur-lined mittens, during her first winter there, when the outside temperature hovered below 0°F, the skin on her fingers went through a series of different color changes. Initially, they felt uncomfortably cold, then became numb, turned white, then blue, and finally a bright red; during this phase, they also felt prickly and increasingly painful. This young person most likely suffered from which one of the following conditions?

(A) Raynaud's phenomenon

(B) Systemic lupus erythematosus

(C) Frostbite

(D) Raynaud disease

(E) Scleroderma

**10** A 66-year-old man with type 2 diabetes has had intractable systolic hypertension for some time. Presently, he is taking the following medications for hypertension: enalapril 20 mg b.i.d., labetalol 100 mg b.i.d., clonidine 0.3 mg t.i.d., doxazosin mesylate 8 mg h.s., amlodipine besylate 10 mg/hs, and hydrochlorothiazide 12.5 mg in the morning. Despite this regime, his systolic blood pressure is not well controlled. It generally is in the 170–190 mm Hg range when he wakes up in the morning. It tends to improve during the day, generally remaining between 140 and 150 mm Hg; however, it rarely gets below the 130 mm Hg desired by his cardiologist. He is 6 feet (1.83 meters) tall and weighs 178 pounds (80.7 kg). In addition to hypertension, he suffers from chronic headache and fatigue, often falling asleep in his chair while watching TV, and his wife complains about his snoring. Which one of the following tests would most likely best elucidate a factor that is at least partially responsible for his intractable systolic hypertension?

(A) A computed tomography scan of the brain
(B) A magnetic resonance study of his chest
(C) A comparison of his ankle and brachial blood pressure
(D) A measurement of his blood percent hemoglobin A1C
(E) A polysomnogram study

**11** A 78-year-old female was walking down the stairway after attending a performance by a symphony orchestra at a prestigious concert hall. Unfortunately, despite the fact that she was concentrating on stepping carefully, she tripped and fell. She was unable to rise and an ambulance was called. When seen in the emergency room, she was in considerable pain. On examination, her temperature was 36.5°C (97.7°F), pulse 100/min and irregular due to atrial fibrillation, blood pressure 102/80 mm Hg, and respirations 20/min. Her right thigh was swollen, and her right leg shortened and externally rotated. She is on anticoagulants for her cardiac problems. The most likely reason for her fall is which one of the following?

(A) She was distracted and not paying attention.
(B) Diminished reflex response due to aging
(C) Lack of depth perception
(D) Irregular cardiac rhythm
(E) Gait problems

**12** A 36-year-old man complains of stomach pain. When the physician tries to ask him questions, he answers, "You're the doctor; you figure it out." He also states that he does not like the physician's attitude and will sue if he is not treated appropriately. "If you make me leave the hospital," he adds, "I'll slit my wrists in the parking lot and it will be your fault."

Which of the following is the best first response to this patient?

(A) "Without better cooperation, I'll be forced to order a stat barium enema and then probably have to do exploratory surgery."
(B) "You make me feel unable to help you, and that hurts me personally."
(C) "You seem angry with me, and I'd like to know why."
(D) "You're an irritating person, and that makes me angry."
(E) "I'm sure that you'd like my colleague better— I'll page him right away."

**13** A mother becomes concerned as her daughter approaches puberty, because her husband has always played a prominent role in raising her and she always looks to him for signs of affection. The mother fears that their obvious intimacy will lead to sexual abuse, particularly as the girl develops more prominent womanly attributes. As a consequence of her fears, she attends a seminar concerning childhood sexual abuse with her husband, during which they learned about many facets of the subject. Which of the following statements did they learn is the most accurate?

(A) Increased involvement of fathers in raising children decreases the risk of sexual abuse.
(B) More men than women have a history of being abused.
(C) More traditional, less democratic families are associated with a decreased risk of childhood sexual abuse.
(D) Mothers who sexually abuse children are often gregarious and socially active.
(E) Most abused children were abused by fathers or stepfathers.

**14** A 20-year-old male complained of chest pains and difficulty in breathing. He was seen in the emergency room, and his vital signs were as follows: temperature, 37°C (98.6°F); pulse, 88/min, regular; blood pressure, mm Hg, 110/70; respirations 20/min; and, $O_2$ saturation on room air, 94%. Physical examination revealed a rather anxious patient with no pallor, icterus, or cyanosis. Jugular venous pressure (JVP) was normal. The apical pulse was in the fifth intercostal space in the mid-clavicular line, and a murmur was heard that extended throughout the cardiac cycle. The most likely cause for this murmur is which of the following?

(A) Aortic stenosis
(B) Mitral regurgitation
(C) Pericarditis
(D) Mitral stenosis
(E) Patent ductus arteriosus

**15** A 32-year-old soccer player has been hit hard on the right breast. Subsequently, while showering, she notes that a firm mass had developed. Worried, she makes an appointment with her gynecologist for further observation. Physical examination reveals a firm, nontender mass with no evidence of involvement of the overlying skin. Lymph nodes and the contralateral breast are normal. A biopsy reveals evidence of an in situ lobular carcinoma. Which one of the following best characterizes this breast cancer?

(A) Increased incidence of negative estrogen- and progesterone-receptor assays
(B) Aggressive natural history with early invasion of the breast stroma
(C) Increased likelihood of cancer developing in the other breast
(D) Increased incidence of chest wall involvement by this tumor
(E) Increased incidence of breast cancer in first- and second-degree relatives

**16** A married couple has been trying to have children of their own for the past 10 years; they are seriously considering adoption at this time. They think they may be getting a little old to adopt a newborn infant and consider an older child, but they worry about the psychologic stability of a child who may have been (or at least believe) he or she was abandoned by a biologic parent, or who may have been overlooked in the past by other couples wishing to adopt. Which one of the following statements about adoptees is most accurate?

(A) About 50% of adoptions are considered "successful."
(B) Improved family environments rarely raise IQ scores in such individuals.
(C) Narcissistic injury is a significant psychologic issue in such individuals.
(D) Rates of psychopathology among adopted individuals are comparable to the rates among individuals reared by their biologic parents.
(E) The relationships of adoptees with their adoptive parents are generally no more troubled than the relationships of individuals with their biologic parents.

**17** A mentally challenged 18-year-old man who had been calmly walking down a street suddenly cried out, fell to the ground, and started to have jerky movements of his right arm and leg accompanied by a twitching of the face. Passersby stopped to help and noticed that he was frothing from the mouth, had wet his trousers, and bitten his tongue. The paramedics were called, and they swiftly transported him to the emergency room. The attending physician

noted he had some small firm swellings around the nose, as well as freckle-like dark spots on his face. The clinical condition affecting this patient can result in the development of which one of the following conditions?

(A) Oligodendroglioma
(B) Melanoma
(C) Renal failure
(D) Peripheral vascular disease
(E) Hepatic failure

**18** A 45-year-old man sees his primary care physician for a persistent cough with a recent history of sputum tinged with blood. He smokes one pack of cigarettes a day and has tried to kick the habit several times, but failed. Physical examination was unremarkable. The physician ordered a chest x-ray. This was reported by the radiologist as showing a "suspicious lesion in the periphery of the right lower lobe, recommend rule out malignancy." The best way to confirm a diagnosis in this patient would be which one of the following?

(A) Sputum cytology
(B) Flexible bronchoscopy and bronchial brushings
(C) Flexible bronchoscopy and biopsy
(D) Mediastinoscopy
(E) Transthoracic needle biopsy

**19** A 55-year-old man with a 20-year history of smoking two packs of cigarettes per day presents to the emergency room with a history of a sudden, severe, and unrelenting substernal chest pain. He informs the attending physician that he is taking medication for hyperlipidemia and diabetes mellitus type 2. Upon examination, he was found to be diaphoretic, hypotensive, and tachycardic. An electrocardiogram (EKG) confirmed a myocardial infarction, and he was transferred to the cardiac intensive care unit. A few days later, he developed a cardiac murmur. The most likely cause for this murmur was which one of the following?

(A) Papillary muscle rupture
(B) Pericarditis
(C) Free wall rupture
(D) Ventricular aneurysm
(E) Ventricular septal defect

**20** A 52-year-old man who is a cattle rancher complains that he has become terrified of flying in private planes since an acquaintance of his was killed in one. However, flying is a necessary part of running his enterprise. He knows his fear is irrational, but no matter how important to him, he fears that he will not be able to make himself fly. An amateur psychologist friend tells him his problem reflects a fear of being abandoned because his father abandoned the family when he was a child. Which one of the following would indicate a specific phobia in this patient?

(A) Patient believes his fear is irrational.
(B) Patient has a history of separation anxiety from childhood.
(C) Patient's fear represents unconscious symbolism.
(D) Patient is not able to fly even when absolutely necessary.
(E) Patient's fears are well grounded in reality.

**21** A 35-year-old woman came to see her family physician because she suddenly lost conscious, but recovered a few minutes thereafter. Her vital signs were as follows: temperature 37°C (98.6°F), pulse 86/min regular, respirations 18/min, blood pressure 110/70 mm Hg, and 98% oxygen saturation on room air. The physician suspected syncope. Which one of the following choices represents the best way to diagnose the underlying cause for this?

(A) A 12-lead electrocardiogram (ECG)
(B) A 24-hour Holter monitoring
(C) History and physical examination
(D) Tilt table test
(E) Echocardiography

**22** A 62-year-old man who worked as a journeyman carpenter for the past three decades makes an appointment with a family practice physician because he can hardly bend his fourth and fifth fingers on both hands. In providing a history, he states that the first relevant problem he noted was about 10–15 years ago, when a small, hard, painless nodule appeared in the palm of his left hand; he adds he is right-handed. This presented no problem, and he ignored it. A couple of years later, a similar nodule formed in the right palm. Somewhat more annoying, it still did not really interfere with his work. A band of firm tissue then developed under the skin from these nodules, which extended up to the ring finger. As time passed this band grew stiffer, making it more and more difficult to bend his ring and pinky fingers, greatly inhibiting his ability to work. As part of his examination, the doctor asked him to flatten his hand, palm down, on a table top; he was unable to perform this maneuver—in fact, he was unable to flatten his hand out even if the physician pushed it down. The physician asked if his patient had any relatives with similar problems. The patient responded that he knew little about his blood relatives because

he is an orphan who immigrated from Norway at the age of 19. The disease in question most likely is which one of the following?

(A) Dupuytren's contracture
(B) Plantar fibromatosis
(C) Peyronie disease
(D) Knuckle pads (Garrod's nodes)
(E) Ledderhose disease

**23** A 55-year-old man, a known alcoholic, was shaving after breakfast in the shower. While shaving, he turned his head far toward the left. He suddenly lost consciousness and fell to the floor. He awoke a few minutes later and noticed that he had cut his head. He had a short episode of blurry vision, but had no nausea, vomiting, or headache. After seeing him emerge from the shower befuddled and bleeding from his forehead, his wife became concerned and called 911. The paramedics took him to the nearest emergency facility, where the patient volunteered that he had had similar episodes on previous occasions but managed to avoid a fall. The emergency physician noted that his vital signs were stable, ruled out intracranial trauma via a computed tomography (CT) scan, obtained a normal 12-lead electrocardiographic (ECG) study, and also found that a complete blood count, urine examination, and comprehensive metabolic panel were normal. He then sutured the laceration. Which one of the following is the most likely cause for this patient's attack?

(A) Carotid sinus sensitivity
(B) Hypoglycemia
(C) Vertebrobasilar attack
(D) Tonic-clonic seizure
(E) Head trauma

**24** An 8-year-old patient presents to her pediatrician complaining of profuse, watery rhinorrhea, difficulty breathing, and itching of the nose and palate. There is a family history of atopy. During the physical examination, the child has paroxysmal sneezing. The physician suspects that the patient has allergic rhinitis. To substantiate the diagnosis, the physician should perform which of the following tests?

(A) A radioallergosorbent test (RAST)
(B) A Coombs' test
(C) A nasal smear for eosinophils
(D) A scratch test
(E) Immunoglobulin E (IgE) levels

**25** A 55-year-old man who recently moved from another part of the country went in for an annual physical examination. He informed the physician that he recently passed a pre-employment physical, had no prior illness, and was not on any medications. He did not drink, smoke, or take recreational drugs. Physical examination was normal. However, he had a friend who had peripheral arterial disease (PAD), and he worried if he was a candidate for it, as he was informed that it could occur to "anyone anytime." The physician described the disorder to him, explaining that PAD most commonly involves the:

(A) Abdominal aorta
(B) Iliac arteries
(C) Peroneal and tibial arteries
(D) Pedal arteries
(E) Femoral and popliteal arteries

**26** A 17-year-old woman, gravida 1, para 0, has come to the outpatient office for a routine prenatal visit. She is currently at 25 weeks' gestation with a singleton pregnancy. She has a 10-year history of asthma but is not requiring any pharmacologic bronchodilator therapy. She is not currently having respiratory complaints or symptoms. An obstetric sonogram performed 3 weeks ago showed a female fetus with grossly normal anatomic findings and appropriate size for gestational age. The patient is scheduled to undergo pulmonary evaluation and spirometry testing today. Which of the following statements regarding her current spirometry findings are most likely to be true when compared with her last pulmonary assessment prior to pregnancy?

(A) Respiratory rate is increased.
(B) Vital capacity is decreased.
(C) Minute ventilation is increased.
(D) Function residual capacity remains unchanged.
(E) Tidal volume is decreased.

**27** A 53-year-old mother obsessed with the idea of teenage pregnancy put her 13-year-old daughter on birth control pills, choosing the progesterone-only "mini-pill." Subsequently, the daughter continued using this form of contraception and, although she was sexually active, she never became pregnant nor did she ever menstruate; she attributed both of these facts to the pill. She eventually married at the age of 22. At that time, she desired to become pregnant and stopped taking the mini-pill. However after having normal sexual intercourse for a full year without practicing any form of birth control, she neither became pregnant nor did she start menstruating. Concerned, she consulted a family physician who

gave her a physical. He found her general appearance to be that of a normal female 5 foot 6 inches (1.68 m) tall and 130 pounds (59 kg), with well-developed breasts and a normal, albeit somewhat sparse, female hair pattern. Other than what he suspected was an abnormally shallow vagina he could not find any gross abnormalities. At the end his examination, he said he thought he knew the cause of her infertility and amenorrhea but recommended further studies by a gynecologist who specialized in such problems. More detailed studies by such a specialist would most likely discover which one of the following additional findings?

(A) An XO genotype
(B) An XXX genotype
(C) An XXY genotype
(D) An XY genotype
(E) The presence of two Barr bodies

**28** A 16-year-old boy has the onset over several weeks of disorganized thinking. His utterances are clearly enunciated but impossible to understand, and he seems perplexed by events around him. He seems agitated, unable to sit or stand still, and suspicious of the actions and thoughts of others. Which one of the following would best suggest that the boy's symptoms include a flight of ideas?

(A) The sudden disappearance of thoughts from consciousness
(B) Catatonic excitement
(C) Illogical thought processes
(D) Rapid shifting from one thought to another
(E) An irrational belief that one has special powers

**29** A 33-year-old man with a history of bipolar I disorder is brought into the hospital with a self-inflicted stab wound. He admits to suicidal intent. He had been on valproic acid therapy for the past 4 years. However, because he had been doing well since starting therapy, he decided he was cured and stopped taking the drug 2 months ago. For purposes of determining treatment for this acute mood episode, which of the following will best distinguish mania from depression?

(A) An altered level of activity
(B) The presence of psychosis
(C) The quality of mood
(D) The presence of insomnia
(E) The presence of known pathophysiology

**30** A 24-year-old woman, gravida 1, para 0, is 20 weeks' pregnant. She recently had a mononucleosis-like syndrome with right upper quadrant tenderness. Laboratory testing showed elevation of liver enzymes. While working as a nurse in a neonatal intensive care unit, she had been taking care of a newborn who was small for gestational age and had hepatosplenomegaly. Workup of the neonate showed chorioretinitis, microcephaly, and intracranial calcifications. Which of the following statements is true regarding the probable infection this woman acquired from the neonate?

(A) No specific treatment exists.
(B) Cesarean delivery of her baby is recommended.
(C) Risk of fetal infection is highest during the first trimester.
(D) γ-Globulin is useful for prophylaxis after exposure.
(E) Most infected infants are asymptomatic.

**31** A 52-year-old woman, gravida 4, para 4, comes to the outpatient office complaining of hot flashes, which occur without warning. At night, the episodes result in profuse diaphoresis, leaving her nightgown and bed sheets wet. She is experiencing less lubrication and vaginal secretions with intercourse, leading to pain and discomfort. She also is having mood swings and difficulty concentrating. Her last menstrual period was 3 months ago. She is 168 cm (66 in) tall and weighs 61 kg (135 lb). She smokes one pack of cigarettes a day and is a social user of alcohol. Which of the following is most likely to be found on laboratory blood testing?

(A) Elevated cortisol
(B) Decreased luteinizing hormone (LH)
(C) Elevated follicle-stimulating hormone (FSH)
(D) Decreased free thyroxin
(E) Elevated androstenedione

**32** A 24-year-old woman complains of chronic and diffuse body pain since a bicycle accident 6 months ago in which she sustained abrasions and a wrist sprain. Despite lack of objective findings, she refuses to engage in even minimal exercise and says that she can't drive. Which of the following features would be most important in making a diagnosis of pain disorder?

(A) The pain is largely mediated by psychologic factors.
(B) A physical lesion will be determined by imaging studies.
(C) No personality pathology is present.
(D) There is not a good response to biofeedback therapy.
(E) Worker's compensation and legal issues are not involved.

**33** A low-birth-weight infant presents to his pediatrician at 2 months of age. The mother states that the infant has not been eating well. Upon physical examination, the infant is noted to be pale and tachycardic. The lungs are clear to auscultation, and there is no hepatosplenomegaly. A complete blood count (CBC) shows a hemoglobin level of 6 g/dL. Which of the following is the most likely cause of anemia in this infant?

(A) Megaloblastic anemia
(B) Sickle cell anemia
(C) Anemia of prematurity
(D) α-Thalassemia
(E) Homozygous β-thalassemia

**34** A 55-year-old male was seen by his physician for pain in the upper abdomen, which he described as burning in character. He also complained of nausea and feeling rather tired. The pain had been present on and off over the past year; he had been taking several over-the-counter pain killers to relieve the pain, but they did not seem to work. He also stated that the pain became worse after eating, and that he had lost weight. He had no other relevant symptoms or medical history. He did not smoke; he drank beer in the past, but stopped about a year ago. On examination, his vital signs were normal. He was slightly below his average weight range. He had some pallor but no icterus. There was tenderness in the epigastric area, but no guarding or rigidity. No hepatosplenomegaly was noted, and bowel sounds were present. The most likely cause for his pain was:

(A) Cholecystitis
(B) Duodenal ulcer
(C) Hiatal hernia
(D) Gastric ulcer
(E) Chronic pancreatitis

**35** A child was in her usual state of good health when she developed a focal seizure while playing with her sister. The mother, a registered nurse, states that the seizure lasted approximately 5 minutes. 911 emergency services were called, and the child arrived postictal to the emergency department approximately 1 hour after the seizure first occurred. On physical examination, the vital signs are stable, but the patient is noted to have weakness and hemiparesis. Remarkably, within 24 hours the weakness and neurologic deficits disappear. Which one of the following is the most likely diagnosis?

(A) Hemiplegia complicating a migraine headache
(B) Spastic hemiplegia
(C) Postviral encephalitis
(D) Todd's paralysis
(E) Infratentorial tumor

**36** A 3-year-old boy with puffy eyes presents to the pediatric emergency department. His physician had treated the patient for allergies, but symptoms have not improved. Upon physical examination, the patient is noted to have edema. The physician suspects nephrotic syndrome. Which of the following characteristics would support the diagnosis of nephrotic syndrome?

(A) Hyperproteinemia
(B) Heavy proteinuria
(C) Hypolipidemia
(D) Hyperalbuminemia
(E) Hypertension

**37** A 53-year-old man of Scotch-Irish ancestry consults a physician because, in the past few months, he has developed joint and abdominal pains. Moreover, he lacks energy, feeling so tired that even getting up in the morning is difficult. He has lost interest in sex, and he also has had chronic diarrhea with greasy stools. Physical examination reveals a patient with pale grayish bronze skin color, hepatosplenomegaly, and an irregular heart rhythm. A finger stick glucose analysis shows a serum glucose value of 452 mg/dL. Which one of the following laboratory findings will also most likely be present?

(A) Decreased serum ceruloplasmin synthesis
(B) Decreased serum iron concentration
(C) Decreased small bowel reabsorption of D-xylose
(D) Increased serum ferritin levels
(E) Increased total iron-binding capacity

**38** Sigmund Freud is often described as the father of modern psychiatry. Throughout most of the 20th century, his theories were refined by others such as Jung and Klein, all of whom used the process of psychoanalysis to root out and treat subconscious factors underlying psychological problems. During the last third of the 20th century, other schools of therapy became more common, including somatic, psychodynamic, behavioral, cognitive, and humanistic. Which of the following is the most common component shared by the various schools of psychotherapy and psychoanalysis?

(A) An explanation of pathologic behavior
(B) A firm concept of the unconscious
(C) A long duration of treatment
(D) A dependency on drugs to alter behavior
(E) A belief that the primacy of the interpersonal experience must take precedence over other considerations

**39** A 14-year-old previously well patient is diagnosed with clinical sinusitis by his physician. A prescription for antibiotics was made out for the patient and given to his parents to treat this condition. The patient's parents had the prescription filled at the pharmacy. Unfortunately, the teenager, who does not like to take medication, was not always compliant and missed many doses. Presently, he is being evaluated in the emergency department for fever, confusion, extraocular palsies, and proptosis of the eye. Which of the following is the most likely diagnosis?

(A) Hand-Schüller-Christian disease
(B) Graves disease
(C) Cavernous sinus thrombosis
(D) Acute bacterial conjunctivitis
(E) Temporal lobe abscess

**40** A 36-year-old man suffered a fracture of his vertebrae in a motorcycle accident. As a consequence, his spinal cord was severed, and he was paralyzed from the waist down and confined to a wheelchair. He became depressed and started drinking alcohol as an escape mechanism, spending much time wheeling from his residence to various bars. Consequently, he did not practice optimum hygiene and self-care and developed an infected pressure sore (aka, a decubitus ulcer) on his sacrum. He eventually sought help at an emergency facility. Upon examination, the attending physician found his blood pressure to be 108/80 mm Hg; pulse, 76/min and regular; and temperature, 39.5°C (103.1°F). He found an 8 × 6 cm decubitii on the sacrum that emitted a purulent and foul-smelling discharge. Which one of the following is true concerning decubitus ulcers?

(A) Decubitus ulcers are more likely to occur in bedridden patients than in patients whose mobility is compromised in any other way.
(B) Erythema may progress to ulceration quickly.
(C) A decubitus ulcer is unlikely to ever be located on the heel.
(D) Decubitus ulcer infections are almost always caused by *Staphylococcus aureus*.
(E) A decubitus ulcer should be treated with a topical antiseptic such as hypochlorite solutions, povidone–iodine, acetic acid iodophor, or hydrogen peroxide.

*Directions for Matching Questions (41 through 50):* *Each set of matching questions is preceded by a list of 4 to 26 lettered options followed by a brief explanation of the required task and then by a series of numbered statements. For each lettered statement, you are to select ONE lettered option that best fulfills the task as it relates to that statement. Remember that each of the listed options might be correctly selected once, more than once, or not at all.*

## Questions 41–50

(A) Acetaminophen
(B) Diazepam
(C) Scopolamine
(D) Ethanol
(E) Amitriptyline
(F) Barbiturates
(G) Nicotine
(H) Sertraline
(I) Amphetamines
(J) Cocaine

*Match each numbered description below with the ONE lettered drug or agent above.*

**41** In acute oral overdose, signs and symptoms may include dilated pupils; nystagmus; hot, dry skin; decreased bowel sounds; confusion; hallucinations; and seizures. Characteristic cardiotoxic effects include tachycardia, QRS prolongation, hypotension, and cardiac arrhythmias.

**42** Symptoms of acute oral overdose include diarrhea, myoclonus, diaphoresis, elevated temperature, facial flushing, and tremor. Depending on the dose ingested, the patient may become agitated, confused, and hypertensive. Hyperreflexia can occur and progress to seizures. These symptoms may occur at conventional doses if the patient is also using monoamine oxidase inhibitors.

**43** An over-the-counter drug that is the most common cause of hepatic failure in the United States.

**44** A fat-soluble substance that crosses the blood–brain barrier, where it acts on the limbic system to potentiate dopamine transmission in the basal nuclei. The rush obtained from this substance lasts for less than 30 minutes when it is smoked.

**45** An anticholinergic substance commonly used to combat motion sickness.

**46** The drug that indirectly results in the greatest drug-related medical expenditure in the United States.

**47** The number-one drug problem in the Unites States in terms of direct observable effects.

**48** A potentially habit-forming drug that is the prototype of a family of drugs presently having widespread medical use including treatment of anxiety, panic, posttraumatic stress, and sleep disorders, as well as in substance withdrawal symptoms.

**49** The first member of this class of so-called sedative, hypnotic drugs was synthesized in 1903, and until the 1970s, members of this class were the primary drugs used as sedatives to treat anxiety and epilepsy. Taking an overdose was a favored means of committing suicide, particularly among women. They still have medical use but have in large part been replaced by newer, safer drugs.

**50** Their medical use includes appetite suppression in weight loss programs, treatment of narcolepsy and depression, and in children, treatment of attention deficit and hyperactivity syndrome. Despite profound health hazards, they also are gaining popularity as recreational drugs because they are easily synthesized from readily available materials.

# Answer Key

| | | | | | | | | | |
|---|---|---|---|---|---|---|---|---|---|
| **1** | B | **11** | C | **21** | C | **31** | C | **41** | E |
| **2** | D | **12** | C | **22** | A | **32** | A | **42** | H |
| **3** | C | **13** | A | **23** | A | **33** | C | **43** | A |
| **4** | A | **14** | E | **24** | C | **34** | D | **44** | J |
| **5** | C | **15** | C | **25** | E | **35** | D | **45** | C |
| **6** | C | **16** | C | **26** | C | **36** | B | **46** | G |
| **7** | B | **17** | C | **27** | D | **37** | D | **47** | D |
| **8** | C | **18** | E | **28** | D | **38** | A | **48** | B |
| **9** | D | **19** | E | **29** | C | **39** | C | **49** | F |
| **10** | E | **20** | A | **30** | E | **40** | B | **50** | I |

# Answers and Explanations

**1** **The answer is B** *Obstetrics and Gynecology*

This woman has the classic symptoms of endometriosis, namely dysmenorrhea (painful menses), dyspareunia (painful intercourse), dyschezia (painful defecation), and infertility. Endometriosis is a benign condition in which the endometrial glands and stroma are present outside the uterus and uterine cavity. The most common sites of occurrence, in order of frequency, are ovaries (choice **B**), cul-de-sac, uterosacral ligaments (choice **A**), broad ligaments, and oviducts. Currently, surgery is the only definitive treatment; medical treatment is seldom curative.

This condition typically occurs in the early reproductive years, not after 35 years of age (choice **C**). Endometriosis is not associated with endometrioid carcinoma of the ovary or a high chance of malignant transformation (choice **D**). Nor is endometriosis associated with uterine leiomyomata (choice **E**); however, in 15% of cases, it is associated with adenomyosis, a benign condition in which islands of endometrial glands and stroma are found within the myometrium, without a direct connection to the endometrial cavity.

**2** **The answer is D** *Medicine*

A normal diurnal response retained in diabetics is to produce increased levels of cortisol and growth hormone shortly before dawn (choice **D**). These hormones act antagonistically to insulin, causing an increase in the serum glucose level; this is called the "dawn phenomenon," and it must be taken into account when calculating insulin requirements in patients on insulin therapy. In normal individuals, this spike in glucogenic hormones is counteracted by a corresponding increase in insulin secretion. However, in type 1 diabetics, this increase in glucogenic hormones is only opposed by whatever insulin remains from the last insulin injection, whereas in type 2 diabetics, it is insulin resistance that prevents serum glucose levels from returning to normal fasting levels.

The livers of diabetic individuals are exposed to glucagon levels that are lower than normal; thus decreased gluconeogenesis (choice **A**) is incorrect because glucagon levels tend to be higher in diabetics, not lower. Both nondiabetics and diabetics produce increased levels of cortisol and growth hormone early in the morning, thus choice **B** is incorrect. The rise in serum glucose levels, the dawn phenomenon, is largely blunted by increased insulin secretion in normal individuals. Insulin resistance does not vary in a diurnal manner (choice **C** is incorrect). The liver does not become loaded with glucose (choice **E**); excess glucose would be stored as glycogen, hence this choice is wrong.

**3** **The answer is C** *Pediatrics*

Reye syndrome (choice **C**) is a secondary mitochondrial hepatopathy that, in genetically susceptible individuals, has a very high association with the ingestion of aspirin-containing medicines during influenza-like illnesses or varicella. Its incidence peaked in the 1970s, with mortality rates of greater than 40%, and although the prevalence today has significantly decreased, the mortality rate has not changed. Reye syndrome has a biphasic course. It usually presents in a previously healthy child who had an upper respiratory infection or varicella. After the child seems to have recovered, the symptoms of vomiting, lethargy, and confusion can appear and progress quickly. The patient may also be combative. Liver enzymes and ammonia level are elevated. Treatment requires early recognition and control of increased intracranial pressure. Prognosis depends on the duration of disordered cerebral function. Early diagnosis and treatment increases the likelihood for recovery to 90%.

Hepatitis A virus (HAV; choice **A**) is an RNA-containing virus. It is a member of the Picornaviridae family and is spread predominantly by the fecal–oral route. In the United States, there is increased risk of infection with HAV in day care centers, in contacts of children who attend day care centers, and in the homosexual population. The diagnosis of HAV infection should be considered when a history of jaundice exists in the patient's contacts, or if the patient or his or her family has traveled to an endemic area. The acute infection is diagnosed by the presence of immunoglobulin M (IgM) anti-HAV. Although elevation may be found in the bilirubin and serum transaminase levels, they do not help to differentiate the cause. Drug-induced hepatitis (choice **B**) is not the correct answer, because the patient in this scenario has a history of aspirin usage, and aspirin is excreted by the kidney. Infectious mononucleosis (choice **D**) is a clinical syndrome caused by the Epstein-Barr virus (EBV). Clinical symptoms in children are often mild, but patients may have fatigue, fever, sore throat, and generalized lymphadenopathy. Splenomegaly may be prominent, causing left upper quadrant abdominal tenderness. Hepatomegaly may be present in a small number of patients. Symptomatic hepatitis or jaundice is uncommon. A mononuclear lymphocytosis with atypical-appearing lymphocytes is associated with infectious mononucleosis. Gilbert syndrome (choice **E**) is an inherited, benign, unconjugated hyper-bilirubinemia that is transmitted as an autosomal dominant disease. The hyperbilirubinemia is mild, and the bilirubin level may fluctuate. Jaundice is intermittent and may be noted on routine physical examination. Results of liver biopsy and other liver function tests are normal.

## 4 The answer is A *Psychiatry*

The distinguishing feature of autistic disorder is a qualitative disturbance in development (choice **A**), as opposed to retardation of development. Qualitative disturbances include lack of attachment to others; restrictive, repetitive, and stereotyped behavior patterns; and peculiar use of speech. The onset of such deficits occurs before the age of 3 years, and it occurs at a 5:1 male-to-female ratio.

Although autistic individuals may have normal intelligence (choice **E**) or may even be gifted in certain areas (choice **D**), 75% have concurrent mental retardation. The prognosis for autistic disorder is most severe when associated with mental retardation or failure to speak by age 5. Depending on the cause of the disorder, there may, but need not, be progressive deterioration of function (choice **B**). Autistic disorder has multiple causes, including intrauterine infection, errors of metabolism (choice **C**), and encephalitis. A genetic component in at least some cases is suggested by the observation of an increased incidence of autism among family members.

## 5 The answer is C *Pediatrics*

The infectious disease that the physician would be most concerned about is meningitis. The treatment must be designed to prevent or, if already fulminating, cure this disease. *Streptococcus agalactiae* (group B streptococcus) is a common inhabitant of the maternal genitourinary tract. It is acquired by newborns via vertical transmission, and it is the most common cause of neonatal meningitis, followed by *Escherichia coli* and *Listeria monocytogenes*. Early-onset disease is associated with sepsis; late onset is associated with meningitis. Consequently, *S. agalactiae, E. coli,* and *L. monocytogenes* (choice **C**) is the correct answer.

*Streptococcus pneumoniae* (part of choice **A, B,** and **E**) and *Neisseria meningitidis* (part of choice **B, D,** and **E**) are seen in older age groups; therefore, these are incorrect responses.

## 6 The answer is C *Surgery*

A ruptured Achillis tendon (choice C) most commonly occurs in the so-called "weekend warrior," who engages in a strenuous sport after permitting him- or herself to get out of shape. The immediate symptoms are similar to those described. Following these initial signs and symptoms, the area around the attachment of the tendon to the calcaneus will swell and bruise. Often one can feel a gap where the tendon has pulled away from the bone. It is important to see an orthopedic surgeon immediately because early treatment leads to the best results. Surgery is typically recommended.

Clearly, a repetitive strain injury (choice **A**) is incorrect since the man had not been participating in active sports for some time. Tendinitis (choice **B**) describes inflammation of a tendon usually caused by overuse; its onset tends to be gradual not acute. Tendinosis (choice **D**) describes a condition in which a tendon is chronically damaged by overuse or some other injury resulting in formation of scar tissue; typically, in its earlier stages, it presented as tendinitis. A case of paratenonitis (choice **E**) refers to injuries primarily limited to the outer sheath covering a tendon.

## 7 The answer is B *Pediatrics*

Werdnig-Hoffmann disease (choice **B**) is a spinal muscular atrophy caused by a pathologic continuation of a process of programmed cell death that occurs in embryonic life, but normally not postnatally. It is inherited in an autosomal recessive fashion. Infants can be symptomatic at birth. Sparing of the extraocular muscles and sphincters is characteristic. Fasciculations are a sign of denervation of muscle and are best seen in the tongue. Infants assume a flaccid "frog-leg" posture. Most die by 2 years of age.

A neonatal form of myotonic dystrophy (choice **A**) appears in infants born to mothers with myotonic dystrophy. Clubfoot and contractures are common. Fasciculations are not seen. Infant botulism (choice **C**) has a peak onset at 2–6 months of age. Sources for spores include honey, corn syrup, soil, and dust. Infantile myasthenia gravis (choice **D**) can be transient—as in those infants born of mothers with myasthenia gravis—or, very rarely, a congenital manifestation of the disease itself. Fasciculations are not seen, and the extraocular muscles are not spared. Duchenne's muscular dystrophy (choice **E**) is rarely symptomatic at birth.

### 8 The answer is C *Medicine*

Rheumatoid arthritis (RA) is a common affliction estimated to affect some 1% of the population; it may occur at any age but symptoms most commonly first manifest themselves between the ages of 40 and 60 years. Women are affected about 3 times more often than men. It is a chronic, systemic disorder that generally primarily attacks specific joints by producing an inflammatory synovitis. Usually, smaller joints are the first to be attacked, often the fingers and wrists; it may then progress to affect other body parts. As a rule, the symptoms occur in a symmetrical fashion (e.g., both wrists will be affected simultaneously). The patient described is in the earlier stages of developing RA, as evidenced by the facts that symptoms first became severe enough for her to consult her chiropractor after a month, and one can estimate that she then consulted a rheumatologist within 2 additional months. The anticyclic citrullinated peptide antibody test (choice **C**), also referred to as anticitrulline antibody or as citrulline antibody, provides positive results early in the course of the disease and has a reported sensitivity of 67% and a specificity of 95%.

The erythrocyte sedimentation rate (choice **A**) and the C-reactive protein test (choice **B**) are nonspecific tests for inflammation. Negative results would not be consistent for RA, but a positive result would be expected from many conditions. Antinuclear antibody (choice **D**) is not a viable test for RA, with a sensitivity of less than 30%. It is more sensitive for systemic lupus erythematosus (present is about 80%–90% of cases) and Sjögren disease (found in about 60% of cases). Rheumatoid factor (choice **E**) has a sensitivity of about 80% in well-developed cases of RA but is slow to develop. In many cases, it does not appear until a year after the appearance of early symptoms; thus, it may not yet have developed in the case described. Nor is rheumatoid factor specific for RA; it is actually more specific for Sjögren disease, where its sensitivity approaches 100%.

### 9 The answer is D *Medicine*

Raynaud disease (choice **D**) results from arterial spasm that block the flow of blood to the finger tips. The spasm typically is caused by exposure to cold (sometimes emotion or other stimuli may also induce a spasm), and the white coloration is due to blockage of normal blood flow. The blue color results from prolonged hypo-oxygenation, and the red color occurs as the spasm relaxes and blood flow is reestablished. A primary Raynaud's phenomenon, generally called Raynaud disease, is not associated with any other condition and usually occurs in younger persons, those under the age of 30 years (most often those between 15 and 25). About 80% of affected individuals are female, and the disorder may be found in several family members. Although uncomfortable and tending to limit outdoor activity in cold climates, as a rule, the condition is self-limiting and causes no permanent damage. However, constant repeated exposure to the inducing factor may eventually cause tissue damage; thus, common sense suggests excess exposure to the cold should be avoided.

Raynaud's phenomenon (choice **A**), also known as secondary Raynaud disease, is a similar condition generally found in association with any one of several autoimmune conditions. It again generally affects females but usually those older than 40 years of age. Often, the Raynaud's phenomenon shows up before the more serious manifestations of the underlying autoimmune disease. Systemic lupus erythematosus (choice **B**) and scleroderma (choice **E**) are two autoimmune conditions that often bring about Raynaud's phenomenon. Frostbite (choice **C**) is initially marked by sensations of cold then burning, numbness, tingling, and itching; the affected areas tend to turn white and appear frozen, but they retain resistance to pressure. Tissues in such a condition are said to have undergone superficial frostbite. As freezing continues, sensation becomes lost, and swelling and blood filled blisters are noted. The area is hard, has no resistance to pressure, and may appear blackened and dead. This is called deep frostbite.

### 10 The answer is E *Medicine*

A common factor contributing to systolic hypertension is sleep apnea, a condition in which breathing repetitively stops during sleep for periods of time varying from seconds to even a minute or two. Normally, throat muscles work to maintain an open passage for air. However, in persons with obstructive sleep apnea (OSA), these muscles relax more than normal during sleep, inhibiting the flow of air into the lungs. Such inhibition may be facilitated if the diameter of the patient's trachea is relatively small, if the patient is overweight, or if neuropathy associated with age or disease inhibits the neural signals keeping the glottis open. These restrictions of air flow induce frequent drops in oxygen saturation, which in turn trigger the release of stress hormones that promote hyperglycemia and induction of obesity and diabetes. Bouts of hypertension also occur, leading to cardiac failure. Moreover, low levels of oxygen saturation may lead to cardiac arrhythmia, angina, or even myocardiac infarction. Since OSA raises blood pressure, it is potentially a component in this patient's intractable hypertension. Thus, the diagnosis of OSA is important for treatment of otherwise intractable hypertension. A polysomnogram study (choice **E**) is the most common way to diagnose the possibility of sleep apnea. The patient is admitted to a sleep study center where he or she is allowed to sleep comfortably but is fitted with sensors on the scalp, fingers, chest, face, and limbs. These sensors will record brain activity, eye movement, limb muscle activity, heart and breathing activity, movement of air in and out of the lungs, and the degree of oxygen saturation while the patient is asleep. The most common treatment for sleep apnea is continuous positive air pressure (CPAP) delivered via a CPAP machine.

Brain computed tomography scans (choice **A**), magnetic resonance images of the chest (choice **B**), comparison of the ankle and brachial blood pressure (choice **C**), or measurement of the percentage of hemoglobin A1C (choice **D**) will not help elucidate the cause of his systolic hypertension.

### 11 The answer is C *Medicine*

Falls are the leading cause of trauma-related death in people over 75 years of age, and the most common cause for tripping and falling in the elderly is the lack of depth perception (choice **C**). Of all the tests available to assess vision, the best predictor for falling and subsequent injury is poor depth perception. Patients with good vision in both eyes are at low risk, but those who have diminished vision in one eye, even when the other is normal, have the same risk of falling as those with moderate or poor vision in both eyes. This is because the ability to judge distances and spatial relationships is impaired. Even though she was concentrating, the woman in this question could not tell exactly where the next step was.

A younger person with quicker reflexes would have probably grabbed onto a rail or corrected this error even if such an event did occur. While diminished reflex response due to aging does occur (choice **B**), it usually is not the primary reason for a fall and is an incorrect response. Distraction (choice **A**) can play a role in an inadvertent fall, but again this is not the most likely cause for this fall. Although she has atrial fibrillation, which would cause an irregular cardiac rhythm (choice **D**), there is no reason to assume that she had a transient ischemic attack (TIA) or syncope, either of which could have led to a fall. Furthermore, neither TIA nor syncope is a common cause for falls among the elderly. The elderly may have problems with balance, and therefore may find it difficult to react to sudden stresses affecting balance, but problems with gait (choice **E**) per se are not among the more common cause for falls.

### 12 The answer is C *Psychiatry*

This man is demonstrating passive-aggressiveness, which is described as covert aggression expressed through passivity, masochism, and self-defeating behavior. Such an individual often is angry—and often angers others. The usual result is further deterioration of the interaction, with even greater anger and passive-aggressiveness. The most effective way to deal with covert communication is to bring it into the open and discuss it (choice **C**). The psychological term for this technique is called "identifying the process."

Threats (choice **A**) and expressions of anger (choice **D**) or hurt (choice **B**) are generally not useful. Because personality traits are generally stable in various environments, it is unlikely that a different clinician (choice **E**) would be spared this patient's passive-aggressiveness.

### 13 The answer is A *Psychiatry*

Increased involvement of fathers in raising children decreases the risk of sexual abuse (choice **A**).

More women than men have a history of being abused (choice **B**). More traditional, less democratic families are associated with an increased, not decreased (choice **C**) risk of abuse. Mothers who sexually abuse children are often lonely and emotionally deprived, not gregarious and socially active (choice **D**). Contrary to popular wisdom, only a minority of childhood sexual abuse is perpetrated by fathers and stepfathers (choice **E**). However, the abuser is often another relative or family member.

### 14 The answer is E *Medicine*

This patient has a continuous murmur that straddles the entire spectrum of the cardiac cycle. Such a murmur is called a "machinery murmur," and is observed in patients having patent ductus arteriosus (PDA; choice **E**) or an arteriovenous fistula. The ductus arteriosus normally closes shortly after birth. However, if it is left untreated, it may persist into adulthood with few if any untoward symptoms until discovered—usually because of this machinery murmur. Other late presentations include heart failure, pulmonary hypertension, and endocarditis or occasionally a calcified ductus arterious is discovered upon x-ray. Mortality rates among untreated patients have been estimated to be as high as 4% per year, with two-third dying before the age of 64 years.

The murmur associated with aortic stenosis (choice **A**) is ejection systolic. A holosystolic murmur is associated mitral regurgitation (choice **B**). Pericarditis (choice **C**) is associated with a pericardial friction rub. This is a grating or scratching sound that varies with respiration. It can be mistaken for either a systolic or a diastolic murmur. Mitral stenosis (choice **D**) is associated with an opening snap and a diastolic rumble that has presystolic accentuation.

### 15 The answer is C *Obstetrics and Gynecology*

Lobular carcinoma, the most common malignancy of the terminal lobule, is usually nonpalpable on self-examination; in this case, her injury probably induced a lump caused by fat necrosis, which in turn led to an early diagnosis. Lobular carcinoma accounts for 5%–10% of all breast cancers and, if left untreated, becomes invasive in 20%–30% of patients over a prolonged period of time (10–15 years; not early invasion choice **B**). It is most commonly associated with a high degree of bilaterality in the same quadrant of the contralateral breast (choice **C**), which underscores the need for mammography. The contralateral breast may develop another lobular cancer or a ductal carcinoma. Simultaneous bilateral breast carcinoma occurs in less than 1% of cases.

The majority of in-situ lobular carcinomas are estrogen- and progesterone-receptor positive, not negative (choice **A**). Chest wall involvement is uncommon in cases of lobular carcinoma, this choice **D** is incorrect. There is an increased incidence of breast cancer in first-degree relatives, but not in second-degree relatives (not in both first- and second-degree relatives; choice **E**).

### 16 The answer is C *Psychiatry*

Narcissistic injury (choice **C**), the emotional pain from having been rejected as a child, often plays a significant role in the emotional life of adoptees. It sometimes manifests itself as insecurity about acceptance by others and requires sensitive care and patience on the part of new adoptee parents.

Over 80% (not about 50%, choice **A**) of adoptions are considered successful, and IQ scores have been demonstrated to rise in adoptive environments that provide enriched intellectual and social stimulation (choice **B**). However, the rate of psychopathology is higher among adoptees (choice **D**), as is the rate of parent–child problems (choice **E**).

### 17 The answer is C *Medicine*

This patient is suffering from tuberous sclerosis complex (TSC), an autosomal dominant disease with variable penetrance, in which there is a genetic mutation involving two genes, *TSC1* and *TSC2*; these turn on two tumor-suppressor proteins, tuberin and hamartin, located on chromosome 16 and 9, respectively. As a result, tumors, most often benign, and cysts may develop. The disease affects various organs with variable severity. The features of this syndrome include mental retardation, seizures, and adenoma sebaceum, characterized by firm nodules on the face in a butterfly distribution. Patients with this disease may have renal cysts (angiomyolipomas) that could lead to hematuria, and renal failure could supervene (choice **C** is correct).

Patients with this disorder can develop tubers on the cortex (hence the name); these are subependymal nodules of glial or neuronal origin, as well as subependymal giant cell astrocytomas that can block the foramen of Munro. This may lead to acute hydrocephalus, with a tragic outcome if not recognized and treated; however, since oligodendroglioma (choice **A**) are tumors in their own right, they are not expected to be present in patients suffering from TSC. Melanomas do not present with café au lait spots on the face, nor is there any reason to suspect that this patient has a melanoma (choice **B**). Other skin manifestations of the disease may include the Shagreen patch, wherein the skin has the texture of leather (often seen on the lower back or over the back of the neck), and "ash leaf spots," which are hypomelanotic patches that can occur in various parts of the body. Peripheral vascular disease (choice **D**) is not a manifestation of this disease, although these patients can develop cardiovascular problems such as rhabdomyomas, cardiac murmurs, arrhythmias, and cardiac failure in early infancy and childhood, and sometimes during their adult years. Hepatic failure (choice **E**) is not a feature of this disease.

### 18 The answer is E  *Surgery*

This patient has a peripheral lung lesion, the diagnosis of which can be best confirmed by transthoracic needle biopsy (choice **E**) under CT guidance.

Sputum cytology, especially from the first morning sample, can confirm the diagnosis in some but not all cases and is less likely to be helpful in peripheral lesions (choice **A** is incorrect). It is more effective at diagnosing central squamous cell carcinomas than peripheral adenocarcinomas. This is because, when a patient coughs, he is more likely to produce sputum from the larger central parts of the bronchial tree (where squamous cell carcinomas abound) than from the smaller peripheral airways where adenocarcinomas typically reside. Flexible bronchoscopy and bronchial brushings, washings, or biopsy cannot be done for lesions that are located peripherally, as the flexible bronchoscope can penetrate only as far as the secondary branches of the bronchial tree (hence choices **B** and **C** are incorrect). Likewise, choice **D** is incorrect since mediastinoscopy is a procedure performed via an incision in the suprasternal notch to gain access to the mediastinum via a mediastinoscope. This procedure is undertaken to obtain a lymph node biopsy.

### 19 The answer is E  *Medicine*

Over 90% of new murmurs following a myocardial infarction (MI) are due to a ventricular septal defect (VSD; choice **E**). Such murmurs are usually present between the third and fifth day post MI. The murmur is holosystolic and harsh. It is often associated with a precordial thrill. These patients can rapidly develop pulmonary embolus and hemodynamic collapse; survival rate is less than 50%. Twenty-five percent of patients have a history of a previous MI.

Papillary muscle rupture (choice **A**) is seen in some 50% of cases involving a relatively small infarction. These patients develop a mitral regurgitation murmur that is heard between the third and fifth day post MI. Like patients with VSD following an MI, the murmur is holosystolic and harsh but, unlike VSD, a precordial thrill is rarely present. However, similar to patients with VSD, these patients can develop pulmonary embolus and hemodynamic collapse. A history of previous MI is present in around 30% of cases. Survival rate is less than 50%. Pericarditis (choice **B**) is not associated with a murmur but with a rub. It is due to inflammation of the pericardium at the site where myocardial necrosis has occurred. It can occur in the early post infarct period, or several weeks later due to autoimmune pleuropericarditis. Fever and an elevated erythrocyte sedimentation rate are present; this condition is known as Dressler syndrome. Free wall rupture (choice **C**) is associated with a murmur in less than 25% of cases and usually occurs around the third to sixth day following MI. Patients may complain of recurrent chest pains, and they may develop pericardial tamponade and even sudden death. A pericardial effusion may be present on echocardiography. Survival following a free wall rupture is extremely rare, and a history of a previous MI may be present in approximately 25% of cases. Ventricular aneurysm (choice **D**) is not associated with a murmur. These are located at regions where myocardial necrosis has occurred. They can be visualized on echocardiography and an electrocardiogram may show persistent ST elevation. Although pseudo aneurysms are more prone to rupture, true aneurysms are not.

### 20 The answer is A  *Psychiatry*

Adults with specific phobia believe that their fear is irrational (choice **A**). Other features of specific phobia include fear of an object or situation that is excessive or unreasonable, efforts to avoid the feared object or situation, and extreme anxiety if the object or situation cannot be avoided. The objective or actual degree of danger is not relevant to a diagnosis of phobia.

It is often difficult to determine whether or not a particular fear has associated unconscious symbolism, and the presence or absence of symbolism does not indicate a phobia (choice **C**). A history of separation anxiety in childhood (choice **B**) is not associated with specific phobia; however, it is associated with the later development of panic disorder. Individuals may be able to force themselves to confront the feared situation (choice **D**) but will experience severe anxiety in such instances. While some phobias make logical sense, many have no basis in reality (choice **E**).

### 21 The answer is C  *Medicine*

The diagnosis of syncope is best made by taking a good history and performing a careful physical examination (choice **C**). The underlying cause can be picked up in over 50% of cases by this alone. Of the remaining cases, in roughly half, the etiology will be remain unknown, while in the rest it will be established via a history of stress, chest pain, palpitations, medication, relationship to Valsalva maneuvers, positional change, prior episodes of syncope, history of neurologic/psychiatric/endocrine/metabolic/hemopoietic disorder, or family history. Never forget to rule out pregnancy in a woman of childbearing age. Physical examination should include neurological, cardiovascular, endocrine, and other systems.

A 12-lead electrocardiogram (ECG; choice **A**) is the initial test performed. It may reveal tachyarrhythmias and other abnormalities. However, in other cases of syncope, the ECG will be normal. Additional tests that should be done for all patients at this time include a complete blood count (CBC), comprehensive metabolic panel, urine examination, and where indicated, a pregnancy test. A 24-hour Holter monitoring (choice **B**) is indicated in patients who are suspected to have a cardiogenic cause for syncope when the 12-lead ECG has been normal. The tilt table test (choice **D**) would only be helpful in ruling out vasovagal syncope, and not for the other potential causes. Echocardiography (choice **E**) would only be indicated when there is a structural cause that prevents adequate ventricular outflow, such as valve stenosis or cardiomyopathy.

### 22 The answer is A  *Medicine*

Dupuytren's contracture (choice **A**) also known as Dupuytren disease or Dupuytren's diathesis, was once believed to be a very rare disease. More recently, it has been found to be common among certain ethnic groups, including Scandinavians and other Northern Europeans—so much so that it has called the "Viking disease." It is believed to be a genetic condition, since 27%–68% of patients report a positive family history. The prevailing belief is that the condition is inherited in an autosomal dominant manner with variable penetrance; this variability in expression, plus the fact that mild cases are nothing more than a nuisance, has led to a wide variance in the reported incidence. In the United States, the frequency is reported at between 5% and 15% of males older than 50 years of age; prevalence among Americans with a northern European lineage will be higher since this condition is rarely found among Hispanics, African Americans, Asians, or Native Americans. In males, the condition generally first shows up at about the age of 50; initially in the form of fibroblast-rich nodules that synthesize collagen, primarily type 3. These are then replaced by myofibroblasts, which line up linearly to form cords that grow to the base of the fourth and fifth fingers. As they age, these myofibroblast contract, causing the cords to stiffen, eventually immobilizing these fingers and, in severe cases, causing them to lock at a near 90 degree angle from the palm. Although the process may start on either hand, within a short time, it generally affects both hands. In more severe cases, the two affected fingers are useless, so much so that at one time amputation was the recommended treatment. The process starts some years later in females, and consequently, cases are reported less often and are usually less severe than in males. The disease has also been reported to be more common among manual laborers, likely because such individuals are more dependent upon functional hands. Classically, treatment has been to surgically severe the fibrous cords by some mechanism, but recently the U.S. Food and Drug Administration approved a nonsurgical treatment in which collagenase derived from *Clostridium histolyticum* is injected directly into the cords. This softens the cord and improves function.

Plantar fibromatosis (choice **B**) is similar to Dupuytren's contracture, but it occurs on the sole of the foot. Nodules and cords of tissue form on the sole, and these cords tend to pull the toes down, making it difficult to walk. This condition is often associated with patients having a severe form of Dupuytren's contracture. Peyronie disease (choice **C**) is a rare tissue disease affecting the penis. Bands of connective tissue form under the skin, causing the erect penis to bend. In severe cases, it may interfere with intercourse. Knuckle pads (Garrod's nodes; choice **D**) are pads of tissue that form above the proximal interphalangeal joints. Ledderhose disease (choice **E**) is an alterative name for plantar fibromatosis.

### 23 The answer is A  *Medicine*

The fact that this patient has fainted or almost passed out several times with little trauma and with few consequences strongly suggests that he has carotid sinus sensitivity (choice **A**). Consequently, the episode described was a vasovagal attack leading to syncope. Loss of consciousness is induced by a combination of bradycardia and vasodilatation. Patients commonly induce an attack usually by turning their head to the side, as occurred in this case. Gentle pressure over the carotid artery will replicate the symptoms. However, before doing so, it is important to auscultate over the artery to ensure that the patient does not have a carotid artery bruit.

Hypoglycemia is known to occur in alcoholics. If the patient had not eaten anything in the morning, this could have induced syncope. However, in this patient, the problem occurred after breakfast, only when he turned his head during shaving, and he had earlier episodes with a similar genesis. Therefore, hypoglycemia (choice **B**) is not likely to have been the inducing factor. Vertebrobasilar attack/syncope (choice **C**) is a possible mechanism, but it usually occurs in patients when they extend their necks. Patients may have a history of neck pain due to osteoarthritis. Narrowing of the vertebral foramina in the cervical vertebrae through which the vertebral arteries traverse cranially can contribute to ischemia of the brainstem when the neck is extended and lead to transient loss of consciousness. A tonic-clonic seizure should certainly be considered in the differential diagnosis of syncope—especially in this patient, who is an alcoholic as well. Turning the head to the side will not cause a seizure. However, a patient who has a tonic-clonic seizure (choice **D**) may have an aura, cry out, fall to the ground, seize, and then become unconscious. The patient in this scenario became unconscious and *then* fell. The timing of the fall in relationship to coma is a very important distinction that should be borne in mind while taking a history in a patient who presents with sudden loss of consciousness. While it is true that alcoholics are prone to head trauma due to falls as a result of inebriation or ataxia secondary to involvement of the cerebellum, head trauma is incorrect (choice **E**) because head trauma is followed by coma, and not preceded by it.

### 24 The answer is C  *Pediatrics*

Finding a predominance of eosinophils on nasal smear (choice **C**) substantiates the diagnosis of allergic rhinitis. Neutrophils are indicative of infectious rhinitis.

The Coombs' test (choice **B**) is used to detect hemolytic anemia due to blood group incompatibility. The radioallergosorbent test (RAST) (choice **A**) helps determine antigen-specific immunoglobulin E (IgE) concentrations in serum. The RAST is less sensitive than direct skin testing but brings no risk of allergic reactions. A scratch test (choice **D**) is used to determine sensitivity to certain allergens (e.g., foods, drugs). The side of a beveled, sterile needle is used to break the skin with a scratch that is 1 cm long. A drop of test material is then placed on the scratch. A positive reaction is a wheal-and-flare response, usually obvious 15–20 minutes after application. IgE levels (choice **E**) are increased in allergic disease.

### 25 The answer is E  *Medicine*

Peripheral arterial disease (PAD) is the most common manifestation of atherosclerosis. Atherosclerotic lesions tend to occur at junctions where vessels branch off. This is due to increased shearing forces and turbulence that occurs at these sites. Around 90% of PAD involves the femoral and popliteal arteries (choice **E**). Decrease in blood flow proximally leads to tissue ischemia and symptoms downstream. Patients complain of fatigue, aches, and pain due to claudication. The pain gets worse as the occlusive process progresses, and eventually lingers on even at rest. The location of pain depends on the distribution sites of vessels involved. In the case of femoral-popliteal involvement, pain occurs in the calf.

The abdominal aorta and iliac vessels are involved in around 30% of cases (choices **A** and **B** are incorrect). Patients complain of pain in the gluteal area and may have impotence as well. Involvement of the peroneal, tibial, and pedal arteries occurs much later than that of the femoral and popliteal arteries (choices **C** and **D** are incorrect). These arteries are involved in around 40%–50% of cases.

### 26 The answer is C  *Obstetrics and Gynecology*

This patient does not currently have any respiratory complaints or symptoms; therefore, she will undergo the normal changes in pulmonary physiology that occur during pregnancy. Respiratory rate is unchanged (not increased choice **A**). Tidal volume is increased (not decreased choice **E**). Minute ventilation is the product of respiratory rate and tidal volume, thus it increases. This is the correct answer (choice **C**). Vital capacity (the sum of inspiratory reserve volume, tidal volume, and expiratory reserve volume) remains unchanged (not decreased choice **B**). The enlarging uterus elevates the resting position of the diaphragm, resulting in the functional residual capacity decreasing (not remaining unchanged choice **D**).

### 27 The answer is D  *Medicine*

Genetically speaking, this woman is a male (choice **D**). She has complete androgen insensitivity syndrome (CAIS), formerly known as testicular feminization syndrome. This is an X-linked recessive disorder that has been estimated to affect 2–5 per 100,000 genetic males and is defined by the complete absence of androgen receptors. Consequently, even though concentrations of testosterone and dehydrotestosterone are in the normal range, the absence of androgen receptors prevents development of male secondary sex characteristics, including the external genitalia. Excess circulating testosterone is converted into estradiol, and since estrogen receptors are present, secondary sexual female traits develop. Thus, externally, the genetic male appears to be a phenotypic female. Internal structures do not develop normally: for example, undescended rudimentary testes form and these are able to synthesize antimüllerian hormone, which prevents the upper third of the vagina, and the ovaries, fallopian tubes, cervix, and uterus from forming. As a result, a CIAS individual has a vagina that ends as a blind pouch, is amenorrheic, and infertile. Therefore, the initial clue that most often leads to the discovery of CIAS is the lack of menstrual flow; in this case, that symptom was obscured by use of the mini pill. Partial androgen insensitivity, including Reifenstein syndrome, is thought to be at least as common as CIAS and leads to difficulties in gender identification as well as other problems.

About 1 in 2,500 females are 45 XO (choice **A**). These females have Turner syndrome, usually characterized by a short stature, increased distance between the nipples, low hairline, low set ears, a webbed neck, amenorrhea, and sterility. They also tend to suffer from several health problems including heart disease, hypothyroidism, diabetes, vision and/or hearing problems, autoimmune disease, and some specific types of cognitive problems. It has been estimated that about 1 in 1,000 females are born with an extra X chromosome (choice **B**); this is a noninherited trait usually caused by a nondisjunction error during cell division. These "super females" tend to be slightly taller than their XX siblings, but are otherwise essentially indistinguishable. Klinefelter syndrome is a condition in which males have an extra X chromosome in most of their cells (choice **C**). This is the most common chromosomal aberration; about 1 in 500 males have an extra X chromosome, and 1 in 1,000 have the full-blown syndrome. Generally, Klinefelter men are taller, less muscular, and less aggressive than the typical XY male, and over 90% are sterile. The case describes a genetic male and, like all males, he/she should not have any Barr bodies, let alone two (choice **E**).

### 28 The answer is D *Psychiatry*

Flight of ideas refers to a rapid flow of thoughts (choice **D**), often unconnected or tenuously related to one another. This condition is commonly associated with pathologically accelerated psychomotor activity, as is seen in the manic phase of bipolar I disorder.

Catatonic excitement (choice **B**) and illogical thought processes (choice **C**), examples of disorganized thinking and behavior, are seen in many psychotic disorders. The sudden disappearance of thoughts from consciousness (choice **A**) is called thought blocking and may represent unconscious psychologic conflict. An irrational belief about possessing special powers (choice **E**) is an example of a grandiose delusion, often associated with psychotic episodes in schizophrenia or bipolar I disorder, manic phase.

### 29 The answer is C *Psychiatry*

The quality of mood distinguishes mania from depression (choice **C**). Mood pathology during a manic episode includes elation, expansiveness, and irritability. Mood pathology during a depressive episode includes dysphoria and loss of the ability to experience pleasure.

Sleep disturbances (e.g., insomnia; choice **D**), psychotic symptoms (choice **B**), and altered levels of activity (choice **A**) may be present during both manic and depressive episodes. Both mania and depression may be caused by known pathophysiology (choice **E**), such as endocrinopathies and steroid use.

### 30 The answer is E *Obstetrics and Gynecology*

Cytomegalovirus (CMV) is the most common congenital viral syndrome in the United States. The triad of chorioretinitis, microcephaly, and intracranial calcifications is characteristic for neonatal CMV infection. Specific treatment does exist (choice **A**) in the form of ganciclovir. Cesarean delivery is not effective in the prevention of transmission of CMV to the fetus (choice **B**). The risk of fetal infection from a maternal primary infection is the same in all trimesters (choice **C**), approximately 40%–50%. γ-Globulin prophylaxis is ineffective (choice **D**). However, 85% of infected infants are asymptomatic, with only 5% of them later developing symptoms (choice **E**).

### 31 The answer is C *Obstetrics and Gynecology*

The case scenario is characteristic of perimenopause. It is caused by increasing depletion of ovarian follicles and decreasing estrogen levels. With decreased estrogen and inhibin feedback to the anterior pituitary, there is an increase in follicle-stimulating hormone (FSH) levels (choice **C**), the correct answer. In addition, the other gonadotropin hormone, luteinizing hormone (LH), will also increase (not decrease, as in choice **B**). The concentrations of cortisol (choice **A**), thyroxine (choice **D**), and androstenedione (choice **E**) do not change after menopause.

## 32 The answer is A *Psychiatry*

By definition, pain disorder is characterized by pain that is largely mediated by psychologic factors (choice **A**). There is often an underlying physical lesion; psychological factors are considered to be primary when the resultant pain is disproportional to the nature of the lesion.

In individuals with chronic, physiologically mediated physical pain, as in individuals with pain disorder, physical lesions may be difficult to find (choice **B**), personality pathology may emerge (choice **C**), there is often a good response to biofeedback therapy (choice **D**), and economic and legal issues are involved (choice **E**). Consequently, none of these factors clearly discriminates between pain disorder and physiologically mediated pain conditions. Worker's compensation issues may raise additional concerns about malingering.

## 33 The answer is C *Pediatrics*

Anemia of prematurity (choice **C**) occurs in low-birthweight infants approximately 1–3 months after birth. It is caused by the physiologic effects of the transition from fetal to neonatal life, as well as by factors such as shortened red blood cell survival, rapid growth, and frequent phlebotomy for blood tests. Hemoglobin (Hb) levels in anemia of prematurity are below 7–10 g/dL. Clinical manifestations may include feeding problems, tachypnea, tachycardia, and pallor.

Megaloblastic anemia of infancy (choice **A**) usually is caused by a deficiency of folic acid and has its peak incidence between 4 and 7 months of age. Infants with folate deficiency are irritable, have poor weight gain, and have chronic diarrhea. Newborns with sickle cell anemia (choice **B**) rarely exhibit clinical manifestations until 5–6 months of age, when the γ-globin of fetal Hb is replaced by the β-globin of adult Hb. Acute sickle dactylitis (i.e., painful swelling of the fingers and toes) is usually the first evidence that sickle cell disease is present in an infant. The thalassemias are a group of heritable, hypochromic anemias. α-Thalassemia (choice **D**) is caused by abnormalities in the synthesis of the α chains of Hb and is manifested as microcytosis of the newborn (mean corpuscular volume [MCV] <95 pg). Homozygous β-thalassemia (choice **E**) usually manifests as a severe, progressive hemolytic anemia in the second 6 months of life (after Hb A replaces Hb F) and requires regular blood transfusion.

## 34 The answer is D *Surgery*

This patient has a gastric ulcer (choice **D**). Gastric ulcers most commonly are found in men over the age of 50. Patients generally complain of pain getting worse during or after eating. They often take over-the-counter nonsteroidal analgesics (NSAIDs), which only aggravates the situation. This patient's complaint of being tired, and the pallor noted on clinical examination is due to upper gastrointestinal (GI) bleed. Consumption of NSAIDs, such as aspirin, will only lead to increased bleeding from the site of the ulcer. Production of hydrochloric acid is normal or even low.

Cholecystitis (choice **A**) is an inflammation of the gall bladder that is associated with fever, nausea, vomiting, and right upper quadrant pain. Tenderness and guarding in the area will be present, a positive Murphy's sign may be elicited, and leucocytosis will be present. Duodenal ulcers (choice **B**) are more common in men in the third and fourth decade of life. Unlike gastric ulcer pain, abdominal pain commences some time after eating. This is because food has to enter the duodenum to trigger it. Production of hydrochloric acid is normal or increased. Hiatal hernia (choice **C**) is usually associated with upper abdominal pain, and gastroesophageal reflux may be present. Chronic pancreatitis (choice **E**), although a possibility, causes pain some time after consuming food. Moreover, pain is usually in the back, and gastrointestinal bleeding is not a feature.

## 35 The answer is D *Pediatrics*

Todd's paralysis (choice **D**) commonly occurs after a seizure. The hemiparesis lasts minutes to hours but resolves within 24 hours. It can easily be confused with a stroke except for its duration.

Hemiplegia complicating migraine headaches (choice **A**) also shows recovery within a few hours, without seizures, but with residual neurologic effects associated with transient hemiparesis/plegia. The disorder usually involves a strong maternal history of classic migraine. Neurologic deficits would not disappear after 24 hours in patients with infratentorial tumor (choice **E**). In postviral encephalitis (choice **C**), focal neurologic signs may be stationary, fluctuating, or progressive. Spastic hemiplegia (choice **B**) occurs in patients with cerebral palsy who have decreased spontaneous movements on one side of their body. These patients may also demonstrate hand preference at a very early age. This problem is not transient.

## 36 The answer is B *Pediatrics*

Nephrotic syndrome is characterized by hypoproteinemia (serum albumin <2.5 g/dL) (not hyperproteinemia; choice **A**), heavy proteinuria (choice **B**) (>40 mg/m$^2$/h in a 24-hour urine sample), edema, and hyperlipidemia (predominantly triglycerides and cholesterol) (not hypolipidemia; choice **C**). *Primary nephrotic syndrome* is the term applied to diseases limited to the kidney. *Secondary nephrotic syndrome* is the term applied to a multisystem disease in which the kidney is involved. Hypertension (choice **E**) is rarely seen in nephrotic syndrome. Diarrhea is commonly seen. Patients with nephrotic syndrome have hypoalbuminemia, not hyperalbuminemia (choice **D**).

## 37 The answer is D *Medicine*

The patient has hemochromatosis, an autosomal recessive disease that is relatively common among individuals of northern European ancestry. Most cases are due to a mutation in *HFE* on chromosome 6. About 7% of northern Europeans carry the defective gene, with a 0.5% prevalence of the homozygous condition; it is diagnosed five times more often in men than in women, and is rarely found in Asian or African Americans. The homozygous condition causes unrestricted reabsorption of iron from the small intestine, leading to iron overload in the liver (where it causes cirrhosis), pancreas (where it causes type 1 diabetes and malabsorption leading to diarrhea), and skin (where it increases the production of melanin, causing increased skin pigmentation). The term "bronze diabetes" is often applied to this condition because affected patients tend to present with type 1 diabetes and a bronze skin color. The disease has a slow onset and is not generally diagnosed in men until the fifth decade and later in women because menstrual blood loss protects them. It is postulated that, in former times, it had survival value when it helped protect against iron deficiency anemia and the diseases of late middle-age were of less consequence because of the shorter life expectancy. Once diagnosed, it is treated by phlebotomy and, as long as the secondary organ damage described has not yet reached an irreversible stage, prognosis is good. An excellent screening test is the serum ferritin level. Ferritin is a soluble iron–protein complex that reflects the iron stores in bone marrow macrophages; in iron overload diseases, serum ferritin levels are increased (choice **D**).

Patients with iron overload diseases such as hemochromatosis also have an increase in serum iron concentration (not decreased; choice **B**) and percentage saturation of transferrin (>50% transferrin saturation after an overnight fast). Transferrin is the iron-binding protein. A decreased synthesis of ceruloplasmin (choice **A**) is found in Wilson disease, which is an autosomal recessive disorder characterized by defective secretion of copper into bile and reduced synthesis of ceruloplasmin in the liver. The accumulation of excess copper in the tissues causes chronic liver disease and a movement disorder. Although excess copper deposition in tissues does not cause skin discoloration or pancreatic insufficiency, it does cause cirrhosis, a finding that is also present in hemochromatosis. D-Xylose absorption is an excellent screening test for malabsorption caused by small-bowel disease. Decreased absorption of orally administered D-xylose into the blood occurs in small-bowel disease (e.g., celiac disease) because of flattening of the villi. The reabsorption of D-xylose (choice **C**) is normal in pancreatic disease associated with hemochromatosis, because pancreatic enzymes are not required to degrade xylose for reabsorption by the small bowel. Patients with iron overload diseases have a decrease in total iron-binding capacity (not increased; choice **E**). The total iron binding capacity (TIBC) is decreased, because increased iron stores in the bone marrow cause decreased synthesis of transferrin (binding protein of iron) in the liver. An increase in serum TIBC is only present in iron deficiency, because decreased iron stores in the bone marrow cause increased synthesis of transferrin by the liver.

## 38 The answer is A *Psychiatry*

Most effective psychotherapies and psychoanalyses have specific explanations for the genesis of pathologic behavior (choice **A**). However psychoanalysis tends to focus on subconscious factors initiated during early childhood, whereas the modern psychotherapies focus on specific factors directly affecting behavior in the present.

Since psychoanalysis requires exploration of the subconscious, it is often a lengthy process (choice **C**), but since the brief psychotherapies focus on the immediate, they are often completed more quickly. Moreover, the explanations and treatment techniques differ between psychoanalysis and psychotherapy, as well as among schools of psychotherapy. For instance, interpersonal psychotherapies may emphasize interpersonal experiences over unconscious conflicts or biologic factors (choice **E**); psychodynamic psychotherapy, such as psychoanalysis, may center on a concept of unconscious processes (choice **B**); and cognitive psychotherapy focuses on ways to change a person's way of looking at problems. In general, use of drugs in therapy is limited to certain conditions such as the psychoses, bipolar disorders, anxiety states, and depression, and therapies for substance abuse that are based on the recovery model often include a warning to avoid drug treatment (choice **D**).

### 39 The answer is C *Pediatrics*

Cavernous sinus thrombosis (choice **C**) is a complication of sinusitis. Symptoms of cavernous sinus thrombosis include ophthalmoplegia and loss of accommodation. Sinusitis also can be complicated by meningitis, epidural or subdural abscesses, optic neuritis, periorbital and orbital cellulitis and abscess, and osteomyelitis of surrounding bones. Complications develop secondary to local extension of the infection.

Hand-Schüller-Christian disease (choice **A**) has a variable presentation. It may involve skeletal abnormalities, skin lesions, exophthalmos, hepatosplenomegaly, or pituitary dysfunction. Proptosis is not a feature. Graves disease (choice **B**) is a hyperthyroid state characterized by irritability, excitability, crying easily, restlessness, and tremors of the fingers. Acute bacterial conjunctivitis (choice **D**) presents with generalized conjunctival hyperemia, edema, mucopurulent exudate, and various degrees of ocular discomfort. Temporal lobe abscess (choice **E**) does not present with proptosis.

### 40 The answer is B *Surgery*

Decubitii also known as decubitus ulcers and commonly called bed sores, are generally associated with bedridden elderly individuals. However, they occur in persons of any age whenever there is prolonged pressure of the skin against an external object. However, those who are aged, debilitated, paralyzed, or unconscious are more susceptible. To avoid ulcer formation, prolonged pressure on any given area of the skin must be avoided. This requires frequent rotation of immobilized bedridden patients and changing the position of wheelchair-bound individuals. Friction must also be avoided, since friction is liable to occur on the sacrum, buttocks, and upper legs of patients in wheelchairs who drive around, as in the patient described. Once erythema develops, it may progress to ulceration quickly, and a small ulcer can progress to a large ulcer within 24–48 hours (choice **B**). The progression is caused by local edema or infection. Severe infection must be recognized and treated with appropriate therapy before it leads to more generalized problems.

Although pressure in medical parlance sores are commonly thought of as a problem unique to bedridden patients (as demonstrated by the alternative name of bed sores), persons who sit in a given position are just as prone to develop an ulcer as are those who lies still in bed (choice **A** is incorrect). The most common sites for pressure sores to develop are the sacrum, the trochanters, the heels (choice **C** is incorrect), the lateral malleoli, and the buttocks over the ischium. The heel is susceptible in bed because it may press upon the mattress, in wheelchairs because it may press upon the back of the footrest; a distinctive type of ulcer may develop on the heels of diabetic individuals with neuropathy who do not realize that their shoes are rubbing against the back of their heels.

Gram-positive cocci are found in fewer than 40% of infected ulcers; consequently, decubitus ulcer infections are not almost always caused by *Staphylococcus aureus* (choice **D** is incorrect). Other organisms commonly found in such infections include *Pseudomonas aeruginosa, Providencia* species, *Proteus* species, and *Bacteroides fragilis,* and other anaerobic species. The best combination of antibiotics, therefore, is one that will treat gram-positive aerobic cocci, gram-negative aerobic rods, and anaerobic bacteria. A recommended drug combination is clindamycin and gentamicin, with the warning to monitor renal function carefully while the patient is on gentamicin.

In addition to using systemic antibiotics, the ulcer itself must be treated. An infected decubitis ulcer should not be treated with topical antiseptics that may irritate the wound because this might inhibit healing; thus, choice **E** is incorrect. However, clearing up the infection is critical, since otherwise septicemia, bacterial cellulitis, osteomyelitis, or septic arthritis may develop. In the United States most hospitals have wound teams employed in treatment of decubities ulcers. The first step in treatment is cleaning and débridement. Cleaning is best done by rinsing with a sterile isotonic saline solution. The débridement may be facilitated by use of enzymatic agents such as collagenase, fibrinolysin, deoxyribonuclease, streptokinase, and streptodornase, augmented by hydrophilic polymers such as dextranomer. Once an ulcer is clean and granulation or epithelialization begins to occur, then a moist wound environment should be maintained without disturbing the healing tissue.

**41** **The answer is E** *Preventive Medicine and Public Health*

The "3 Cs"—cardiotoxicity, convulsions, and coma—are the most common causes of death after overdose of tricyclic antidepressants, such as amitriptyline (choice **E**). Many of the signs and symptoms of poisoning caused by a tricyclic antidepressant are similar to those seen with drugs that have atropine-like actions, including scopolamine (choice **C**) and the phenothiazines. However, widening of the QRS complex to more than 1 second on the electrocardiogram (ECG) is an important diagnostic feature of tricyclic overdose. Multiple dosing with activated charcoal may prevent absorption of tricyclics. Key interventions include correction of the acidosis with bicarbonate, control of cardiotoxicity with phenytoin, and use of intravenous diazepam or lorazepam for control of seizures.

**42** **The answer is H** *Preventive Medicine and Public Health*

Given the widespread use of selective serotonin reuptake inhibitors (SSRIs) in the management of major depressive disorders, it is hardly surprising that their toxicity in overdose has been designated "serotonin syndrome." Diaphoresis, diarrhea, myoclonus, tremor, and confusion are characteristics of overdoses of fluoxetine, sertraline (choice **H**), and most other SSRIs. In extreme situations, the toxic syndrome may be life-threatening, with seizures, marked hyperthermia, and possible ventricular arrhythmias. The syndrome may occur at conventional doses of the SSRIs with concomitant administration of monoamine oxidase inhibitors, levodopa, meperidine, lithium, or dextromethorphan (in over-the-counter cough medications). Management is supportive, with the possible use of phenytoin or lidocaine for cardiac arrhythmias and benzodiazepines for seizures.

**43** **The answer is A** *Preventive Medicine and Public Health*

Acetaminophen is the most widely used analgesic in the United States. In addition to being sold as an individual product under several trade names, the most common being Tylenol, it is found as an ingredient in at least 100 compounded products. Its widespread use makes it one of the most common causes of accidental poisoning. When ingested at a toxic level, either as a single dose or because of accumulation associated with long-term consumption, acetaminophen (choice **A**) is a hepatotoxin and is the most common cause of liver failure requiring transplantation in the United States and Great Britain. Normally, acetaminophen is conjugated in the liver and excreted in the urine. However, if the amount of acetaminophen exceeds the liver's ability to conjugate it, the excess is oxidized by a P450 mixed oxidase to *N*-acetyl-*p*-benzoquinone-imine (NAPQI), a toxic byproduct that binds with SH groups on glutathione, vital enzymes, and membrane proteins; the result being centrilobular liver necrosis. *N*-Acetylcysteine is used as an antidote. Most vulnerable to being overdosed are children given adult doses, individuals with renal problems, alcoholics with already compromised livers, and arthritic elders with concomitant memory problems.

**44** **The answer is J** *Preventive Medicine and Public Health*

Cocaine (choice **J**) is a drug that is available in many forms, can be ingested in many ways, and has many physiologic effects. A strong psychologic addiction is primarily caused by its effect on the limbic system, which results in irresistible feelings of euphoria and pleasure. These effects last for a limited time—when snorted or swallowed with ethanol, usually for less than 4 hours and when smoked or taken intravenously, for less than 30 minutes (the latter modes of consumption are popular because they induce an almost immediate high). The profound feelings of well-being that are induced and its limited duration leads to a desire to repeat the experience as soon as possible, causing "bingeing." In addition to these pleasant central nervous system (CNS) effects, cocaine has several other physiologic effects. A primary one is blockade of norepinephrine reuptake, resulting in release of norepinephrine and α-adrenergic hyperactivity, causing hypertension. β-Receptor stimulation via epinephrine causes tachycardia and vasoconstriction. The net result is an increase in myocardial infarcts, aortic dissections, and other medical emergencies, making cocaine abuse the most frequent drug-related cause of visits to emergency departments. Use of cocaine among pregnant mothers, particularly during the first trimester, when many don't even realize they are pregnant, can have disastrous effects on the fetus. The vasoconstrictor properties of cocaine still find medical use as a way to stop nose bleeds, and it also still finds limited use as a local anesthetic. The latter effect is due to the drug's blockade of voltage-gated fast sodium channels, which reduces permeability to sodium and results in increasing the threshold of excitability and decreasing the rise rate of the action potential. Cocaine, when used recreationally, is commonly taken in conjunction with other drugs, including alcohol, diazepam, or heroin. The latter combination is called speed balling; the heroin is used to increase the length of a pleasant experience.

**45** **The answer is C** *Preventive Medicine and Public Health*

Scopolamine (choice **C**) is an anticholinergic drug commonly used to combat motion sickness and is provided as a dime-sized patch, usually worn behind the ear. It causes dry mouth in most users and may also induce temporary blurred vision and dilation of the pupils. Other medical uses include treatment of ataxia in Parkinson disease, muscle spasms of the stomach and intestines, and irritable bowel syndrome.

**46** **The answer is G** *Preventive Medicine and Public Health*

Nicotine, primarily in the form of cigarettes, has been estimated to cost more than $150 billion per year in direct medical costs, as well as an even greater amount in indirect cost, making its use the greatest drug-related medical expenditure in the United States (choice **G**). It is also the leading preventable cause of health problems in the United States, if not in the world. Diseases to which tobacco consumption has been linked include carcinoma of the lung, larynx, mouth, pharynx, stomach, liver, pancreas, bladder, uterine cervix, and brain; emphysema; chronic bronchitis; asthma; bacterial pneumonia; tubercular pneumonia; asbestosis; coronary artery disease; hypertension; aortic aneurysm; arterial thrombosis; stroke; carotid artery atherosclerosis; intrauterine growth retardation; spontaneous abortion; fetal and neonatal death; abruptio placenta; bleeding in pregnancy not yet discovered; placenta previa; premature rupture of the membranes; prolonged rupture of the membranes; preterm labor; preeclampsia; sudden infant death syndrome; congenital malformations; low birth weight; frequent respiratory and ear infections in children; higher incidence of mental retardation; peptic ulcer disease; osteoporosis; Alzheimer disease; wrinkling of the skin ("crow's feet" appearance on the face); and impotence. However, on the optimistic side, the 2009 survey conducted annually by the National Institute on Drug Abuse (NIDA) found cigarette smoking to be at its lowest point in the history of the survey among students in grades 8, 10, and 12.

**47** **The answer is D** *Preventive Medicine and Public Health*

Although tobacco is a greater problem in terms of diseases induced and cost for medical care, ethanol abuse (choice **D**) is certainly the greatest problem in terms of directly observable effects. In any given year, 5%–7% of the population has an alcohol-related problem, and some 13% have had a problem during their lifetime. Two levels of problems are recognized. The initial level is alcohol abuse, in which alcohol consumption continues even though use has already caused failure to meet obligations, accidents (automobile being paramount), legal problems, and/or relationship problems. The next level is alcohol dependency. At this stage, withdrawal causes severe physiologic symptoms (said to be more severe than those in heroin withdrawal). Ethanol-dependent individuals also take extreme actions to avoid withdrawal symptoms, such as drinking early in the morning or, in desperation, drinking anything they think may contain ethanol as an ingredient. Another symptom of alcohol dependence is a change in tolerance, either increased or decreased. Environmental issues and genetic imprinting play a role in determining if a person will have alcohol-related problems. Concordance studies show that the rate of alcoholism between fathers and sons, brothers, and identical twins is very high. A potentially optimistic observation for the future is the report of the National Institute on Drug Abuse (NIDA) in its 2009 survey of alcohol use among high school students that, from 2004 to 2009, decreases were observed in lifetime, past-year, past-month, and binge use of alcohol among students in grades 8, 10, and 12.

**48** **The answer is B** *Preventive Medicine and Public Health*

Diazepam (choice **B**), the generic name for Valium, was put on the market in the 1960s as the prototype member of the benzodiazepine family of anxiolytics. Presently, there are about 15 commonly prescribed drugs in this family, the choice of which is often determined by the length of action. All potentiate the action of $\gamma$-aminobutyric acid (GABA) as a neurotransmitter by binding to its receptor. The major resultant effect is sedation, anxiolysis, and striated muscular relaxation; the latter effect makes them useful as anticonvulsants. In psychiatry, they are used to treat anxiety, panic, posttraumatic stress, and sleep disorders, as well as symptoms due to substance withdrawal. All have adverse effects, including impairment of concentration and memory and possible induction of confusion, ataxia, hypotension, bradycardia, and vertigo. Although rarely fatal alone, they may cause respiratory depression and cardiac arrest, particularly in the elderly. All are also potentially addictive, and withdrawal symptoms include anxiety, insomnia, and tremors. After withdrawal from prolonged use, delirium and seizures may also occur. In the United States during 2008, there were 78,443 emergency department visits related to single-substance benzodiazepine exposure, of which 332 (0.004%) resulted in major toxicity and 8 (0.0001%) resulted in death, most of which involved use of a benzodiazepine in conjunction with another drug, often ethanol.

**49** **The answer is F** *Preventive Medicine and Public Health*

Veronal, the first barbiturate, was synthesized in 1903. During most of the 20th century, the barbiturates (choice **F**) were widely prescribed as sedatives, anxiolytics, and antiseizure drugs. Although largely replaced by the benzodiazepines, phenytoin, or other drugs, they still have medical uses today. Commonly used barbiturates include phenobarbital, seconal, and mephobarbital. Like the benzodiazepines, they act by binding to the γ-aminobutyric acid (GABA) receptors to cause central nervous system inhibition. They also are highly addictive, with profound withdrawal symptoms including irritability, fainting, nervousness, nausea, and convulsions, and they are commonly abused, either because they provide a feeling of euphoria or because withdrawal is uncomfortable. Long-term use causes impaired thinking, poor reflexes, depression, reduced sex drive, and deterioration of the liver, pancreas, and brain. They have been implicated in many suicides. On the street, they are often used in combination with caffeine, heroin, or methamphetamine to enhance the euphoric effects of these drugs.

**50** **The answer is I** *Preventive Medicine and Public Health*

The amphetamines (choice I; amphetamine, dextroamphetamine, and especially methamphetamine) are central nervous system stimulants that act by releasing dopamine. Their medical use includes control of excessive appetite in weight-loss programs, and in the treatment of narcolepsy and depression. Paradoxically, their widest use is to calm children who have attention deficit and hyperactivity (ADH) syndrome. They were first introduced to the general public during World War II, when the German army used them during the invasions of Poland and France. The Allies could not understand how the German troops kept going without dropping from exhaustion. Following the German example, the U.S. army also used them to keep tired and hungry soldiers going after the invasion of France and during the Battle of the Bulge. After the war, returning GIs introduced these drugs to college and university campuses, where they became popular as drugs to permit late-night cramming. Some students continued to use them because of the feeling of euphoria produced and because they could be purchased relatively cheaply; the amphetamines can be synthesized in "kitchen" laboratories, and during the past decades, there has been a virtual explosion in use. According to the National Institute on Drug Abuse (NIDA) survey during 2009, 1.2% of high school seniors, 1.6% of 10th graders, and 1.0% of 8th graders used methamphetamine during that year. This was a significant drop in use since 2003. However, once hooked, persons become addicted and tolerance builds, causing them to consume increasing quantities. Side effects include loss of appetite, aggressiveness, delusions, paranoid personality disorder, hallucinations, and eventually, true paranoid psychotic events. In addition to these negative psychologic manifestations, they also have profound physical effects: they wreak havoc within the circulatory system, damaging blood vessels and causing arrhythmias and hypertension, all of which may induce a cerebrovascular accident or cardiac failure. To get "better highs," an amphetamine is often "speed-balled" by mixing with other drugs, usually a barbiturate, cocaine, or heroin, and sometimes lysergic acid (LSD) or phencyclidine (aka, PCP, angel dust, peace pill, or hog).

# Discipline Index

## Medicine

**Test 1:** 1, 3, 8, 9, 10, 12, 13, 15, 18, 20, 22, 27, 29, 30, 31, 32, 35

**Test 2:** 12, 13, 17, 20, 23, 25, 28, 29, 31, 34, 37, 43, 44, 45, 46, 47, 48

**Test 3:** 1, 4, 8, 14, 18, 22, 25, 27, 28, 38, 43,44, 45, 46, 47, 48

**Test 4:** 4, 6, 7, 10, 11, 14, 15, 16, 20, 21, 27, 30, 31, 34, 35, 40

**Test 5:** 3, 8, 9, 17, 19, 22, 28, 29, 35, 36, 38, 39, 40

**Test 6:** 2, 4, 6, 8, 9, 11, 13, 16, 17, 18, 19, 22, 25, 27, 28, 30, 36, 37

**Test 7:** 2, 11, 13, 17, 20, 27, 30, 31, 33, 35

**Test 8:** 4, 8, 12, 14, 16, 18, 20, 22, 24, 27, 32, 40, 41, 42, 43, 44, 45, 46, 47, 48, 49, 50

**Test 9:** 2, 3, 5, 7, 8, 11, 19, 20, 21, 25, 26, 32, 36

**Test 10:** 3, 5, 7, 8, 14, 15, 18, 29, 34, 44, 45, 46, 47, 48, 49, 50

**Test 11:** 1, 5, 10, 12, 14, 16, 17, 22, 23, 29, 30, 37, 39, 40

**Test 12:** 2, 8, 9, 10, 11, 14, 17, 19, 21, 22, 23, 25, 27, 37

## Obstetrics and Genecology

**Test 1:** 4, 19, 21, 24, 37, 39, 40

**Test 2:** 3, 9, 10, 16, 18, 21, 32

**Test 3:** 2, 7, 11, 26, 30, 34, 39

**Test 4:** 2, 8, 13, 22, 26, 37, 38

**Test 5:** 41, 42, 43, 44, 45, 46, 47, 48, 49, 50

**Test 6:** 40, 41, 42, 43, 44, 45, 46

**Test 7:** 9, 18, 29, 39, 40, 41, 42, 43, 44, 45, 46

**Test 8:** 1, 11, 21, 30, 31, 37

**Test 9:** 12, 18, 23, 27, 35, 38

**Test 10:** 11, 28, 37, 38, 39, 40, 41, 42, 43

**Test 11:** 18, 24, 25, 28, 33, 35

**Test 12:** 1, 15, 26, 30, 31

## Pediatrics

**Test 1:** 36, 41, 42, 43, 44, 45

**Test 2:** 4, 7, 22, 33, 38

**Test 3:** 3, 9, 12, 19, 24, 31, 32, 35

**Test 4:** 1, 19, 23, 24, 28, 29, 32, 39

**Test 5:** 2, 6, 11, 14, 24

**Test 6:** 3, 5, 23, 24, 31, 33, 34, 39

**Test 7:** 7, 12, 14, 19, 22, 25, 28, 34

**Test 8:** 2, 5, 10, 13, 15, 19, 23, 36

**Test 9:** 6, 10, 13, 17, 29, 34, 40

**Test 10:** 1, 17, 21, 22, 25, 26, 33

**Test 11:** 41, 42, 43, 44, 45, 46, 47, 48, 49, 50

**Test 12:** 3, 5, 7, 24, 33, 35, 36, 39

## Preventive Medicine and Public Health

**Test 1:** (0)

**Test 2:** 1, 8, 19, 30

**Test 3:** 17, 23, 29, 36

**Test 4:** 36, 48, 49, 50

**Test 5:** 4, 20, 25, 27, 30, 37

**Test 6:** (0)

**Test 7:** 4, 23, 38

**Test 8:** 3, 25, 28

**Test 9:** 41, 42, 43, 44, 45, 46, 47, 48, 49, 50

**Test 10:** 2, 9, 13, 23, 30

**Test 11:** 7, 19, 32, 38

**Test 12:** 41, 42, 43, 44, 45, 46, 47, 48, 49, 50

## Psychiatry

**Test 1:** 5, 7, 11, 14, 17, 23, 34, 38

**Test 2:** 2, 11, 15, 36, 40, 41, 42, 49, 50

**Test 3:** 6, 13, 15, 21, 49, 50

**Test 4:** 3, 5, 9, 12, 17, 18, 25, 33

**Test 5:** 7, 13, 15, 21, 26, 31, 32, 34

**Test 6:** 20, 21, 32, 38, 47, 48, 49, 50

**Test 7:** 1, 3, 5, 21, 24, 36, 47, 48, 49, 50

**Test 8:** 6, 17, 33, 38, 39

**Test 9:** 1, 14, 16, 22, 31, 33, 37

**Test 10:** 4, 6, 12, 16, 20, 27, 31, 36

**Test 11:** 2, 8, 9, 11, 20, 26, 27, 36

**Test 12:** 4, 12, 13, 16, 20, 28, 29, 32, 38

## Surgery

**Test 1:** 2, 6, 25, 26, 28, 33, 46, 47, 48, 49, 50

**Test 2:** 5, 6, 14, 24, 26, 27, 35, 39

**Test 3:** 5, 10, 16, 20, 33, 37, 40, 41, 42

**Test 4:** 41, 42, 43, 44, 45, 46, 47

**Test 5:** 1, 5, 10, 12, 16, 18, 23, 33

**Test 6:** 1, 7, 10, 12, 14, 15, 26, 29, 35

**Test 7:** 6, 8, 10, 15, 16, 26, 32, 37

**Test 8:** 7, 9, 26, 29, 34, 25

**Test 9:** 4, 9, 15, 24, 28, 30, 39

**Test 10:** 10, 19, 24, 32, 35

**Test 11:** 3, 4, 6, 13, 15, 21, 31, 34

**Test 12:** 6, 18, 34, 40

# *Index*

Note: Page numbers followed by *f* indicate figures and those followed by a *t* indicate tables.

Ruptured aortic aneurysm, 75
Ruptured duodenum, 69, 88
Ruptured esophageal varices, 161, 178–179
Russell-Silver syndrome, 256

## S

St. Louis encephalitis virus, 108
Salicylates, 260
*Salmonella paratyphi*, 139
Salpingitis isthmica nodosa, 116
Sapropterin, 157, 171
Sarcoidosis, 229
Sarcoma botryoides, 135, 152
*Sarcoptes scabei*, 172
Sarin, 119
Saturated solution of potassium iodide (SSKI), 230
Scarlet fever, 88, 205
Schatzki ring, 80
Schilling test, 200
*Schistosoma hematobium*, 285
Schizoaffective disorder, 17, 181
Schizoid personality disorder, 189, 205, 289
Schizophrenia, 95, 107, 144, 146, 197, 237, 273, 280, 288, 315
    family history of, 196
    paranoid type251
    residual type, 289
Schizophrenia disorder, 196
Schizophreniform disorder, 196
Schizotypal personality disorder, 205, 274, 289
Scleroderma, 234, 335
Sclerosing mediastinitis, 237
Sclerosing pericholangitis, 313
Scopolamine, 331, 346
Scorpion sting, 317
Screening test, new
    test the efficacy of, 221, 235
*Scrub typhus*, 58
SEB. *See* Staphylococcal enterotoxin B (SEB)
Seconal, 347
Second-degree burns, 287
Secondary amine tricyclic antidepressant, 210
Secondary dysmenorrheal, 152
Secondary nephrotic syndrome, 343
Secondary optic atrophy, 91
Secondary Raynaud disease, 335
Sedation and sialorrhea (drooling), 282
Seizure disorder, 1, 13, 259, 316
Selective serotonin reuptake inhibitors (SSRIs), 192, 210, 345
Selegiline, 203
Selenium, 149
Separation anxiety disorder, 146
Sepsis, 204
Septic arthritis, of knee, 232
Serologic analysis, of blood, 150
Serologic test, for febrile agglutinins, 231
Serotonin, 2, 15
Serous cystadenoma, 236, 313
Sertoli-Leydig cell tumor, 9, 25, 194, 212
Sertraline (Zoloft), 160, 176, 210, 331, 345
Serum sickness, 14
Seventh-Day Adventist, 190, 206
Severe preeclampsia, 5, 19
Sevoflurane, 262
Sexual abuse, 325, 336
Sexually transmitted disease (STD), 232
Shaken baby syndrome, 201, 227, 237
Shared psychotic disorder, 141

Sheehan syndrome, 26
Shingles, 58
Shock, 281
Shy-Drager syndrome, 178
SIADH. *See* Syndrome of inappropriate ADH secretion (SIADH)
Sickle cell disease, 139, 179, 259
Sickle cell trait, 236
Sideroblastic anemia, 201
Side-to-side portacaval shunt, 306
SIDS. *See* Sudden infant death syndrome (SIDS)
Sigmoidoscopy, 142
Sinemet, 203
Sinus tachycardia, 54, 229
Sinusitis, 163, 182
Sitagliptin, 276, 288, 293
Sitagliptin phosphate, 175
Six P's, 56
Sjögren syndrome, 74
*SLC12A3* gene, 85
SLE. *See* Systemic lupus erythematosus (SLE)
Sleep apnea, 335–336
Slipped capital femoral epiphysis, 232
Small- (oat) cell cancers, 78
Social phobia, 40, 58–59
Social withdrawal, premorbid history of, 196
Sociocultural deprivation, 262
Sodium bicarbonate, 283
Sodium nitrite, 116
Sodium restriction and systolic blood pressure, 267
Sodium thiosulfate, 116
Solitary ulcer syndrome, 142
Somatization disorder, 102, 120–121, 183, 238, 280, 285, 316
Sound, increased sensitivity to, 231
Spastic hemiplegia, 181
Specific phobias, 197
Spinal cord astrocytoma, 197
Spinal cord tumor, 145
Spleen, rupture of, 222, 237
Splenectomy, 286
Splitting, 63, 79
Spondylitis, ankylosing, 209
Spontaneous pneumothorax, 264
*Sporothrix schenckii*, 230
Sprains, 27
Sputum cytology, 338
Squamous cell carcinoma, 63, 64, 78, 79, 81
SSKI. *See* Saturated solution of potassium iodide (SSKI)
SSRIs. *See* Selective serotonin reuptake inhibitors (SSRIs)
*Staphylococcal enterocolitis*, 103, 121
Staphylococcal enterotoxin B (SEB), 117
*Staphylococcus aureus*, 8, 24, 70, 87, 92, 147, 148, 230, 282, 289, 311, 344
*Staphylococcus saprophyticus*, 93
Stasis dermatitis, 198
Status epilepticus, 13
STD. *See* Sexually transmitted disease (STD)
"Steakhouse syndrome", 80
Stickler syndrome, 279
Stool, blood in
    of newborn, 217, 229
Stool examination, for ova and parasites, 231
Stool, impacted, 201
Strains, 27
Strawberry tongue, 205
*Streptococcus agalactiae*, 53, 156, 169, 324, 334
*Streptococcus bovis*, 147
*Streptococcus pneumoniae*, 68, 87, 97, 111, 275, 287, 289, 290, 297, 309, 334